APPLIED BIOLOGICAL ENGINEERING – PRINCIPLES AND PRACTICE

Edited by **Ganesh R. Naik**

INTECHOPEN.COM

Applied Biological Engineering – Principles and Practice
Edited by Ganesh R. Naik

Published by InTech

Janeza Trdine 9, 51000 Rijeka, Croatia

Edition 2014

Publishing Process Manager Martina Durovic

Technical Editor Teodora Smiljanic

Cover Designer InTech Design Team

Additional hard copies can be obtained from orders@intechopen.com

Applied Biological Engineering – Principles and Practice, Edited by Ganesh R. Naik
p. cm.
ISBN 978-953-51-0412-4

INTECH

open science | open minds

Contents

Preface

Background and Motivation

Biological and medical phenomena are complex and intelligent. Our observations and understanding of some of these phenomena have inspired the development of creative theories and technologies in science. Biological engineering (also known as bioengineering) represents an exciting, broad-based discipline that ties together the engineering, medical and biological sciences, with slight help from physics, chemistry, mathematics and computer science. The key objective is to benefit human-kind, animal and plant life - in other words, it is *"engineering for life"*.

In all different areas of biological engineering, the ultimate objectives in research and education are to improve the quality life, reduce the impact of disease on the everyday life of individuals, and provide an appropriate infrastructure to promote and enhance the interaction of biomedical engineering researchers. Biological engineering has a base that applies the principles of engineering to a wide range of systems and complexities including the molecular level such as biochemistry, molecular biology, pharmacology, microbiology, cytology, protein chemistry and neurobiology.

The most important trend in biological engineering is the dynamic range of scales at which biotechnology is now able to integrate with biological processes. An explosion in micro/nanoscale technology is allowing the manufacture of nanoparticles for drug delivery into cells, miniaturized implantable microsensors for medical diagnostics, and micro-engineered robots for on-board tissue repairs. This book aims to provide an up-to-date overview of the recent developments in biological engineering from diverse aspects and various applications in clinical and experimental research.

Intended Readership

This book covers some of the most important current research related to biological engineering. It is partly a textbook and partly a monograph. It is a textbook because it gives a detailed introduction to biological engineering techniques and applications. It is simultaneously a monograph because it presents and brings together several new results, concepts and further developments. Furthermore, the research results previously scattered throughout many scientific journals and conference papers worldwide, are methodically collected and presented in the book in a unified form.

As a result of its twofold character the book is likely to be of interest to graduate and postgraduate students, engineers and scientists in the field of biomedical and biological engineering. This book can also be used as handbook for students and professionals seeking to gain a better understanding of where bioengineering stands today. One can read this book through sequentially but it is not necessary since each chapter is essentially self-contained, with as few cross-references as possible. So, browsing is encouraged.

As an editor and also an author in this field, I am honoured to be editing a book with such fascinating and exciting content, written by a select group of gifted researchers. I would like to thank the authors, who have committed so much effort to the publication of this work.

Dr Ganesh R. Naik
RMIT University, Melbourne
Australia

Part 1

Computational Methods in Bioengineering

1

Efficient Computational Techniques in Bioimpedance Spectroscopy

Aleksander Paterno, Lucas Hermann Negri and Pedro Bertemes-Filho
Department of Electrical Engineering, Center of Technological Sciences
Santa Catarina State University, Joinville,
Brazil

1. Introduction

Electrical Bioimpedance Analysis (BIA) is an important tool in the characterization of organic and biological material. For instance, its use may be mainly observed in the characterization of biological tissues in medical diagnosis (Brown, 2003), in the evaluation of organic and biological material suspensions in biophysics (Cole, 1968; Grimnes & Martinsen, 2008), in the determination of fat-water content in the body (Kyle et al., 2004) and in *in vivo* identification of cancerous tissues (Aberg et al., 2004), to name a few important works. It is also natural to have different computational approaches to bioimpedance systems since more complex computational techniques are required to reconstruct images in electrical impedance tomography (Holder, 2004), and this would open a myriad of other computational and mathematical questions based on inverse reconstruction problems.

In many practical cases, the obtained bioimpedance spectrum requires that the produced signal be computationally processed to guarantee the quality of the information contained in it, or to extract the information in a more convenient way. Such algorithms would allow the removal of redundant data or even the suppression of invalid data caused by artifacts in the data acquisition process. Many of the discussed computational methods are also applied in other areas that use electrical impedance spectroscopy, as in chemistry, materials sciences and biomedical engineering (Barsoukov & Macdonald, 2005).

BIA systems allow the measurement of an unknown impedance across a predetermined frequency interval. In a typical BIA system, the organic or biological material suspension or tissue sample to be characterized is excited by a constant amplitude sine voltage or current and the impedance is calculated at each frequency after the other parameter, current or voltage, is measured. This technique is called sine-correlation response analysis and can provide a high degree of accuracy in the determination of impedances. By using the sine-correlation technique, the spectrum is determined either by obtaining the impedance real and imaginary parts, or by directly obtaining its modulus and phase. For this purpose, analog precision amplifiers and phase detectors provide signals proportional to modulus and phase at each frequency, and the interrogated frequency range is usually between 100 Hz up to 10 MHz. In such BIA systems the current signal used in the sample excitation is band-limited, because the output impedance of the current source and the open-loop gain of its amplifiers are low, especially at high frequencies (Bertemes-Filho, 2002). Some of these limitations may be avoided by using digital signal processing techniques that may take the place of the electronic circuitry that have frequency constraints.

In the BIA electronics, when considering the phase detection part of analog circuits used, a high-precision analog multiplier provides a constant signal proportional to the phase of its input. However, the frequency response of the circuit is usually limited, for example, to 1 MHz and such multipliers require the excitation source signal as a reference. A software solution would provide an alternative to the use of such phase detectors, where in some cases an algorithm may be capable of calculating the phase spectrum from the acquired modulus values. With this system configuration, phase/modulus retrieval algorithms may be used to obtain the phase or modulus of an impedance, considering that one of these sets of values has been electronically obtained.

In electrical bioimpedance spectroscopy applied to medical diagnosis, research groups cite the use of the Kramers-Kronig causality relations Kronig (1929) to obtain the imaginary part from the real part (or equivalently phase/modulus from modulus/phase parts) of a causal spectrum (Brown, 2003; Nordbotten et al., 2011; Riu & Lapaz, 1999; Waterworth, 2000). A similar procedure occurs when obtaining the modulus from the phase, or vice-versa, using the Hilbert transform in a causal signal (Hayes et al., 1980). With constraints on the characteristics of the acquired phase or modulus spectrum, the use of these algorithms may allow the calculation of the missing part of an electrical bioimpedance spectrum. In addition, such algorithms may be used to validate the obtained experimental impedance spectrum (Riu & Lapaz, 1999). However, there may be restrictions to the signals that can be processed with these techniques, specifically with the Fourier-transform based phase/modulus-retrieval algorithms (Paterno et al., 2009), even though it may provide a computationally efficient solution to the problem.

Still related to the multi-frequency BIA systems, after the raw non-processed information is acquired, the choice of an appropriate numerical model function to fit the experimental data and generate a summary of the information in the spectrum condensed in a few parameters is also another niche where computational techniques may be used. The choice of an efficient fitting method to be used with experimental data and with a non-linear function, as the Cole-Cole function, is a problem that has been previously discussed in the literature (Halter et al., 2008; Kun et al., 2003; 1999). It is natural to think that once such algorithms work for the fitting with a non-linear Cole-Cole function, they will also work with other different non-linear functions in bioimpedance experimental data. With this in focus, an algorithm is demonstrated that shows novelties in terms of computational performance while fitting experimental data using the Cole-Cole function as part of the fitness function and particle-swarm optimization techniques to optimally adjust the model function parameters (Negri et al., 2010). Other computational intelligence algorithms are also used for comparison purposes and a methodology to evaluate the results of the fitting algorithms is proposed that uses a neural network.

The experimental data in this work were obtained with a custom-made multi-frequency bioimpedance spectrometer (Bertemes-Filho et al., 2009; Stiz et al., 2009). Samples of biological materials were used like bovine flesh tissue and also raw milk, that may constitute a suspension of cells, since the samples of raw milk may have cells, for example, due to mastitis infection in sick animals. Other characteristics of milk, which are currently important in the dairy industry, could be evaluated, as, for instance, a change in the water content or even the presence of an illegal adulterant, like hydrogen peroxide (Belloque et al., 2008). The problem was then to characterize the raw milk with such adulterants using the bioimpedance spectrum either fitted to a Cole-Cole function or not (Bertemes-Filho, Valicheski, Pereira & Paterno, 2010). The neural network algorithm may be in this particular case a useful technique to classify the milk with hydrogen peroxide (Bertemes-Filho, Negri & Paterno, 2010).

As a summary, the authors provided a compilation of problems into which computational intelligence and digital signal processing techniques may be used, as well as the illustration of new methodologies to evaluate the processed data and consequently the proposed computational techniques in bioimpedance spectroscopy.

2. Materials and methods

2.1 The BIA system to interrogate bioimpedances

The used BIA system is based on a bioimpedance spectrometer consisting of a current source that injects a variable frequency signal into a load by means of two electrodes. It then measures the resulting potential in the biological material sample with two other electrodes and calculates the transfer impedance of the sample. The complete block diagram of the spectrometer system is shown in fig. 1. A waveform generator (FGEN) board supplies a sinusoidal signal with amplitude of $1\,V_{pp}$ (peak-to-peak) in the frequency range of 100 Hz to 1 MHz. The input voltage (V_{input}) is converted to a current ($+I$ and $-I$) by a modified bipolar Howland current source (also known as voltage controlled current source) (Stiz et al., 2009), which injects an output current of $1\,mA_{pp}$ by two electrodes to the biological material under study. The resulting voltage is measured with a differential circuit between the other two electrodes by using a wide bandwidth instrumentation amplifier (Inst. Amp. 02). The amplitude of the injecting current is measured by another instrumentation amplifier (Inst. Amp. 01) while using a precision shunt resistor (R_{shunt}) of $100\,\Omega$. A custom made tetrapolar impedance probe was used to measure the bioimpedance and is composed of 4 triaxial cables. The outer and inner shields of the cables are connected together to the ground of the instrumentation. The tip of the probe has a diameter of 8 mm (D), and the electrode material is a wire of 9 carat gold with a diameter of 1 mm (d). The wires are disposed in a circular formation about the longitudinal axis. Finally, a data acquisition (DAQ) board measures both voltage load and output current by sampling the signals at a maximum sampling frequency of 1.25 MSamples/s for each of the possible 33 frequencies in the range. Data are stored in the computer for the processing of the bioimpedance spectra. Although the modulus and phase of the load are electronically obtained, one of the parameters can be used to experimentally validate the phase/modulus retrieval technique while comparing the calculated and measured values.

For completeness purposes, if one decides to use the bioimpedance spectrum points at frequencies which were not used in the excitation or were not acquired, the value at this frequency can be determined by means of interpolation, since the evaluated spectra are usually well-behaved.

The nature of the experimental bioimpedance spectra is important for the use of the algorithms described in this work. It is assumed here that the experimental sample bioimpedance spectrum may have its points represented by a Cole-Cole function in the interrogated frequency range. This is a plausible supposition, since it is a function that represents well many types of bioimpedance spectra associated with cell suspensions and

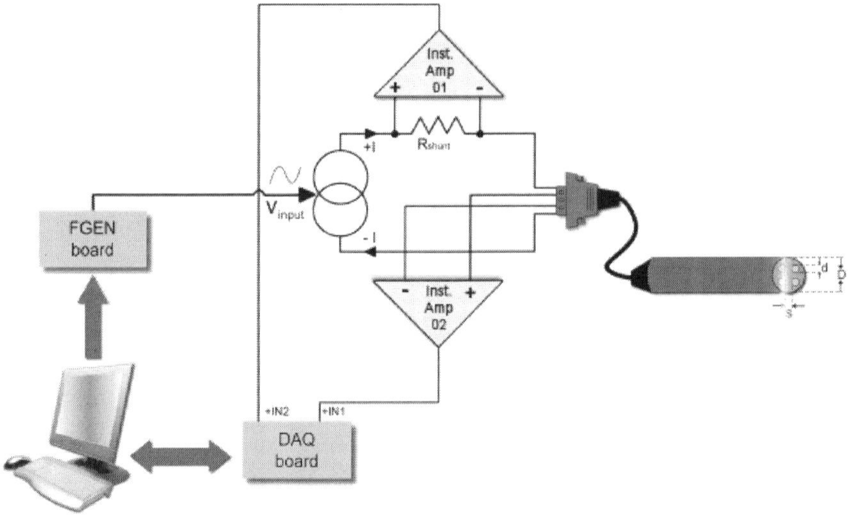

Fig. 1. BIA system complete block diagram for the interrogation of electrical bioimpedances.

many types of organic tissues and materials (Cole, 1940; 1968; Grimnes & Martinsen, 2008). When the Cole-Cole function shown in the following equations is not an appropriate model function to fit the experimental data, the data are not processed with these algorithms and are used in phase/modulus retrieval or in the neural network without further processing.

2.2 Cole-Cole fractional order impedance function

Tissues or non-uniform cell suspensions have bioimpedance spectra that are not well represented by a Debye-type single-pole (single-relaxation) function. In any case, the bioimpedance may be represented as a complex number in polar or cartesian, as in eq. 1:

$$Z(s) = |Z(s)|e^{j\theta} = Z_R(s) + jZ_I(s) \tag{1}$$

where $s = j\omega$, ω represents the angular frequency and $j = \sqrt{-1}$. The cartesian form takes its graphical representation in the complex impedance plane where the ordinate axis is the negative of the impedance imaginary part (-reactance) and the abscissa axis is the real part of the impedance. Usually different configurations of a semi-circular arc in the complex impedance plane may represent the experimental bioimpedances spectra or they may be depicted by plotting the modulus and phase versus frequency.

In addition, the bioimpedance function used in this work is going to be represented within a limited frequency range in terms of a distribution function of relaxation times, τ, which would correspond to the spectrum of cell sizes, particles or molecules in a suspension or tissue. This distribution function approach was proposed by Fuoss and Kirkwood (Fuoss & Kirkwood, 1941) where they extended the Debye theory from which a relation can be obtained between the distribution function, $G(\tau)$, and a transfer function, $Z(s)$, that corresponds in this case to a bioimpedance. This relation is given by:

$$Z(s) = \int_0^\infty \frac{G(\tau)}{1+s\tau} d\tau \tag{2}$$

By using eq.2, the relation between $Z(s)$ and $G(\tau)$ is stressed:

$$Z_{frac}(s) = \frac{R_0 - R_\infty}{1+(s\tau_0)^\alpha} = (R_0 - R_\infty) \int_0^\infty \frac{G(\tau)}{1+s\tau} d\tau \tag{3}$$

In eq. 3, the frequency dependent part of the impedance in the Cole-Cole type model function, $Z_{frac}(s)$, is represented, where R_0 is the impedance resistance at very low frequencies, R_∞ is the resistance at very high frequencies, and the function containing the fractional order term, $(s\tau_0)^\alpha$ can be represented by an integral of the distribution function $G(\tau)$ (Cole & Cole, 1941), and α is a constant in the interval $[0,1]$ and τ_0 is the generalized relaxation time. $G(\tau)$ is a distribution function for the fractional order Cole-Cole model function and is explicitly represented by Cole & Cole (1941):

$$G(\tau) = \frac{1}{2\pi} \left[\frac{\sin\left[(1-\alpha)\pi\right]}{\cosh\left[\alpha \log(\frac{\tau}{\tau_0})\right] - \cos\left[(1-\alpha)\pi\right]} \right] \tag{4}$$

The complete model developed by Cole and Cole consists of an equation, an equivalent circuit and a complex impedance circular arc locus, and in terms of impedances, after integrating eq. 3, one obtains the Cole-Cole function to represent the evaluated impedance spectrum:

$$Z_{Cole}(\omega) = R_\infty + \frac{R_0 - R_\infty}{1+(j\omega\tau_0)^\alpha} \tag{5}$$

In eq. 5, the variable $Z_{Cole}(\omega)$ is a complex impedance and is a function of the angular frequency ω. The Cole-Cole function was obtained by the Cole and Cole brothers when they also introduced the distribution function of eq. (4). It is worth noticing that the function containing the fractional order term, $(s\tau_0)^{1-\alpha}$ instead of the $(s\tau_0)^\alpha$, was originally used in a model for dielectrics (Cole & Cole, 1941).

For the use of the phase/modulus retrieval algorithm in $Z_{Cole}(s)$ the independent term corresponding to the resistance, R_∞, causes the frequency dependent function to satisfy neither the phase- nor the modulus-retrieval algorithm conditions (Hayes et al., 1980; Paterno et al., 2009). In other words, the experimental points to be used with the phase/modulus retrieval algorithm must be previously tested with known bioimpedance spectrum data to verify if the process is applicable. Consequently, the algorithm has limitations of use if the resistance at very high frequencies is not zero, or if the condition of minimum phase in the spectrum is not satisfied. In addition to that, for the reconstruction of phase and modulus of $Z_{Cole}(s)$, the experimental data must correspond to a Cole-Cole spectrum that may be fitted to a specific set of values of α (Paterno et al., 2009), otherwise the algorithm may not converge to the correct values. Fortunately, these values of α with which the algorithm properly works correspond to a broad class of tissues, cell suspensions and organic materials to be evaluated in practical cases. In the limit, when $\alpha \approx 0$, $Z_{frac}(s)$ becomes a pure resistance having minimum-phase. For values of α in the interval $(0,1)$, the modulus retrieval algorithm may be capable of producing a limited error, as demonstrated elsewhere (Paterno et al.,

2009). For the use of instrumentation to characterize the spectrum of organic material, this conditions are usually met, as in the illustration case of bioimpedances obtained from mango, banana, potato and guava, shown in the results in section 3. These are illustrative examples of organic material to have its impedance phase measured and used as input to the algorithm that determines the bioimpedance modulus. In this case, both parameters were measured to validate the results (Paterno & Hoffmann, 2008).

2.3 Phase/modulus retrieval algorithm description

The algorithm is based on the flowchart in fig. 2. It starts by being fed with the modulus sequence vector (in the phase retrieval algorithm) provided by electronic means. In the case of using the modulus retrieval procedure, phase and modulus must be interchanged in the algorithm. A vector containing the N modulus samples equally spaced in frequency is saved in $|Z_{OR}(k)|$ and a vector that contains the estimated phase samples is initialized with random values. The initial impedance Fourier transform spectrum is a vector represented by the N values, $Z_{OR}(k) = |Z_{OR}(k)|\, e^{j\theta_{est}}$. In the following step, the real part of an M-point inverse fast-Fourier transform (IFFT) algorithm is used to produce a sequence in the time-domain, $z_{est}[n]$. An M-point IFFT is used, where the constraint $M \geq 2N$ guarantees the algorithm convergence. Only the real part of the M-point IFFT is used because the input signal is real in the time-domain Quartieri & Oppenheim (1981), and has an even Fourier transform, allowing half of the samples (N samples) to represent the bioimpedance spectrum.

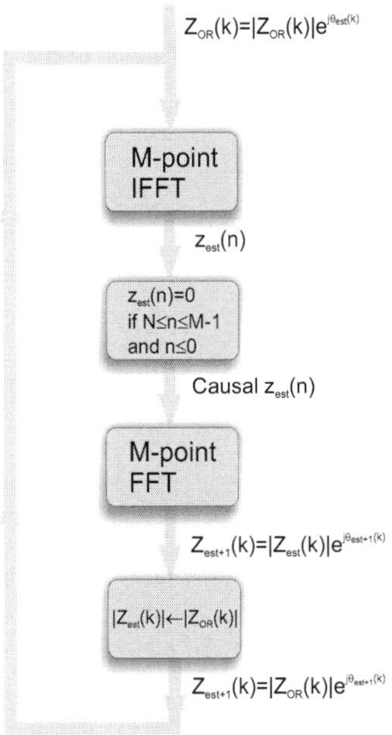

Fig. 2. Flowchart representing the processing steps in the modulus-retrieval algorithm for the BIA system.

Causality is imposed in the fourth block while a finite length constraint on the time-domain sequence sets $z_{est}(n)$ to zero for $n > N - 1$. The M-point FFT of the data set containing $z(n)$ produces the estimates of the bioimpedance spectrum. This flowchart indicates the process that is repeated until the root-mean squared value of the difference between two consecutive estimated vectors is less than a stopping parameter, ϵ. It was set equal to $\epsilon = 10^{-6}$, which is a much lower value than the necessary modulus or phase resolution in BIA systems. The length of the input vector sequences is a power of 2, since the iterative solution uses uniformly spaced samples Quartieri & Oppenheim (1981) and the Fast-Fourier Transform (FFT) radix-2 algorithm (Proakis & Manolakis, 2006).

2.4 Computational intelligence algorithms in electrical bioimpedance spectroscopy

In this section computational intelligence algorithms will be briefly described such as to be used in an application to fit experimental data obtained with BIA systems using particle swarm optimization techniques; additionally, artificial neural networks (ANN) are described to provide a methodology to evaluate the fitting algorithms. The performance testing is implemented by associating the training phase of the ANN to previously known information contained in the bioimpedance spectrum. For example, in the evaluated sample. The presence of different adulterants in raw milk, specifically water and hydrogen peroxide, and the characterization of the type of bovine flesh tissue are samples that were interrogated with the BIA system. The ANN is used to evaluate how much information the fitting process may extract from the experimental data such as to condense it into the parameters of the used function model, namely, the Cole-Cole function that contains four parameters (R_0, R_∞, τ and α) as in eq.5 with the information of the electrical bioimpedance spectrum.

2.4.1 The Particle-Swarm Optimization (PSO) experiment

The particle swarm optimization algorithm was used to extract the Cole-Cole function parameters, R_0, R_∞, τ_0 and α from experimental data. For this experiment, the previously described bioimpedance spectrometer injected a sinusoidal current via the two electrodes of a tetrapolar probe into bovine liver, heart, topside, and back muscle samples. A cow was killed in a slaughterhouse, where the samples were extracted and immediately headed to the laboratory where the bioimpedance measurements were performed. The measured bioimpedance spectrum points contained 32 modulus and phase values at frequencies in the range from 500 Hz up to 1 MHz. A set of 20 pairs of reactance and resistance points corresponding to the lowest frequencies (from 500 Hz up to 60 kHz) was processed with a PSO algorithm.

2.4.1.1 The PSO algorithm

PSO is inspired by bird flocking, where one may consider a group of birds that moves through the space searching for food, and that uses the birds nearer to the goal (food) as references (Xiaohui et al., 2004). PSO algorithms to fit a known function to experimental data is a technique similar to the one using genetic algorithms (GA). PSO has however a faster convergence for unconstrained problems with continuous variables such as the addressed fitting problem of the Cole-Cole function and has a simple arithmetic complexity (Hassan et al., 2005). Briefly, the PSO algorithm can be separated in the following steps:

1. Population initialization;

2. Evaluation of the particles in the population by a heuristic function, where in this case the particles are formed by a vector with the Cole-Cole function parameters;
3. Selection of the fittest particles (set of parameters) to lead the population towards the best set and
4. Update of the position and velocity of each particle by repeating the steps from 2 to 4 until a stopping condition is satisfied (Xiaohui et al., 2004).

Each parameter of the optimized function, in this case the fitting of the Cole-Cole function in eq. 5 to an experimental bioimpedance spectrum, can be represented as one dimension in the search space. The velocity update rule for the i-th particle is given by:

$$v_{id} = w \times v_{id} + c_1 \times rand() \times (p_{id} - x_{id}) + c_2 \times rand() \times (p_{nd} - x_{id}) \tag{6}$$

where v_{id} is the velocity of the i-th particle in the dimension d; w is the inertia weight, in the $[0,1)$ range; c_1 and c_2 are the learning rates, usually in the $[1,3]$ range; $rand()$ is a random number in the $[0,1]$ interval, p_{id} is the best position of the i-th particle for the d-th dimension and p_{nd} is the best neighborhood position for the d-th dimension. The particle position is updated by summing the present position to the velocity.

Each particle is made by a vector with the parameters $[R_0, R_\infty, \tau_0, \alpha]$ of the Cole-Cole function, that are randomly initialized with arbitrary values in an interval corresponding to the physical limits of the system. A parameter restart step for the global search, inspired by the genetic algorithm mutation operator, was added to the code to prevent the premature convergence of the algorithm.

Like a genetic algorithm, the PSO enhances the solution based on a heuristic function named fitness function, that measures the difference between the experimental spectrum and the fitted one. The fitness function is shown in eq. 7

$$fitness(p) = -\frac{1}{N}\sum_{i=1}^{N} abs(Z_i - A_i)^2 \tag{7}$$

It is defined by the modulus of the difference between the original complex bioimpedance experimental points, Z_i, and the fitted spectrum, A_i. As a consequence, resistance and reactance are taken into account in the function, and therefore, in the fitting.

2.4.2 Artificial neural networks and the fitted functions of the bioimpedance spectrum

Artificial neural networks (ANN) were implemented such as to evaluate the behavior of the fitting algorithms to experimental data. This was developed to determine, comparatively, how much information the extracted parameters from the fitted Cole-Cole function may contain that represents correctly the experimental bioimpedances.

2.4.2.1 ANN as used in BIA

One of the important features of a neural network resides in its capability to learn the relationships in a given data mapping, such as the mapping from the bioimpedance spectra to the type of the analyzed sample. This feature allows the network to be trained to perform estimations and classify new samples according to the learned pattern.

An ANN is composed of interconnected artificial neurons, each neuron being a simple computer unit (Haykin, 1999). Although a single neuron can perform only a simple operation, the network computational power is significant (Cybenko, 1989; Gorban, 1998) and can tackle any computable problem (Siegelmann & Sontag, 1991), under certain circumstances.

In a perceptron-like network such as the ones employed in this work, each neuron performs the operation shown in eq. 8, where y is the output value, defined as the result of the activation function ϕ evaluated with the summation of m input signals x_i, each one multiplied by a weight w_i (also seen in fig. 4). All neural networks had neurons using the symmetric sigmoid activation function (Haykin, 1999). It is mathematically represented with its input in eq. 8. In eq. 9, the description of the sigmoid function is shown, and in fig. 3 a graphical illustration of its output is depicted as a function of its input for different steepness parameters. For this work, the steepness parameters were determined empirically. In the classification experiments, the parameter is $s_{tp} = 0.65$ in the bovine flesh classification and $s_{tp} = 0.5$ in the milk classification.

$$y = \phi\left(\sum_{i}^{m} x_i w_i\right) \tag{8}$$

$$\phi(x) = \frac{2}{1 + e^{-2s_{tp}x}} - 1 \tag{9}$$

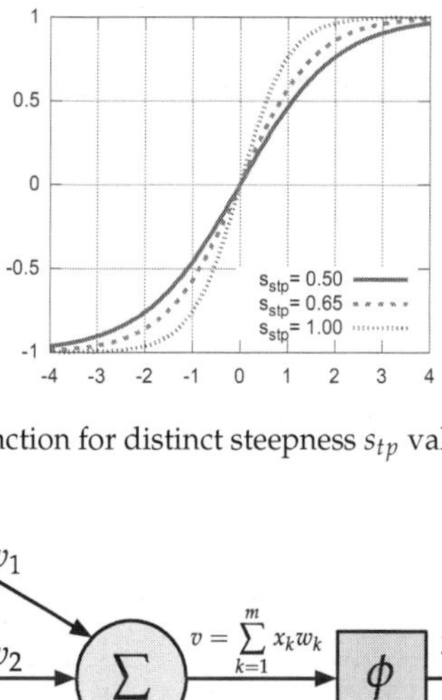

Fig. 3. Symmetric sigmoid function for distinct steepness s_{tp} values. In the experiments, $s_{tp} = 0.65$ and $s_{tp} = 0.5$.

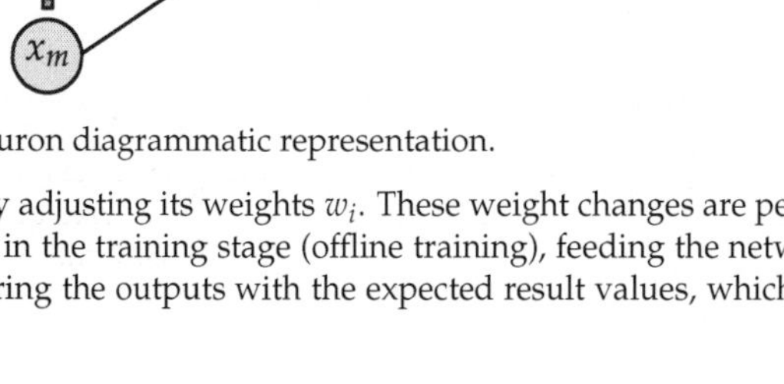

Fig. 4. Artificial neuron diagrammatic representation.

The ANN learns by adjusting its weights w_i. These weight changes are performed by using a training algorithm in the training stage (offline training), feeding the network with the input values and comparing the outputs with the expected result values, which would provide an error measure. The calculated error is the information used to modify the weights of the connections, in order to reduce the errors on the next run. This procedure can be executed many times until the error converges to a minimum. The training procedure for the networks employed in this work are based on the following steps (error backpropagation procedure):

1. Feed the input data (Cole-Cole parameters or raw bioimpedance spectrum points) to the network;
2. Compute the output value of all neurons from the current layer and then propagate the results to the next layer (forward propagation);
3. Compare the network outputs at the output layer with the expected ones to have an error measure;
4. Propagate the measured errors to the previous layers, in a way that each neuron has a local error measure (back propagation);
5. Adjust the connection weights of the network, based on the local errors;

Different training algorithms can be used to adjust the weights of an ANN. It is common to supervised training algorithms to follow the same steps as the error backpropagation procedure, differing only in the weight adjusting step (Haykin, 1999). As an example, while the classical backpropagation has only a centralized learning rate, the iRPROP algorithm (Anastasiadis & Ph, 2003) has a learning rate for each connections and uses only the sign changes in the local error to guide the training. Other algorithms like NBN (Neuron by Neuron) uses the local errors to estimate second-order partial derivatives, which in some cases can lead to a faster training (Wilamowski, 2009).

In the bovine tissue classification experiment, two different fully connected cascade (FCC) topologies were employed. Both topologies had two hidden layers (with one neuron each) and an output layer with 4 neurons. The first one diagrammatically depicted in fig. 5(a) employed only 3 neurons in the input layer, for the R_0, τ and α fitted Cole-Cole parameters, while the other one depicted in fig. 5(b) used 40 input neurons, corresponding to 20 impedance and reactance pairs. Both topologies had the goal of mapping the input data into one of 4 classes. To implement this, 4 output neurons were used, each one corresponding to a class. The NBN training algorithm was used to adjust the synaptic weights for the network to predict the correct beef classes.

The milk adulterant detection experiment employed a multilayer perceptron (MLP) topology (as in fig. 5(c)), with 30 input neurons (15 impedance and reactance pairs), one hidden layer with two neurons and an output layer with 3 neurons. Each output neuron corresponds to one class (one of C classes coding). The ANN was trained with the NBN algorithm.

2.4.2.2 Experiments with the ANN testing

The evaluated experimental data were also added to artificial noise such as to determine the robustness of the ANN classification when trained with the raw experimental points, with and without artificial noise, and also with the extracted parameters using different fitting techniques. Additionally, a genetic algorithm to similarly extract Cole-Cole function parameters (Halter et al., 2008) and the least-squares minimization algorithm for the fitting (Kun et al., 2003; 1999) were implemented to provide comparative results using the same methodology. It is expected that the stochastic algorithms may produce a set of parameters with small variances and with approximately the same mean values when

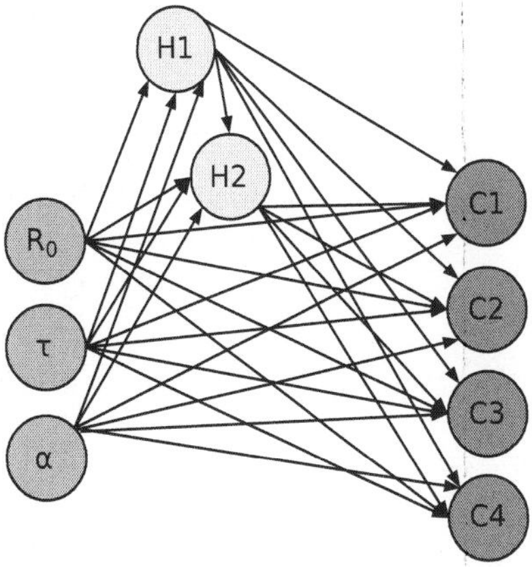

(a) 3–2–4 FCC topology employed in the bovine tissue classification experiment.

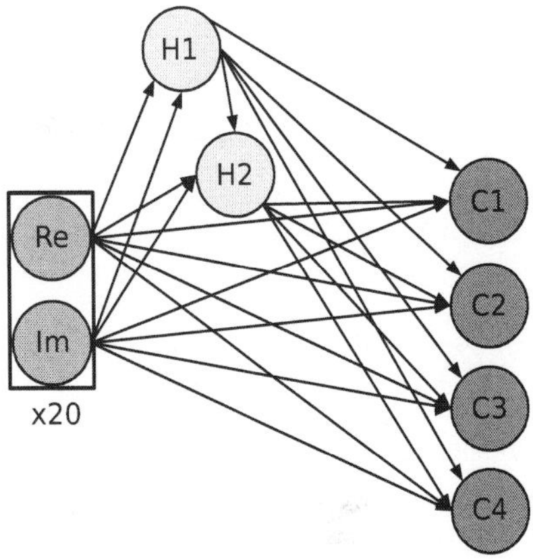

(b) 40–2–4 FCC topology employed in the bovine tissue classification experiment. The input layer has 40 neurons condensed in the box or 20 times 2 ('x20').

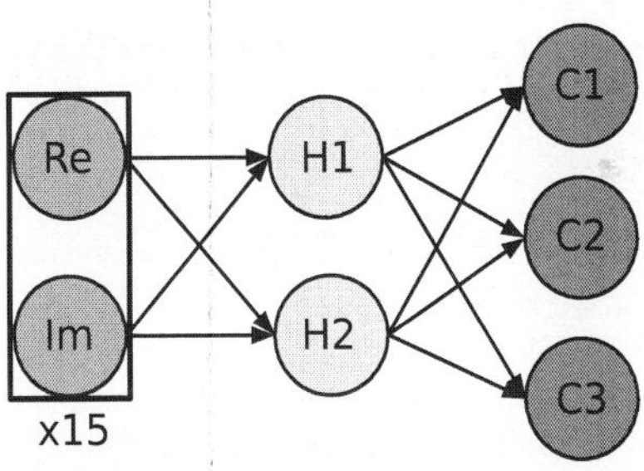

(c) 30–2–4 MLP topology employed in the milk adulterant detection experiment. The input layer has 30 neurons condensed in the box or 15 times 2 ('x15').

Fig. 5. Topology of artificial neural networks used in the experiment of bioimpedance spectra classification with bovine tissue and adulterated milk.

executed several times with the same set of experimental data. This would happen if the Cole-Cole function were an appropriate representation of the acquired bioimpedance spectrum data.

The resulting fitted parameters were used as input to the neural networks such as to classify the data by means of its known type (liver, heart, topside, or back muscle). Another neural network performed the same classification, but using the unprocessed spectrum points as inputs. The input signal was incrementally added to white-gaussian noise (AWGN) such as to produce different signal to noise ratios. A total of 24 electrical impedance measurements were divided into two sets. The first set is formed by 15 measured spectra and is used for the neural network training, while the second set formed by the remaining 9 measurements were used for the neural network validation test. Another 11 sets were created with AWGN having signal-to-noise ratio (SNR) from 2 to 32 dB with steps of 2 dB, forming the base validation set where each spectrum was used more than once to sum a total of 20 spectra in each set. Four ANN were created, one for each fitting algorithm and another for the raw spectra. Each neural network was trained with the spectra from the training set and tested with the validation sets, using the corresponding results from the extracted Cole-Cole parameter output or the raw spectra as input. The neural networks for the use with the testing of fitting algorithms have a $3-2-4$ fully connected cascade (FCC) topology to allow a better generalization in the ANN (Wilamowski, 2009), as diagrammatically illustrated in fig. 5, with the 3 input neurons corresponding to the $[R_0, \tau_0, \alpha]$ parameters and the 4 output neurons corresponding to the confidence level of each bovine tissue type.

The neural network that uses the set of bioimpedance spectrum points as input with a $40-2-4$ FCC topology had the 40 inputs corresponding to the real and imaginary parts of the 20 input spectrum points associated with the lowest frequencies in the experimental spectrum which would correspond to a maximum frequency of 60 kHz.

One ANN was trained with the parameters fitted by the PSO algorithm using the training set, by exposing the ANN to the sample values associated with the input that corresponds to the extracted Cole-Cole parameters. After that, the neural network performance was measured to classify the sample type correctly. The rate of correct classifications was calculated by using the extracted parameters and also the raw data from 11 spectrum and using the corresponding trained ANN.

2.4.3 Raw milk evaluation through bioimpedance spectra

In the dairy industry, conductivity measurements are made to test for abnormal milk. This is somehow similar to the process of obtaining a bioimpedance spectrum from a milk sample. However, in conductivity tests the sample is usually interrogated at a single frequency and the results give false positives and negatives (Belloque et al., 2008). Conductivity, therefore bioimpedance (Piton et al., 1988), and acidity measurements are also used to measure microbial contents of the milk, being indirect and rapid methods (Belloque et al., 2008; Hamann & Zecconi, 1998). The drawbacks of these methods are associated with the lack of sensitivity and specificity. In addition, the conductivity test is also included in screening tests to detect mastitis. Since mastitic milk contains pathogens and spoilage microorganisms, and it is also characterized by an increase in Na^+ and Cl^- as well as leucocytes (Kitchen, 1981), this may be indicated by changes in bioimpedance spectrum (Bertemes-Filho, Negri & Paterno, 2010) as discussed here, and it would also characterize the analysis of raw milk as of a cell suspension.

Other changes in the milk, which may not have its causes in a sick animal, could also be indicated by changes in the bioimpedance spectrum, as when the milk has water or hydrogen peroxide, for example, added to it for fraudulent purposes (Bertemes-Filho et al., 2011). The modulus and phase of the bioimpedance along a frequency range containing more than one frequency point is therefore an extension of the typical measurement of conductivity in the process of milk quality evaluation and is justified by previous published results.

2.4.3.1 Detection of water and hydrogen peroxide in raw milk

Milk may be adulterated by the addition of water, food coloring, conservants and substances used for the milk thickening, as for example the hydrogen peroxide. The commonest method of adulterating milk may be the dilution of water and a common method to detect it is by measuring its freezing point and use this value to calculate the percentage of the diluted water (Belloque et al., 2008). Another indication of water content would be provided by changes of bioimpedance spectra from the milk. To illustrate it, the bioimpedance spectra from raw milk with and without added water and hydrogen peroxide were determined and compared with each other.

An ANN is subsequently used to classify the milk sample by using the points of the bioimpedance spectrum. For this purpose, samples of raw milk from 27 Holstein cows in lactation were obtained in a local farm. The sample sets were divided into two groups. The first group (A) was used to train the neural network with 16 samples. From this set, 4 samples were randomly taken and had distilled water added to them in a volumetric concentration of 10%; other 4 samples had hydrogen peroxide added to them in a volumetric concentration of 3%. In the second group (B), 11 samples were used for the ANN validation, this is, to test if the trained algorithm correctly classifies the samples, that were also equivalently adulterated. Before the measurements, the samples were kept in a refrigerator at a temperature of 4°C for 4 hours.

The ANN used the multilayer perceptron topology of fig.5(c) with 30 neurons corresponding to resistance and reactance input values at 15 different frequency points in the bioimpedance spectrum. The output layer was formed by 3 neurons corresponding to a defined class (raw milk, milk with water and milk with hydrogen peroxide). If the bioimpedance spectrum of a sample containing H_2O_2 is fed to the ANN, this output neuron must have the largest value output among the other two output neurons.

The ANN was trained using the Neuron by Neuron (NBN) algorithm by using 24 spectra, in which 4 samples were adulterated with water and other 4 with H_2O_2. For the ANN validation, 30 milk bioimpedance spectra were measured in a different data set producing another data set different from the one used in the training. The validation spectra were then separated into three different classes associated with the evaluated types of samples and the percentage of correct classifications were calculated.

2.4.3.2 Evaluation of mastitic milk

The bioimpedance spectra of raw milk were acquired in samples from 17 Holstein cows, three of them with mastitis infection. Three milk samples of 100 ml from each animal were collected and stored in a refrigerator at a temperature of 4°C. Four hours later, the bioimpedance spectrum from each sample was collected and the material was sent to an accredited laboratory to characterize the presence of somatic cells and bacteria by using flow cytometry[1]. Selected samples had the acquired bioimpedance spectrum data points processed and the experimental points and Cole-Cole parameters analyzed and shown for illustration purposes of the changes presented in the mastitic and raw milk spectra.

[1] The laboratory managed to follow the International Dairy Federation Standards 148:2008 and 196:2004. These standards specify, respectively, methods for the counting of somatic cells and for the quantitative determination of bacteriological quality in raw milk.

3. Results and discussion

3.1 Retrieving modulus from phase in experimental bioimpedance spectra

In the experiment to illustrate the effectiveness of modulus retrieval from the data acquired by the bioimpedance spectrometer, four vegetables were excited by a signal from the tetrapolar probe. Phase and modulus were acquired in the previously specified range at non-uniformly distributed frequencies. The first procedure in the experimental data was the interpolation to produce uniformly spaced points in the frequency range. The values of phase from the bioimpedance spectrum fed the algorithm to retrieve modulus. It is seen that the impedance at high frequencies is a small value tending to zero in one of the vegetables. However both data allowed the recovery of modulus from phase with an average error as shown in table 1 and as shown in fig. 6, where the behavior of the estimated modulus error is shown with the modulus from phase and the actual acquired phase for mango, banana, potato and guava. A higher error was observe in low frequencies since the lowest measured frequency was 500 Hz. In this experiment, the constraints for the use of the algorithm are such that it allowed the modulus recovery from the phase with a well-behaved error, and one can also infer that depending on the evaluated sample, the response of the algorithm may provide smaller errors.

As a general rule, the resistance at infinite frequencies must tend to zero for the algorithm to converge. In the case of an organic material suspension or a sample with a previously known bioimpedance and whose spectrum are not supposed to change much during its interrogation, the algorithm may be a convenient choice to substitute modulus measurements in bioimpedance interrogations while reading only phase. The resulting magnitude value associated with the modulus is normalized, since it is produced differently from the actual impedance value to a scale factor, requiring calibration.

Vegetable	Mean Error	Deviation σ
Mango	2.34%	2.84%
Banana	1.54%	2.86%
Potato	5.2%	6.06%
Guava	2.94%	1.96%

Table 1. Mean errors in modulus retrieval and standard deviation for the evaluated interval for mango, banana, potato and guava.

3.2 PSO fitting using the Cole-Cole function in bovine flesh bioimpedance

Due to the noise incorporation characteristics (convergence to the mean noise level) caused by the presence of a constant value in the model function, the R_∞ parameter is neither included in the results, nor in the classification experiment. Since the signal-to-noise ratio (SNR) of the experimental data was changed by adding white gaussian noise to the experimental data points, this would be another reason not to include the R_∞ parameter in the performance tests. The R_0 and α parameters did not show any significant fluctuation differences when they resulted from any of the tested fitting algorithms, either the PSO or the Genetic Algorithm or the Least-Squares ordinary fitting, implemented as proposed in the literature (Halter et al., 2008; Kun et al., 2003; 1999). The results of the computational performance experiment depicted in table 2 contains both the mean and sample standard deviation of the required iterations for the convergence of the PSO algorithm and also for comparison purposes, the iterations needed for the convergence of the Genetic Algorithm and for the execution of the

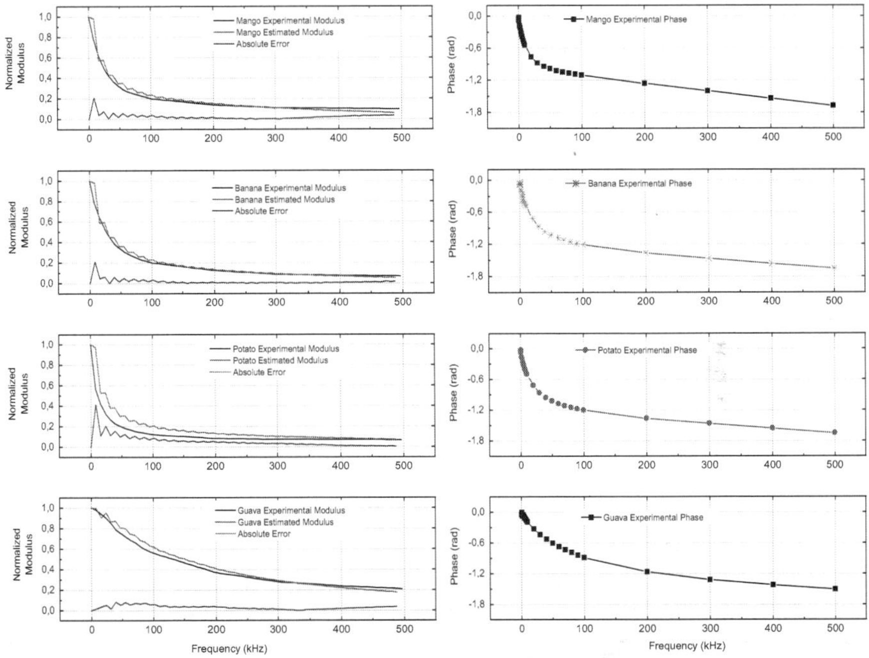

Fig. 6. Modulus retrieval obtained with the phase/modulus retrieval algorithm previously described. The input data was the interpolated 64 points of phase from the mango, banana, potato and guava.

Least-Squares (LS) fitting. Since the LS method is not stochastic, the deviation statistic is not applicable in this case. In fig. 7, the percentage of correct classification rate is depicted for the trained artificial neural networks using as inputs the parameter sets resulting from each of the fitting methods. The unprocessed bioimpedance spectrum points (raw) were used as inputs to an ANN with 40 input neurons, and the classification rate is also depicted in fig.7 together with the results from the testing of the PSO, LS and GA for an ANN with three input neurons.

Fitting Method	$\bar{n}$	σ_n
PSO	30	5.63
LS	134	Not applicable
GA	600	402.33

Table 2. Mean number of iterations, $\bar{n}$, for convergence of each fitting method producing a parameter set for the ANN input and its standard deviation for the stochastic fitting methods, σ_n.

From fig. 7, one may infer that the GA and proposed PSO methods demonstrate a higher accuracy and noise tolerance than the LS method, since under a higher SNR the used parameters provide the information for the correct classification of the samples. The LS method does not provide a better accuracy since for higher values of SNR, the experimental

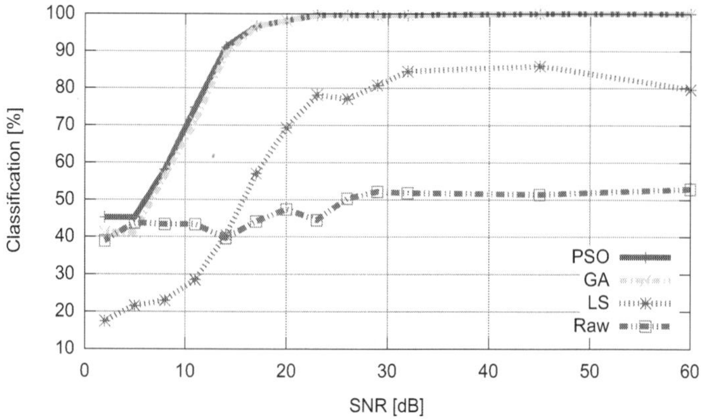

Fig. 7. Neural network classification rate when using as inputs the parameters from the fitting methods (PSO, GA and LS) and also the unprocessed bioimpedance spectrum points (Raw).

data still have distortions caused by artifacts or external effects in the system that may cause its parameters to provide a wrong guess in the classification. The Cole-Cole parameters with any fitting technique also produce improved results than when using a data set with the raw spectrum points in the classification. The quality of the LS fitting performance is influenced by its noise sensitivity. When tested with experimental points that have distortions from the electronic system or errors caused during the acquisition process from the material sample, the LS algorithm converged prematurely, producing parameter sets that deteriorated the classification. As the inputs provided by the PSO and GA methods produced a better classification rate and resulted in networks with reduced neurons and synaptic connections than using the full spectrum points, it is possible to recommend their use for bioimpedance classification systems even under worse SNR then usual.

In addition, the used model function was such that it was appropriate for the proposed methodology and allowed the verification of a conformity between the experimental bioimpedance spectrum and the Cole-Cole function to a certain degree, even with AWGN and other unavoidable artifacts. In the case of the experimental points without artificial AWGN added to the data, the results of the fitted spectra are depicted in fig. 8. In this case, it is also observed that the PSO/GA methods produce a better approximation to the experimental data, intrinsic distortion of the used BIA system notwithstanding.

It is equivalently shown in table 2, about the performance of the algorithms, that the PSO method converges faster, requiring less iterations than the GA method. The PSO algorithm also has a linear complexity per iteration with respect to the input data vector size. Due to implementation characteristics and its deterministic nature, the LS algorithm has the fastest performance, two orders of magnitude faster than what is obtained with the PSO and GA. It is possible to infer that the LS method has a superior computational performance than the other two fitting methods, and is followed respectively by the PSO and GA methods.

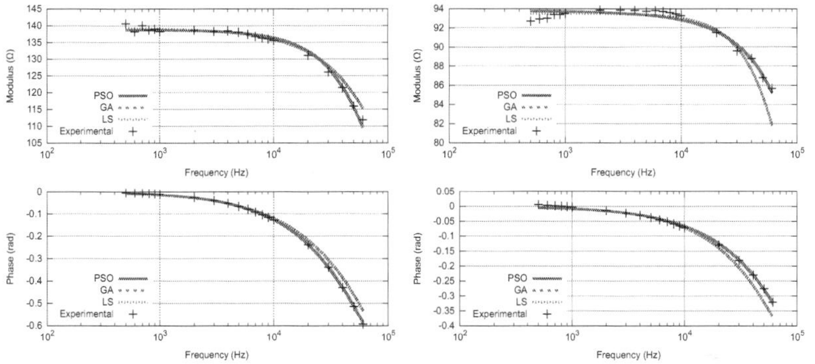

(a) Modulus and Phase of bovine liver bioimpedance spectrum

(b) Modulus and Phase of bovine heart bioimpedance spectrum

Fig. 8. Experimental data points containing modulus and phase of bioimpedance spectra of liver and heart samples from bovine flesh tissue. Experimental points are shown with the curves associated with the fitted Cole-Cole functions using PSO, LS and GA.

3.3 Abnormal milk testing with bioimpedance

3.3.1 Spectra of adulterated milk

In fig. 9(a),(b) and (c), the bioimpedance spectra from the pure raw milk, and raw milk adulterated with water and hydrogen peroxide are depicted. The data were processed with the three fitting algorithms, and it is evidenced that the LS algorithm did not allow a proper fitting to the experimental points since one may observe a larger error along a wide frequency interval in the fitting. Since the PSO and GA have an equivalent qualitative performance, but a better computational performance in the PSO, the Cole-Cole parameters may represent more properly the information contained in the bioimpedance spectra. For higher frequencies, the Cole-Cole function is not capable of representing the experimental points characteristics in the phase spectrum, due to non-ideal characteristics and intrinsic artifacts and distortions inserted by the BIA system and the probe.

Comparatively one can observe some improvement in the fitting while using the PSO/GA algorithms in these data. However, distortions and artifacts produced by stray capacitance may cause a deviation in the resistance at high frequencies while obtaining the Cole-Cole parameters. Such changes may be observed in the complex impedance arc locus diagram plotted as the imaginary part of the bioimpedance as a function of its real part. The capacitive effect causes a hook like form in this diagram and the fitting process it may also produce a set of Cole-Cole parameters with negative resistances at high frequencies, as illustrated in fig. 9 (d).

In fig.10(a), the proportion of correct classification when using the raw data points to the trained ANN that classify adulterated milk is depicted and the average value of correct classifications is depicted as the total rate. It is observed that, if no other substance in the milk is related to the bioimpedance changes, except for the adulterants, the ANN is capable of properly characterizing the presence of water or hydrogen peroxide with a low error rate. The

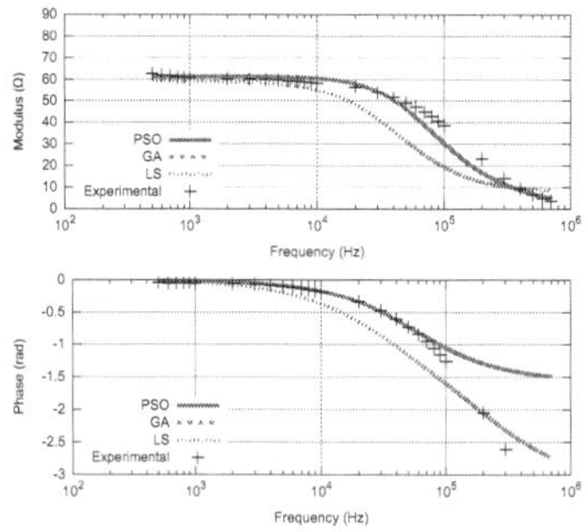

(a) Modulus and Phase of bioimpedance spectrum from raw milk

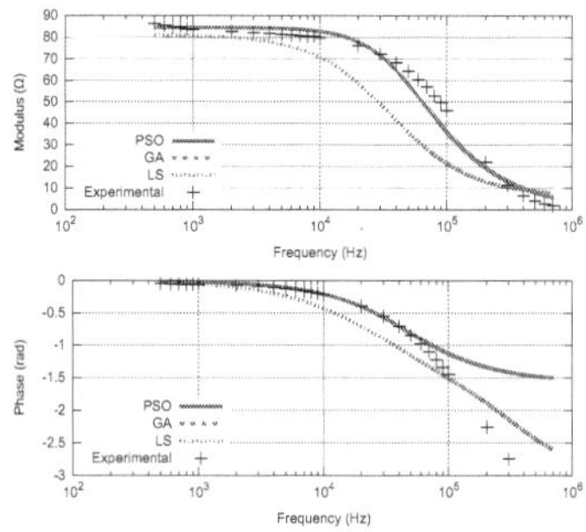

(b) Modulus and Phase of the bioimpedance spectrum from milk adulterated with water

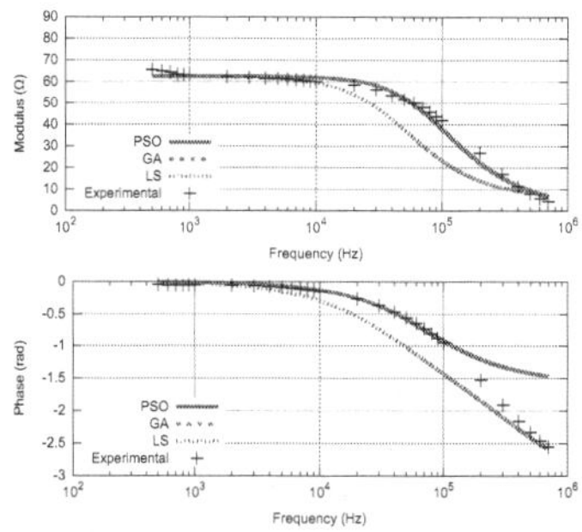

(c) Modulus and Phase of the bioimpedance spectrum from milk adulterated with hydrogen peroxide

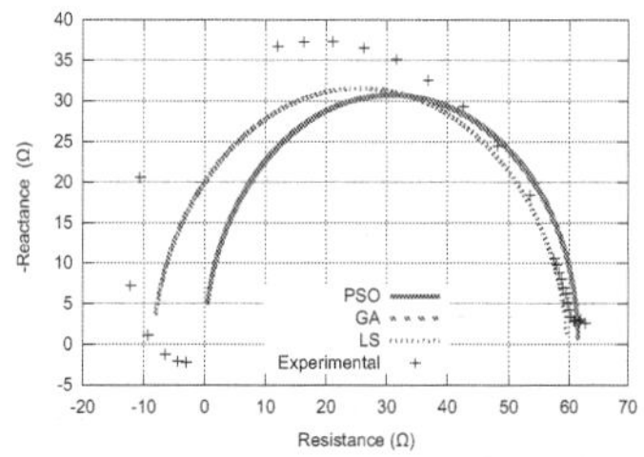

(d) Complex impedance arc locus plot example of the bioimpedance spectrum from raw milk

Fig. 9. Experimental bioimpedance spectrum and the results from the fitting with PSO, GA and LS algorithms. Data were obtained from raw milk and from raw milk adulterated with distilled water and with hydrogen peroxide. The complex impedance arc locus plot is depicted in fig. 9(d) associated with the raw milk sample.

used bioimpedance data have artifacts that were not corrected, and this was partly responsible for the non-null error in the classification rate.

In this evaluation of raw milk, it is possible to evidence the presence of artifacts that may invalidate the bioimpedance spectra. In order to avoid discarding spectra that may be corrupted mainly by impedance stray effects, usually the experimental data shown to have a hook-like form in the impedance plot at high frequencies requires that the data points be multiplied by a linear phase factor corresponding to a delay in the time domain. This would fit the experimental data with such distortions by multiplying the impedance function, i.e., an exponential factor $e^{-j\omega T_d}$ (De Lorenzo et al., 1997). It would be equivalent to a delay of T_d s in the impedance time domain function if T_d is real and it would partly compensate the high frequency artifacts. The only problem in this compensation resides in the choice of the optimal T_d value, which is usually done on a trial-and-error basis.

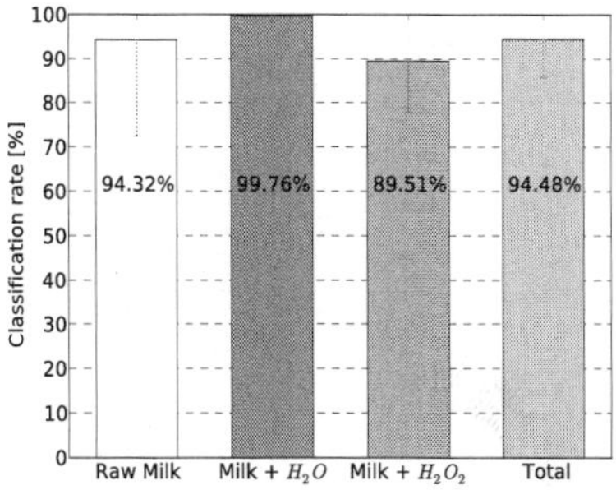

Fig. 10. ANN correct classification rate for adulterated milk when using raw spectrum points as inputs to the ANN.

3.3.2 Spectra of mastitic milk

In the evaluation of the mastitic milk with different concentrations of cells, the graphs showing two examples of complex impedance arc locus are depicted in fig.11 (a) and (b). The somatic cell concentration (SCC) of the 17 milk samples as obtained from the accredited laboratory is shown in fig.11(c). The concentrations of 3000 cells per milliliter and 1.274 millions of cells per milliliter, as determined by the characterization in the laboratory, illustrate that the impedance spectra may confirm the differences between a mastitic milk sample with low cell concentration and mastitic milk. The impedance spectrum differences may be observed in the Cole-Cole parameters obtained in the fitting with the PSO technique while using also the compensation to reduce stray impedance effects, as depicted in fig. 11(a) and (b). The values of the fitting are depicted in table 3 for illustration purposes only and not to be used as references of mastitic milk bioimpedances. The compensation of stray impedance effects, however, may be used in any bioimpedance spectrum containing distortions due to stray impedances at high frequencies. The technique that shows how the optimal time delay for this compensation is obtained will be published elsewhere. The used T_d s are also shown in table 3 together with the mean squared error after the convergence of the algorithm and visually shows that the mean squared error between experimental points and fitted curves are reduced after correction. The resistances obtained by the model function fitting are also naturally reduced to zero, as observed in table 3. The parameters that change after time delay compensation may be

Parameters	Mastitic milk	Compensated mastitic milk	Raw milk	Compensated raw milk
R_∞ [Ω]	−14.6	0	−11.7	0
R_0 [Ω]	94.9	94.8	100.3	100.7
α	1	1	0.99	0.96
τ [μs]	0.552	0.515	0.711	0.672
T_d [μs]	0	0.100726	0	0.110161
Mean Squared Error	14.6	9.2	31.6	26.9

Table 3. Cole-Cole parameters and final fitting mean squared error from the fitting with PSO algorithm for the spectra of mastitic milk samples and the bioimpedance from the raw milk sample, also containing the parameters from the fitted spectra compensated with specific time delays T_d.

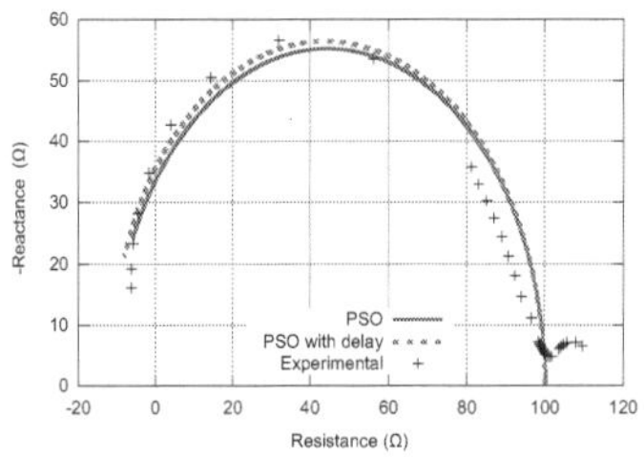

(a) Complex impedance diagram of mastitic milk with 3000 cells per milliliter

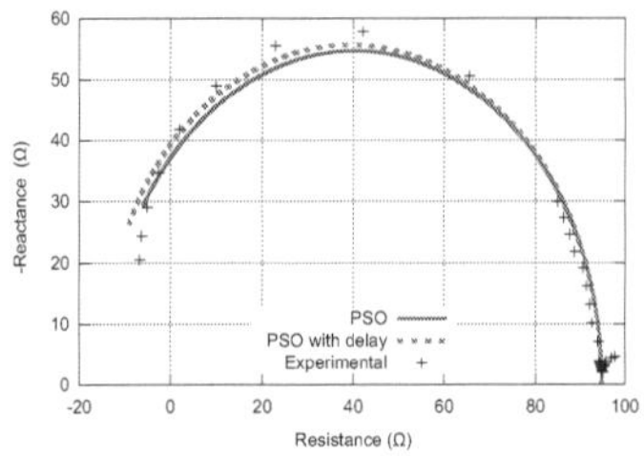

(b) Complex impedance diagram of mastitic milk with 1, 274 millions of cells per milliliter

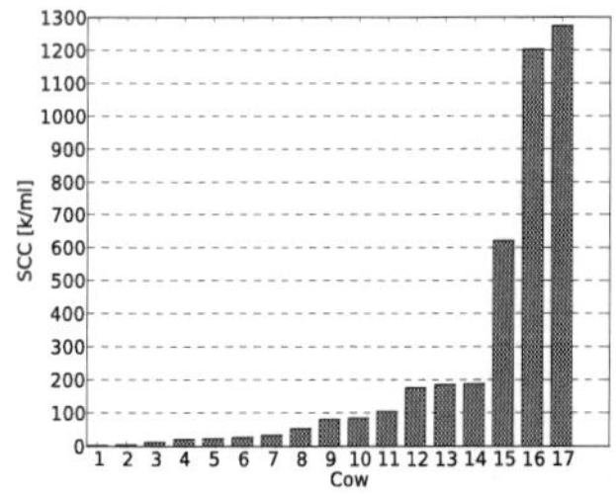

(c) Somatic cells concentration (SCC) for the 17 Holstein cows milk samples, given in thousands of cells per milliliter for each cow sample.

Fig. 11. The complex impedance arc locus diagram for two samples of milk with tolerable concentration of mastitis cells in fig. 11(a), a concentration above the limit characterizing mastitic milk in fig. 11(b). Experimental points and fitted curves with PSO and with the modified model function using the T_d parameter. In fig. 11(c), SCC for the evaluated samples.

markedly observed in the relaxation constant in the Cole-Cole function. The reciprocal of the relaxation constant would be related to the characteristic frequency of the sample that changes from 1.811 MHz to 1.941 MHz in the mastitic milk and in the compensated parameters. This indicates also that the experimental bioimpedance spectrum does not contain this frequency, requiring a wider frequency interval to evaluate more accurately the characteristics of the sample. In the low cell concentration mastitic milk, the parameters reflect a change in the frequency from 1.406 MHz to 1.488 MHz, that shows the same limitation in the experimental points, requiring a more detailed study where the spectrum will be analyzed with an analyzer in a wider frequency spectrum range.

In the results shown in table 4, the same compensation with a proper chosen time delay is applied to the Cole-Cole fitting and is compared to the parameters fitted with the PSO algorithm without compensation. One may observe that the low frequency resistance and the dispersion parameter α is not affected by the compensation, but the compensated high frequency resistances are no longer negative. The improvement in the mean squared error of the final fitting procedure is significantly reduced, more than in the case of the compensation

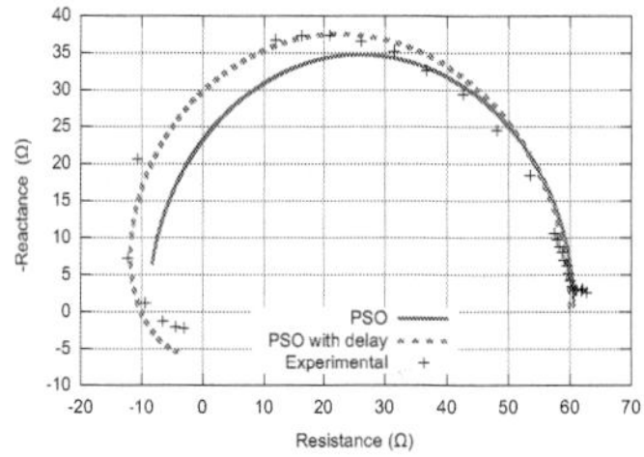

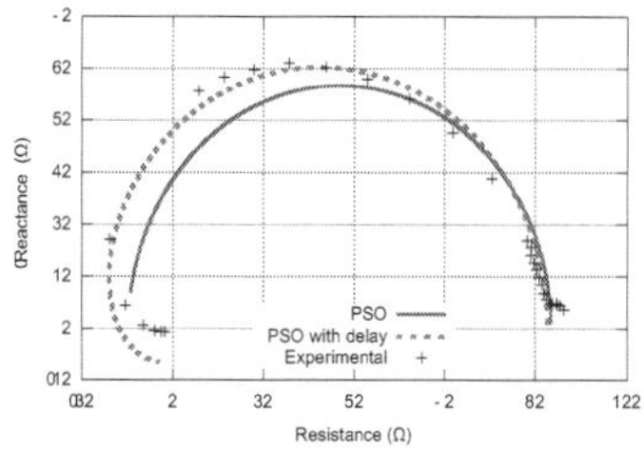

(a) Complex impedance diagram of raw milk (b) Complex impedance diagram of milk with water

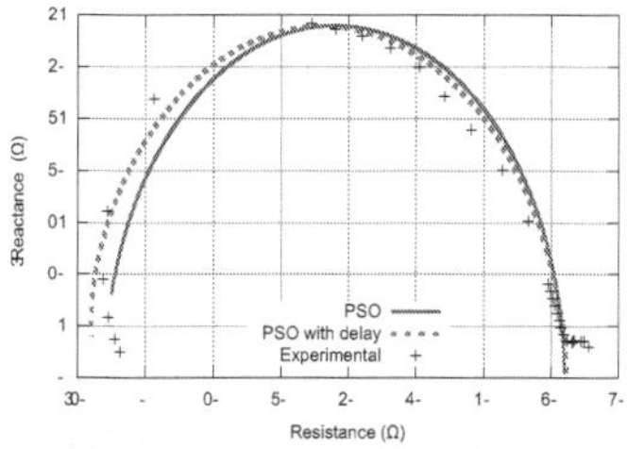

(c) Complex impedance diagram of milk with hydrogen peroxide

Fig. 12. The complex impedance arc locus diagram for samples of milk adulterated with water and hydrogen peroxide. The plots show the experimental points, the curve fitting with the Cole-Cole model function, and also the curve fitting containing the phase factor with the properly chosen time delay parameter.

Parameters	Raw milk	Compensated Raw Milk	Milk + H_2O	Compensated Milk + H_2O	Milk + H_2O_2	Compensated Milk + H_2O_2
R_∞ [Ω]	−8.8	0	−9.7	0	−5.9	0
R_0 [Ω]	60.6	59.9	83.5	82.7	62	62.4
α	1	1	1	1	1	0.95
τ [μs]	2.446	2.014	3.019	2.575	1.882	1.733
T_d [μs]	0	0.595	0	0.631	0	0.301
Mean Squared Error	24	4.7	39.3	13.4	10.8	6.7

Table 4. Cole-Cole parameters and final fitting mean squared error from the fitting with PSO algorithm for the spectra of adulterated milk samples and the bioimpedance from a raw milk sample, also containing the parameters from the fitted spectra compensated with specific time delays T_d.

of the mastitic milk data. The complex impedance arc locus of the evaluated cases can be seen in fig. 12. It is evident from fig. 12 that the compensating time delay improves the fitting, indicating that the stray impedance effect is responsible for an important contribution to the hook-like behavior of the complex impedance arc locus. Observing the dispersion parameter α, it is usually close to unity in every sample, compensated or not. This is an indication that the milk may be modeled by a single pole function with fitting errors of the same order of magnitude as shown in table 4 and 3. Differently from the mastitic milk analysis, the reciprocal of the relaxation constant is in the experimental frequency interval obtained with the BIA system. The characteristic frequency of the samples in the raw milk changes from 408 kHz to 496 kHz after compensation. Equivalently for adulterated milk with water and hydrogen peroxide, the changes occur from 331 kHz to 388 kHz and from 531 kHz to 577 kHz, respectively. These variations indicate an increase in the compensated characteristic frequency when the stray effects are compensated this way.

4. Conclusion

The authors report the use of computational intelligence and also well known digital signal processing algorithms in bioimpedance spectroscopy. The BIA analysis of data obtained from a custom made spectrometer were processed with a modulus retrieval algorithm from phase of bioimpedance spectra of vegetables showing the feasibility of using this specific and well known algorithm in a practical case. This would also allow the BIA system hardware to be simplified. In this case, since only the phase of the bioimpedance is going to be acquired to obtain the complete modulus of the bioimpedance spectrum, the involved electronic circuitry, as expected, may be reduced and the instrumentation amplifiers to measure modulus would be unnecessary. This would pave the way to embed algorithms in a much more simplified electronics for bioimpedance systems designed for specific applications as in the characterization of fruits, for example.

The bioimpedance data may also be processed with computational intelligence techniques. The authors improved already known techniques to fit experimental bioimpedance spectrum data to a specific model function. This is common practice in bioimpedance spectroscopy and is already implemented in commercial systems, however they do not use the techniques proposed here, only the least-squares algorithms, but no other more elaborate algorithms, like evolutionary techniques and particle-swarm optimization procedures. It is shown that the PSO technique has advantages over the already proposed procedures. The comparison of such techniques was implemented and artificial neural networks were used for the specific purpose of comparing them. The use of an Artificial Neural Network that receives as input the parameters produced by the fitting illustrates that different techniques, specifically the least-square fitting, simply would not be capable of allowing the identification of the correct tissue or the sample experimentally evaluated. The genetic algorithm and the particle-swarm optimization were capable of allowing the correct classification of the samples with experimental data added to noise in a much better proportion than the least-squares algorithm. Considering that the number of iterations in the PSO is much less than the genetic algorithm, and since they provide the same qualitative results in terms of classification, the PSO shows a superiority with respect to performance. The arithmetic complexity of the PSO is also an important characteristic that could facilitate embedded implementations.

Still in the dairy food applications, the idea of using bioimpedance to classify milk with the previously described techniques was also illustrated. Milk with different concentrations of mastitis cells were evaluated and the differences in the phase and modulus of the bioimpedance spectrum are noticed. However, the selectivity of the BIA system could not be demonstrated, and this would force one to use other additional sensing systems to evidence the interesting characteristic. During the evaluation of adulterated milk with typical adulterants, like water and hydrogen peroxide, the information would be present in the bioimpedance spectrum, but an identification of the exact adulterant or its quantity would require other sensing systems.

The experimental data produced with the milk evaluation have also other characteristics not related to the sample itself, but to the instrumentation and also to reactions occurring between the sample and the electrode. The hook like figure in the complex plane arc locus in the milk measurements demonstrate the effect. Such a behavior may be considered due to adsorption in the impedance electrode in some types of samples. However, the hook-like characteristic of the spectrum may be due to impedance stray effects, either from the cables, electrodes or the electronic circuitry. This may be corrected in some cases with a change in the model, by considering the effect of a phase corresponding to a complex exponential in the model function. The optimal values were determined for the correction and the error in the fitting was significantly reduced in those sets of data. Specifically in the raw mastitic and adulterated milk, the Cole-Cole parameters were compared and the fitting algorithms are once again shown to be efficient in illustrating the computational power of the techniques in bioimpedance spectroscopy.

5. Future directions

The idea of determining efficient and simple algorithms to process bioimpedance spectra is a topic that may allow the implementation of sophisticated algorithms in embedded systems and could also improve the quality of the analysis produced by simple equipment. One can mention that in the case of the phase/modulus retrieval algorithms, since the technique is based on the use of the well-known fast-Fourier transform algorithm, it would be natural to implement it in embedded systems. However, the applications could not be restricted to such systems, since the use of the proposed algorithms may help improve the bioimpedance spectrum analysis while correcting experimental data and retrieving the more convenient information from the improved fitting algorithms. The methodology that uses artificial neural networks to evaluate the performance of the algorithms could also be used in systems that require automated analysis of bioimpedance spectra, as in an industrial environment to characterize samples of milk or beef, for example.

As a direction to the future research efforts, a final goal for the use of such algorithms would be their implementation in reconfigurable hardware, more specifically, in field-programmable gate arrays (FPGA). Commercial systems already use such technologies, like the FPGA in bioimpedance spectrometers (Nacke et al., 2011). Therefore the evaluated techniques are suggested to be implemented in hardware, since the particle swarm optimization algorithms would be a good choice for this purpose. The arithmetic operations in the particle-swarm optimization update step requires only random number generation, and a series of summations and multiplications. In the phase/modulus retrieval algorithm case, the FFT could also be easily instantiated from the core provided by the FPGA company.

6. Acknowledgements

The authors gratefully acknowledge the experimental data collected by Rogerio Martins Pereira, Rodrigo Stiz and Guilherme Martignago Zilli as students supervised in the Laboratories of the Santa Catarina State University in Joinville City.

7. References

Aberg, P., Nicander, I., Hansson, J., Geladi, P., Holmgren, U. & Ollmar, S. (2004). Skin cancer identification using multifrequency electrical impedance - a potential screening tool, *IEEE Transactions on Biomedical Engineering* 51(12): 2097–2102.

Anastasiadis, A. D. & Ph, U. U. (2003). An efficient improvement of the RPROP algorithm, *In Proceedings of the First International Workshop on Artificial Neural Networks in Pattern Recognition*.

Barsoukov, E. & Macdonald, J. R. (eds) (2005). *Impedance spectroscopy: theory, experiment and applications*, 2 edn, Wiley, New York.

Belloque, J., Chicon, R. & Recio, I. (2008). *Milk Processing and Quality Management*, 1 edn, Wiley-Blackwell, West Sussex, United Kingdom.

Bertemes-Filho, P. (2002). *Tissue Characterisation using an Impedance Spectroscopy Probe*, PhD Thesis, The University of Sheffield, UK.

Bertemes-Filho, P., Negri, L. H. & Paterno, A. S. (2010). Mastitis characterization of bovine milk using electrical impedance spectroscopy, *Congresso Brasileiro de Engenharia Biomédica (CBEB) – Biomedical Engineering Brazilian Congress*, pp. 1351–1353.

Bertemes-Filho, P., Negri, L. & Paterno, A. (2011). Detection of bovine milk adulterants using bioimpedance measurements and artificial neural network, *in* Ákos Jobbágy (ed.), *5th European Conference of the International Federation for Medical and Biological Engineering*, Vol. 37 of *IFMBE Proceedings*, Springer, pp. 1275–1278.

Bertemes-Filho, P., Paterno, A. S. & Pereira, R. M. (2009). Multichannel bipolar current source used in electrical impedance spectroscopy: Preliminary results, *in* O. Dössel, W. C. Schlegel & R. Magjarevic (eds), *World Congress on Medical Physics and Biomedical Engineering, September 7 - 12, 2009, Munich, Germany*, Vol. 25/7 of *IFMBE Proceedings*, Springer Berlin Heidelberg, pp. 657–660.
URL: *http://dx.doi.org/10.1007/978-3-642-03885-3_182*

Bertemes-Filho, P., Valicheski, R., Pereira, R. M. & Paterno, A. S. (2010). Bioelectrical impedance analysis for bovine milk: Preliminary results, *Journal of Physics: Conference Series* 224(1): 012133.
URL: *http://stacks.iop.org/1742-6596/224/i=1/a=012133*

Brown, B. H. (2003). Electrical impedance tomography (EIE): a review, *J. Med. Eng. Technol.* 3: 97–108.

Cole, K. S. (1940). Permeability and impermeability of cell membranes for ions, *Cold Spring Harb. Symp. Quant. Biol.* 8: 110.

Cole, K. S. (1968). *Membranes, Ions and Impulses: A Chapter of Classical Biophysics*, Biophysics Series, first edn, University of California Press.

Cole, K. S. & Cole, R. H. (1941). Dispersion and Absorption in Dielectrics I. Alternating Current Characteristics, *The Journal of Chemical Physics* 9(4): 341–351.
URL: *http://link.aip.org/link/doi/10.1063/1.1750906*

Cybenko, G. (1989). Approximation by superpositions of a sigmoidal function, *Mathematics of Control, Signals, and Systems (MCSS)* 2: 303–314.

De Lorenzo, A., Andreoli, A., Matthie, J. & Withers, P. (1997). Predicting body cell mass with bioimpedance by using theoretical methods: a technological review, *Journal of Applied Physiology* 82(5): 1542–1558. URL: *http://jap.physiology.org/content/82/5/1542.abstract*

Fuoss, R. M. & Kirkwood, J. G. (1941). Electrical properties of solids. viii. dipole moments in polyvinyl chloride-diphenyl systems*, *Journal of the American Chemical Society* 63(2): 385–394. URL: *http://pubs.acs.org/doi/abs/10.1021/ja01847a013*

Gorban, A. (1998). Approximation of continuous functions of several variables by an arbitrary nonlinear continuous function of one variable, linear functions, and their superpositions, *Applied Mathematics Letters* 11(3): 45 – 49.
URL: *http://www.sciencedirect.com/science/article/pii/S0893965998000329*

Grimnes, S. & Martinsen, O. G. (2008). *Bioimpedance & Bioelectricity BASICS*, 2 edn, Academic Press.

Halter, R. J., Hartov, A., Paulsen, K. D., Schned, A. & Heaney, J. (2008). Genetic and least squares algorithms for estimating spectral eis parameters of prostatic tissues, *Physiological Measurement* 29(6): S111.
URL: *http://stacks.iop.org/0967-3334/29/i=6/a=S10*

Hamann, J. & Zecconi, A. (1998). Bulletin 334, *Evaluation of the Electrical Conductivity of Milk as a Mastitis Indicator*, International Dairy Federation, pp. 1–23.

Hassan, R., Cohanim, B., Weck, O. D. & Venter, G. (2005). A comparison of particle swarm optimization and the genetic algorithm, *46th AIAA/ASME/ASCE/AHS/ASC Structures, Structural Dynamics, and Materials Conference*, pp. 1–13.

Hayes, M., Lin, J. S. & Oppenheim, A. V. (1980). Signal Reconstruction from Phase or Magnitude, *IEEE Transactions on Acoustics, Speech and Signal Processing* 28(6): 672–680.
URL: *http://dx.doi.org/10.1109/TASSP.1980.1163463*

Haykin, S. (1999). *Neural Networks*, Prentice-Hall, New Jersey.

Holder, D. S. (2004). *Electrical impedance tomography: methods, history and applications*, 1st edn, Taylor and Francis, New York.

Kitchen, B. J. (1981). Bovine mastitis: milk compositional changes and related diagnostic tests, *Journal of Dairy Research* 48(01): 167–188.
URL: *http://dx.doi.org/10.1017/S0022029900021580*

Kronig, R. D. L. (1929). The theory of dispersion of x-rays, *Journal of the Optical Society of America* 12(6): 547.
URL: *http://dx.doi.org/10.1364/JOSA.12.000547*

Kun, S., Ristić, B., Peura, R. A. & Dunn, R. M. (2003). Algorithm for tissue ischemia estimation based on electrical impedance spectroscopy, *IEEE Transactions on Biomedical Engineering* 50(12): 1352–9.

Kun, S., Ristic, B., Peura, R. & Dunn, R. (1999). Real-time extraction of tissue impedance model parameters for electrical impedance spectrometer, *Medical and Biological Engineering and Computing* 37: 428–432.
URL: *http://dx.doi.org/10.1007/BF02513325*

Kyle, U. G., Bosaeus, I., Lorenzo, A. D. D., Deurenberg, P., Elia, M., Gómez, J. M., Heitmann, B. L., Kent-Smith, L., Melchior, J.-C., Pirlich, M., Scharfetter, H., Schols, A. M. & Pichard, C. (2004). Bioelectrical impedance analysis: part i. Review of principles and methods, *Clinical Nutrition* 23(5): 1226.

Nacke, T., Barthel, A., Beckmann, D., Pliquett, U., Friedrich, J., Peyerl, P., Helbig, M. & Sachs, J. (2011). Messsystem für die impedanzspektroskopische breitband-prozessmesstechnik – broadband impedance spectrometer for process instrumentation, *Technisches Messen* 78(1): 3–14.
URL: *http://www.oldenbourg-link.com/doi/abs/10.1524/teme.2011.0077*

Negri, L. H., Bertemes-Filho, P. & Paterno, A. S. (2010). Extração dos parâmetros da função de Cole-Cole utilizando otimização por enxame de partículas, *XXII Congresso Brasileiro de Engenharia Biomédica (CBEB) – Biomedical Engineering Brazilian Congress*, pp. 928–931.

Nordbotten, B. J., Tronstad, C., Ørjan G Martinsen & Grimnes, S. (2011). Evaluation of algorithms for calculating bioimpedance phase angle values from measured whole-body impedance modulus, *Physiological Measurement* 32(7): 755.
URL: *http://stacks.iop.org/0967-3334/32/i=7/a=S03*

Paterno, A. S. & Hoffmann, M. (2008). Reconstrução de sinais em espectroscopia de bioimpedância elétrica, *XXI Congresso Brasileiro de Engenharia Biomédica (CBEB) – Biomedical Engineering Brazilian Congress*, pp. 1–4.

Paterno, A., Stiz, R. & Bertemes-Filho, P. (2009). Frequency-domain reconstruction of signals in electrical bioimpedance spectroscopy, *Medical and Biological Engineering and Computing* 47: 1093–1102.
URL: *http://dx.doi.org/10.1007/s11517-009-0533-1*

Piton, C., Dasen, A. & Bardoux, I. (1988). Evaluation de la mesure d'impédance comme technique rapide d'appréciation de la qualité bactériologique du lait cru, *Lait* 68(4): 467–484.
URL: *http://dx.doi.org/10.1051/lait:1988430*

Proakis, J. G. & Manolakis, D. K. (2006). *Digital Signal Processing*, 4 edn, Prentice Hall.

Quartieri, T. & Oppenheim, A. V. (1981). Iterative techniques for minimum phase signal reconstruction from phase or magnitude, *IEEE Transactions on Acoustics, Speech and Signal Processing* 29(6): 1187–1193.
URL: *http://dx.doi.org/10.1109/TASSP.1981.1163714*

Riu, P. J. & Lapaz, C. (1999). Practical limits of the Kramers-Kronig relationships applied to experimental bioimpedance data, *Annals of the New York Academy of Sciences* 873(1): 374–380.
URL: *http://dx.doi.org/10.1111/j.1749-6632.1999.tb09486.x*

Siegelmann, H. T. & Sontag, E. D. (1991). Turing computability with neural nets, *Applied Mathematics Letters* 4(6): 77 – 80.
URL: *http://www.sciencedirect.com/science/article/pii/089396599190080F*

Stiz, R. A., Bertemes, P., Ramos, A. & Vincence, V. C. (2009). Wide band Howland bipolar current source using AGC amplifier, *IEEE Latin America Transactions* 7(5): 514–518.

Waterworth, A. R. (2000). *Data Analysis Techniques of Measured Biological Impedance*, Phd Thesis, The University of Sheffield, UK.

Wilamowski, B. M. (2009). Neural network architectures and learning algorithms, *IEEE Industrial Electronics Magazine* 3: 56–63.

Xiaohui, H., Yuhui, S. & Eberhart, R. (2004). *Congress on Evolutionary Computation, 2004 – CEC2004*, Vol. 1, IEEE, pp. 90–97.
URL: *http://ieeexplore.ieee.org/xpl/freeabs_all.jsp?arnumber=1330842*

2

Computer Simulation and Analysis of Three-Dimensional Tumor Geometry in Radiotherapy

Seishin Takao, Shigeru Tadano,
Hiroshi Taguchi and Hiroki Shirato
Hokkaido University
Japan

1. Introduction

Radiotherapy plays an important role in the treatment for patients with solid tumors. Recently, the advantages in high-precision radiotherapy enable focusing of higher radiation energy (dose) to the tumor region while minimizing unwanted radiation exposure to surrounding normal tissue to avoid radiation injury. Intensity-modulated radiation therapy (IMRT) varies the intensities and profiles of beams from various directions to fit the tumor size and shape. This technique greatly improves dose concentration on target region and normal tissue sparing. Image-guided radiation therapy (IGRT) uses advanced imaging technology such as on-board imaging system to achieve precise and accurate dose delivery. Many studies have reported inter-fractional organ motions and efficacy of IGRT in reducing targeting errors using daily CT images (Den et al. 2009, Wang et al. 2009, Houghton et al. 2009, Pawlowski et al. 2010, Varadhan et al. 2009, Greene et al. 2009). Owing to these techniques, errors in patient set-up and dose delivery can be reduced to some extent. However, as radiotherapy typically takes several weeks, tumor and normal tissues may deform due to therapeutic effect or loss of body weight during treatment period. Shapes and locations of the tumor and the surrounding organs would be quite different from those when the treatment was planned. This results in overdosage of surrounding normal tissue or underdosage of target region. To overcome this issue, it would be useful to precisely analyse and predict the changes in three-dimensional (3D) geometries of tumors and normal tissues through the treatment.

However, even methodology to evaluate 3D tumor shapes has not been established yet. At present, tumor diameter is commonly used as an indicator to evaluate therapeutic response in cancer patients. Since the 1970s, the World Health Organization (WHO) had suggested to assess tumor response by measurement of maximum diameter and largest perpendicular diameter (World Health Organization, 1979). The response evaluation criteria in solid tumor (RECIST) guideline proposed to use only maximum diameter in categorizing therapeutic response (Therasse et al. 2000, Werner-Wasik et al. 2001). Some researchers have reported that this difference in diagnostic criteria often resulted in different categorization of therapeutic response. Rohbe et al. stated that volumetric measurement with CT might help to evaluate therapeutic response more accurately (Rohbe et al. 2007). For more precise assessment, it would be useful to examine 3D tumor morphological features.

For the purpose of prediction of therapeutic effect, various computational methods have been proposed for simulation of tumor growth and shrinkage as the effects of radiotherapy. Almost all of these method consider tumor as concentration of huge number of cancer cells and calculate the death or birth of these cells pursuant to some rules based on the cell biology (Dionysiou et al. 2004, Stamatakos et al. 2010, Kolokotroni et al. 2011). These approaches look attractive, however it seems to be difficult to implement them into clinical situation because therapeutic effect cannot be evaluated accurately only by the number of cancer cells. Usable method for prediction and evaluation of therapeutic response of tumors has been required strongly.

Authors have proposed novel numerical simulation method to predict changes in tumor volume in radiotherapy (Takao et al. 2009a). We have also established the methodology to evaluate 3D tumor shape visually using color map called surface geometry map (Takao et al. 2009b and 2011). From these knowledge, we proposed simulation method to predict changes in 3D tumor shape through the treatment duration and evaluated tumor geometry visually and quantitatively.

2. Analysis of three-dimensional tumor geometry

It would be valuable if changes in 3D tumor shapes during treatment can be evaluated visually and quantitatively. Quantitative evaluation could be performed using geometric factors such as volume, surface area, and radius. For visual evaluation, we introduce some color map called surface geometry map to represent 3D tumor geometry (shape) into two-dimensional plane. The volume of tumor is also represented as size of the map. Therefore, this surface geometry map is useful to understand how the tumor shrinks during treatment.

2.1 Geometric factor

For quantitative (or numerical) analysis of tumor geometry, volume V, surface area S were measured and evaluated based on the 3D surface models of the tumors constructed from CT image sets taken once a week during treatment. From the values of V and S, spherical shape factor (SSF) which represents degree of sphericity was calculated by following equation (Choia HJ and Choi HK 2007).

$$SSF = \frac{36\pi V^2}{S^3} \tag{1}$$

If SSF=1, the tumor has a perfect sphere. As surface roughness increase, the value of SSF decreases. Tumor radius $R(\theta, \varphi)$ was also measured in all directions from the gravitational canter of the tumor.

2.2 Surface geometry map

We introduced surface geometry map like a global map to visualyze changes in 3D tumor shape (Takao et al. 2009a). Distances from the center of the gravity to its surface, i.e. radius $R(\theta, \varphi)$ were measured in the spherical coordinate system $O\text{-}R\theta\varphi$, with the origin is set at the tumor center. The angle θ represents the azimuthal angle ($-180° \le \theta \le 180°$), and the angle φ

represents the polar angle (-90° ≤ φ ≤ 90°). Radius $R(\theta, \varphi)$ was sampled at 10° intervals in both the polar and azimuthal directions. To enable a visual understanding of the features of the 3D geometry of the tumor, the values of radius $R(\theta, \varphi)$ were represented in a color scale and plotted in the θ-ϕ plane: red indicates the maximum radius and blue the minimum within the tumor. The warm colors (red and yellow) represent convex region and cool colors (blue) represents concave areas (Fig. 1).

Further, to evaluate changes in tumor geometry quantitatively, the image correlation was analyzed. Surface geometry maps were converted into grayscale, therefore the intensities in the maps represented the tumor radius. The intensities at every position in the maps created from CT images taken during the treatment were compared with those of the corresponding position in the map before the treatment, and correlation coefficient was calculated. Similar analysis was performed to evaluate our simulation method, especially calculation considering tumor heterogeneity (discussed later).

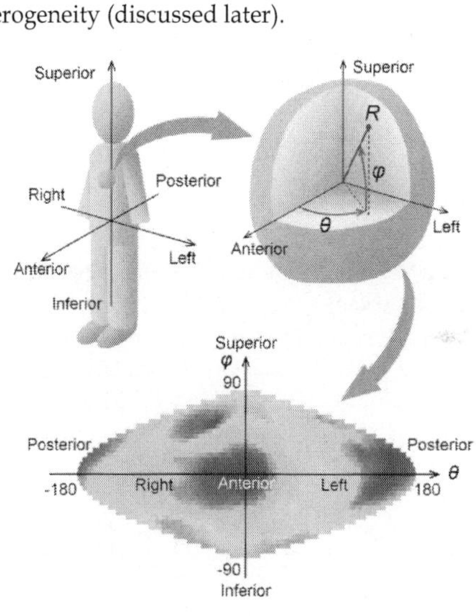

Fig. 1. Coordinate system in radiotherapy and representation of 3D tumor geometry using 2D surface geometry map

3. Simulation of changes in tumor geometry

3.1 Equations for tumor deformation

Equations for describing changes in 3D tumor geometry were established using analogy with deformation of continuous body in solid mechanics (Takao et al. 2009b) (Fig. 2). The relationship between radiation dose D and cell mortality fraction M is described as follows,

$$dM_{ij} = C_{ijkl} dD_{kl} \tag{2}$$

Radiation dose and mortality fraction are tentatively treated as tensor quantities in formulation process so that direction of shrinkage can be considered. C_{ijkl} is the parameter of radioresistance and varies as the function of radiation dose.

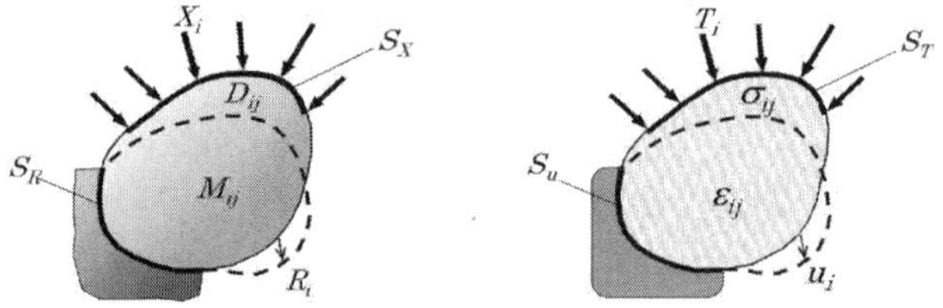

Fig. 2. Tumor deformation due to radiotherapy estimated from solid mechanics.
X_i: Exposure dose, D_{ij}: absorbed dose, M_{ij}: cell mortality, R_i: therapeutic displacement, T_i: external force, σ_{ij}: stress, ε_{ij}: strain, u_i: displacement. Absorbed dose and cell mortality are defined as tensor quantities. Boundary conditions are prescribed on area S_X and S_R.

Radiation dose D should obey following equations in accordance with the rule in solid mechanics.

$$\frac{\partial(D_{ij})}{\partial x_j} = 0 \tag{3}$$

Assuming that cancer cells killed by irradiation are removed from the tumor, decrease in the number of cancer cells, i.e., cell mortality directly relates to the changes in tumor volume and shape. The relationship between cell mortality M and the displacement of tumor boundary R is formulated as follows,

$$dM_{ij} = \frac{1}{2}\left[\frac{\partial(dR_i)}{\partial x_j} + \frac{\partial(dR_j)}{\partial x_i}\right] \tag{4}$$

The boundary condition that prescribes the amount of radiation dose transmitted through the tumor boundary is given by

$$d\overline{X}_i = dD_{ij}n_j \quad \text{(on } S_X, S_X\text{; irradiation boundary)} \tag{5}$$

The geometrical boundary condition is given by

$$d\overline{R}_i = dR_i \quad \text{(on } S_R, S_R\text{; geometrical boundary)} \tag{6}$$

Equations (2)-(6) express tumor response to irradiation in clinical situation. These equations can be solved numerically by means of discretization method such as finite element method (FEM). Assuming that tumors locally (in a sub-millimeter scale) have an isotropic property, C_{ijkl} parameter in Eq. (2) for radioresistance is represented by two parameters; reduction resistance E and reduction ratio ν. The values of E and ν should be determined based on the radiobiological model describing the relationship between radiation dose and therapeutic effect. Here we use the linear-quadratic (LQ) model, which is widely accepted and used in the field of radiobiology. According to the LQ model, cell survival fraction S is expressed by following equation,

$$S = \exp(-\alpha D - \beta D^2) \tag{7}$$

where α and β are parameters of radiosensitivity. In standard radiotherapy, fractionated irradiation, which gives small radiation dose in many times, is performed for reducing radiation damage to normal tissue. Cell survival after n times irradiation (total dose of D, administered in fractionated dose of d) is denoted as follows,

$$S = \exp\{-(\alpha + \beta d)D\} \tag{8}$$

This formula is rewritten as the relationship between radiation dose and mortality fraction and in incremental form as,

$$dM = (\alpha + \beta d)\exp\{-(\alpha + \beta d)D\}dD \tag{9}$$

Equation (9) denotes mortality fraction as the function of radiation dose in terms of radiobiology. Equally equation (2) represents same quantity based on the analogy with solid mechanics. Therefore, right-hand sides of both two equations can be equated and following relationship can be derived.

$$\frac{3(1-2\nu)}{E}\left(1-\frac{1-2\nu}{E}D\right)^2 = (\alpha + \beta d)\exp\{-(\alpha + \beta d)D\} \tag{10}$$

Equation (10) gives the condition that the parameters E and ν must satisfy. When the values of E and ν are determined, therapeutic displacement Ri can be calculated by means of numerical discretization method such as finite element method.

3.2 Heterogeneity of tumor radiosensitivity

Tumor shows internal heterogeneity of radiosensitivity, and it may result in uneven tumor shrinkage. For example, cancer cells under hypoxic environment are likely to be radioresistant, therefore tumor tissue in this region usually does not shrink obviously. Tumor radiosensitivity also varies depend on many other factors such as cell cycle phase or growth rate of each cell. Because of its complexity, it still seems difficult to measure or estimate the distribution of radiosensitivity in tumor tissue. In this study, intratumoral distribution of radiosensitivity is estimated from the degree of tumor shrinkage in the early stage of treatment. The site where tumor radius decreases greatly is considered to be more radiosensitive, and the site where tumor radius decrease slightly is more radioresistant. Therefore tumor radiosensitivity can be represented as the function of position within the tumor. As radiosensitivity is represented by E parameter in this model, heterogeneity of radiosensitivity can be expressed by the distribution of the values of E.

3.3 Simulation procedure

Simulation flow-chart for calculation of tumor geometry is shown in Fig. 3. First, finite element (FE) models of the tumor at the start of the treatment was constructed from the CT images taken for the purpose of treatment planning. Next the values of parameters for tumor radiosensitivity in LQ model, α and β, were set as $\alpha = 0.1$ and $\beta = 0.01$ (α/β=10.0) as suggested by Thames et al. (Thames et al. 1990). Other simulations parameters were consecutively determined The reduction resistance ν was tentatively set to 0 assuming that the relationship between tumor response and radiation dose would entirely obey the LQ model. After then, the reduction resistance E was calculated from Eq. (10) using α, β, cumulative dose D, and daily dose d. The E parameter was initially considered to be uniform throughout the tumor. Using these parameters, changes in tumor volume was calculated by means of FE analysis software. Calculated tumor volumes were compared with corresponding tumor volumes measured from CT image sets for treatment follow-up. Followed by this process, the value of reduction ratio ν, which represents interpatient variation in radiosensitivity, was adjusted for each case so that the discrepancy between the calculated and the actual tumor volumes obtained from follow-up CT would decrease. If the calculated volume was less than the actual volume, the value of ν was incremented and then the tumor volume was recalculated. This iterative process was continued till the root mean square (RMS) error of the calculated and actual tumor volumes reached a minimum.

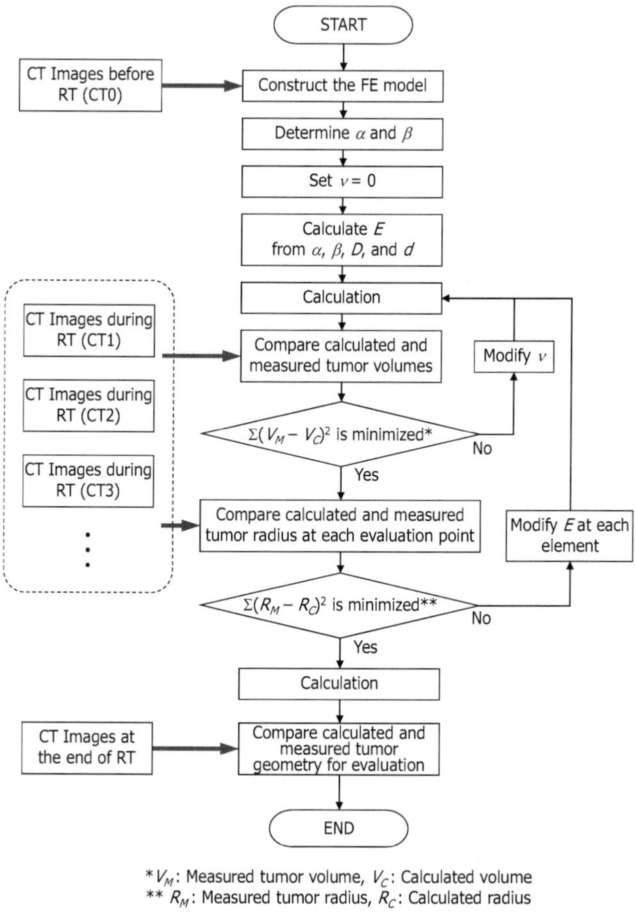

Fig. 3. Flow chart illustrating simulation steps to calculate and predict changes in 3D tumor shape during radiotherapy.

After that, similar process was performed to determine the distribution of the parameter *E* (reduction resistance) to represent intratumoral heterogeneity of radiosensitivity. The *E* parameter was so far considered to be uniform throughout the tumor. In following calculation, the value of *E* parameter was set for each element, which constitutes the whole 3D tumor model for FEA calculation, as the function of azimuthal angle and polar angle φ. Depending on the distance from the gravity center of the tumor to surface, the value of *E* at (θ, φ) was determined by following equation.

$$E(\theta,\varphi)^{n+1} = \frac{R(\theta,\varphi)_M}{R(\theta,\varphi)_C} E(\theta,\varphi)^n \tag{11}$$

where, superscript represents the number of iteration, $R(\theta, \varphi)_M$ is measured tumor radius at (θ, φ), and $R(\theta, \varphi)_C$ is calculated tumor radius at the corresponding point.

4. Clinical cases

4.1 Patient characteristics

The subjects of this study were three clinical cases (case A, B, and C) of metastatic cervical lymph nodes in three patients with nasopharyngeal cancer treated at the Hokkaido University Hospital, Sapporo, Japan between February 2007 and August 2007. Of the patients, case A and B were undifferentiated carcinoma and case C was squamous cell carcinoma. Initial volumes of lymph nodes were 3.5, 55.1, and 10.4 cm^3, respectively. Case A and C were treated with IMRT; patient B received conventional radiotherapy. The dose distribution before radiotherapy intended each node in this study to be homogeneously irradiated with a dose of 66 Gy (case A) to 70 Gy (case B, C) in 2.0 Gy fractions delivered five times a week.

Pre-treatment CT images (CT0) were taken for the treatment planning. The slice thickness of the pre-treatment CT images was 2 mm. After the start of treatment, follow-up CT images were taken at weekly intervals (CT1, CT2, CT3, etc). The slice thickness of the follow-up CT images was 5 mm. All patients were immobilized by thermoplastic masks during the CT scanning and treatment. Additionally, in the head and neck IMRT treatments in our hospital, A mouthpiece with three fiducial markers (2 mm diameter gold pellets) was used for the fluoroscopic verification of the patient set-up by means of real-time tumor-tracking radiotherapy (RTRT) system. This study was conducted with written informed consent obtained from all patients and was approved by the institutional ethical committee at Hokkaido University Hospital.

4.2 Finite element modeling of tumors

Three-dimensional finite element (FE) models of tumors were constructed based on the CT images taken before and during treatment (Fig. 4). One radiation oncologist determined and contoured the boundary of metastatic cervical lymph nodes on the CT images by means of a treatment planning system (Xio). A group of sequential cross-sectional profiles of the tumor was then loaded into biomedical imaging software and interpolated to 1 mm intervals. After file format conversion with in-house software, the data was imported into the finite element analysis software (ANSYS 11.0), and the 3D FE models of the tumors were constructed.

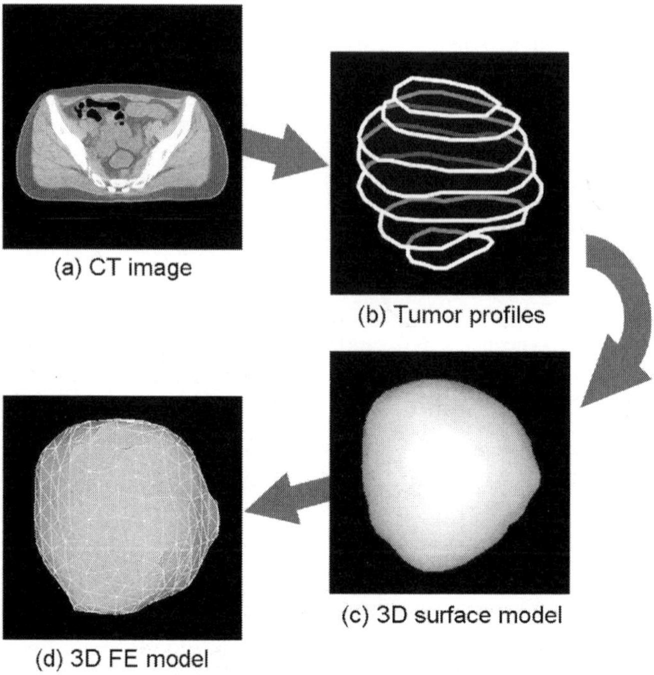

Fig. 4. Process of finite element modelling of tumor. (a) tumor region (red edging) on CT images (b) tumor profiles in each sectional image (c) 3D surface model (d) 3D finite element model

5. Results

This study first aimed to evaluate changes in 3D tumor shapes during treatment visually and quantitatively. We constructed surface model of tumors and then analysed the 3D shapes by geometric factors for quantitative evaluation. Two-dimensional surface geometry map was also proposed for visual evaluation of 3D morphological features of tumors. Other main aims of this study was to propose simulation method to predict changes in 3D tumor shape during radiotherapy.

5.1 Analysis of three-dimensional tumor geometry

5.1.1 Geometric factors

This study investigated geometric factors to accurately evaluate therapeutic response in radiotherapy. Tumor volume, surface area, radius, and spherical shape factor (SSF) were used to quantitatively evaluate tumor geometry. Fig. 5-7 show changes in geometric factors of tumors through treatment duration for quantitative analysis of 3D tumor morphology. Changes in tumor volume and surface area are shown in Fig. 5 and 6. Tumor volume at the end of the treatment period was 8.7% of its initial volume in case A, 15% in case B, and 23% in case C. Changes in tumor surface area showed similar tendency with changes in tumor volume. Tumor surface areas at the end of the treatment were 20%, 28%, and 37% for case A, B, and C, respectively. Changes in SSF are shown in Fig. 7. The values of SSF were about 0.8 through the treatment duration and did not vary widely in all three cases.

Fig. 8 shows changes in average, maximum, and minimum tumor radius through the treatment period. At the start of treatment, each average radius was 9.8 mm, 24.6 mm, and 14.4 mm in tumor A, B, and C. The tumor radius ranged from 7.3 mm to 13.3 mm (75 % to 137 % of average radius) in tumor A, 17.4 mm to 34.4 mm (71 % to 140 %) in tumor B, 9.2 mm to 20.3 mm (64 % to 142 %) in tumor C, respectively. At the end of the treatment, average radius decreased to 4.5 mm, 13.5 mm, and 8.9 mm, respectively. The ranges of radius were 3.3 mm to 5.8 mm (73 % to 129 % of the average radius at the end of the treatment) in tumor A, 9.4 mm to 18.2 mm (70 % to 135 %) in tumor B, 6.3 mm to 12.5 mm (71 % to 140 %) in tumor C, respectively. In Fig. 8, all values are represented as percentages of each initial average radius.

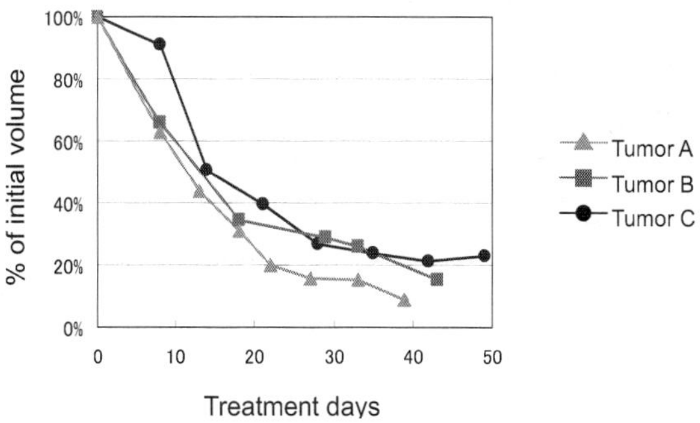

Fig. 5. Changes in tumor volume during radiotherapy. Tumor volumes at each evaluation point are represented as the percentage of initial volume.

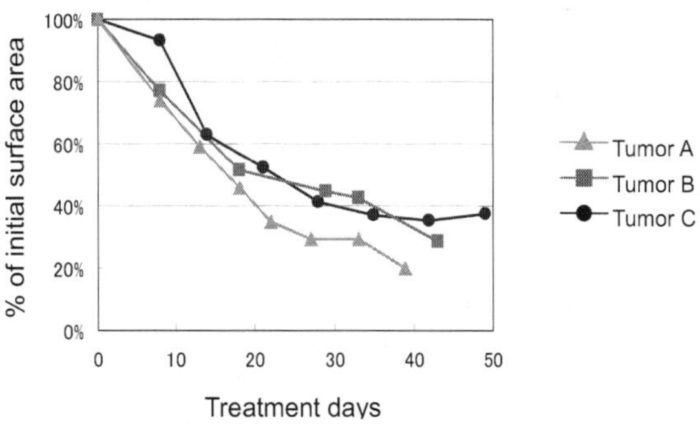

Fig. 6. Changes in tumor surface are during radiotherapy. Tumor surface area at each evaluation point are represented as the percentage of initial surface area.

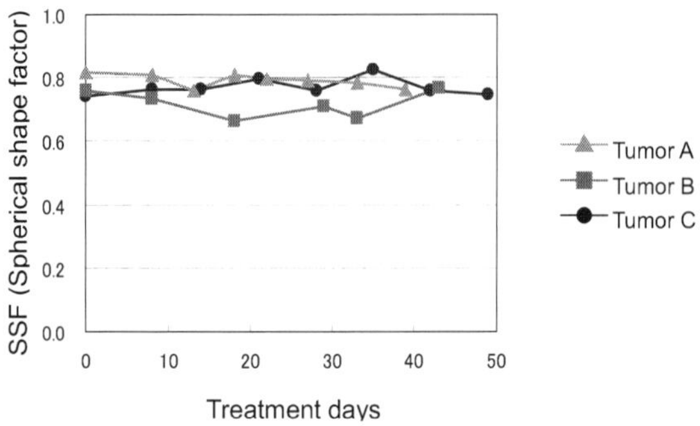

Fig. 7. Changes in spherical shape factors in radiotherapy.

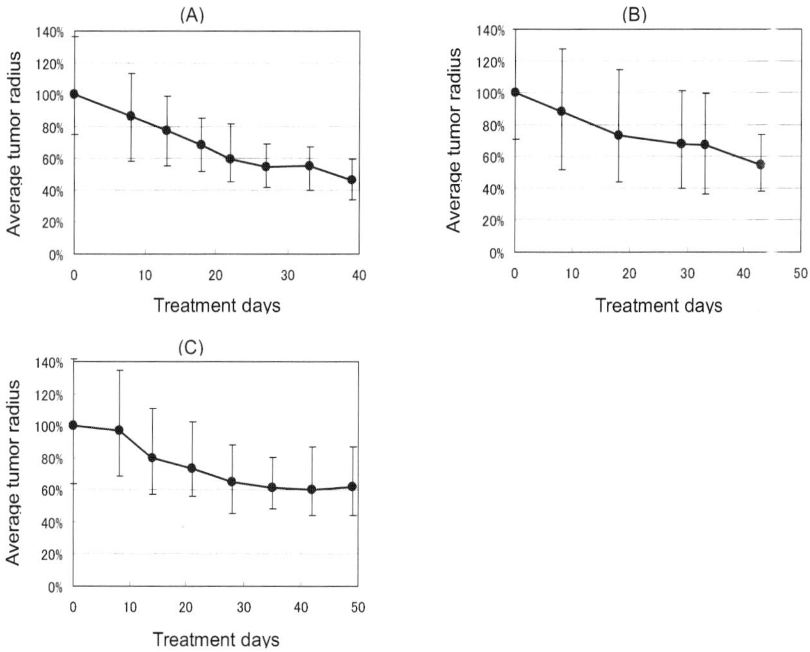

Fig. 8. Changes of average tumor radius during the treatment in tumor A, B, and C. Vertical lines represent ranges from minimum to maximum.

5.1.2 Surface geometry map

This study also proposed representation and evaluation method for changes in 3D tumor geometry using 2D surface geometry map. Distances from the geometrical center to surface were represented in color scale for visual understanding of 3D tumor shape. Fig. 9

shows the changes in tumor geometry through treatment duration using surface geometry map. The red end of the color scale is convex region and blue is concave region. Therefore surface geometry map can provide information about 3D geometrical feature of the tumor. The patterns of color distribution are found to be similar in each case. This result means that tumor shrunk uniformly keeping their original morphological features through the treatment duration.

5.2 Simulation of changes in tumor geometry

A computational simulation method to predict changes in 3D tumor geometry during radiotherapy was proposed. Simulation parameters were determined based on the changes in tumor geometry in the early stage of the treatment (first 19 days in case A and B, 22 days in case C). Using these parameters, tumor geometries in the latter half of the treatment period were calculated sequentially.

Simulation results are shown in Fig. 10-12. Simulation could represent tendencies of tumor geometrical changes in the first 19 or 22 days in each case. Calculation to predict tumor geometries in the rest of the treatment was performed subsequently. The predicted tumor geometries were compared with corresponding actual tumor geometries by surface geometry maps. The calculated tumor geometry at the end of the treatment was found to conform to actual tumor geometry. The discrepancy between calculated and actual tumor geometry could be quantitatively evaluated by tumor radius $R(\theta, \varphi)$. The discrepancies between calculated and actual tumor radius (calculated tumor radius - actual tumor radius) at the end of the treatment were 0.2 mm (maximum), -1.4 mm (minimum), and 0.5 mm (average absolute value) for tumor A, 3.4 mm, -6.3 mm, and 2.1 mm for tumor B, 0.4 mm, -4.3 mm, and 1.3 mm for tumor C, respectively, while average of actual tumor radius was 5.4 mm for tumor A, and 13.2 mm for tumor B, 8.4 mm tumor C, respectively.

6. Discussion

Precise assessment of therapeutic response in radiotherapy has been an important issue in the field of radiation oncology. To understand how tumor geometries change during the treatment would be useful for not only determination of prognosis but for treatment plans as well. However, there has been no research which visualized 3D tumor geometries and evaluated the therapeutic response based on the changes of tumor geometries. In this study, we proposed a method to represent 3D tumor geometry in 2D color map, and evaluated therapeutic response through the treatment period, as well as geometric factors representing therapeutic response quantitatively.

Surface geometry map introduced in this study could indicate 3D morphological features of the tumors in color scale. These figures show that tumors shrank evenly maintaining their original shape. This would be valuable information for determining the optimal radiation field in the latter half of the treatment. The degree of tumor shrinkage, i.e. decrease in tumor radius (shown in Fig. 8), varied approximately plus or minus 20 % depending on tumor region. This variation was considered to represent intratumoral heterogeneity. These findings cannot be obtained from commonly-used geometric factor, i. e., tumor volume or maximum diameter measured on CT images.

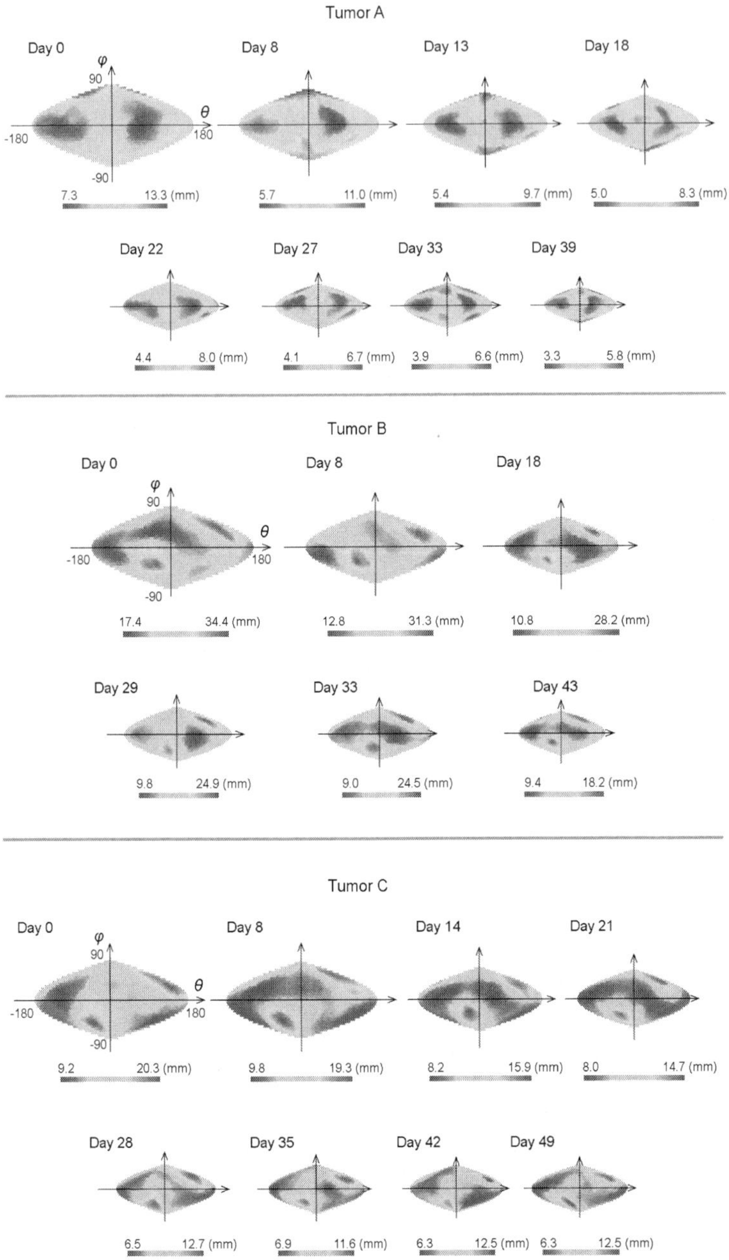

Fig. 9. Changes in 3D tumor geometries represented in surface geometry maps.

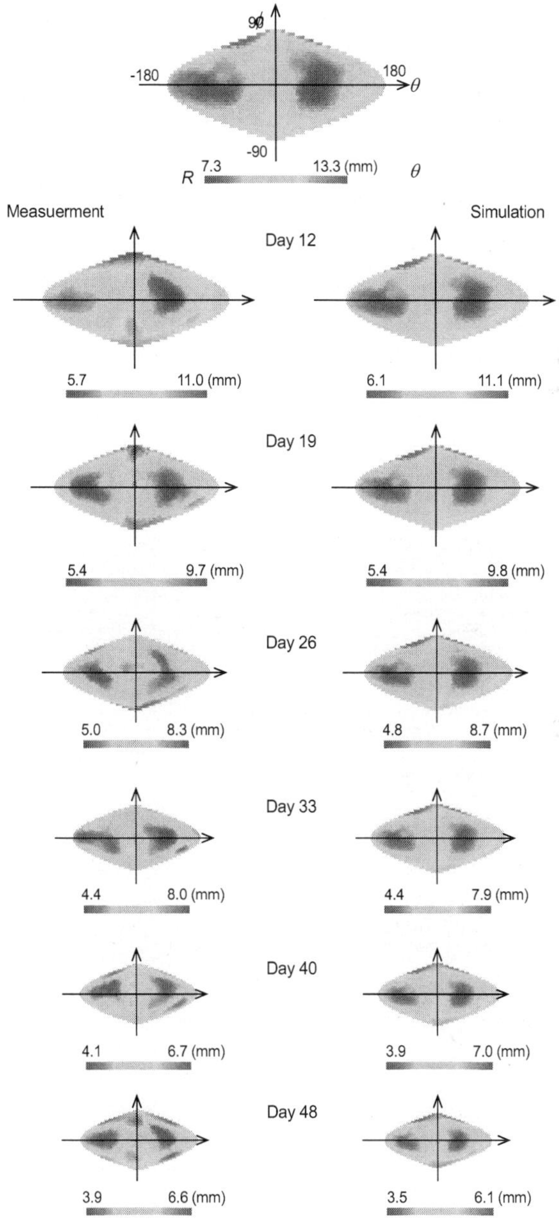

Fig. 10. Comparison of tumor geometries calculated in this method with actual tumor geometries using 2D surface geometry map (case A).

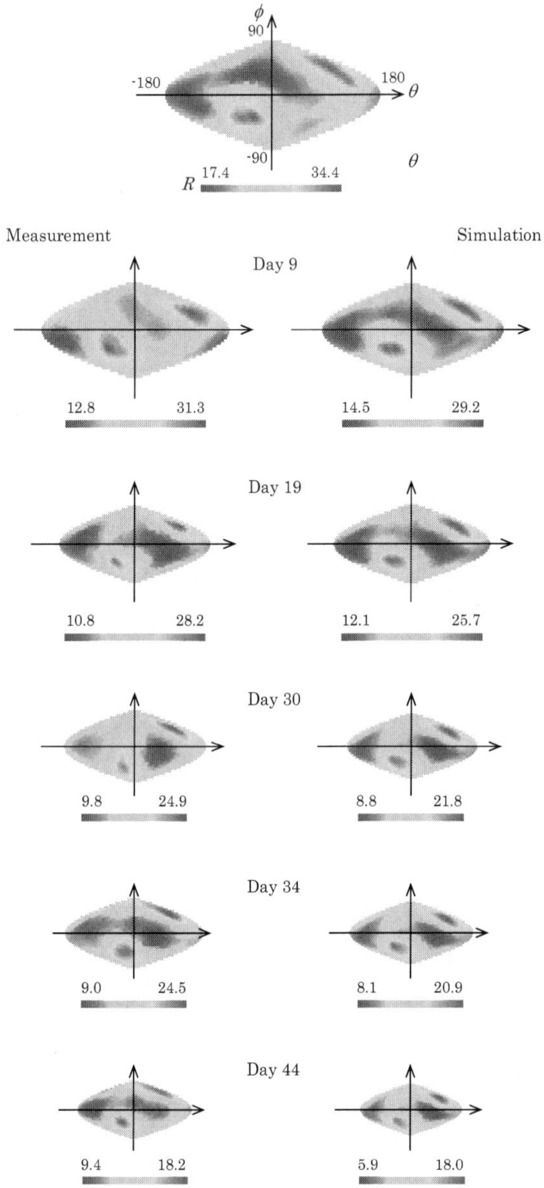

Fig. 11. Comparison of tumor geometries calculated in this method with actual tumor geometries using 2D surface geometry map (case B).

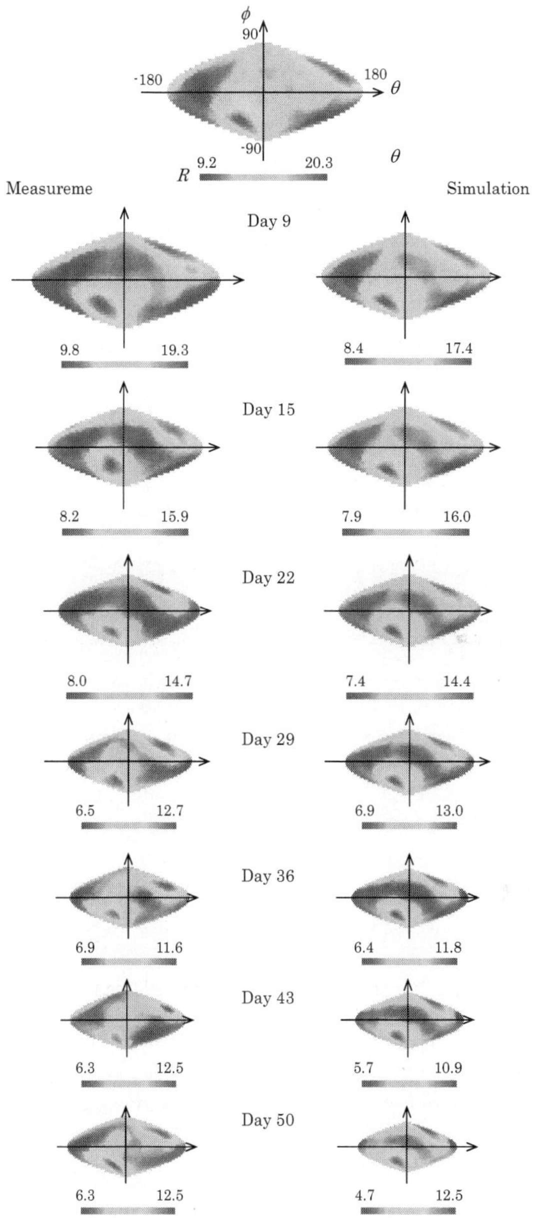

Fig. 12. Comparison of tumor geometries calculated in this method with actual tumor geomet ies using 2D surface geometry map (case B).

A simulation method proposed here enabled to predict changes in 3D tumor geometry considering intratumoral heterogeneity of radiosensitivity therefore would be more valuable for treatment planning or diagnosis of prognosis. The simulation method could predict tumor shapes at the end of the treatment within 2.1 mm discrepancy in radius (absolute average) by considering tumor heterogeneity. As the limitation of present method, these calculations were performed on the assumption that tumors were irradiated evenly. Although dose distribution in IMRT is considered to be uniform to a certain extent, actual dose distribution should be taken into consideration for more precise calculation.

Calculated tumor geometries in the latter half of the treatment strongly depended on changes in tumor geometries in the early stage of the treatment, because values of parameter E were determined only from early tumor geometries. Our present method cannot handle the cases that tumor geometry changes drastically during treatment. We should investigate factors affecting tumor radiosensitivity e.g. angiogenesis, hypoxia, or cell cycle, and appropriately determine the values of E parameter considering these factors.

7. Conclusion

In this work, tumor geometries were analysed visually and quantitatively from several perspectives. The effectiveness of surface geometry map proposed here was confirmed as the tool for precise assessment of therapeutic response based on the 3D tumor geometry. It was revealed that tumors shrunk uniformly keeping their initial morphological features during radiotherapy. This finding cannot be obtained from traditional evaluation by measuring diameters of the tumors on CT images. This study also proposed a novel simulation method to predict changes in 3D tumor geometries during radiotherapy considering intratumoral heterogeneity of radiosensitivity. The simulation results were found to conform to actual changes in tumor geometry. Although some difficulties still remain to be solved, tumor geometries could be predicted using our approach. It would lead to the idea of "Computer associated radiotherapy (CART)", which is the highly-advanced integration of computational technology and radiotherapy to achieve more precise and safety treatment.

8. Future directions

The role of computer technology in recent advanced radiotherapy has rapidly increased. Calculation of 3D dose distribution in patient is indispensable for precise treatment. Imaging techniques, especially image registration technique, are expected as tools for adaptive radiotherapy, which modifies original treatment plan to fit the actual patient condition. Through this research, great contribution of our computational analysis and simulation method for changes in 3D tumor geometry has been confirmed. These methods are expected to play a great important role in putting adaptive radiotherapy into practice. It would be a first step for achievement of computer associated radiotherapy (CART), and attainment of more effective and safety treatment.

9. Acknowledgment

This research is partly granted by the Japan Society for the Promotion of Science (JSPS) through the "Funding Program for World-Leading Innovative R&D on Science and

Technology (FIRST Program)," initiated by the Council for Science and Technology Policy (CSTP), Grant-in-Aid for JSPS Fellows (NO. 09J02587), and Grant-in-Aid for Scientific Research (A), MEXT (NO. 21249065).

10. References

Choia, H.J. and Choi, H.K. (2007), Grading of renal cell carcinoma by 3D morphological analysis of cell nuclei. *Comput Biol Med*,Vol. 37 (2007), pp. 1334–1341

Den, R.B., et al. (2010). Daily image guidance with cone-beam computed tomography for head-and-neck cancer intensity-modulated radiotherapy: A prospective study. *Int J Radiat Oncol Biol Phys*, Vol.76 (2010), pp. 1353–1359.

Dionysiou, D.D., et al. (2004), A four-dimensional simulation model of tumour response to radiotherapy in vivo: parametric validation considering radiosensitivity, genetic profile and fractionation. *J theor Biol*, Vol.230 (2004), pp. 1-20.

Greene,W.H., et al. (2009). Constrained non-rigid registration for use in image-guided adaptive radiotherapy. *Med Image Anal*, Vol.13 (2009), pp. 809–817.

Houghton, F., et al. (2009). An assessment of action levels in imaging strategies in head and neck cancer using TomoTherapy: Are our margins adequate in the absence of image guidance?. *Clin Oncol*, Vol.21 (2009), pp. 720–727.

Kolokotroni, E.A., et al. (2011). Studying the growth kinetics of untreated clinical tumors by using an advanced discrete simulation model. *Math Comp Model*, Vol.54 (2011), pp. 1989-2006.

Pawlowski, J.M., et al. (2010). Reduction of dose delivered to organs at risk in prostate cancer patients via image-guided radiation therapy. *Int J Radiat Oncol Biol Phys*, Vol.76 (2010), pp. 924–934.

Stamatakos, G.S., et al. (2010). An advanced discrete state-discrete event multiscale simulation model of the response of a solid tumor to chemotherapy: Mimicking a clinical study. *J Theor Biol*, Vol.266(2010), pp. 124-139.

Takao, S., et al. (2009a). Analysis of three-dimensional characteristics in tumor morphology. *J Biomech Sci Eng*, Vol.4 (2009), pp. 221-229.

Takao, S., et al. (2009b). Computer simulation of radiotherapy for malignant tumor - A mechanical analogy method -. *J Biomech Sci Eng*, Vol.4 (2009), pp. 576-588.

Takao, S., et al. (2011). Accurate analysis of the change in volume, location, and shape of metastatic cervical lymph nodes during radiotherapy. *Int J Radiat Oncol Biol Phys*, Vol.81 (2011), pp. 871–879.

Thames, H.D., et al. (1990). Time-dose factors in radiotherapy: a review of the human data, *Radiother Oncol*, Vol.19 (1990), pp. 219-235.

Therasse, P., et al. (2000). New Guidelines to Evaluate the Response to Treatment in Solid Tumors, *J Nat Can Inst*, Vol.92 (2000), pp. 205–216.

Varadhan, R., et al. (2009). Assessing prostate, bladder and rectal doses during image guided radiation therapy: Need for plan adaptation?. *J Appl Clin Med Phys*, Vol.10 (2009), pp. 56–74.

Wang, J., et al. (2009). The clinical feasibility and effect of online cone beam computer tomography-guided intensity-modulated radiotherapy for nasopharyngeal cancer. *Radiother Oncol*, Vol.90 (2009), pp. 221–227.

Werner-Wasik, M., et al. (2001). Assessment of lung cancer response after nonoperative therapy: tumor diameter, bidimensional product, and volume. A serial CT scan-based study. *Int J Radiat Oncol Biol Phys*, Vol.51 (2001), pp. 56–61.

World Health Organization (1979). *WHO handbook for reporting results of cancer treatment*, pp. 48, Offset Publication, Geneva, Switzerland.

3

Frequency-Domain Objective Response Detection Techniques Applied to Evoked Potentials: A Review

Danilo Barbosa Melges[1,2], Antonio Mauricio Ferreira Leite Miranda de Sá[1] and Antonio Fernando Catelli Infantosi[1]

[1]*Biomedical Engineering Program, Federal University of Rio de Janeiro (UFRJ)*

[2]*Electrical Engineering Department, Federal University of Minas Gerais (UFMG)*

Brazil

1. Introduction

The Electroencephalogram (EEG) is the biological signal collected at the scalp as a summation result of ionic currents generated from the post-synaptic potentials of the brain neurons. Differently from some other biosignals such as the electrocardiogram, which presents a visual identifiable pattern - particularly the QRS complex, the EEG exhibits a very large random variability. It is indeed quite often assumed to be a white Gaussian noise, and this stochastic behavior turns the analysis of EEG signals by visual inspection a very difficult task. In spite of this, the EEG is known to be correlated with sensorial information processing, and it is widely used for neurophysiologic assessment and neuropathies diagnosis.

The cortical response obtained by sensorial excitation consists of a neurological evaluation paradigm that produces a pattern related to a stimulation that is often rhythmic, such as electric pulses, auditory clicks or intermittent light. The elicited cortical activity is usually synchronized with the stimulation, but it is embedded in the spontaneous EEG, which has much higher amplitude values. An estimation of this evoked response is frequently obtained by averaging EEG epochs stimuli-synchronized. The resulting waveform is visually inspected and evaluated by a neurologist or a technical specialist for both diagnosis/prognosis and surgical monitoring purposes. Such response is locked in time and phase with the stimulation, which can lead to a clear pattern that is usually called evoked potential (EP).

The most employed evoked potentials are the visual (VEP) - elicited by intermittent photic stimuli-, the auditory (AEP) - obtained by tones or clicks-, and the somatosensory ones (SEP), evoked by electric current pulses. Among many applications, the VEP is commonly applied for visual acuity evaluation of infants and newborns (Linden *et al.*, 1997); the AEP is often used for monitoring the depth of anesthesia (Cagy, 2003) and auditory screening of newborns (Ramos *et al.*, 2000); whilst the SEP is frequently employed for monitoring spine (Cruccu *et al.*, 2008) and vascular surgeries (Keyhani *et al.*, 2009).

Although the EP has been widely applied, the conventional procedure is based on the physician experience and ability, as well as in informal criteria (Dobie and Wilson, 1993). The analysis is also hampered by the EEG recording quality, anesthesia regimen, and the high variability inter-observer and inter-patient (Martin *et al.*, 2002). In order to overcome these limitations and aiming at widening the employment of the evoked potentials, the use of Objective Response Detection (ORD) techniques has been proposed. One of the first works applying the ORD to evoked potentials was described in Galambos *et al.* (1984 apud Stapells *et al.*, 1987), which introduced the Phase Coherence. Since then, many other ORD techniques have been investigated.

These methods are based on statistical tests that allow inferring about the presence (or absence) of sensory response with a maximum false-positive rate previously established, which is the significance level of the statistical test. The ORD techniques at the frequency domain are useful, particularly in the presence of narrow band noises, such as network noise and its harmonics. This kind of noise corrupts the EP waveform, yielding to a misleading analysis and, consequently, to a mistaken diagnose or monitoring. However, it only affects the frequency-domain ORD in specific frequencies that can be disregarded in the analysis. Hence, these techniques are more suitable for medical environments (hospitals and intensive care units), which are usually electrically noisy, due to the presence of many electrical and electro-mechanical devices.

Although the ORD allows reducing the subjectivity of neurophysiologic assessment, the probability and rapidness of detection are still aspects to be optimized. The fast detection with high hit rate is a requirement specially for intra-operative monitoring, since it can help the physicians to avoid iatrogenic neurological damages. Methods to accelerate the detection such as the application of a decreasing exponential (Tierra-Criollo *et al.*, 1998) to the ORD techniques have been proposed. More recently, the employment of more than one EEG derivation in a multivariate ORD approach has been suggested in order to improve the detection probability (Miranda de Sá and Felix, 2002). These techniques constitute the state of the art for objectively identify sensorial responses to a stimulation.

This work aims at reviewing the most employed frequency-domain techniques applied to evoked potentials. Besides the Introduction, this chapter will be subdivided into six sections. The second one introduces the model of evoked response generation. Section 3 presents a brief description of the principal applications of the cortical (brain) responses obtained by different types of stimulation (visual, auditory and somatosensory). Both clinical diagnosis and surgical monitoring references are included. In the next section, the mathematical definition of uni- and multivariate techniques is provided. A chronological literature review of applying the ORD to EP is described in Section 5. The subsequent section presents examples of using these techniques, including recent findings. Finally, the last section discloses a discussion about ORD.

2. The model of evoked potential generation and the coherent average

The evoked potential (EP) generation model is shown in Figure 1, where $v[k]$ is the response elicited by the sensory stimulation $x[k]$, $b[k]$ is the spontaneous EEG and $H(f)$ is the transfer function of the sensory pathways. The evoked response v[k] is considered to be identical from stimulus-to-stimulus (i.e. $H(f)$ is assumed to be deterministic) and the background EEG is assumed to be a zero-mean white Gaussian noise. Hence, the measured EEG $y[k]$ is composed by evoked and background activities. In this linear model, a correlation between stimulus and EEG is expected at the stimulation frequency and its multiples.

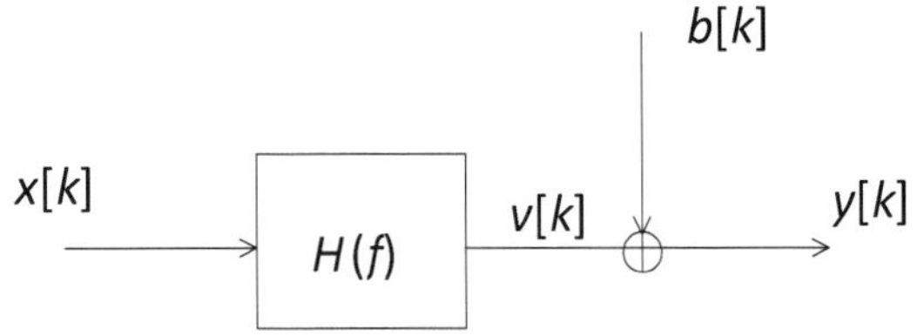

Fig. 1. Linear Model of evoked potential generation: $x[k]$ is the stimulus, $H(f)$ is the frequency-domain transfer function of the sensory pathways, $v[k]$ is the stimuli-response, $b[k]$ is the background EEG and $y[k]$ is the measured EEG.

This model reflects the scalp electrical activity registration, where the evoked potentials are usually embedded in the spontaneous (or background) EEG. Since the EP is tens of times lower than the background EEG, it cannot be visualized; therefore, it is common to perform the averaging of many epochs, taken the stimulus instant as the fiducial point. As mentioned above, assuming that the background EEG is a zero-mean Gaussian noise and the responses are synchronized with the stimulation and identical from stimulus to stimulus (Lopes da Silva, 1999), this procedure, known as coherent average, leads to an increase in the signal-to-noise ratio as shown next.

Considering the linear model presented in Figure 1, the ith EEG epoch during stimulation can be given by:

$$y_i[k] = v[k] + n_i[k]$$

where $v[k]$ is the evoked response and $n[k]$ is the background EEG. The coherent average provides an estimate of the evoked potential, being calculated by:

$$\hat{v}[k] = \frac{1}{M}\sum_{i=1}^{M} y_i[k] = \frac{1}{M}\sum_{i=1}^{M} v[k] + \frac{1}{M}\sum_{i=1}^{M} n_i[k]$$

where the superscript ^ denotes estimation and M is the number of EEG epochs. When M tends to infinity, $\hat{v}[k]$ tends to $v[k]$, since the parcel due to summation involving the $n_i[k]$ terms will vanish.

3. Clinical and surgical application of the evoked potentials

The evoked potentials obtained by different kinds of stimulation have been applied to a broad range of clinical and intra-operative conditions. It is increasing the number of studies that shows the advantages of EP application for supporting the diagnosis of neuropathies and the continuous neuromonitoring in order to avoid neurological damages.

The Brainstem Auditory Evoked Potential (BAEP), elicited by click (sound pulses), is an important tool in the child auditory screening (Ramos *et al.*, 2000, Infantosi *et al.*, 2004), since it can assess the auditory pathways down to the brainstem. It is usually performed by obtaining the auditory neurophysiologic threshold by means of the BERA (Brainstem Evoked Response Audiometry). The most widely employed screening method is the optoacoustic emission (OE). Although this latter has been applied in many hospital units, due to its technical and operational facility (Zaeyen, 2005), the OE evaluate the integrity only up to the cochlea, whereas the BAEP can access the auditory pathways up to the brainstem. Moreover, there are cases in which the BAEP is absent or impaired, but the OE are preserved (Infantosi *et al.*, 2004). Thus, a question that naturally arises is whether the OE is a suitable method for auditory screening in newborn intensive care units (Infantosi *et al.*, 2004).

On the other hand, the BAEP has been also employed for intra-operative monitoring during removal of cerebello-pontine tumors, microvascular decompression of cranial nerves and ischemic complications due the manipulation of the posterior fossa circulation, since this potential is stable to a variety of anesthetics and pharmacological agents and presents adequate reproducibility (Linden *et al.*, 1997).

When the impairment is located in structures above the brainstem, the investigation of late potentials such as the Middle Latency Auditory Evoked Potential (MLAEP) can be suitable for functional evaluation up to the primary auditory cortex (Zaeyen, 2005). The MLAEP has been also applied for monitoring the depth anesthetic plan (Nayak and Roy, 1998, Gemal, 1999, Cagy and Infantosi, 2002, Cagy, 2003), because it presents changes that are dose-dependent with the anesthesia. The anesthetic plan monitoring is particularly important because the clinical signs usually applied for this purpose are masked by the employment of vasodilators, vasoconstrictors, calcium channel blockers and neuromuscular blockers during surgeries (Nayak and Roy, 1998).

The application of the Visual Evoked Potential (VEP) for monitoring is limited due to the need of controlling parameters such as surgical room light and distance between the eye and the stimulator. Although it has been used during surgeries of pituitary tumors and brain aneurisms, the recording of VEP for intra-operative functional evaluation presents low success rate (Linden et al., 1997). Flash-VEP is one of the potentials with the highest signal-to-noise ratio (SNR) , some characteristics of its waveform can be even visually identified with only 100 stimuli. Nevertheless, this potential shows high inter- and intra-observer variability, which makes difficult its evaluation with the administration of anesthetics. Moreover, since the quantity of light is a function of the pupil size, agents causing mydriasis (pupil dilatation) should be applied when anesthetics are administered (Linden et al., 1997). On the other hand, the VEP has been used, especially in pediatrics, for evaluating the visual acuity, detecting amblyopia, and as a useful tool for prognosis of comatose patients, newborn asphyxia and cortical blindness (Linden et al., 1997). Other applications of VEP includes diagnosis of migraine in children and adolescents (Jancic-Stefanovic *et al.*, 2003), childhood optical glioma (Trisciuzzi *et al.*, 2004) and functional visual loss (Xu *et al.*, 2001). It has also been used in studies of dyslexia (Schulte-Körne *et al.*, 2004), periventricular leukomalacia (Kato *et al.*, 2005), retinitis pigmentosa (Holopigian *et al.*, 2005), macular degeneration (Nemoto *et al.*, 2002), schizophrenia (Krishnan *et al.*, 2005), glaucoma (Parisi *et al.*, 2001) and nystagmus (Hoffmann *et al.*, 2004).

The somatosensory evoked potential (SEP) is often obtained by applying electric current pulses and is useful for detecting peripheral nerve lesions, plexopathies and radiculopathies (Linden *et al.*, 1997), and for monitoring vascular and spine surgeries such as desobstruction of the carotid artery (Liu *et al.*, 2010), aortic aneurism repair (Keyhani *et al.*, 2009, Van Dongen *et al.*, 2001), aortic coarctation repair (Faberowski *et al.*, 1999), scoliosis correction procedures (Cruccu *et al.*, 2008) and lumbar pedicle screw placement for in situ posterior spinal fusion (Gundanna, 2003), due to its sensitivity to mechanical stress, hypotension and ischemia.

The neuromonitoring is considered important in the prevention of immediate and late paraplegia caused by medullary ischemia, since it is capable of detecting the "ischemic penumbra", status pathophysiologic present in the acute ischemia, when the neurons are not at functional state, but alive and recoverable by the application of appropriate procedures (Guérit and Dion, 2002).

Due to its sensitivity to temperature, the SEP has been used as optimal temperature identifier during surgeries that require profound hypothermia (Ghariani *et al.*, 1999), being considered as a secure and efficient method (Ghariani *et al.*, 2000). The hypothermia is employed in order to reduce the cerebral metabolism, during surgeries of ascending aorta and aortic arch repair, which require circulatory arrest (Ghariani *et al.*, 1998). This procedure allows the reduction of neurological sequels arising from hypoxia. On the other hand, excessively low temperatures can lead to iatrogenic complications, such as coagulation disorders, hemolysis, increased blood viscosity, among others (Ghariani *et al.*, 2000).

The need of monitoring upper and lower limbs during surgeries has been reported due to the occurrence of paraplegia by unpredicted intra-operative evaluation of only median nerve SEP (Ghariani et al., 1999). The advantages that the monitoring of the four limbs SEP can provide for a low cost, reducing the occurrence of transient and persistent neurological complications, has been also reported by Jones et al. (2004). In a survey conducted with members of the Scoliosis Research Society, Nuwer et al. (1995) reported that 88% of the north-American surgeons used the SEP in more than a half of the surgeries. According to Bose et al. (2004), the neurophysiologic monitoring during lumbar and thoracic surgery has become a routine procedure for years, but its employment during cervical surgeries is more recent and seems to be a sensitive method for detecting neurological insults caused by mechanical stress, surgical manipulation, hypotension and ischemia.

Since it is related with variations in the cerebral blood flow, the SEP presents identifiable changes associated with variation in the hemodynamics (Florence et al., 2004). Moreover, the SEP is not influenced by muscular blockers and present gradual changes with the increase of anesthetic concentration (Angel et al., 1999). Frequently registered over the somatosensory cortex, region vascularized by the carotid artery, the SEP is often used during the carotid endarterectomy (Florence et al., 2004), performed for the treatment of vascular obstructive disease and that presents potential risk of ischemia for the ipsilateral hemisphere during internal carotid artery occlusion (Linden et al., 1997). The absence of the cortical function and of the subcortical EP, in cases of cerebral hemorrhages, is a negative prognostic predictor, although its preservation does not present prognostic value (Guérit, 1999).

For monitoring intracranial aneurysms repair surgeries, the real time detection of cerebral ischemia can help the surgeon, for example, to determine the duration of the temporary vascular occlusion and the optimal systemic arterial pressure (Martin et al., 2002). The SEP and the cortical EEG are the techniques most frequently employed for this purpose in anterior circulation aneurysm surgeries (Martin et al., 2002).

Apart from the cited surgeries, the SEP monitoring was also successfully applied in many other surgical procedures, such as interventional neuroradiology, stereotaxic surgery of the brainstem, thalamus, cerebral cortex, thalamotomy, cortical localization, brachial plexus surgery and pelvic fracture surgery (Linden et. al, 1997). SEP also presents prognostic value in cases of intracranial hypertension (Giugno et al., 2003) and coma (Logi et al., 2003).

Even when post-operative squeals cannot be avoided by monitoring, the detection of neurophysiologic intra-operative changes can make the surgery staff aware of the risk and avoid the exacerbation of the damage (Bose et al., 2004). However, it is important selecting the patients for whom the EP monitoring can be useful, because if the patient does not present pre-operative EP, this technique is not suitable for intra-operative neuro-evaluation (Linden et al., 1997).

Finally, as the neuromonitoring represents only the current status of the patient, many studies point out the importance of the post-surgery SEP monitoring in order to detect late neurological complications (Guérit and Dion, 2002, Dong et al., 2002, Ghariani et al., 2000).

4. Frequency–domain Objective Response Detection (ORD) techniques

This section describes some of the most used frequency-domain Objective Response Detection (ORD) techniques, both in its univariate and multivariate versions. Details about *a priori* assumptions related to the signals are included.

4.1 Univariate ORD techniques

4.1.1 Phase Coherence

The Phase Coherence (PC) was introduced in the analysis of the evoked potentials by Galambos *et al.* (1984) and can be seen as a statistical measure of the phase variance. It can be mathematically defined by:

$$\hat{\theta}_c(f) = \sqrt{\left(\sum_{i=1}^{M} \sin\phi_i(f)\right)^2 + \left(\sum_{i=1}^{M} \cos\phi_i(f)\right)^2} \Big/ M \tag{1}$$

where $\phi_i(f)$ is the phase angle of the ith Fourier Transformed EEG epoch and M is the number of EEG epochs. This measure supposes that the presence of stimuli-response causes a phase aggregation of the Fourier Transformed EEG epochs in the complex plan. On the other hand, on the absence of response, the phase angle is assumed to be randomly distributed between 0 and 2π, and the probability of obtaining this phase angle configuration is accessed by the Rayleigh test (Mardia, 1972). This techniques only takes into account the phase of the Fourier Transform (FT) of EEG epochs.

4.1.2 Hotelling's T^2 test

According to Picton et al. (1987), the Hotelling T2 Test (HT2) is the multivariate analogue of the Student's t test. If M samples of a uni-variate distribution is taken, one can estimate its mean $\overline{y}$ and standard deviation s. Based on this two parameters, it is possible to calculate the limits for the occurrence of the population mean:

$$\sqrt{M}\frac{\left|\overline{y}-y\right|}{s}\leq t$$

where t are the limits taken from the two-tailed Student's t distribution with M-1 degrees of freedom.

For a bidimensional distribution, the confidence region for the mean vector is given by:

$$M\left(\overline{Y}(f)-Y(f)\right)^{H}S^{-1}\left(\overline{Y}(f)-Y(f)\right)\leq\hat{T}^{2}(f) \tag{2}$$

where the superscript H and ^ denote Hermitian and estimation, respectively, S^{-1} is the inverse of the covariance matrix of the sample, Y(f) is the vector of the M Fourier Transformed EEG epochs and $\overline{Y}(f)$ the mean vector.

The statistics T^2 can be related to the Fisher's F distribution by (Picton et al., 1987):

$$\hat{T}_{crit}^{2}(f)=\frac{(M-1)2}{(M-2)}F_{crit,2,M-2,\alpha} \tag{3}$$

where M is the number of epochs used to calculate the T^2 estimate and $F_{crit,2,M-2,\alpha}$ is the critical value of the F-distribution with 2 and M-2 degrees of freedom at the significance level α.

Considering that the Fourier Transformed EEG epochs are bidimensional variables (complex variables with real and imaginary parts), the confidence region for the mean vector leads to an ellipse of confidence. When the ellipse encompasses the origin of the plan (0,0), which represents the response absence condition, one can assume that there is no response to the stimulation. On the other hand, if the origin is not included in the confidence region, the null hypothesis of response absence can be rejected, and one can assume the response detection.

4.1.3 Spectral F Test (SFT)

The Spectral F Test (SFT) is given by the ratio between the Power Spectrum Density (PSD) of the EEG during stimulation $y[k]$ and the background EEG $b[k]$ (Dobie and Wilson, 1996). For windowed EEG signals, the SFT can be estimated by the ratio of the Bartlett periodograms, as follows:

$$\hat{\phi}(f)=\frac{\frac{1}{M_y}\sum_{i=1}^{M_x}\left|Y_i(f)\right|^2}{\frac{1}{M_b}\sum_{i=1}^{M_y}\left|B_i(f)\right|^2} \tag{4}$$

where the superscript ^denotes estimation, $Y_i(f)$ and $B_i(f)$ are, respectively, the Discrete Fourier Transform (DFT) of the ith EEG epoch of $y[k]$ and $b[k]$, and M_y and M_b, are the number of EEG epochs during stimulation and at the resting condition (background EEG), respectively.

In the null hypothesis (H_0) of no stimulus response, the EEG during stimulation belongs to the same population as the background EEG; hence, both $y[k]$ and $b[k]$ are zero-mean Gaussian noise with equal variance. Hence, it can be shown that the distribution of the SFT can be related to the Fisher F-distribution by:

$$\frac{M_y}{M_b}\hat{\phi}(f) \sim F_{2M_y,2M_b} \tag{5}$$

Thus, the critical value for a given significance level α, M_y and M_b number of EEG epochs is expressed by:

$$\hat{\phi}_{crit}(f) = F_{crit2M_y,2M_b,\alpha} \tag{6}$$

where $F_{crit2M_y,2M_b,\alpha}$ is the critical value of the F-distribution with $2M_y$ and $2M_b$ degrees of freedom.

The above expression for critical values calculation is not valid for DC (direct current) and Nyquist frequency, since, in these frequencies, the Fourier Transform of EEG epoch leads to purely real values.

4.1.4 Magnitude-Squared Coherence (MSC)

The squared modulus of the coherence function (also called Magnitude-squared coherence, MSC), $\gamma_{yx}^2(f)$, corresponds to the parcel of the squared mean value of the measured EEG signal $y[k]$ caused by the stimulation $x[k]$ for a given frequency f (Bendat and Piersol, 2000), and is calculated by (Dobie and Wilson, 1989):

$$\gamma_{yx}^2(f) = \frac{\left|G_{yx}(f)\right|^2}{G_{yy}(f)G_{xx}(f)} \tag{7}$$

where $G_{yx}(f)$ is the cross-spectrum of $x[k]$ and $y[k]$ normalized by the auto-spectra, $G_{yy}(f)$ and $G_{xx}(f)$. It can be shown that the MSC (expression 7) is a real function that varies between 0 and 1.

The estimates of $\gamma_{yx}^2(f)$ for discrete-time, finite-duration and windowed signals can be calculated by (Bendat and Piersol, 2000):

$$\hat{\gamma}_{yx}^2(f) = \frac{\left|\sum_{i=1}^{M} Y_i(f)X_i^*(f)\right|^2}{\sum_{i=1}^{M}\left|Y_i(f)\right|^2 \sum_{i=1}^{M}\left|X_i(f)\right|^2} \tag{8}$$

where "^" superscript denotes estimation, * is the complex conjugate, M is the number of epochs, and $Y_i(f)$ and $X_i(f)$ are the Discrete Fourier Transform (DFT) of the ith epoch of signals $y[k]$ and $x[k]$, respectively.

For the case of a periodic stimulation ($x[k]$), $X_i(f)$ is identical for all epochs and the MSC estimate depends only on the measured EEG $Y_i(f)$, since the contribution of the periodic signal to both the numerator and denominator cancels out (Dobie and Wilson, 1989):

$$\hat{\kappa}^2(f) = \frac{\left|\sum_{i=1}^{M} X(f)Y_i(f)\right|^2}{M\sum_{i=1}^{M}\left|X(f)Y_i(f)\right|^2} = \frac{X^2(f)\left|\sum_{i=1}^{M} Y_i(f)\right|^2}{MX^2(f)\sum_{i=1}^{M}\left|Y_i(f)\right|^2}$$

$$\hat{\kappa}^2(f) = \frac{\left|\sum_{i=1}^{M} Y_i(f)\right|^2}{M\sum_{i=1}^{M}\left|Y_i(f)\right|^2} \tag{9}$$

From expression 9, it can be seen that, when there is no response to stimulation, the numerator corresponds only to background EEG (assumed to be a zero-mean white Gaussian noise) and, therefore, $\hat{\kappa}^2(f)$ tends to zero. On the other hand, if a consistent response is present in all epochs ($Y_i(f) = Y(f)$, $\forall i$), $\hat{\kappa}^2(f)$ tends to the unity.

For the null hypothesis (H_0) of response absence ($\kappa^2(f) = 0$, where $\kappa^2(f)$ is the true value of the MSC), it can be shown that, for M independent epochs of $y[k]$ (zero-mean white Gaussian noise, by assumption), the MSC can be related to the F-distribution by the following expression (Simpson et al., 2000):

$$(M-1)\frac{\hat{\kappa}^2(f)}{(1-\hat{\kappa}^2(f))} \sim F_{2,2M-2} \tag{10}$$

Hence, based on the critical values of the F-distribution, one can calculate the critical values for the MSC estimates for a given significance level α (Simpson et al., 2000):

$$\hat{\kappa}^2_{crit,\alpha} = \frac{F_{crit2,2M-2,\alpha}}{M-1+F_{crit2,2M-2,\alpha}} \tag{11}$$

The critical value constitutes a detection threshold and can be alternatively calculated by the following analytical expression (Miranda de Sá and Infantosi, 2007):

$$\hat{\kappa}^2_{\text{crit}} = 1-\alpha^{\frac{1}{M-1}} \tag{12}$$

The detection is based on rejecting the null hypothesis (H_0) of response absence, which is reached when the estimate values exceed the critical value ($\hat{\kappa}^2(f) > \hat{\kappa}^2 crit$).

Considering the linear model presented in Section 2, the response detection is expected in the stimulation frequency and its harmonics. Even in the no-stimulation condition, the detection is expected at the rate of α, that is, the significance level of the statistical test corresponds to the maximum false positive rate. The above mentioned critical values are not valid for DC and Nyquist frequency, since the DFT of these components are purely real, while $Y_i(f)$ is complex for other frequencies.

4.1.5 Magnitude-Squared Coherence (MSC) with Exponential Forgetting (MSC-EF)

The application of an exponential forgetting to the MSC was proposed by Tierra-Criollo et al. (1998) and consists of the employment of a decreasing exponential to the EEG epochs spectra, as follows:

$$\hat{\kappa}_p^2(i,f) = (1-b)\frac{|Y_i(f) + bS'_{i-1}(f)|^2}{|Y_i(f)|^2 + bS''_{i-1}(f)} \tag{13}$$

being

$$S'_i(f) = Y_i(f) + bS'_{i-1}(f)$$

$$S''_i(f) = |Y_i(f)|^2 + bS''_{i-1}(f)$$

where f is the frequency index, ^ denotes estimation, $Y_i(f)$ represents the DFT of the ith EEG epoch and b is the forgetting factor ($0<b<1$).

According to Tierra-Criollo et al. (1998), for the null hypothesis of response absence (H_0), similarly to the described for the MSC, $\hat{\kappa}_p^2(f)$ can be related to the F-distribution:

$$(M'-1)\frac{\hat{\kappa}_p^2(f)}{(1-\hat{\kappa}_p^2(f))} \sim F_{2,2M'-2} \tag{14}$$

where $F_{2,2M'-2}$ is the F-distribution with 2 and $2M'$-2 degrees of freedom and M' is given by:

$$M' = \frac{1+b}{1-b} \tag{15}$$

Thus, based on the critical values of $F_{2,2M'-2}$, one can obtain the critical values for $\hat{\kappa}_p^2(f)$ with a given significance level α:

$$\hat{\kappa}_{pcrit}^2 = \frac{F_{crit2,2M'-2,\alpha}}{M'-1+F_{crit2,2M'-2,\alpha}} \tag{16}$$

Similarly to the mentioned for MSC, the response detection ($\hat{\kappa}_p^2(f) > \hat{\kappa}_{pcrit}^2$) is expected at the stimulation frequencies and its harmonics. Even in the no-stimulation condition, the detection is expected at the rate of the significance level of the statistical test.

The critical value can be alternatively calculated by the following analytical expression:

$$\hat{\kappa}^2_{\text{crit}} = 1 - \alpha^{\frac{1}{M'-1}} \tag{17}$$

4.1.6 Component Synchrony Measure (CSM)

The Component Synchrony Measure (CSM) or Phase Synchrony Measure (PSM) quantifies the degree of synchronism between frequencies of a signal, taking into account only the phase of its Fourier Transform (Simpson et al., 2000):

$$\hat{\rho}^2(f) = \left[\frac{1}{M}\sum_{i=1}^{M}\cos\phi_i(f)\right]^2 + \left[\frac{1}{M}\sum_{i=1}^{M}\sin\phi_i(f)\right]^2 \tag{18}$$

where $\phi_i(f)$ is the phase of the Fourier Transform of the ith EEG epoch and M is the number of epochs used in the CSM estimation.

Assuming that the phase is uniformly distributed between 0 and 2π (absence of synchronism between stimulus and response), the probability density function is given by 1/2π and the functions $\cos\phi_i$ and $\text{sen}\phi_i$ present zero mean and variance ½ (Miranda de Sá and Felix, 2003), as follows:

$$\mu = \int_0^{2\pi} \cos\phi \frac{1}{2\pi} d\phi = \int_0^{2\pi} sen\phi \frac{1}{2\pi} d\phi = 0$$

$$\sigma^2 = \int_0^{2\pi} \cos^2\phi \frac{1}{2\pi} d\phi = \int_0^{2\pi} sen^2\phi \frac{1}{2\pi} d\phi = \frac{1}{2}$$

According to the Central Limit Theorem, the summation of sins (and co-sins) in the expression 18 tends asymptotically to a normal distribution with zero-mean and variance M/2:

$$\sum_{i=1}^{M}\cos\phi_i \sim N\left(0,\frac{M}{2}\right) \quad and \quad \sum_{i=1}^{M}sen\phi_i \sim N\left(0,\frac{M}{2}\right)$$

Hence, it can be shown that:

$$\frac{\left(\sum_{i=1}^{M}\cos\phi_i\right)^2 + \left(\sum_{i=1}^{M}sen\phi_i\right)^2}{M/2} \sim \chi^2_2$$

where χ^2_2 is the chi-squared distribution with 2 degrees of freedom. From this expression, the CSM can be related to the χ^2_2 distribution by:

$$\hat{\rho}^2(f) \sim \frac{1}{M^2}\frac{M}{2}\chi_2^2 = \frac{\chi_2^2}{2M} \tag{19}$$

Thus, for the null hypothesis of absence of synchronism, the critical value for a given significance level α and *M* EEG epochs can be obtained by (Mardia, 1972):

$$\rho^2_{crit,\alpha} = \frac{\chi^2_{2\,crit,\alpha}}{2M} \tag{20}$$

where $\chi^2_{2\,crit,\alpha}$ is the critical value of the chi-squared distribution for the significance level α. It is worth noting that CSM expression corresponds to the square of the Phase Coherence (PC).

Alternatively, the critical value for CSM can be calculated based on the probability density function of the chi-squared distribution given as:

$$p_{\chi_2^2}(z) = \frac{1}{2}e^{-\frac{z}{2}}.$$

The analytical critical value of χ_2^2 for a given significance level α is obtained from

$$\int_0^{\chi^2_{2crit}} \frac{1}{2}e^{-\frac{z}{2}}dz = 1-\alpha,$$

which yields to:

$$\chi^2_{2\,crit,\alpha} = 2\ln\left(\frac{1}{\alpha}\right). \tag{21}$$

Hence, substituting expression (21) in (20) leads to:

$$\rho^2_{crit,\alpha} = \frac{\ln(1/\alpha)}{M} \tag{22}$$

4.2 Multivariate ORD (MORD) techniques

4.2.1 Multiple Coherence (MC)

The Multiple Coherence (MC) - which is the multivariate version of MSC - between a periodic signal and a set of *N* random ones ($y_j[k]$, j = 1..*N*) is given by (Miranda de Sá et al., 2004):

$$\hat{\kappa}_N^2(f) = \mathbf{V}^H(f)\hat{\mathbf{S}}_{yy}^{-1}(f)\mathbf{V}(f)/M \tag{23}$$

where $\mathbf{V}(f) = \left[\sum_{i=1}^{M} Y_{1i}^*(f) \quad \sum_{i=1}^{M} Y_{2i}^*(f) \quad \cdots \quad \sum_{i=1}^{M} Y_{Ni}^*(f)\right]^T$

being $Y_{ki}(f)$ the Fourier Transform of the ith epoch of the kth EEG derivation; H and T superscripts mean, respectively, Hermitian and the matrix transpose; and the pth-row, q^{th}-column element of $\hat{\mathbf{S}}_{yy}(f)$ is $\hat{\mathbf{S}}_{ypyq}(f)=\sum_{i=1}^{M}Y_{pi}^{*}(f)Y_{qi}(f)$.

The distribution of the MC estimates can related to the F-distribution and the critical value for a significance level α, M epochs and N signals can be expressed as (Miranda de Sá et al., 2004):

$$\hat{\kappa}^2_{N_{crit}} = \frac{F_{crit\alpha,2N,2(M-N)}}{F_{crit\alpha,2N,2(M-N)}+[M-N]/N} \tag{24}$$

where $F_{crit\alpha,2N,2(M-N)}$ is the critical value of the F distribution with $2N$ and $2(M\text{-}N)$ degrees of freedom. The detection is identified based on the rejection of the null hypothesis (H_0) of response absence, which is achieved when the estimate values exceed the critical value ($\hat{\kappa}^2_N(f) > \hat{\kappa}^2_{N_{crit}}$). As a multivariate extension of the MSC, MC quantifies the amount of power of a set of signals that is caused by the stimulation.

4.2.2 Multiple Component Synchrony Measure (MCSM)

A multivariate extension of the CSM was proposed by Miranda de Sá and Felix (2003) as a way of measuring the synchronism of the ith epoch of the Fourier Transform of N EEG derivations ($y_1[k]$, $y_2[k]$,..., $y_N[k]$) caused by a rhythmical stimulation only considering their mean phase angle, $\bar{\theta}_i(f)$. This technique, called Multiple CSM (MCSM), can be used for detecting the evoked response and can be mathematically defined by (Miranda de Sá and Felix, 2003):

$$\hat{\rho}^2_N(f) = \left[\frac{1}{M}\sum_{i=1}^{M}\cos\left(\bar{\theta}_i(f)\right)\right]^2 + \left[\frac{1}{M}\sum_{i=1}^{M}\sin\left(\bar{\theta}_i(f)\right)\right]^2 \tag{25}$$

where the M is the number of EEG epochs and the mean phase angle can be calculated by:

$$\bar{\theta}_i(f) = \begin{cases} \tan^{-1}\left(\bar{S}_i/\bar{C}_i\right) & if \;\; \bar{C}_i \geq 0 \\ \tan^{-1}\left(\bar{S}_i/\bar{C}_i\right)+\pi & if \;\; \bar{C}_i < 0 \end{cases}$$

being

$$\bar{C}_i = \frac{1}{N}\sum_{j=1}^{N}\cos\theta_{ij}(f) \quad \text{and} \quad \bar{S}_i = \frac{1}{N}\sum_{j=1}^{N}\sin\theta_{ij}(f)$$

Assuming that the mean phase angle is uniformly distributed between 0 and 2π, it can be showed, in a similar way to the performed to the CSM, that the asymptotical critical value for the MCSM can be expressed by (Felix et al., 2007):

$$\rho^2_{N\,crit,\alpha} = \frac{\chi^2_{2\,crit,\alpha}}{2M} = \frac{\ln(1/\alpha)}{M} \tag{26}$$

where $\chi^2_{2\,crit,\alpha}$ is the critical value of the chi-squared distribution with 2 degrees of freedom for the significance level a and M is the number of EEG epochs used in the estimation. Also for this technique, the detection is based on the null hypothesis (H_0) rejection of synchronism absence, which is achieved when the estimate values exceed the corresponding critical value ($\hat{\rho}^2_N(f) > \rho^2_{N\,crit}$).

5. A chronological review of ORD applied to the evoked potentials

The waveform analysis of the evoked potential (EP) is based on the physician experience, ability and attention level, as well as in informal criteria (Dobie and Wilson, 1993). For the case of the somatosensory evoked potential used in surgical monitoring, for example, one considers a significant modification in its waveform, a reduction of 30% to 50% in the amplitude, an increase of 5% to 10% in the latency, or a combination of these criteria (Linden *et al.*, 1997). Such criteria, used as parameters of modification on the intra-operative strategy, are clearly subjective once they depend on the EEG recording quality, anesthesia regimen, and are hampered by the high variability inter-observer and inter-patient (Martin et al., 2002).

On the other hand, the techniques known as Objective Response Detection (ORD) have been suggested as a way to overcome this subjectivity and allow the stimuli-response detection with a maximum false positive rate *a priori* established. Dobie and Wilson (1993) numbered the advantages of the ORD application compared to the conventional analysis by visual inspection, such as avoiding the persistence of the trained observer and obtaining relevant information even for experienced observers in the judgment of questionable cases.

5.1 Univariate ORD techniques

In 1984, Galambos *et al.* (apud Stapells, 1987) introduced the ORD technique Phase Coherence (PC) in the analysis of the steady state auditory responses. This technique can be seen as a statistical measure of the phase variance and uses only the phase information of the Fourier Transform of the EEG epochs. Two years later, Stapells *et al.* (1987) have applied the PC for obtaining the auditory threshold of normal adults. This method showed to be accurate to establish the behavioral auditory threshold, being considered as fast as obtaining the brainstem responses by tones. Moreover, these authors pointed out that the PC showed better results for determining the optimal stimulation rate when compared to the amplitude inspection of the coherent average, since the latter presents higher variability than the PC.

Still in 1987, Picton *et al.* have applied the Hotelling T^2 Test (HT2) and the PC to the steady state auditory evoked potential (AEP). The HT2 (Hotelling, 1931) takes into account both amplitude and phase of the Fourier Transformed EEG epochs and allows the calculation of a confidence ellipse for the response vectors (EP). In the case in which the ellipse do not encompass the origin (0,0), which corresponds to the absence response condition, its presence is assumed (Dobie and Wilson, 1993). Since the PC represents a kind of HT2 without considering the amplitude information (Picton *et al.*, 1987), theoretically, HT2 would be statistically more powerful than the PC. However, Picton *et al.* (1987) have found small difference between the two methods when the auditory threshold was measured by means of the steady state AEP. Based on these results, the authors have reported that, for intensities near the threshold, most of the information about the signal is in the phase, since using the amplitude information (HT2) didn't result in an improvement in the response detection. Other studies also found that the phase is more important than magnitude (Greenblat *et al.*, 1985, Beagley *et al.*, 1979).

In 1989, Dobie and Wilson have proposed the use of the Magnitude-Squared Coherence (MSC), an ORD technique that uses magnitude and phase of the Fourier Transform of EEG epochs, for identifying the frequencies that significantly contribute to the auditory EP. In this work, the MSC was considered more sensible than the simple visual inspection of the replicated responses. In a later work, Dobie and Wilson (1990) have applied the coherence (MSC) to the AEP filtered with the "Optimum" Wiener Filtering and, compared to the non-filtered version, it was verified that this procedure can be advantageous for signals with low signal-to-noise ratio, such as the obtained with stimulation near the auditory threshold.

Later, Victor and Mast (1991) have proposed a variant of HT2, named T^2 circular (T2C). This method assumes that the real and imaginary parts of the Fourier Transform of the EEG epochs are independent and present equal variance. This assumption results in a simpler statistical approach, and the ellipse of confidence of HT2 becomes a circle of confidence in T2C. Moreover, in this study, a comparison between the performances of three ORD methods was performed: the HT2, the T2C and the Phase Rayleigh Criterion (PRC) - a technique that uses only the phase of the signal. The comparison was based on simulation and application to the steady state visual evoked potential. As a result, it was observed that, for low signal-to-noise (SNR) ratio values, HT2 and T2C have shown to be superior to the PRC. The authors consider that this result is due to the fact that the first two methods use information of amplitude, while the PRC discard it. Furthermore, it was verified that for low SNR, a high number of EEG epochs is needed in order to achieve statistical significance. On the other hand, for a low number of EEG segments, T2C and PRC presented advantage over HT2 and for intermediate SNR values T2C showed better performance than any technique.

Dobie and Wilson (1993) also compared the performance of T2C, PC and MSC using simulated signals. Additionally, a variant version of the MSC, the MSC-WA (WA, of Weighted Averaging), which consists of the multiplication of each epoch by the inverse of its power, was investigated. This weighting assumes that epochs with high power are the ones that present lower SNR and, therefore, should have their weight reduced. This procedure can be particularly interesting in the cases of non-stationary noises, which can harm the performance of the MSC, leading it to have inferior results to the PC (Dobie and Wilson, 1993). According to these authors, the T2C is mathematically related to the MSC, and it is possible to obtain one estimator from the other, although the MSC is computationally simpler. The MSC (or T2C) weighted averaging was the technique that presented the best performance in the detection of response to the auditory stimulus. In a later study (Dobie and Wilson, 1994a), the MSC, the MSC-WA and the PC were applied to the steady state 40Hz AEP. The three techniques presented similar performance in the response detection, although a slightly advantage for the MSC-WA over the MSC and for the MSC over the PC has been observed (Dobie and Wilson, 1994b).

At the same year, Dobie and Wilson (1994b) have applied the MSC and the MSC-PW (PW, of Phase Weighting) to the steady state 40Hz AEP. In the MSC-PW, a weighting is applied and it is related to the phase error calculated as the difference between the phase of the averaged signal (coherent average) and an expected phase (or target-phase). The target-phase is calculated from the coherent average with a high M number of EEG epochs during stimulation with intensities higher than the commonly used for obtaining the AEP. As a result, it was verified that the phase weighting improved the performance of the MSC. At the same year, Miranda de Sá et al. (1994) investigated the theoretical confidence limits for the coherence estimate (MSC) comparing them to the limits obtained by simulation with random signals.

In 1995, Dobie and Wilson (1995) verified the superior performance for the MSC-WA, when compared to the human inspection. The MSC-WA allowed detecting the responses to auditory stimulation with a lower number of stimuli and with lower stimulation intensity. At the same year, Thakor *et al.* (1995) have proposed an adaptive algorithm for the coherence estimate, in order to detect changes in the somatosensory evoked response. This study showed that, during hypoxia in cats, the MSC presents a sharp decrease, confirming the applicability of the adaptive MSC for monitoring purposes.

In 1996, Dobie and Wilson (1996) compared the Spectral F Test (SFT) and the MSC in the detection of the steady state AEP and concluded that, as they presented the same performance, the choice for using one technique or other would be a convenience issue. Two years later, Liavas *et al.* (1998) used successfully an ORD technique based on the periodogram for detecting the steady state visual evoked potential, aiming at investigating neuropathies related to the visual system.

Applying a decreasing exponential weighting to the spectral estimates of the EEG epochs during somatosensory stimulation used for MSC calculation, Tierra-Criollo *et al.* (1998) showed that this technique leads to the detection of the evoked responses faster than its simple version. This weighting emphasizes the latest spectral estimates, making the MSC more representative of the current status of the patient. This technique was named MSC with exponential forgetting (MSC-EF). Due to its promising results, Tierra-Criollo (2001) suggested the application of both the MSC and MSC-EF to the posterior tibial nerve SEP as a method to be evaluated for real-time monitoring of surgical procedures.

In 2000, Ramos et al. compared the MSC and the CSM (Component Synchrony Measure), which corresponds to the square of the PC (Phase Coherence). They reported that there is no statistical difference in performance for response detection when applied to the EEG of children and newborns during click stimulation. However, the MSC showed higher specificity in the detection of auditory deficiency, which gives to this technique greater clinical interest. Moreover, this method presented higher potentiality for determining the auditory threshold in the studied age group (Ramos et al., 2000). Also in the detection of the somatosensory response, the MSC presented better performance when compared to the CSM and the SFT (Simpson *et al.*, 2000, Tierra-Criollo, 2001). The MSC was also applied to the EEG during intermittent photic stimulation in order to quantify the degree of cortical activation (Miranda de Sá, 2000) and in the identification of inter-hemisphere symmetry between homologues regions of the visual cortex at the stimulation frequency and its harmonics (Miranda de Sá and Infantosi, 2002).

Miranda de Sá *et al.* (2001) proposed a coherence-based method to emphasize the stimuli-synchronized responses and reduce the background EEG influence. Later (Miranda de Sá *et al.*, 2002), the confidence limits for the coherence estimates between one random and one periodic signal were calculated based on a monotonically increasing function of the estimates, which involves the non-central F-distribution. Miranda de Sá (2004) obtained the sampling distribution of this coherence estimate itself and found it to be non-central beta distributed. This allowed further investigations to be carried out (Miranda de Sá *et al.*, 2009) for assessing both bias and variance of the estimate as well as the performance of the normalizing transform in it.

The MSC and the CSM were also applied for monitoring the anesthetic plan (Cagy *et al.*, 2000, Cagy, 2003). These studies showed that, during infusion of anesthetic, a reduction in values of both estimates is verified. Moreover, the results for MSC and CSM were quite similar, indicating the phase to be more important than the magnitude, as previously reported by Dobie and Wilson (1993). The MSC was also used to identify the maximum response band for the Brainstem Auditory Evoked Potential (BAEP) (Pacheco, 2003, Pacheco and Infantosi, 2005).

Infantosi *et al.* (2004) applied the MSC to the Middle Latency Auditory Evoked Potential (MLAEP) of normal individuals for different sound pressure levels aiming at investigating the frequency bands that better characterize this evoked response for distinct stimulation intensities. They have found consistent response detection for frequencies within the gamma band (30-50 Hz). Furthermore, the application of the MSC to the AEP for determining the auditory threshold L, defined as the volunteer response to a click stimulation, resulted in the detection near the visual identification by a specialist of the BAEP waves (L and L+5) or of the MLAEP's (L+15).

Melges *et al.* (2005) employed the methodology suggested by Tierra-Criollo (2001), and used the temporal evolution of the MSC for a given frequency in order to evidence the transitions from tibial nerve somatosensory stimulation to resting condition, and conversely. The transition from a responsive to a no-responsive status is very important for surgical monitoring and this work have mimicked these statuses by presenting and omitting the stimulus. At the same year, Miranda de Sá *et al.* (2005) have investigated the coherence between two EEG derivations due to a visual rhythmic stimulation and the partial coherence (after removing the contribution of the stimulus) applied to the same signals. They concluded that these techniques present complementary role, since the coherence quantifies the degree of synchronism between the derivations, whereas the partial coherence informs about the relationship due to the non-phase locked activities, suggesting its use in ERD/ERS (event related desynchronization/synchronization) studies.

In 2006, Campos *et al.* (2006) applied the SFT to the EEG of epileptic patients during intermittent photic stimulation, and concluded that this technique should be employed as a complement to the traditional identification methods of photo-recruited responses, such as spectral analysis. By using EEG signals during the same type of stimulation, Miranda de Sá *et al.* (2006) studied the SFT applied to the signals of normal individuals. Moreover, they investigated the probability distribution of this test, as well as the confidence limits for its estimates, using simulated signals with different signal-to-noise ratio and M-values. Since the majority of the EP applications use periodic stimulation (intermittent photic stimulation, train of current pulses or clicks), Miranda de Sá (2006a) developed analytical expressions for calculating the trend, variance and probability density function for the coherence (MSC), in the particular case in which the input signal (stimulus) is periodic.

Tierra-Criollo (2001) and Infantosi *et al.* (2006), by applying the MSC to the responses evoked by electric stimulation, identified the low gamma band (30-60 Hz) as the one that better represents the short-latency components of the somatosensory evoked potential. Also in 2006, Klein *et al.* (2006) have introduced a variant of the MSC, the Wavelet Coherence (WC), which allowed obtaining the temporal information that is lost when frequency-domain techniques are used.

Infantosi and Miranda de Sá (2006) proposed a methodology based on the MSC in order to study EEG activities that are synchronized in time (time-locked) with the stimulation signal, but non-synchronized in phase (non phase-locked). Such technique was investigated using the visual evoked potential, elicited by intermittent photic stimulation. In another study, Miranda de Sá (2006b) developed an expression for the partial coherence between two signals, removing the contribution of the stimulation, and showing that this estimates is independent of the stimulus signal. In 2007, Miranda de Sá and Infantosi (2007) introduced a method based on the estimates of the MSC and the Partial Coherence in order to quantify the similarity between two EEG activities that are not synchronized in phase with the stimulation signal. At the same year, Cagy and Infantosi (2007) showed that the MSC is capable of indicating modification both in amplitude and latency of the MLAEP.

Later, Melges *et al.* (2008a) investigated the topographic distribution of the tibial nerve somatosensory evoked potential (SEP) using the MSC and verified that the best regions for SEP recording, in an ORD approach, includes the central and parietal leads at the midline and parasagittal line ipsilateral to the stimulated limb. Two years later, Farina *et al.* (2010) proposed a novel ORD technique based on the Rice distribution, obtaining the analytical critical values and using simulated signals to calculate the probability of detection for different values of signal-to-noise ratio.

More recently, Melges *et al.* (2011a) showed that, although the variation of the stimulation frequency to values higher than 5 Hz produces distortion in the tibial nerve SEP waveform, hampering the visual inspection, the detection rates obtained with the MSC (and CSM) are statistically equivalent for different stimulation frequencies. Hence, higher values can be used in order to fasten the detection. The maximum frequency, however, is limited to about 10 Hz, since higher values could lead to steady state tibial nerve SEP, instead of transient one.

5.2 Multivariate ORD (MORD) techniques

The introduction of the ORD techniques represented an advance in the study of the evoked potentials, since these methods are based in statistical tests for inferring about the absence of stimulus-response (Dobie and Wilson, 1989). These techniques present the advantage (over traditional methods of identification of response), since they have a maximum false-positive rate (false alarm) a priori defined. However, for a fixed signal-to-noise ratio, it is only possible to improve the response detection rates, at the expense of increasing the recording length (number M of EEG epochs). This aspect may limit the application of ORD techniques, especially for surgical monitoring, case in which a fast detection of EP variations is needed, aiming at modifying the intra-operative strategy to avoid the occurrence of neurological damages.

In order to overcome this drawback and improve the detection rates, Miranda de Sá and Felix (2002) suggested the employment of multivariate extensions of the ORD techniques, named MORD (Multivariate ORD), which use information of more than one EEG derivation. In this study, they introduced the Multiple Coherence (MC), a multivariate version of the MSC, and verified that the detection percentages can be improved by augmenting the number of EEG channels used. These authors also verified that, similar to the proved to the uni-variate version (MSC), the estimate of the MC, for a periodic and deterministic stimulation, is independent of the stimulation signal. Moreover, they showed, by means of simulation, that even the addition of a second EEG signal with lower signal to noise-ratio than the first could result in an increase in the probability detection. Since the MORD does not require increasing the number of epochs for obtaining higher detection rates, the MC has been suggested as a useful tool to be applied in the surgical monitoring, allowing a faster detection of the elicited responses.

In the following year, Miranda de Sá and Felix (2003) proposed a multivariate extension for the Component Synchrony Measure (CSM), the MCSM (Multiple CSM), for which it was verified that the detection rates for the intermittent photic stimulation responses increase by augmenting the number of signals used in its calculation. Such results were observed for both simulated and real EEG signals.

In 2004, Miranda de Sá *et al.* (2004) proposed a matrix-based algorithm for the calculation of the Multiple Coherence. The results obtained by simulation showed that for achieving a detection probability of 95%, for example, the signals added to the set of EEG channels used for the MC estimate can present SNR lower than the first one. This can be observed until the 6th signal, from which a signal with SNR higher than the first one should be employed in order to maintain the detection rate (95%). However, in this case it would be more advantageous using only the 6th signal for estimating the MSC.

Later, Ferreira and Miranda de Sá (2005) compared the simple, multiple and partial coherences applied to the EEG during intermittent photic stimulation and consider these techniques promising in the analysis of the EEG during sensory stimulation. In the same year, Infantosi *et al.* (2005) verified, as theoretically predicted (Miranda de Sá and Felix, 2002, Miranda de Sá *et al.*, 2004), a better performance of the MC when compared to the MSC applied to the EEG during somatosensory stimulation of the tibial nerve. In this study, the MSC was applied to the bipolar derivations [Cz'-Fpz'] and [C3'-C4'] (where [Fpz'] is midway between [Fpz] and [Fz]; [Cz'], [C3'], and [C4'] are 2 cm posterior to [Cz], [C3] and [C4], respectively) - very often used for scalp SEP recording - and the MC was applied to both derivations. Using EEG signals from the same derivations during electric stimulation, Melges *et al.* (2006a) have found the MCSM to be useful for tibial nerve SEP detection. At the same year, Melges *et al.* (2006b) compared the performance of the MC and the MCSM, observing higher detection rates for the former. This result was observed for different values of M epochs (100, 200, 400, 800) used in the calculation of the estimates. A comparison between the two techniques applied to the EEG during intermittent photic stimulation (Felix *et al.*, 2007) has also resulted in higher detection percentages for the MC over the MCSM. By means of simulation, it was observed that the presence of noise correlated with the responses degrades the detection rates (Felix *et al.*, 2007).

In 2008, Miranda de Sá *et al.* (2008) derived the probability density function of the MC and a set of evoked responses embedded in additive noise for the zero-coherence case (null hypothesis of response absence). In this work, it was also demonstrated the influence of the number of EEG epochs (M) in both bias and variance of the MC estimates. At the same year, Melges *et al.* (2008b) compared the performance of MSC applied to the bipolar derivations [Cz-Fz] and [C3-C4] with the MC applied to the pairs of unipolar derivations [Cz][Fz] and [C3][C4]. The results showed that if two leads are available, it is better to use the MC of unipolar recordings than the MSC applied to the difference of the leads (bipolar derivation).

Since the use of unipolar derivations seemed to be more adequate, the performance for the MC and MCSM were compared, by applying both techniques to the pairs of unipolar derivations [Cz][Fz] and [C3][C4] (Melges *et al.*, 2010). The comparison was performed for M=100 and 800 epochs. The MC outperformed the MCSM, regardless the pair of derivations or the number of EEG epochs used for the estimates calculation.

More recently, Melges *et al.* (2011b) compared the MSC applied to the unipolar derivations [Cz], [Fz], [C3] and [C4] - usually employed in a bipolar SEP recording, as above mentioned - and the MC applied to the pairs [Cz][Fz] and [C3][C4]. The results evidenced the detection improvement by using synergically the information of two derivations, showing to be more advantageous using the MC than the MSC.

6. Examples and applications of ORD and MORD techniques

This section presents examples of using ORD and MORD techniques to the EEG during somatosensory stimulation. Following, the experimental protocol of EEG acquisition, the pre-processing and processing steps, and some results are shown.

6.1 EEG acquisition, pre-processing and processing

EEG Acquisition: EEG signals during somatosensory stimulation were collected from forty adult volunteers aging from 21 to 41 years old (mean ± standard deviation: 28.6 ± 4.6 years), without history of neurological pathology and with normal SEP. The signals were collected using the EEG BNT-36 (EMSA, Brazil, www.emsamed.com.br) according to the 10-20 International System and all leads referenced to the earlobe average. The volunteers were laid down in the supine position with eyes closed. The stimuli were applied by means of current pulses (200 μs width) to the right posterior tibial nerve using the Atlantis Four (EMSA, Brazil, www.emsamed.com.br). About 1000 to 1400 stimuli were applied at the motor threshold (the lowest intensity that produces toe oscillations) and at the rates of 1.99, 4.83, 6.68, 8.51 Hz (nominal values: 2, 5, 7, 9 Hz). The motor threshold was determined by an accelerometer tied in the toe that allowed the recording of the oscillations. The stimuli in the frequencies of 7 and 9 Hz were applied to 32 of the 40 volunteers. The ground electrode was attached to the poplitea fossa. Surface silver and gold electrodes were used, respectively, for recording and stimulation. An Institutional Review Board approved this research and all volunteers signed informed consent forms.

Pre-processing: The signals were band-filtered (0.5 - 100 Hz) and digitized (16-bits resolution) with BNT-36 at the sampling rate of 600 Hz. Then, the EEG was segmented into epochs of 501, 207, 149 and 117 ms, stimuli-synchronized, leading to spectral resolution of 2.0, 4.83, 6.71 and 8.55 Hz, respectively. In order to minimize the interference of the stimulus artifact in the ORD and MORD techniques we have set to zero the first 5 ms after each stimulus. Furthermore, the final 5 ms were zero padded to ensure window symmetry. A Tukey window with 7 ms rising (falling) time has been next applied to each epoch to ensure that the late components of the artifact are also attenuated. Noisy epochs were next discarded by a semi-automatic artifact rejection algorithm, which rejects epochs with more than 5% of continuous samples or more than 10% of samples exceeding ± 3 SD (where SD is the standard deviation of 20 s of noise-free background EEG selected as reference signal). Details about the windowing and artifact rejection can be found in Infantosi *et al* (2006).

ORD and MORD application: $\hat{\kappa}^2(f)$, $\hat{\kappa}^2_{crit}$, $\hat{\kappa}^2_N(f)$, $\hat{\kappa}^2_{N\,crit}$, $\hat{\rho}^2(f)$, $\hat{\rho}^2_{crit}$, $\hat{\rho}^2_N(f)$, $\hat{\rho}^2_{N\,crit}$ were calculated for the EEG signals using expressions (9),(11),(23),(24),(18),(20), (25), (26), respectively. The significance level $\alpha = 5\%$ was generally adopted, but the *M*-value varied and is cited for each illustration that follows. The detection was achieved when the estimate values exceeded the critical value.

6.2 The tibial nerve somatosensory evoked potential waveform

As mentioned in the Section 2, the waveform quality of SEP is very dependent on the number of stimulus presented. Figure 2 illustrates this characteristic of the analysis performed by visual inspection. For the coherent average obtained with *M*=50 epochs for derivation Cz of volunteer #35, the tibial nerve SEP waveform is very noisy and it is difficult to identify its characteristic waves. For *M*=200 epochs, the P37 (at 40 ms) and N45 (at 52 ms) are visible, respectively with amplitudes equal to -2.86 µV and 0.86 µV. However, it can be seen that, when a higher number of epochs (*M* = 500 epochs) is used, the waveform is smoother and the identification of the short-latency SEP components can be easily pointed even for an untrained observer at 40 ms and 50 ms.

Even for the SEP obtained with high signal-to-noise ratio, the components P37 and N45 presents high amplitude and latency (time duration from the stimulus to a peak or valley occurrence) variability, as it can be observed in Figure 3, which presents the SEP for six individuals calculated by averaging 500 epochs. This variability, associated with low signal-to-noise SEP recording obtained in hospital units, reinforces the subjectivity of such analysis.

6.3 ORD techniques applied to the somatosensory evoked response detection

The application of MSC to the EEG of volunteer #40 (stimulated at 6 mA) is illustrated in Figure 4. The horizontal black dashed line represents the detection threshold; when the corresponding MSC tracing surpasses its critical value, the detection is assumed for that (those) specific frequency (frequencies). As it can be observed, the MSC presents low values for derivation [C3] and higher values for [C4], that is, the higher response effects occur ipsilateral to the stimulated limb (the well known paradoxical lateralization (Cruse et al., 1982)). For derivation [C4], the detection is evident, predominantly at the frequencies from 30 to 65 Hz. On the other hand, for [C3], MSC exceeds the critical value only for the frequencies 29.0 and 33.8 Hz (nominal values: 30 and 35 Hz).

Both the CSM and MSC of derivation [C4] of volunteer #38 are showed in Figure 5, in which it can be visualized the similarity of values of $\hat{\rho}^2[C4]$ and $\hat{\kappa}^2[C4]$. Since the CSM can be obtained from the MSC when the amplitude information is discarded, this similarity evidences the importance of phase in the Objective Detection.

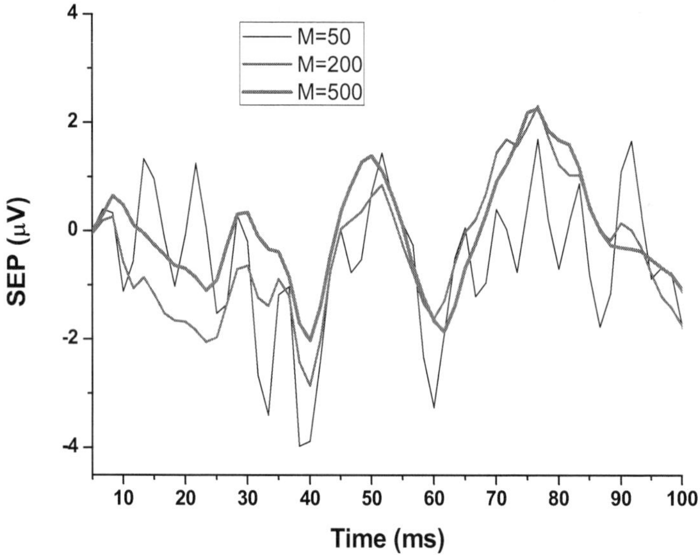

Fig. 2. Coherent Average (M = 50, 200 and 500 epochs) of derivation [Cz] of volunteer #35, stimulated at 24 mA and 5 Hz.

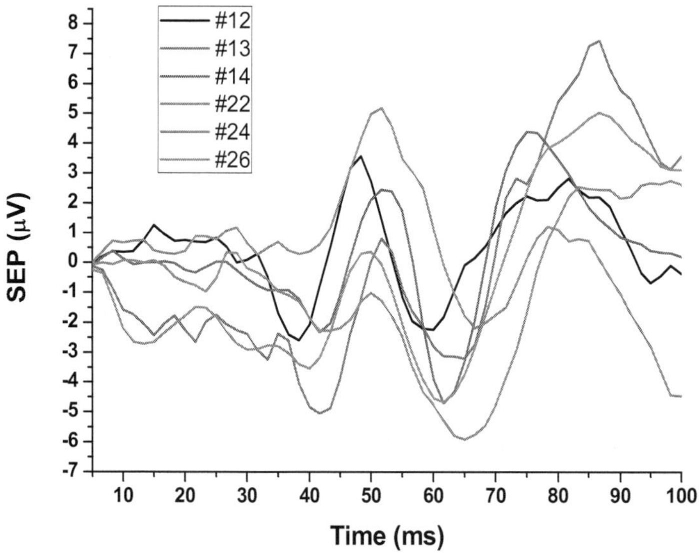

Fig. 3. Coherent Average (M = 500 epochs) of derivation [Cz] of volunteers #12, #13, #14, #22, #24, #26, respectively stimulated at 10, 10.5, 18, 12.5, 16 and 15 mA (these currents correspond to the individual motor threshold) and 5 Hz.

As it should be clear, establishing a statistical threshold for identifying the response detection reduces the subjectivity of the analysis. It is worth noting that the maximum false positive alarm can be as lower as desired, setting up α for the corresponding value.

6.4 Topographic distribution of the evoked responses

The localization on the scalp of the response to a specific kind of stimulation is a critical issue for the detection performance, since it determines the best regions for the evoked potential recording. In Melges et al. (2008), we have described that the leads with best signal-to-noise ratio for electrical stimulation of the right posterior tibial nerve are [Pz], [P4], [Cz], [C4] that is, leads at the parietal and central regions midsagital and ipsilateral to the stimulated limb. The results were obtained with the MSC applied to the SEP using 5 Hz as frequency of stimulation (f_{stim}). In fact, although the SEP is known to change its waveform characteristics with the stimulation frequency, the best detection percentages were obtained in the same leads for all investigated frequencies (2, 5, 7 and 9 Hz). Figure 6 shows the performance of the MSC for all the casuistry stimulated at the motor threshold and with f_{stim} = 9 Hz. As it can be seen, the same leads [Pz], [P4], [Cz], [C4] present the best detection rates. The ordinate presents the percentage of volunteers for whom it was possible to detect the evoked response for each frequency from the 1st to 12nd harmonics of the stimulation frequency.

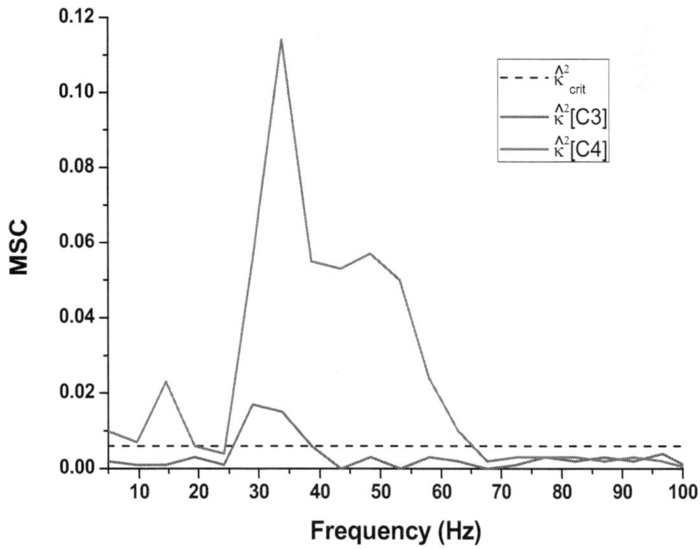

Fig. 4. $\hat{\kappa}^2$[C3] and $\hat{\kappa}^2$[C4] of volunteer #40, stimulated at 6 mA and 5 Hz. Horizontal line represent the critical value: $\hat{\kappa}^2_{crit} = 0.006$ (M = 500 epochs and α=0.05). Vertical axis (MSC) is dimensionless.

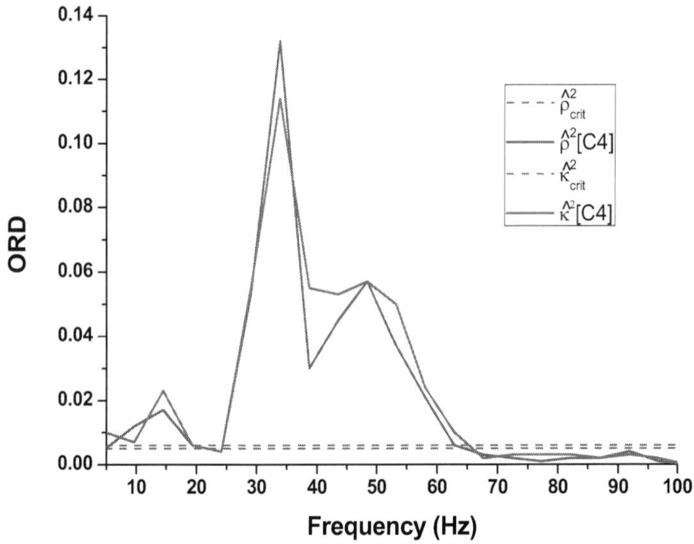

Fig. 5. $\hat{\rho}^2$[C4] and $\hat{\kappa}^2$[C4] of volunteer #38, stimulated at 14 mA and 5 Hz. Horizontal lines represent the critical values: $\hat{\rho}^2_{crit} = 0.005$ and $\hat{\kappa}^2_{crit} = 0.006$ (M = 500 epochs and α=0.05). Vertical axis (ORD) is dimensionless.

6.5 Maximum response frequency band

Apart from choosing suitable sites for EP recording, selecting the frequencies that are more responsive to a specific kind of stimulation is also important, since it leads to a more reliable objective neurophysiologic evaluation during surgical procedures.

From Figure 6, it is also possible to identify, in the derivations with best detection percentages, that the frequency range that includes from 2nd to the 6th harmonics of the stimulation frequency (9Hz) - frequencies from 18 to 54 Hz - is the more responsive. Hence, the presence of stimuli-response leads to positive detection in these frequencies, which were classified as the maximum response frequency band (Tierra-Criollo, 2001, Infantosi *et al.*, 2006); that is, frequencies within this range should be selected in order to augment the probability and rapidness of detection.

6.6 Stimulation frequency

The increase of the stimulation frequency is the simplest way of obtaining faster the response to a set of M stimuli, and enhances the time of detection. However, this frequency increase is known to cause changes in the SEP waveform (Chiappa, 1997, p. 307 and 323), whose characteristics are the basis for neurophysiologic monitoring. Fortunately, the detection rates obtained with an ORD approach is not statistically modified for different stimulation frequencies, as it was shown in a recent study of ours

(Melges *et al.*, 2011a). In this case, the use of the higher investigated frequency 9 Hz, represent a gain of 9:5 in the time of detection, if we consider the very often used stimulation frequency (5 Hz). Figure 7 presents the detection rates for derivation [Cz] and M = 200 epochs. In this figure it is possible to visualize the similarity in the profile of the detection percentage tracings, showed to be statistically equivalent for the maximum response frequency band, for both M = 100 and 500 epochs (Melges *et al.*, 2011a).

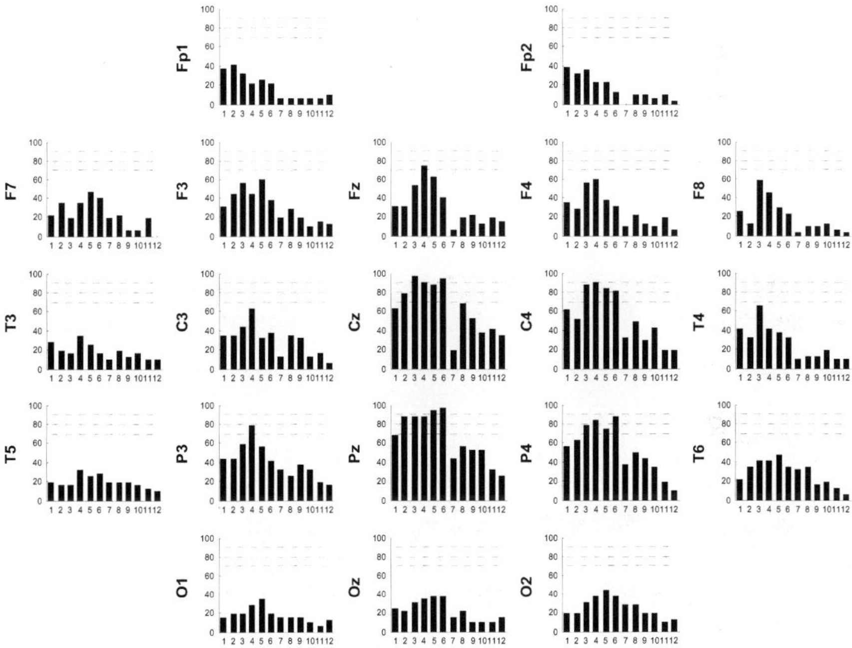

Fig. 6. Percentage of volunteers whose response to the stimulation could be detected using the MSC for multiples from 1 to 12 (9 to 100 Hz) of the stimulation frequency (9 Hz). Horizontal lines indicate 70, 80 and 90% of detection. For derivations Fp2 (31), F8 (31) and C4 (31), it was not possible to obtain 500 artifact-free epochs for the 32 volunteers, hence, the percentages were calculated with the number of volunteers in parenthesis.

6.7 ORD temporal evolution

After identifying the more responsive frequencies and have optimized the stimulation frequency aiming the fast detection, it is possible to choose one or some frequencies for monitoring its temporal evolution. In Figure 8A, a modulus of a Virtual Instrument (software) for Evoked Potential Objective Detection developed in Melges (2005) is shown, containing the temporal evolution of the MSC for the frequency of 36.8 Hz (Horizontal line represents the detection threshold). This signal was collected from volunteer #6, using parameters very commonly applied during surgical procedures. That is, the EEG was collected from derivation [Fpz'-Cz'] and with stimulation frequency of 5 Hz. In order to evaluate the capability of the MSC to reflect the transition of a responsive status to a no-responsive one, these conditions were mimicked by periods with and without electrical stimulation, respectively. Moreover, four periods with stimulation (S) were alternated with no-stimulation (NS) periods (starting without stimulation). The first S-period corresponds to the stimulation with the motor threshold intensity level (MT). In the following three S-periods, an intermediary intensity (IT) level was used; this intensity value was obtained by the arithmetic mean between MT and the sensitivity threshold, which corresponds to the lowest current level that is felt by the individual.

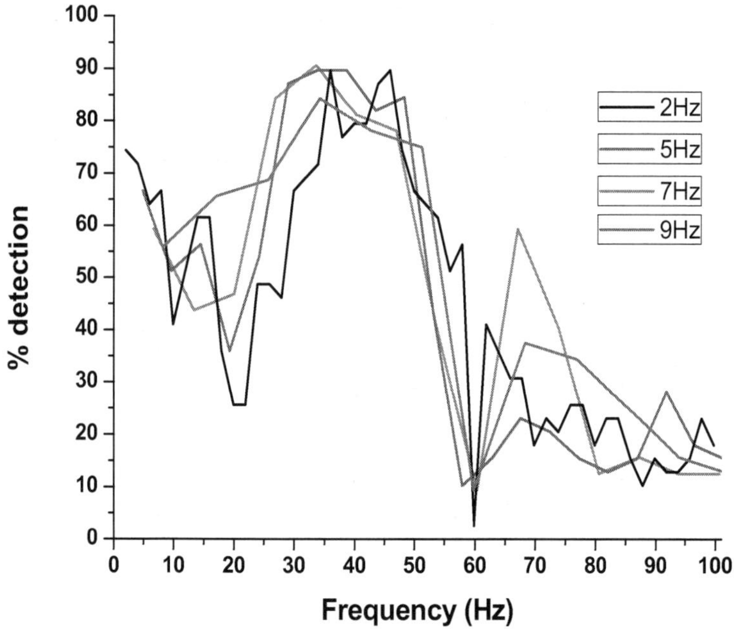

Fig. 7. Percentage of volunteers for whom the stimulation response was detected using the MSC (M = 200 epochs) for the frequencies from 2 to 100 Hz at the derivation [Cz] for the stimulation frequencies 2, 5, 7, 9 Hz.

The MSC estimates can be dynamically estimate as follows: 1) Store M EEG epochs in a matrix (A_{EEG}); 2) Calculate the MSC estimate using the M EEG epochs of A_{EEG} and expression 9; 3) When a new EEG epoch is acquired, substitute the older EEG epoch of A_{EEG}, i.e., the first line of it, by the new epoch and return to step 1.

From Figure 8A, one can note that even for a low *M*-value (*M*=50 epochs), the MSC was capable to follow the transition from rest to stimulated condition (Figure legend indicates the instant when the stimulus started and stopped), and conversely. Since the increase of *M* is known to improve the detection rate, the time evolution of MSC was also evaluated using *M*=400 epochs (Figure 8B). As it can be noted, the MSC estimate with *M*=50 epochs (MSC_{M50}) presents higher variability than the obtained with *M*=400 epochs (MSC_{M400}). On the other hand, MSC_{400} presents a higher inertia to change from one status to the other. Hence, the *M*-value should be parsimoniously chosen for the clinical or intra-operative application.

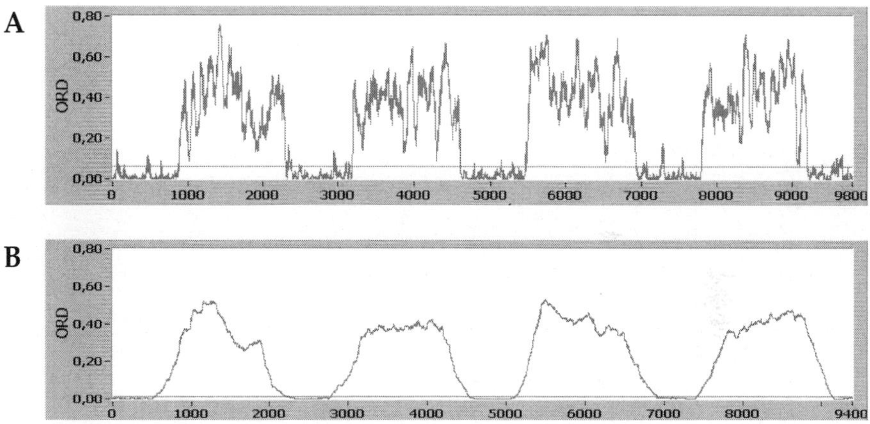

Fig. 8. $\hat{\kappa}^2(f)$ of the frequency 36.8 Hz (α=0.05) for derivation [Fpz'-Cz'] of volunteer stimulated at MT and IT for A) *M*=50 epochs (Horizontal orange line: $\hat{\kappa}^2_{crit} = 0.0593$); B) *M*=400 epochs ($\hat{\kappa}^2_{crit} = 0.0075$). Transitions from/to stimulated to/from no-stimulated condition at: A) t=830, 2296, 3164, 4591, 5459, 6889, 7781 and 9204 elapsed epochs. B) t=480, 1946, 2814, 4241, 5109, 6539, 7431 and 8854 elapsed epochs. Horizontal scale in elapsed epochs. Vertical axis (ORD-MSC) is dimensionless. The decimal separator in the coordinates scale is "comma", since the virtual instrument was developed using Brazilian Portuguese Regional Settings.

6.8 MORD techniques applied to SEP

The use of more than one derivation, as suggested by Miranda de Sá and Felix (2002), can improve the detection rates without the need of augmenting the exam duration (the number of EEG epochs used for ORD estimation). Figure 9 shows the MSC (*M* = 100 epochs) for [C3] and [C4], and the MC (*M* = 100 epochs) using both leads of volunteer #17. Since the somatosensory region on the contralateral hemisphere presents SEP with very low amplitude, as expected, the MSC values are low and under the detection threshold. On the other hand, the lead ipsilateral to the stimulated limb, [C4], shows detection for the nominal frequencies 35, 40, 50-60 Hz. It is worth noting that the employment of the $\hat{\kappa}_2^2[C3][C4]$ resulted in estimate values higher than $\hat{\kappa}^2[C3]$ and $\hat{\kappa}^2[C4]$, and the MC tracing surpasses its corresponding critical value for 35-60 Hz.

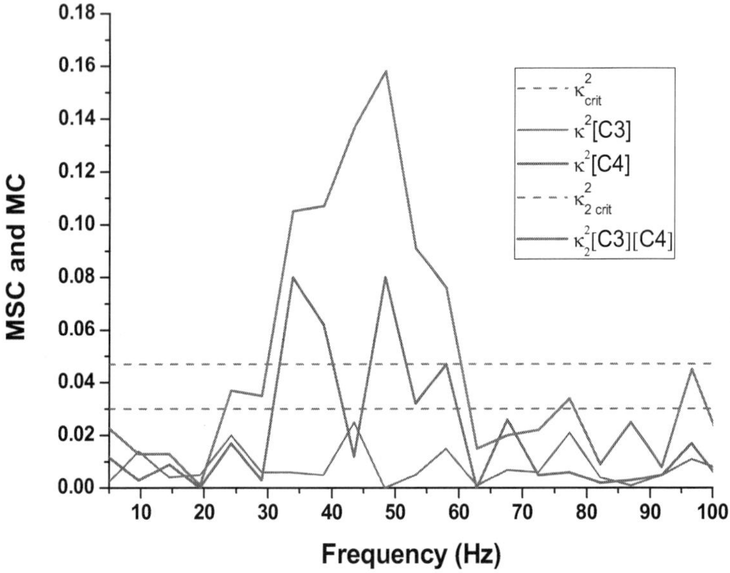

Fig. 9. $\hat{\kappa}^2[C3]$, $\hat{\kappa}^2[C4]$ and $\hat{\kappa}_2^2[C3][C4]$ of volunteer #17, stimulated at 10 mA and 5 Hz. Horizontal lines represent the critical values: $\hat{\kappa}_{crit}^2 = 0.0300$ and $\hat{\kappa}_{2crit}^2 = 0.0470$ for α=0.05, M = 100 epochs and N=2. Vertical axis (MSC and MC) is dimensionless.

The detection rates for the MSC applied to [Cz] and [C4] and for MC applied to [Cz][C4] is showed in Figure 10A. It is easy to note that the percentages for $\hat{\kappa}^2[Cz]$ are higher than the observed for $\hat{\kappa}^2[C4]$, and both are lower than $\hat{\kappa}_2^2[Cz][C4]$. Hence, "adding" the information from [Cz] to the [C4] resulted in an increase in the overall response detection performance.

In fact, even when a derivation with lower signal-to-noise ratio ([C3]) is added to the estimation of the Multiple Coherence, the detection rates can be improved (Figure 10B), as theoretically predicted by Miranda de Sá and Félix (2002).

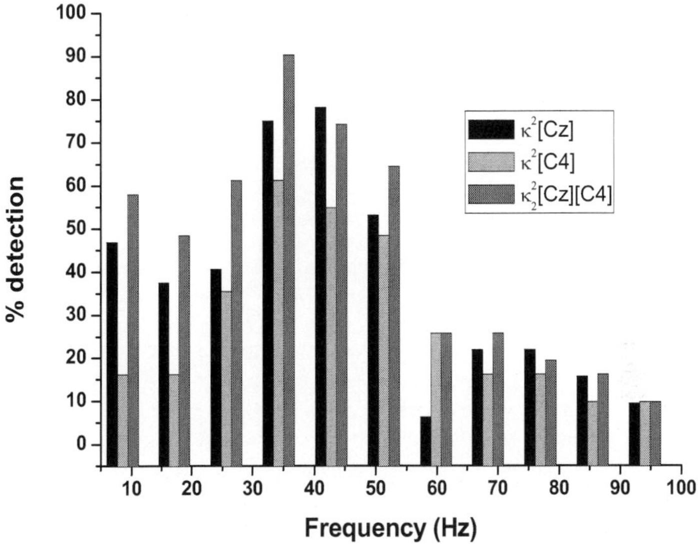

A

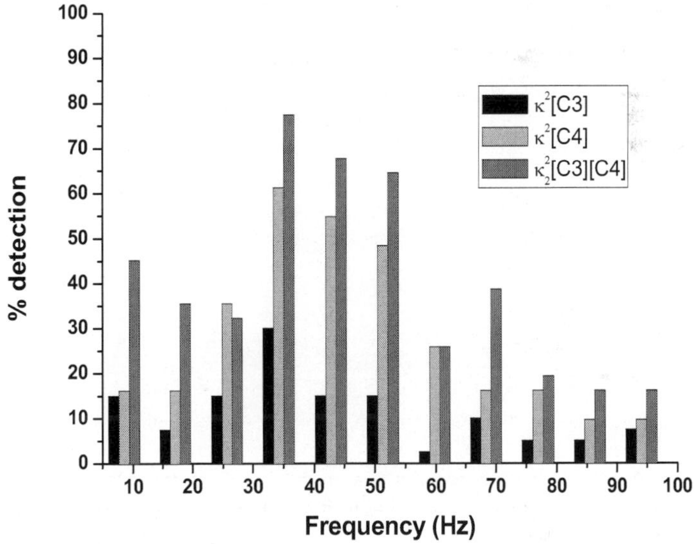

B

Fig. 10. Detection rates ($M = 100$ epochs) for A) $\hat{\kappa}^2[Cz]$, $\hat{\kappa}^2[C4]$ and $\hat{\kappa}_2^2[Cz][C4]$; B) $\hat{\kappa}^2[C3]$, $\hat{\kappa}^2[C4]$ and $\hat{\kappa}_2^2[C3][C4]$. For derivation [Cz], it was only possible to obtain 100 artifact-free epochs for 39 from the 40 volunteers, hence, the percentages of detection for [Cz] and [Cz][C4] were calculated over 39.

7. Conclusion

The ORD approach allows the detection of sensory response with a maximum false-positive rate (α) that can be defined as strict as desired. This leads to techniques that can be employed for a variety of occasions ranging from children auditory screening to the fast intra-operative monitoring in order to avoid early or late neurological sequels, including the ones arising from surgical manipulation. The wide applicability of the ORD comes from its computational simplicity, being usually based on the calculation of parameters derived from the Fourier Transform of EEG epochs.

When a very low signal-to-noise ratio is observed, which is the circumstance expected in hospital units due to the presence of electrical/electro-mechanic devices that generate electrical/electromagnetic interference, the use of more than one derivation, in a multivariate ORD approach, may improve the probability of detection without increasing in the exam duration. For this purpose, both scalp regions and frequencies more responsive should be employed in the objective detection. Moreover, in order to obtain faster response detection, the most higher stimulation frequency that does not result in decrease in the detection rates should be used.

For the right posterior tibial nerve SEP, presented as an illustration in this review, the maximum response frequency range is within the high beta and low gamma band (20-60 Hz); the best regions for SEP recording includes the central and parietal leads at the midline and parasagital line ipsilateral to the stimulated limb ([Cz], [C4] [Pz] and [P4]). The stimulation frequency of 9 Hz, instead of the often employed 5 Hz, can be used without diminishes the probability of detection. Hence, once the application of MORD produces an increase in the detection percentages compared to the MSC for the same M-value, it can, on the other hand, be employed to reduce the exam duration (M), whereas the detection probability is maintained.

Analogue results are expected for SEP obtained for the left tibial nerve and even for upper limbs, since the anatomical pathways follow similar routes, including decussation and somatotopic mapping. However, it should be effectively measured.

This review presented the theoretical background of ORD and MORD techniques applied to the Evoked Potential field. The historical aspects together with the included examples may be useful to many researches, since they encompass applications ranging from elementary goals up to the state of art in biosignal detection.

8. Future directions

Based on the prominent results found by using multivariate objective response detection techniques, it would be useful to investigate it for a number of derivations higher than $N = 2$. The MCSM critical value does not vary with N, as stated on expression (26) (Felix and Miranda de Sá, 2003). Thus, augmenting the number of derivations would imply increasing the detection rate. However, it did not occur in practical applications (Melges, 2009, Felix *et al.*, 2007). This could be explained by the fact that the background activities are correlated and hence there would be no improvement by continuously adding new derivations. However, this hypothesis of correlated activities should be verified for different kinds of evoked potentials. Additionally, it would be worth to identify the optimal number of derivations to be employed for both MC and MCSM estimation for each kind of stimulation, since the presence of a massive number of leads is undesirable for clinical and surgical monitoring purposes. Moreover, the exponential forgetting, suggested by Tierra-Criollo *et al.* (1998), should be applied for multivariate ORD in order to increase the rapidness of response detection. Finally, both ORD and MORD techniques should be incorporated in the EP analysis software to have their efficacy evaluated for diagnosis and neuro-monitoring.

9. Abbreviations

EEG - Electroencephalogram; EP - Evoked Potential; AEP - auditory EP; SEP - somatosensory EP; VEP - Visual EP; ORD - Objective Response Detection; MORD - Multivariate ORD.

10. Acknowledgements

To the Brazilian research and education agencies, the Rio de Janeiro State Research Council (FAPERJ), the National Council for Scientific and Technological Development (CNPq - Ministry of Science and Technology) and CAPES (Ministry of Education) for the financial support. We also acknowledge the Military Police Central Hospital of Rio de Janeiro for providing infrastructure support.

11. References

Angel, A, Linkens, DA, Ting, CH. 1999. Estimation of latency changes and relative amplitudes in somatosensory evoked potentials using wavelets and regression, *Comput Biomed Res*, Vol. 32, No. 3, Jun, pp. 209-251.

Beagley, HA, Sayers, BMcA, Ross, AJ. 1979. Fully objective ERA by phase spectral analysis, *Acta otolaryngol*, Vol. 87, No. 3, Jan, pp. 270-278.

Bendat, JS, Piersol, AG. 2000. *Random Data Analysis and Measurement Procedures* (3 ed), New York, Wiley-Interscience.

Bose, B, Sestokas, AK, Schwartz, DM. 2004. Neuropsychological monitoring of spinal cord function during instrumented anterior cervical fusion, *Spine J*, Vol. 4, No. 2, Mar/Apr, pp. 202-207.

Cagy, M, Infantosi, AFC, Gemal, AE. 2000. Monitoring depth of anaesthesia by frequency-domain statistical techniques, *Braz J Biomed Eng*, Vol. 16, No. 2, pp. 95-107.

Cagy, M, Infantosi, AFC. 2002. Unconsciousness indication using time-domain parameters extracted from mid-latency auditory evoked potentials, *J Clin Monit Comput*, Vol. 17, No.6, pp. 362-366.

Cagy, M., 2003, Monitorização do plano anestésico usando o potencial evocado auditivo de média latência: técnicas no domínio do tempo e coerência espectral. D.Sc. Thesis., COPPE/UFRJ, Rio de Janeiro, Rio de Janeiro, Brazil.

Cagy, M, Infantosi, AFC. 2007. Objective response detection technique in frequency-domain for reflecting changes in MLAEP, Medl Eng Phy, Vol 29, No 8, Oct, pp. 910-917.

Campos, DV, Infantosi, AFC, Lazarev, VV. 2006. Aplicação do Teste F spectral na detecção de respostas fotorecrutantes no eletroencefalograma multicanal de pacientes epilépticos, *Anais do XX Congresso Brasileiro de Engenharia Biomédica - CBEB2006* (CDROM), pp. 318-321, São Pedro, São Paulo, Brazil, Oct 2006.

Cruccu, G, Aminoff, MJ, Curio, G, Guerit, JM, Kakigi, R, Mauguière, F, Rossini, PM, Treede, R-D, Garcia-Larrea, L. 2008. Recommendations for the clinical use of somatosensory-evoked potentials, *Clin Neurophysiol*, Vol. 119, pp. 1705–1719.

Cruse R, Klem G, Lesser RP, Leuders H. 1982. Paradoxical lateralization of cortical potentials evoked by stimulation of posterior tibial nerve, *Arch Neurol*, Vol. 39, pp. 222-225.

Dobie, RA, Wilson, MJ. 1989. Analysis of auditory evoked potentials by Magnitude-Squared Coherence. *Ear Hear*, Vol. 10, No. 1, Fev, pp. 2-13.

Dobie, RA, Wilson, MJ. 1990. Optimal ('Wiener') digital filtering of auditory evoked potentials: use of coherence estimates. *Electroencephalogr Clin Neurophysiol*, Vol. 77, No. 3, May/Jun, pp. 205-213.

Dobie, RA, Wilson, MJ. 1993. Objective response detection in the frequency domain, *Electroencephalogr Clin Neurophysiol*, Vol. 88, No. 6, Nov/Dec, pp. 516-524.

Dobie, RA, Wilson, MJ. 1994a. Objective detection of 40Hz auditory evoked potentials: phase coherence vs. magnitude-squared coherence, *Electroencephalogr Clin Neurophysiol*, Vol. 92, No. 5, Set, pp. 405-413.

Dobie, RA, Wilson, MJ. 1994b. Phase weighting: a method to improve objective detection of steady-state evoked potentials, *Hear Res*, Vol. 79, No. 1-2, Set, pp. 94-98.

Dobie, RA, Wilson, M J. 1995. Objective versus human observer detection of 40 Hz auditory-evoked potentials, *J Acoustic Soc Am*, Vol. 97, No. 5, Mai, pp. 3042-3050.

Dobie, RA, Wilson, MJ. 1996. A comparison t test, F test and coherence methods of detecting steady-state auditory-evoked potentials, distortion product otoacoustic emissions, or other sinusoids, *J Acoustic Soc Am*, Vol. 100, No. 4, Out, pp. 2236-2246.

Dong, CC, MacDonald, DB, Janusz, MT. 2002. Intraoperative spinal cord monitoring during descending thoracic and thoracoabdominal aneurysm surgery, *Ann Thorac Surg*, Vol. 74, pp. S1873-S1876.

Faberowski, LW, Black S., Trankina, M.F., Polland, RJ, Clarck, RK, Mahla, ME. 1999. Somatosensory-evoked potentials during aortic coarctation repair, *J Cardiothorac Vasc Anesth*, Vol. 13, No. 5, Out, pp. 538-543.

Farina Jr, PD, Melges, DB, Miranda de Sá, AMFL, Infantosi, AFC. 2010. Técnica de detecção objetiva de resposta baseada na distribuição de Rice, *Anais do XXII Congresso Brasileiro de Engenharia Biomédica - CBEB2010*, [ISSN: 2179-3220], pp. 915-918, Tiradentes, Minas Gerais, Brazil, Nov 2010.

Felix, LB, Miranda de Sá, AMFL, Infantosi, AFC, Yehia, HC. 2007. Multivariate objective response detectors (MORD): statistical tools for multichannel EEG analysis, Ann Biomed Eng, Vol. 35, No. 3, Mar, pp. 443-452.

Ferreira, DD, Miranda de Sá, AMFL. 2005. Análise do EEG durante estimulação sensorial baseada nas funções de coerência simples, múltipla e parcial, *Braz J Biomed Eng*, Vol. 21, No. 1, pp. 5-14.

Florence, G, Guérit, J-M, Gueguen, B. 2004. Electroencephalography and somatosensory evoked potentials to prevent cerebral ischaemia in the operating room, Clin Neurophysiol, Vol. 34, No. 1, Fev, pp. 17-32.

Galambos, R, Makeig, S, Stapells, DR. 1984. The phase aggregation of steady state (40Hz) event related potentials: its use in estimating hearing thresholds. *XVII International Congress of Audiology*, Santa Barbara, California, Aug 1984.

Ghariani, S, Spaey, J, Liard, L, Verhelst, R., El Khoury, G, Noirhomme, P, D'udekem, Y., Matta, A, Dion, R, Guérit, J-M. 1998. Sensibilité, specificité et impact sur la stratégie chirurgicale du neuromonitorage peropératoire par potentiels évoqués somesthésiques em chirurgie vasculaire pratiquée avec arrêt circulatoire sous hypothermie profonde, *Neurohpisiol Clin*, Vol. 28, No. 4, Set, pp. 335-342.

Ghariani, S, Liard, L, Spacy, J, Noirhomme, PH, Khoury, GAE, Tourtchaninoff, M, Dion, RA, Guérit, J-M. 1999. Retrospective study if somatosensory evoked potential monitoring in deep hypothermic circulatory arrest, *Ann Thorac Surg*, Vol. 67, No. 6, Jun, pp. 1915-1918.

Ghariani, S, Matta, A, Dion, R, Guérit, J-M. 2000. Intra- and postoperative factors determining neurological complications after surgery under deep hypothermic circulatory arrest: a retrospective somatosensory evoked potential study, *Clin Neurophysiol*, Vol. 111, No. 6, Jun, pp. 1082-1094.

Gemal, AE. 1999. Changes in the auditory middle latency response to propofol infusions. Ph.D. Thesis, University of Bristol, Bristol, England.

Giugno, K M, Maia, TR, Kunrath, CL, Bizzi, JJ. 2003. Tratamento da hipertensão intracraniana, *Jornal de Pediatria*, Vol. 79, No. 4, Jul/Aug, pp. 287-296.

Greenblatt, E, Zapulla, RA, Kaye, S, Friedman, J. 1985. Response threshold determination of the brain stem auditory evoked response: a comparison of the phase versus magnitude derived from the Fast Fourier Transform, *Int J Audiol*, Vol. 24, No. 4, Jan, pp. 288-296.

Guérit, J-M. 1999. Medical technology assessment EEG and evoked potentials in the intensive care unit, *Clin Neurophysiol*, Vol. 29, No. 4, Sep, pp. 301-317.

Guérit, J-M, Dion, RA. 2002. State-of-the art of neuromonitoring for prevention of immediate and delayed paraplegia in thoracic and thoracoabdominal aorta surgery, *Ann Thorac Surg*, No. 74, pp. S1867-S1869.

Gundanna, M, Eskenasi, M, Bendo, J, Spivak, J, Moskovich, R. 2003. Somatosensory evoked potential monitoring of lumbar pedicle screw placement for in situ posterior spinal fusion, *Spine J*, Vol. 3, No. 5, Sep/Oct, pp. 370-376.

Hotelling, H. 1931. The generalization of Student's ratio, *Ann Math Stat*, Vol. 2, pp. 360-378.

Infantosi, AFC, Cagy, M, Zaeyen, EJB. 2004. Aplicação da Magnitude Quadrática da Coerência ao MLAEP com estimulação a baixos níveis de pressão sonora. *IFMBE Proceedings - III Congreso Latinoamericano de Ingeniería Biomédica – CLAIB2004 (CDROM)*, Vol. 5, pp. 1111-1114, João Pessoa, Paraíba, Brazil, 2004.

Infantosi, AFC, Melges, DB, Miranda de Sá, AMFL, Cagy, M. 2005. Uni- and multi-variate coherence-based detection applied to EEG during somatosensory stimulation, *IFMBE Proceedings - 3rd. European Medical & Biological Engineering Conference - EMBEC'2005 (CDROM)*, Vol. 11, pp. 1-4 (578F.pdf), Prague, Czech Republic, 2005.

Infantosi, AFC, Melges, DB, Tierra-Criollo, CJ. 2006. Use of magnitude-squared coherence to identify the maximum driving response band of the somatosensory evoked potential, *Braz J Med Biol Res*, Vol. 39, pp. 1593-1603.

Infantosi, AFC, Miranda de Sá, AMFL. 2006. A coherence-based technique for separating phase-locked from non-phase-locked power spectrum estimates during intermittent stimulation, *J Neurosci Methods*, Vol. 156, No. 1-2, Set, pp. 267-274.

Hoffmann, MB, Seufert, PS, Bach, M. 2004. Simulated nystagmus suppresses pattern-reversal but not pattern-onset visual evoked potentials, *Clin Neurophysiol*, Vol. 115, No. 11, Nov, pp. 2659-2665.

Holopigian, K, Shuwairi, SM, Greenstein, VC, Winn, BJ, Zhang, X., Carr, RE, Hood, DC. 2005. Multifocal visualevokedpotentials to cone specific stimuli in patients with retinitis pigmentosa, Vision Research, Vol. 45, No. 25-26, Nov, pp. 3244-3252

Jancic-Stefanovic, JB, Stefanovic, DM, Obradovic, D, Cetkovic, MV. 2003. Visual-evokedpotentials as additional diagnostic procedure in migraine headaches in childhood and adolescence, *International Congress Series*, Vol. 1240, Oct, pp. 1395-1398.

Jones, SC, Fernau, R, Woeltjen, BL. 2004. Use of somatosensory evoked potentials to detect peripheral ischemia and potential injury resulting from positioning of the surgical patient: case reports and discussion, *Spine J*, Vol. 4, No. 4, May/Jun, pp. 360-362.

Kato, T, Okumura, A, Hayakawa, F, Kuno, K, Watanabe, K. 2005. The evolutionary change of flash visual evoked potentials in preterm infants with periventricular leukomalacia, *Clin Neurophysiol*, Vol. 116, No. 3, Mar, pp. 690-695.

Keyhani, K, Miller III, CC, Estrera, AL, Wegryn, T, Sheinbaum, R, Safi, HJ. 2009. Analysis of motor and somatosensory evoked potentials during thoracic and thoracoabdominal aortic aneurysm repair, *J Vasc Surg* 49 p. 36-41.

Klein, A, Sauer, T, Jedynak, A, Skrandies, W. 2006. Conventional and Wavelet Coherence applied to sensory-evoked electrical brain activity, *IEEE Trans Biomed Eng*, Vol. 53, No. 2, Fev, pp. 266-272.

Krishnan, GP, Vohs, JL, Hetrick, WP, Carroll, CA, Shekhar,A, Bockbrader, MA, O'Donnell, BF. 2005. Steady state visual evoked potential abnormalities in schizophrenia, *Clin Neurophysiol*, Vol. 116, No. 3, Mar, pp. 614-624.

Liavas, AP, Moustakides, GV, Henning, G, Psarakis, EZ, Husar, P. 1998. A periodogram-based method for the detection of steady-state visually evoked potentials, *IEEE Trans Biomed Eng*, Vol. 45, No. 2, Fev, pp. 242-248.

Linden, RD, Zappula, R, Shields, CB. 1997. Intraoperative evoked potential monitoring. In: *Evoked Potentials in Clinical Medicine*, Chiappa, KH, pp. 601-638, Raven Press, New York, USA.

Liu, H, Di Giorgio, AM, Williams, ES, Evans, W, Russell, MJ. 2010. Protocol for electrophysiological monitoring of carotid endarterectomies, *J Biomed Res.*, Vol. 24, pp. 460-466.

Logi, F, Fisher, C, Murri, L, Mauguière, F. 2003. The prognostic value of evoked responses from primary somatosensory and auditory in comatose patients, *Clin Neurophysiol*, Vol. 114, No. 9, Set, pp. 1615-1627.

Lopes da Silva, F. 1999. Event-Related Potentials: Methodology and Quantification. In: *Electroencephalography - Basic Principles, Clinical Applications, and Related Fields*, Niedermeyer, E, Lopes da Silva, FH (eds), 4 ed., chapter 52, Baltimore, USA, Williams &Wilkins.

Mardia, KV. 1972. *Statistics of Directional Data.* 1 ed. London, Academic Press.

Martin, CJ, Sinson, G, Patterson, T, Zager, EL, Stecker MM. 2002. Sensitivity of scalp EEG, cortical EEG, and somatosensory evoked responses during surgery for intracranial aneurysms, *Surg Neurol*, Vol. 58, No. 5, Nov, pp. 317-321.

Melges, DB, 2005, A Virtual Instrument for Somatosensory stimulation response monitoring. M.Sc. Dissertation, COPPE/UFRJ, Rio de Janeiro, Rio de Janeiro, Brazil. (Available at: http://www.dominiopublico.gov.br/)

Melges, DB, Infantosi, A FC, Cagy, M, Miranda de Sá, AMFL. 2005. The Magnitude-Squared Coherence in the Detection of Stimulation/No-Stimulation Transitions, *IFMBE Proceedings - 13th Nordic Baltic Conference - Biomedical Engineering and Medical Physics*, [ISSN 1680-0737], Vol. 9, pp. 58-59, Umea, Suécia, 2005.

Melges, DB, Miranda de Sá, AMFL, Infantosi, AFC. 2006a. Using Component Synchrony Measure for somatosensory evoked potential detection, *Proceedings of the 28 th Annual International Conference IEEE - Engineering in Medicine and Biology Society-EMBC' 2006* [ISSN: 1557-170X], pp. 4572-4575, New York, USA, Aug/Sept 2006.

Melges, DB, Miranda de Sá, AMFL, Infantosi, AFC. 2006b. Técnicas multivariadas de detecção objetiva aplicadas ao EEG durante estimulação somato-sensitiva, *Anais do XX Congresso Brasileiro de Engenharia Biomédica - CBEB2006 (CDROM)*, pp. 338-341, São Pedro, São Paulo, Brazil, Oct 2006.

Melges, DB, Infantosi, AFC, Miranda de Sá, AMFL. 2008a. Topographic distribution of the tibial somatosensory evoked potential using coherence, *Braz J Med Biol Res*, Vol. 41, No. 12, Dec, pp. 1059-1066.

Melges, DB, Infantosi, AFC, Miranda de Sá, AMFL. 2008b. Detecção da resposta somato-sensitiva: coerência simples (derivações bipolares) vs múltipla (unipolares), *Anais do XXI Congresso Brasileiro de Engenharia Biomédica - CBEB' 2008* [ISBN: 978-85-60064-13-7], Vol. 1, pp. 1671-1674, Salvador, Bahia, Brazil, Nov 2008.

Melges, DB, 2009, Uni and multivariate frequency-domain objective response detection techniques application to the EEG during somatosensory stimulation. D.Sc. Thesis, COPPE/UFRJ, Rio de Janeiro, Rio de Janeiro, Brazil. (Available at: http://www.dominiopublico.gov.br/)

Melges, DB, Miranda de Sá, AMFL, Infantosi, AFC. 2010. Multiple Coherence vs Multiple Component Synchrony Measure for somatosensory evoked response detection, *Proceedings of the 32nd Annual International Conference of the IEEE Engineering in Medicine and Biology Society - EMBC' 2010* [ISSN: 1557-170X], pp. 1662-1665, Buenos Aires, Argentina, Aug/Sep 2010.

Melges, DB, Infantosi, AFC, Miranda de Sá, AMFL. 2011a. Using Objective Response Detection techniques for detecting the tibial somatosensory evoked response with different stimulation rates, *J Neurosci Methods*, Vol. 195, pp.255-260.

Melges, DB, Miranda de Sá, AMFL, Infantosi, AFC. 2011b. Tibial nerve somatosensory evoked response detection using uni and multivariate coherence. *Biomed Signal Process Control (in press)*.

Miranda de Sá, AMFL, Simpson, DM, Infantosi, AFC. 1994. Estudo da função de coerência aplicada a sinais EEG, *Braz J Biomed Eng*, Vol. 10, No. 2, pp. 39-55.

Miranda de Sá, AMFL. 2000. Desenvolvimento de técnicas para o estudo da coerência no EEG durante foto-estimulação intermitente. D.Sc. Thesis, COPPE/UFRJ, Rio de Janeiro, Rio de Janeiro, Brazil.

Miranda de Sá, AMFL, Infantosi, AFC, Simpson, DM. 2001. A statistical technique for measuring synchronism between cortical regions in the EEG during rhythmic stimulation, *IEEE Trans Biomed Eng*, Vol. 48, No. 10, Oct, pp. 1211-1215.

Miranda de Sá, AMFL, Felix, LB. 2002. Improving the detection of evoked responses to periodic stimulation by using multiple coherence - application during photic stimulation, *Med Eng Phys*, Vol. 24, No. 4, May, pp. 245-252.

Miranda de Sá, AMFL, Infantosi, AFC. 2002. A coherence-based technique for evaluating the degree of synchronism in the EEG during sensory stimulation, *Braz J Biomed Eng*, Vol. 18, No. 1, Jan/Apr, pp. 39-49.

Miranda de Sá, AMFL, Infantosi, AFC, Simpson, DM. 2002. Coherence between one random and one periodic signal for measuring the strength of responses in the EEG during sensory stimulation, *Med Biol Eng Comput,* Vol. 40, pp. 99-104.

Miranda de Sá, AMFL, Felix, LB. 2003. Multi-channel evoked response detection using only phase information, *J Neurosci Methods*, Vol. 129, No. 1, Oct, pp. 1-10.

Miranda de Sá, AMFL. 2004. A note on the sampling distribution of coherence estimate for the detection of periodic signals, *IEEE Signal Process Lett*, Vol. 11, No. 3, Mar, pp. 323-325.

Miranda de Sá, AMFL, Felix, LB, Infantosi, AFC. 2004. A matrix-based algorithm for estimating multiple coherence of periodic signal and its application to the multichannel EEG during sensory stimulation, *IEEE Trans Biomed Eng*, Vol. 51, No. 7, Jul, pp. 1140-1146.

Miranda de Sá, AMFL, Cagy, M, Melges, DB, Infantosi, AFC. 2005. Multivariate spectral analysis applied to the EEG during rhythmic stimulation - a coherence-based approach, *IFMBE Proceedings - 13th Nordic Baltic Conference - Biomedical Engineering and Medical Physics* [ISSN 1680-0737], Vol. 9, pp. 60-61, Umea, Suécia, Jun 2005.

Miranda de Sá, AMFL. 2006a, A note on the coherence-based signal-to-noise ratio estimation in systems with periodic inputs, *J Franklin Institute*, Vol. 343, No. 7, Nov, pp. 688-698.

Miranda de Sá, AMFL. 2006b. Evaluating spectral relationships between signals by removing the contribution of a common, periodic source - a partial coherence-based approach, *Inter J Biomed Sci*, Vol. 1, No. 1, pp. 15-18.

Miranda de Sá, AMFL, Cagy, M, Lazarev, VV, Infantosi, AFC. 2006. Spectral F-test power evaluation in the EEG during intermittent photic stimulation, *Arq Neuropsiquiatr*, Vol. 64, n. 2-A, Jun, pp. 228-232.

Miranda de Sá, AMFL, Infantosi, AFC. 2007. Evaluating the relationship of non-phase locked activities in the electroencephalogram during intermittent stimulation: a partial coherence-based approach, *Med Biol Eng Comput*, Vol. 45, pp. 635-642.

Miranda de Sá, AMFL, Infantosi, AFC, Melges, DB. 2008. A multiple coherence-based detector for evoked responses in the EEG during sensory stimulation, *Proceedings of the 30th Annual International Conference of the IEEE Engineering in Medicine and Biology Society- EMBC' 2008* [ISSN: 1557-170X], p. 3516-3519, Vancouver, Canada, Aug 2008.

Miranda de Sá, AMFL, Ferreira, DD, Dias, EW, Mendes, EMAM, Felix, LB. 2009. Coherence estimate between a random and a periodic signal: bias, variance, analytical critical values and normalizing transforms, *J Franklin Institute*, Vol. 346, pp. 841-853.

Nayak, A, Roy, RJ. 1998. Anesthesia control using midlatency auditory evoked potentials, *IEEE Trans Biomed Eng*, Vol. 45, No. 4, Apr, pp. 409-421.

Nemoto, N, Mori, H, Kiyosawa, M, Wang, WF, Mochizuki, M, Momose, K. 2002. Visual Evoked Potentials Elicited by Pseudorandom Stimulation from Patients with Macular Degeneration, *Japanese Journal of Ophthalmology*, Vol. 46, No. 1, pp. 108-113.

Nuwer, MR, Dawson, EG, Carlson, LG, Kanim, Le, A, Sherman, JE. 1995. Somatosensory evoked potential spinal cord monitoring reduces neurologic deficits after scoliosis surgery: results of a large multicenter survey, *Electroencephalogr Clin Neurophysiol*, Vol. 96, No. 1, Jan, pp. 6-11.

Pacheco, EA. 2003. Determinação da banda de máxima resposta do potencial evocado auditivo de curta latência por meio da magnitude quadrática da coerência. M.Sc. Dissertation, COPPE/UFRJ, Rio de Janeiro, Rio de Janeiro, Brazil.

Pacheco, EA, Infantosi, AFC. 2005. Determinação das Bandas de Máxima Resposta Espectral do Potencial Evocado Auditivo de Tronco Cerebral Utilizando a Magnitude Quadrática da Coerência, *Braz J Biomed Eng*, Vol. 21, No. 3, pp. 105-113.

Parisi, V, Manni, G, Centofanti, M, Gandolfi, SA, Olzi, D, Bucci, MG. 2001. Correlation between optical coherence tomography, pattern electroretinogram, and visual evoked potentials in open-angle glaucoma patients, *Ophthalmology*, Vol. 108, No. 5, May, pp. 905-912.

Picton, TW, Vajsar, J, Rodriguez, R, Campbell, KB. 1987. Reliability estimates for steady-state evoked potentials, *Electroencephalogr Clin Neurophysiol/Evoked Potentials Section*, Vol. 68, No. 2, Mar, pp. 119-131.

Ramos, EG, Zaeyen, EJB, Simpson, DM, Infantosi, AFC. 2000. Detecção da resposta auditiva no EEG de crianças utilizando técnicas no domínio da freqüência, *Braz J Biomed Eng*, Vol. 16, No. 3, Sep/Dec, pp. 127-137.

Simpson, DM, Tierra-Criollo, CJ, Leite, RT, Zaeyen, EJB, Infantosi, AFC. 2000. Objective response detection in an electroencephalogram during somatosensory stimulation, *Ann Biomed Eng*, Vol. 28, No. 6, Jun, pp. 691-698.

Schulte-Körne, G, Bartling, J, Deimel, W, Remschmidt, H. 2004. Visual evoked potentials elicited by coherently moving dots in dyslexic children, Clin Neurophysiol, Vol. 115, No. 3, Mar, pp. 207-120.

Stapells, DR, Makeig, S, Galambos, R. 1987. Auditory steady state responses: threshold prediction using phase coherence, *Electroencephalogr Clin Neurophysiol*, Vol. 67, No. 3, Sep, pp. 260-270.

Thakor, NV, Kong, X, Handley, DF. 1995. Nonlinear changes in brain's response in the event of injury as detected by adaptive coherence estimation of evoked potentials, *IEEE Trans Biomed Eng*, Vol. 42, No. 1, Jan, pp. 42-51.

Tierra-Criollo, CJ, Zaeyen, EJB, Simpson, DM, Infantosi, AFC. 1998. Detecção da resposta à estimulação somato-sensitiva no EEG utilizando a Magnitude Quadrada da Coerência Ponderada, *Anais do IV Fórum Nacional de Ciência e Tecnologia em Saúde*, pp. 441-442, Curitiba, Paraná, Brazil, Oct 1998.

Tierra-Criollo, CJ. 2001. Monitorização objetiva da resposta à estimulação somato-sensitiva utilizando parâmetros espectrais. D.Sc. Thesis, COPPE/UFRJ, Rio de Janeiro, Rio de Janeiro, Brazil.

Trisciuzzi, MTS, Riccardi, R, Piccardi, M, Iarossi, G, Buzzonetti, L, Dickmann, A, Colosimo, C, Ruggiero, A, Di Rocco, C, Falsini, B. 2004. A fast visualevokedpotential method for functional assessment and follow-up of childhood optic gliomas, Clin Neurophysiol, Vol. 115, No. 1, Jan, pp. 217-226

Van Dongen, EP, Schepens, MA, Morshuis, WJ, Ter Beek, HT, Aarts, LP, De Boer, A, Boezeman, EH. 2001. Thoracic and thoracoabdominal aortic aneurysm repair: Use of evoked potential monitoring in 118 patients, J Vasc Surg, Vol. 34, No. 6, Dec, pp. 1035-1040.

Victor, JD, Mast, J. 1991. A new statistic for steady-state evoked potentials, Electroencephalogr Clin Neurophysiol, Vol. 78, No. 5, May, pp. 378-388.

Xu, S, Meyer, D, Yoser, S, Mathews, D, Elfervig, JL. 2001.Pattern visual evoked potential in the diagnosis of functional visual loss, *Ophthalmology*, Vol. 108, No. 1, Jan, pp. 76-80.

Zaeyen, EJB. 2005. Aplicação da Coerência ao eletroencefalograma para investigar características do Potencial Evocado Auditivo de Média Latência. M.Sc. Dissertation, COPPE/UFRJ, Rio de Janeiro, Rio de Janeiro, Brazil. (Available at: http://www.dominiopublico.gov.br/)

4

Extraction of 3D Geometrical Features of Biological Objects with 3D PCA Analysis and Applications of Results

Michal Rychlik and Witold Stankiewicz
Poznan University of Technology
Division of Machine Design Methods
Poland

1. Introduction

The Computer Aided Design (CAD) systems are very well known by designers in their every day practice and numerical analysis. Computer models of real objects with advanced numerical tools, significantly improves the quality and reduce time of design process. In addition to the three-dimensional modeling systems, there are many other tools and techniques (such as reverse engineering, rapid prototyping), which will further enhance the capabilities of engineers.

Many of those engineering technologies, especially CAD/CAM techniques, have an application not only in mechanical design. These tools also can be used in different disciplines, like biomechanics, bioengineering, biometrics, etc. This interdisciplinary area of knowledge takes advantage of Reverse Engineering, three-dimensional modeling and simulation, FEM[1] analysis and is equipped with Rapid Prototyping and CNC machines. The acquisition and processing of three-dimensional models with complicated shapes becomes the important issue in applications mentioned above. The 3D virtual models have numerous applications, simply such as visualization, but also more advanced like medical diagnostics (virtual endoscopes), pre-surgical planning (simulations of surgical operations), FEM and CFD[2] analysis, CNC machining, Rapid Prototyping, preparation and fabrication of implants, etc. Several engineering technologies and tools can be used for advanced analysis of biological objects.

The first step in computer analysis of biological/medical objects is to obtain the correct and high accurate 3D model. This 3D modeling generally is made by reconstruction procedure. 3D reconstruction can be done by usage of medical imagining systems (such as CT, NMR) or 3D scanning systems. Reconstruction of 3D model based on DICOM[3] images must be supported by image processing (segmentation of the region of interest) to extract 3D shape of the object. Dependent on the area of interest the bones, blood vessels or other soft tissues can be searched.

---

[1]FEM - finite element method

[2]CFD - computational fluid dynamics

[3]DICOM - Digital Imaging in Communications in Medicine

The main objective of this chapter is to present the possibility of a new use of "tools", known from engineering area, in the biomedical applications. One of the useful tools, known from technical applications (mainly in images and signal analysis) is Principal Component Analysis. This method is usually used for one or two dimensional "statistical" analysis, but three or more dimensions also can be analyzed. That multidimensional PCA analysis supported by other "high-tech" technologies (Reverse Engineering - 3D scanners, thermal camera, CT or NMR imagining), can generate very interesting results especially for 3D biomedical objects. In further sections the three applications (in anthropometrics, biometricsand for 3D geometry reconstruction procedure) of three-dimensional PCA analysis of biological objects will be presented and discussed.

2. Methods of modal analysis

In this chapter authors present modal analysis methods which can be used for geometry description of three dimensional objects. This methods are used for simplify and minimize the number of parameters which describe 3D objects.

The kinds of modal method (mathematical, physical or empirical) which are applied to analysis have a fundamental importance onto results. One of the method which based on modal decomposition is PCA (Principal Component Analysis, known also as POD - Proper Orthogonal Decomposition). If empirical modes (PCA) are optimal from viewpoint of information included inside of the each modes [Holmes, Lumley and Berkooz, 1998], also others decompositions based on mathematical (e.g. spherical harmonics) or physical modes (vibration modes) are also used.

The goal of using mathematical modes is conversion physical features onto mathematical features (synthetic form). In the event of the mathematical modes usually the features which describing geometry of 3D object is save as the vectors. Each vector is obtained through splitting of the 3D model on the several classes (different diameter spheres) and calculates common areas for 3D object and surface of individual spheres. All areas are described by set of vectors (spherical functions). For spherical functions Fourier transformation is used. After this operation the new unit is inserting. Goal of unit is made easier multidimensional description of features vectors. For representation of features vectors spherical harmonics are used (Fig. 1.).

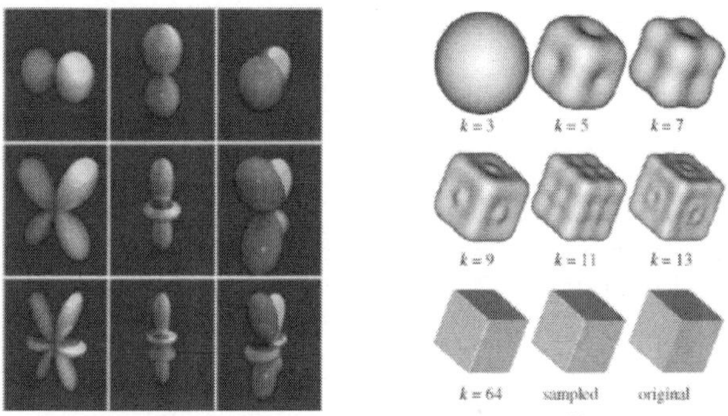

(a) (b)

Fig. 1. Example of spherical harmonics of 3D model of plane (a) and application spherical harmonic to reconstruction of geometry of the cube (b) [Vranic and Saupe, 2002]

Application of spherical modes is not "optimal" solution and sometimes cause of increasing complication of the computation because all objects are approximated by deformed sphere. Reconstruction of cube geometry can be done by very many numbers of spherical harmonics. This problem is analogous to Fourier decomposition of rectangular signal.

The second group of modal decomposition of 3D objects is present by physical modes (mechanical modes). This modes - known also as the vibration modes - are obtained by solution of equitation of own issue for resilience model of analyzing object. Vibration modal decomposition provides alternative parameterization of degree of freedom of the structure (only translation of the nodes in x, y, z directions) based on proper vibration of the objects and correlated frequencies. The most often are used low frequencies of the modes which described vectors of deformations for individual nodes of FEM grid. This way is possible the deformation of geometry of basic object and to fit it into searched object. Vibration modes compute for rigid body are responsible for translations and rotations of 3D model. Vibration modes compute for spring body describe different variation of the shape of basic model (Fig. 2.).

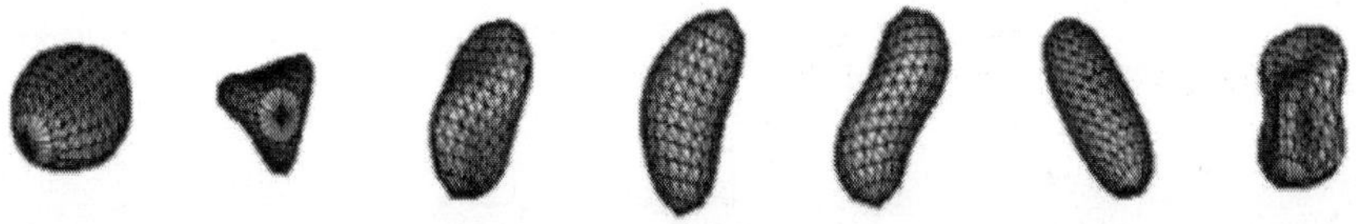

Fig. 2. Graphical representation of seven low frequencies vibration modes for surface model of ellipsoids [Syn and Prager, 1994]

PCA transformation gives orthogonal directions of principal variation of input data. Principal component which are connected with the largest eigenvalue[4], represent factor (direction) of the largest variation of data in data space. Variation is described by eigenvalue connected with the first principal component. The second principal component describes the next in order, orthogonal direction in the space with the next largest variation of data. Usually only few first principal components are responsible for a majority variations of the data. Data projected onto other principal components often have small amplitude and don't cross a amplitude of measurement noise. Therefore they can be deleted, without dangerous of decreasing of the accuracy.

3. Principal Component Analysis (empirical modes)

For reconstruction of the 3D geometry, "low-dimensional" decomposition based on Principal Component Analysis (PCA) can be used [Benameur S., Mignote M., Parent S., Labelle H., Skalli W., De Gusie J., 2001]. PCA provides a "relevant" set of basis functions, which allow identification of a low-dimensional subspace [Holmes, Lumley and Berkooz, 1996].

The used algorithm is based on statistical representation of the random variables.

---

[4]The prefix **eigen-** is adopted from the German word "eigen" for "own" in the sense of a characteristic description

The shape of the each object is represented in the data base as the set of 3D point clouds. Each point clouds is described by a vector (1):

$$S_i = \left[s_{i1}, s_{i2}, \ldots, s_{iN}\right]^T,\ i = 1,2,\ldots,M, \tag{1}$$

where $s_{ij} = (x,y,z)$ describes coordinates of the points in Cartesian system, M is the number of the objects which are in database, N is the number of the points in single point cloud. In the next step the mean shape $\overline{S}$ and covariance matrix C are computed (2):

$$\overline{S} = \frac{1}{M}\sum_{i=1}^{M} S_i,\ C = \frac{1}{M}\sum_{i=1}^{M} \tilde{S}_i \tilde{S}_i^T, \tag{2}$$

The difference between mean and object that is in data base are describe by the deformation vector $\tilde{S}_i = S_i - \overline{S}$. The statistical analysis of the deformation vectors gives us the information about the empirical modes. Modes represent the geometrical features (shape) but also can carry other information like texture, map of temperature and others. Only few first modes contains most information, therefore each original object S_i is reconstructed by using some K principal components (3):

$$S_i = \overline{S} + \sum_{k=1}^{K} a_{ki}\Psi_k,\ i = 1,2,\ldots,M, \tag{3}$$

where Ψ_k is an eigenvector representing the orthogonal mode (the feature computed from data base), a_{ki} is coefficient of eigenvector.

Energy (equivalent of quantity of information) transmitted by eigenvector m is appointed on following equation:

$$E = \frac{\Psi_m}{\sum_{k=1}^{M} \Psi_k}, \tag{4}$$

The example of the low dimensional reconstruction for three different values of the coefficients is presented on the Figure 3. Every manipulations of coefficients value of the modes, changing geometry of the objects.

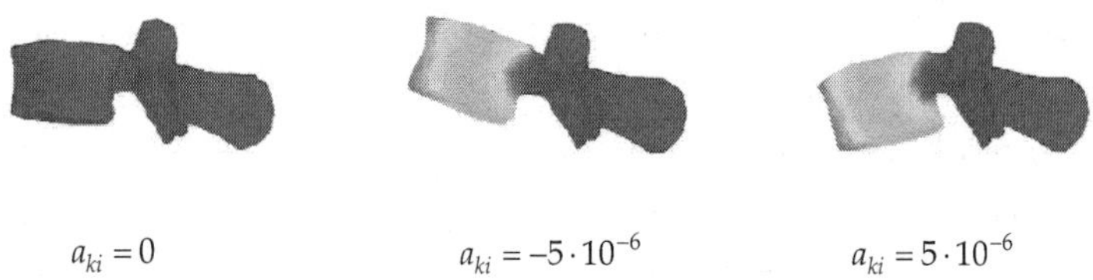

Fig. 3. The visualization ofthe low dimensional reconstruction for L4 vertebra: average value (left side) and two different deformation which are compute for different values of the coefficients (middle and right side).

4. Applications of Principal Component Analysis of 3D biological objects

Several engineering technologies can be used for advanced analysis of biological objects. In further chapters the three applications, anthropometric (femur bones), biometric (human faces), geometry reconstruction (lumbar vertebra) of three-dimensional models will be presented and discussed. For biometric database the thermal (infrared) images was tested as support information.

4.1 Biometric application of 3D PCA

The security and access systems are very important and rapidly advancing, not only in computer vision. Such systems are used obviously during passenger control on the airport or boundary crossing [Schneider W., 2007]. Biometrics identify people by measuring some aspects of individual anatomy or physiology - such as hand geometry or fingerprint, some deeply ingrained skill, or other behavioral characteristic - handwritten signature, or something that is a combination of the two - voice [Anderson, R. J., 2008]. In generally the biometrics can be sorted into two types [Mainguet J-F. , 2004]:

a. physical - face, fingerprint, hand/finger, iris, ear, retinal, DNA, vein, blood pulse, dental, lips, nail;
b. behavioral - voice, gait, tapping, signature, keystroke dynamics, mouse dynamics.

The face recognition method is the oldest and the most "natural" method of identification person's. Recognizing people by their facial features is going back at least to our early primate ancestors.

The disadvantage of the most commonly used recognition techniques is their insufficient reliability. A 2D dimensional photo cannot be measured like a landscape and simply doesn't contain the same amount of information as the 3D "photo" [Xiaoguang Lu, 2006]. This problem is especially essential for twins, when the similarity of face shape is very high [Anil K. J., at al., 2002].

Facial identification reads the peaks and valleys of facial features. These peaks and valleys are known as nodal points (80 nodal points exist in a human face, but usually only 15-20 are used for identification - known as „Golden triangle" region between the temples and the lips.

4.1.1 Materials – Acquisition of input data

For obtain the 3D input data the 3D scanning system (the structural light scanner) was used. The two groups of biological models were measured: set of human faces and set of femur bones. Each input object was scanned and 3D surface model was computed.

To increase the accuracy of PCA analysis, each face was described (Fig. 4.) by individual points cloud (40k points) instead of few markers from "Golden triangle" area.

Database for biometric PCA analysis is prepared onto the multiple human faces. There are 39 faces (Fig. 5.) with neutral expression of different persons. To improve sensitivity of presented method, three sets (6 faces) of the twin's faces in the database were included. There are two sets of identical - monozygotic twins and one set of fraternal - dizygotic twins.

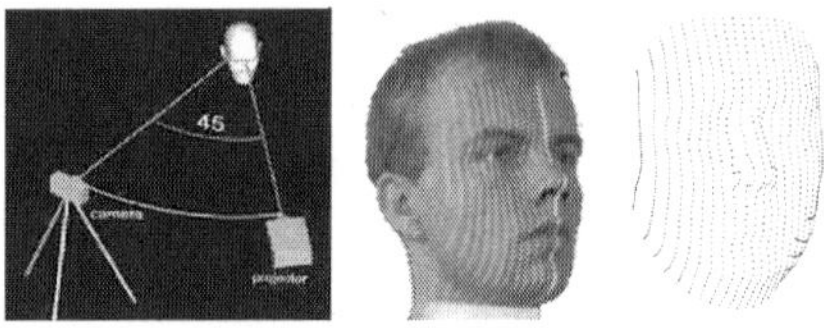

Fig. 4. Data acquisition process (from left): hardware configuration, captured image, input data set (points cloud).

Second part of input data for biometric database is set of two-dimensional infrared images (thermal images). In this research the thermal images of 17 different persons were collected (Fig. 5.). For acquisition of infrared images the thermal camera was used. All pictures were collected in the same conditions of the measurement: room ($+22^{0}$C) and camera settings: matrix VOx 320x240 pixels, thermal resolution +/0.03^{0}C, range of measured temperature: 26-40^{0}C.

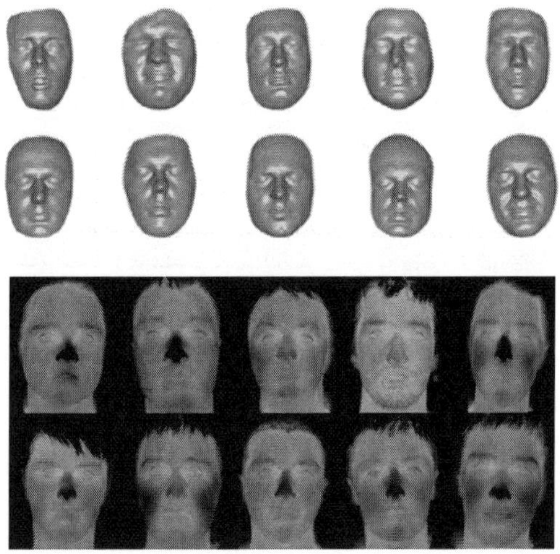

Fig. 5. An example of the models in database (from the left): 3D faces, 2D thermal images.

4.1.2 Data registration

The Principal Component Analysis requires the same position, orientation and topology of the data input (the same number of nodes, matrix connection, etc.) for all objects. To achieve this, each new object added to database must be registered.

For face the origin point (0, 0, 0) of coordinate system is arranged in cross section of two lines: vertical middle line on the face, horizontal - eyes line. The registration is made in two steps. First step (preliminary registration) is the rigid registration. It consists of simple, affine geometrical transformation of object in three-dimensional space (rotation and transformation). For control of this process three points are used: two points in the centers of the eyes, one on the top of the nose (Fig.6.).

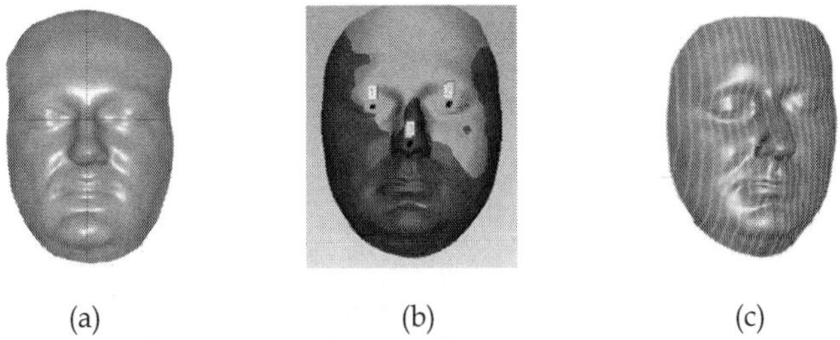

Fig. 6. Data registration: a) origin point, b) three point of rigid registration, c) 3D curves network.

The second step is connected with curves extraction. Independently from face size, always 201 curves on face are only. To achieve this, scaling of space between curves is used. For infrared images only the first step of registration was done.

4.1.3 Results of 3D PCA analysis – Face print

For prepared database of human faces (39 faces of young persons) the PCA analysis was performed. The result of this operation is the mean object, thirty nine modes (Fig. 7) and coefficients (Tab. 1.).

The first thirty eight modes include one hundred percent of information about decomposed geometry. Mode thirty nine contains only a numerical noise. For further reconstruction of face geometry only first twenty five modes are used.

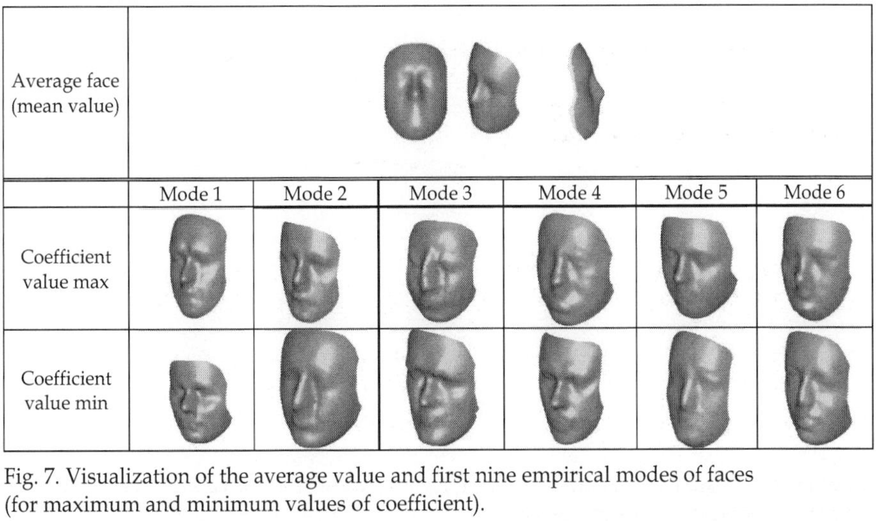

Fig. 7. Visualization of the average value and first nine empirical modes of faces (for maximum and minimum values of coefficient).

Number of the mode	Participation of the mode [%]	Total participation of the modes [%]
1	57,2010066	57,2010066
2	13,4976482	70,6986548
3	5,9128812	76,6115360
4	4,3703630	80,9818990
5	4,0161309	84,9980299
6	3,1945602	88,1925901
7	2,6277538	90,8203439
8	1,3584618	92,1788057
9	1,2914768	93,4702825
10	0,9734244	94,4437069
11	0,8401794	95,2838863
12	0,6097119	95,8935982
13	0,4819451	96,3755433
14	0,4433567	96,8189000
15	0,3511382	97,1700382
16	0,3001483	97,4701865
17	0,2681638	97,7383503
18	0,2577919	97,9961422
19	0,2179374	98,2140797
20	0,1973631	98,4114428
21	0,1767063	98,5881491
22	0,1608646	98,7490137
23	0,1512224	98,9002361
24	0,1311154	99,0313516
25	0,1250506	99,1564022

Table 1. Participation of the modes in faces geometry reconstruction.

Modes describe the features of the faces. Two first modes characterize global transformation: first mode changing of the face size in vertical direction, second mode changing the size in horizontal direction. Further modes describe more complex, local deformations. For example third mode is responsible for changes in nose and eyes areas. Results of the statistical analysis (empirical modes) can be used for reconstruction of geometry (in CAD systems) of individual features of the object. Those 3D models of faces can be used in many applications: 3D visualizations, Rapid Prototyping technologies, surgical planning, archivisation and many others.

Each face in database has unique set of coefficient values "faceprint" (Fig. 8.) - individual ID code like fingerprints. As the authorization key the set of coefficient values for the faces can be used. Each key describes individual shape of face and can be decoded and compared with the original data of user to obtain access to restricted area or data files.

Faces of different people

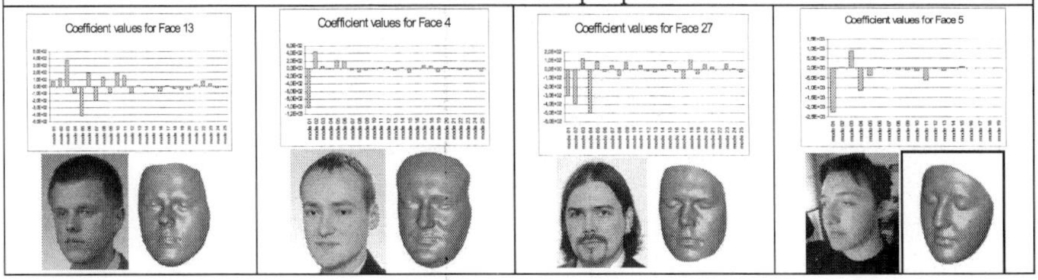

Fig. 8. Faceprints (ID codes) for few faces from database (for each object is presented - graph of coefficient values, original photo and 3D face model).

4.1.4 Results of 2D PCA analysis – Thermal images

As a support for three-dimensional face recognition, additional information - the thermal images - can be used [Akhloufi, M, Bendada A., 2008, Prokoski. F., 2000]. The two-dimensional infrared images can be added to database as a "fourth" dimension. For prepared infrared images of human faces the 2D PCA analysis was done. The result of this operation is the mean face (Fig. 9.), seventeen modes and set of coefficients.

Mean face	Mode 1	Mode 2	Mode 3	Mode 4

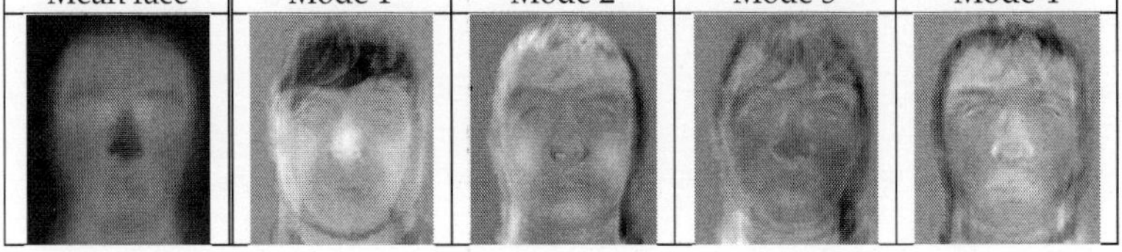

Fig. 9. Visualization of the mean face and first four empirical modes of infrared images.

For presented analysis the sixteen modes include one hundred percent of information about decomposed thermal images (Table 2.). Seventeenth mode contains only a numerical noise.

Number of the mode	Participation of the mode [%]	Total participation of the modes [%]
1	26.4191478	26.4191478
2	16.7302890	43.1494367
3	10.9104597	54.0598965
4	8.3397586	62.3996550
5	6.5525733	68.9522283
6	5.6298384	74.5820668
7	4.4142731	78.9963398
8	3.6441677	82.6405075
9	3.3063140	85.9468215
10	2.7908036	88.7376251

Table 2. Participation of the first 10 modes PCA decomposition of thermal images.

Similarly to 3D data, each infrared image of the face in database has unique set of coefficient values - "thermal faceprints" (Fig. 10.). This additional information can be associated with 3D data to increase the level of security and can complicate the trials of fake the system.

Thermal faceprint of few faces of different person

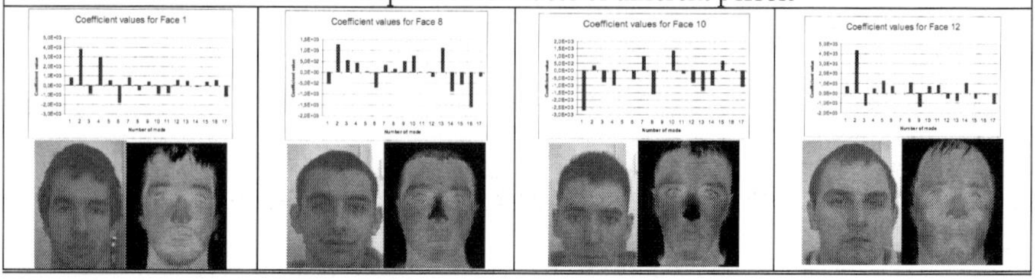

Fig. 10. Thermal faceprint for few faces from infrared database (for each object is presented - graph of coefficient values, original photo and thermal image).

4.1.5 Analysis of similarity and differences of twin's faces

For testing of sensitivity level of presented faceprint method the twin's faces was used. For numerical experiment the database with 19 faces (which include three couples of twins - two couples of monozygotic twins and one couple of dizygotic twins) was prepared.

For better comparison and computation of similarity of twin's faces the additional analysis was done. PCA analysis give information about common shape and differences between each face of twins couple. Results of this analysis (surface map of differences are presented) is presented for one monozigotic and one dizygotic twins (Fig. 11., Fig. 12.).

Faces of monozygotic twins

Common shape	Differences Max	Differences Min	Surface map of differences

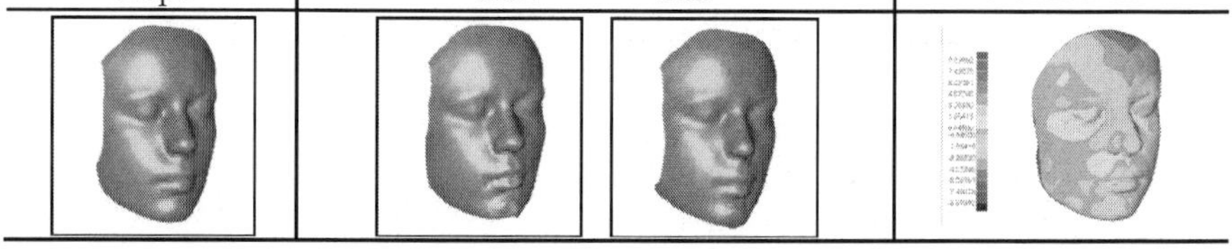

Fig. 11. Visualizations of the common shape (average face) and differences (empirical mode and surface map of difference) for monozygotic twins (gender: female).

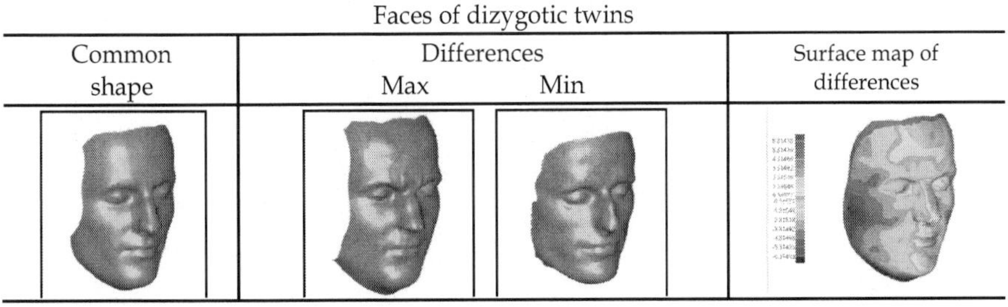

Fig. 12. Visualizations of the common shape (mean face) and differences (empirical mode and surface map of difference) for dizygotic twins (gender: male).

For comparison of similarity of twins faces the value of surface deviation was done. For faces of monozygotic couple the value of standard deviation was 1,19mm and average distance 0,29mm. For faces of dizygotic twins standard deviation is near 1,79mm and average distance 0,83. Each twin's face in database has unique set of coefficient values - "ID code" (Fig. 13.).

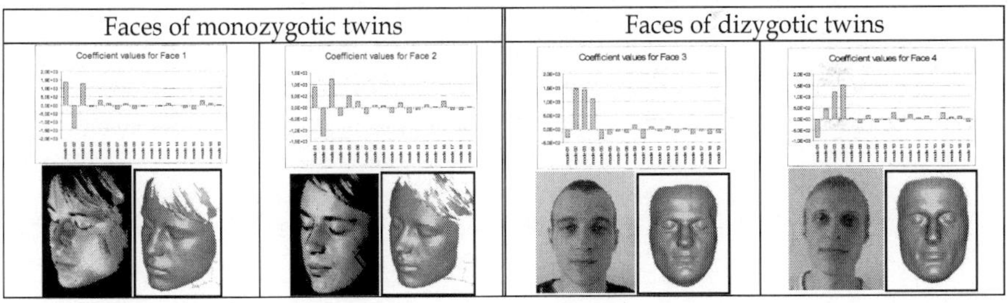

Fig. 13. Face ID code for faces of two types of twins (from upper left): face code - coefficient values, original photo, 3D face mode.

Also for identical (for human eye view) monozygotic twins this "face-code" is incomparable for each one face similar like for fingerprints (Anil K., 2002).

Trend curves (Fig. 14) of coefficients values showing how faces of twins are similar between each other. In general shape, curves (trends) are the same but in local values they have small differences. By this way the description ofsimilarity level between faces of the same couple of twins. As much faces are different from each other, than curves are automatically more far from each other.

When we try comparing two trends curves from different couple of twins, we can observe very big difference. Each face have own unique trend curve even for twins.

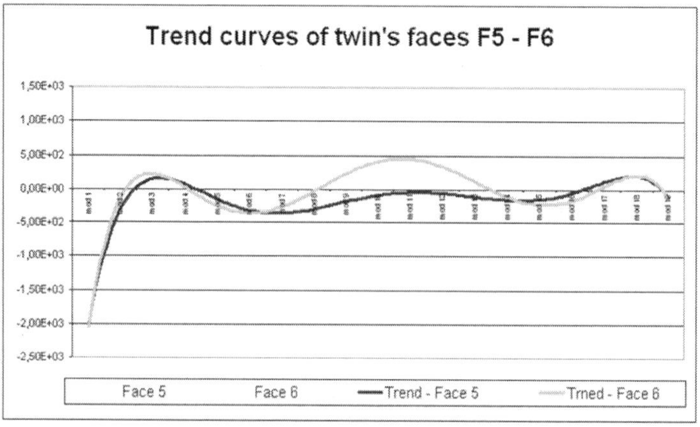

(a)

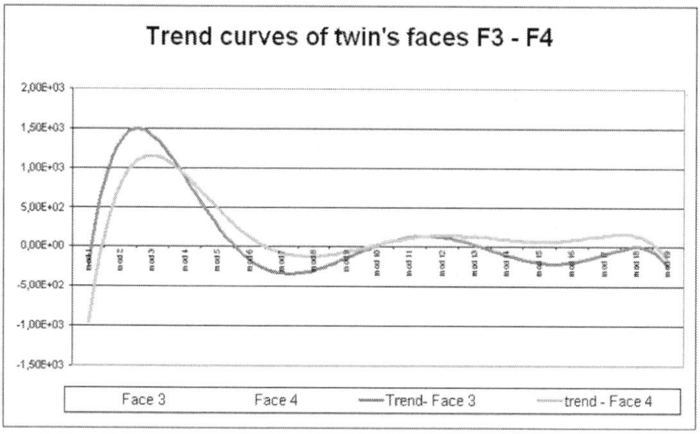

(b)

Fig. 14. Comparison of trend curves of coefficient values of modes: a) monozygotic twins, b) dizygotic twins.

4.1.6 Results of 3D PCA analysis – Hand shape biometrics

For identity of persons as a input data the many different information can be used. One of them is the hand shape. Hand geometry verification systems use geometric measurements of hand as the features for the verification of individuals. Usually they measure and analyze the overall structure, 2D shape (silhouette) and proportions of the hand e.g. length, width and thickness of hand, fingers and joints [Sanchez-Reillo R. at al., 2000]. Hand geometry biometrics systems measure up to 90 parameters (Fig. 15). Hand biometrics systems have some limitations, especially for people with severe arthristis who cannot spread their hands on the special hand reader.

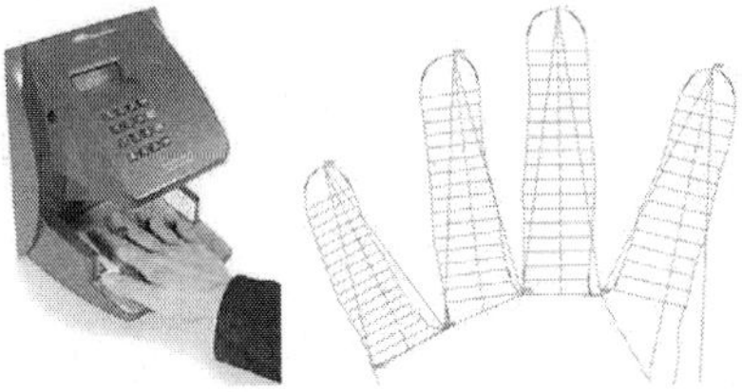

Fig. 15. Hand biometrics (from left): 2D biometric hand reader, segmentation of length and weight of the hand fingers features [Sanchez-Reillo R. at al., 2000].

Basis on faceprint methodology (described in chapter 4.1.3.) the 3D hand biometric identification system was prepared and tested.

The data input for numerical experiment was obtained by using the 3D optical scanner analogues to obtain the geometry of the bones. Measurements of hand geometry are easy to collect but for obtain full 3D information the special platform with mirrors was created. The system of mirrors and settings for localization of fingers (Fig. 16.) are comparable like used in regular 2D silhouette scanners [Jain A.K., at al., 1999].

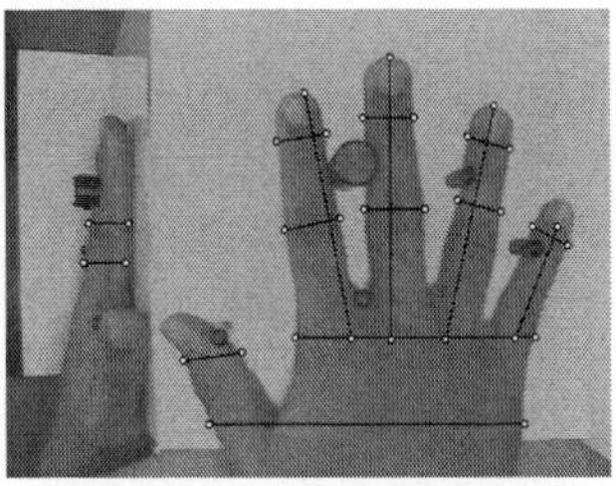

Fig. 16. Hand positioning system with mirror [Jain A.K., at al., 1999]

For test the database contains of 10 different 3D models of human hand (Fig. 17.). For each hand the registration procedure was done. As final result the set of polygon meshes (6,5k triangles) describing hands was obtained and used in further 3D PCA analysis.

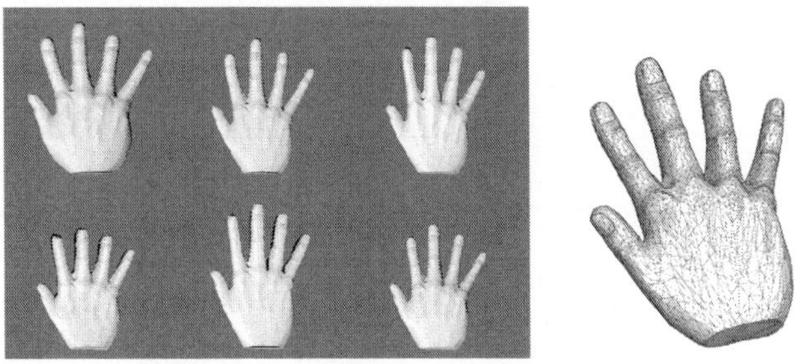

Fig. 17. Input data for 3D hand PCA analysis: five 3D models of different hands, example of mesh grid.

For this analysis the nine modes include one hundred percent of information about hand geometry (Table 3.). The last, tenth mode, contain only a numerical noise.

Number of the mode	Participation of the mode [%]	Total participation of the modes [%]
1	94.2193186	94.2193186
2	1.9215473	96.1408659
3	1.4766160	97.6174819
4	0.8838991	98.5013809
5	0.8546490	99.3560300
6	0.3615261	99.7175561
7	0.1225032	99.8400593
8	0.0912159	99.9312752
9	0.0687248	100.0000000
10	0.0000000	100.0000000

Table 3. Participation of the first 10 modes PCA decomposition of handgeometry.

Comparable like it was for 3D faces, the same situation is for hands. Individual modes characterize principal features of hand: size of hand, length of fingers, thickness of fingers and shape of hand regions (Fig. 18).

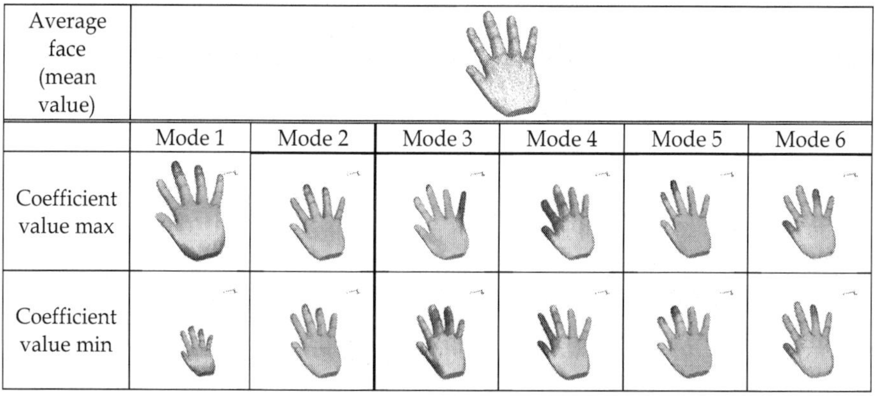

Fig. 18. Visualization of the average value and first nine empirical modes of faces (for maximum and minimum values of coefficient).

Each hand in database has unique set of coefficient values "handprint" (Fig. 19.) - individual ID code like fingerprints just based on full 3D hand geometry. As the authorization key the set of coefficient values for the hands can be used. Each key describes individual 3D geometry of hand and can be decoded and compared with the original data of user to obtain access to restricted area or data files.

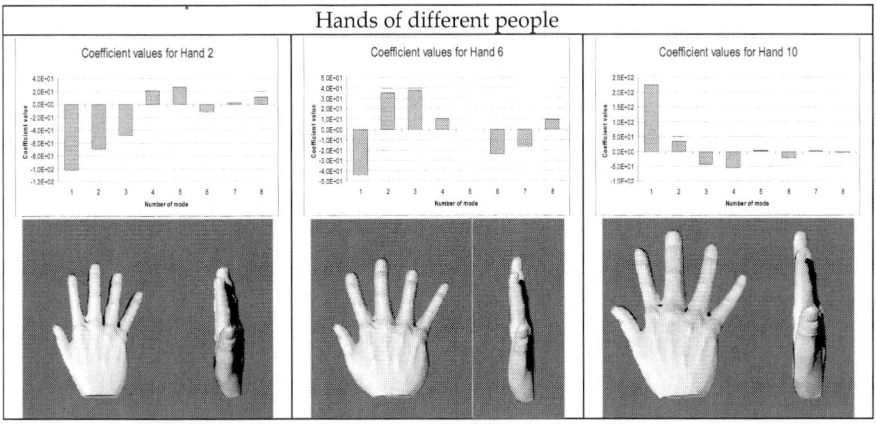

Fig. 19. Handprints (ID codes) for few hands from database (for each object is presented - graph of coefficient values, two views of 3D hand model).

4.2 Anthropometric application of 3D PCA

Anthropometry is the science of measuring the human body (e.g. height, weight) and size of component parts, including skinfold thickness, to study and compare the relative proportions. Measurements can be done under normal and abnormal conditions. The results of measurements done for group or population of people are organised in special databases. The basic problem which exists in most of databases is not enough information. Most of them are old and not includes all interesting dimensions. Traditional anthropometric database contains information only about some characteristic points (other parameters are not described). The set of the bones are described only in two dimensional space [Jantz, R.L. and P.H. Moore-Jansen, 1988], by the collection of linear and angular dimensions (Fig.20.).

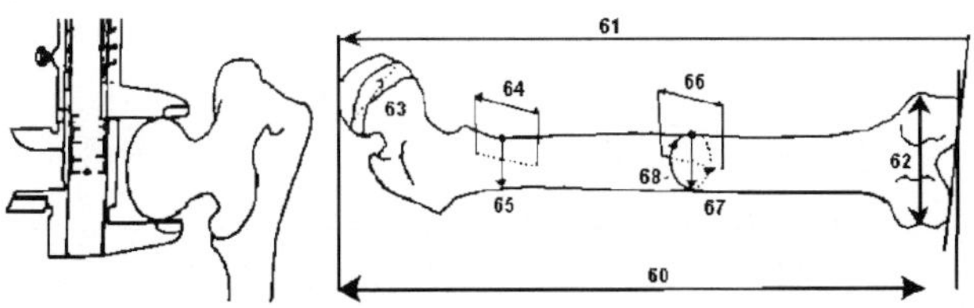

Fig. 20. Example of measurement process and view on a few characteristic points for femur bone [Moore-Jansen at al., 1994]

Three dimensional knowledge about mean geometry of the bones are not exist. Usually data acquisition process is prepared with usage of the conventional osteological instruments (measurements equipment like: caliper, spreading calliper, or osteometric board - Fig.21.).

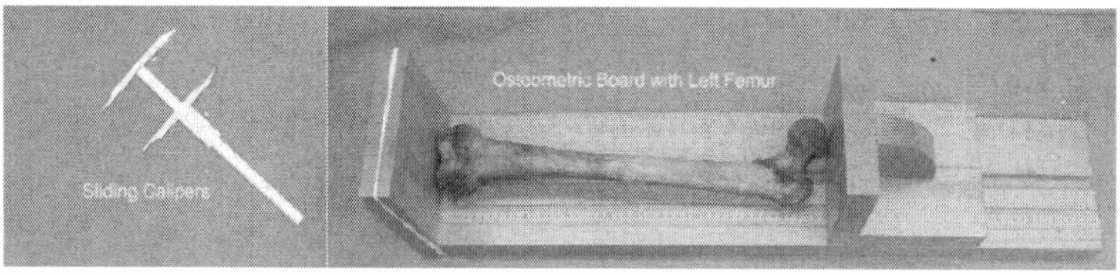

Fig. 21. Osteological instruments usually used for measuring the femur bone [Vitek C., 2005]

The solution of presented problem is proposition to use the Reverse Engineering techniques for measurement process (to achieve precision 3D data) and modal analysis (PCA) to compute the 3D anthropometric database. These aspects are presented further in details.

4.2.1 Acquisition of input data

For creation of database, the set of real bones was used. In this work was used the 15 femur bones (Fig. 22) - 6 female, 9 male - which are obtained from Poznan University of Medical Science.

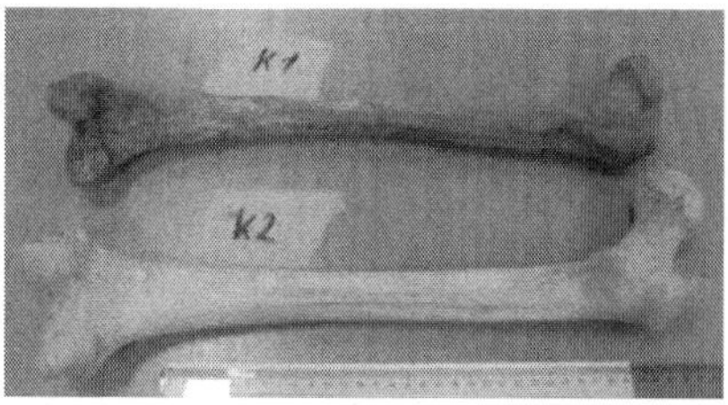

Fig. 22. View of two different female femur bones.

For acquisition of data the 3D structural light scanner was used (Fig. 23.). To acquire full 3D geometry, each bone was measured from 15 different directions with accuracy 0,05mm. Effect of measure process, is set of 3D points clouds (Fig. 23). All points clouds must be registered (orientation and connection between clouds).

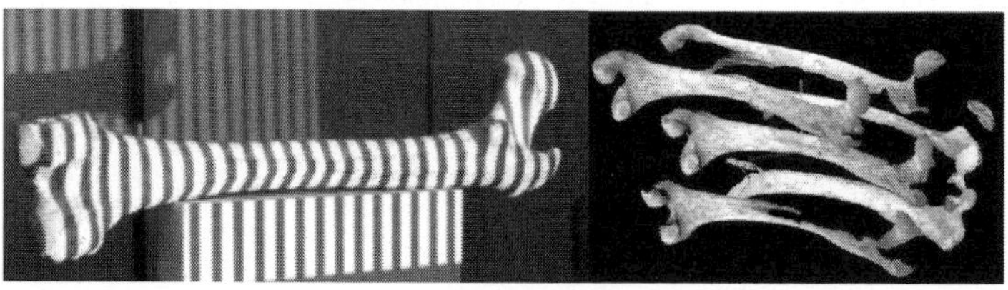

Fig. 23. Data acquisition process on 3D structural light scanner and set of points clouds.

The result of registration is one points cloud which consist about 1,5 mln points (Fig. 24). As the final step is generated 3D triangle surface grid.

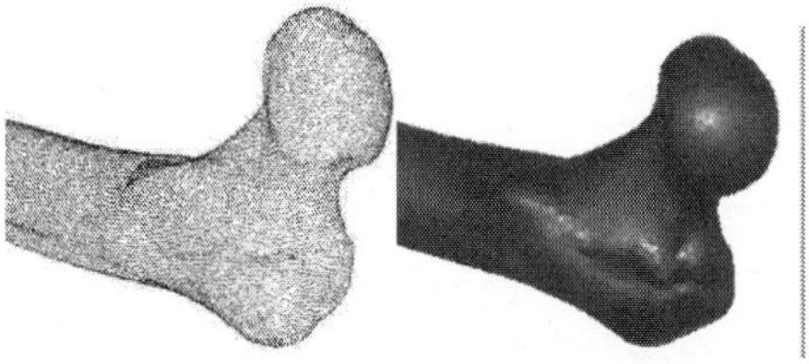

Fig. 24. Complete points cloud (1,5 mln points) and final triangle surface grid.

4.2.2 Data registration

The registration procedure forbones was made also in two steps. First step (preliminary registration) is simply rigid registration. The second step is the viscous fluid registration. For this registration the modified Navier-Stokes equation in penalty function formulation (existing numerical code [Morzynski M., at al., 1999]; source segment [Bro-Nielsen, M., Gramkow, C., 1996]) is used (5):

$$\underbrace{\dot{V}_i + V_{i,j}V_j - \frac{1}{\mathrm{Re}}V_{i,jj} + \frac{\varepsilon - \lambda}{\rho}V_{j,ji}}_{existing\ numerical\ code} + \underbrace{(f-g)f_{,i}}_{source\ segment} = 0 \qquad (5)$$

where ρ - is fluid density, V_i - velocity component, Re - Reynolds number, λ - bulk viscosity. In this application, parameters ε and λ are used to control the fluid compressibility, f is the base object and g is the target object (input model). The object is described by the grid nodes (FEM grid). The displacements of the nodes are computed from integration of the velocity field.

Every based and new model is represented by several cross-sections with the same transfer area (Fig. 25.). The transfer area is needed for topology conservation.

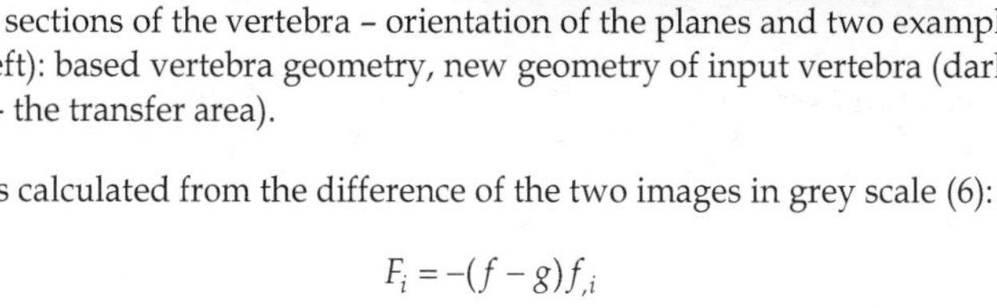

Fig. 25. Cross sections of the vertebra - orientation of the planes and two examples of 2D slices (from left): based vertebra geometry, new geometry of input vertebra (dark colour around bone- the transfer area).

Source term is calculated from the difference of the two images in grey scale (6):

$$F_i = -(f-g)f_{,i} \qquad (6)$$

where f and g are areas in grayscale f - base image (base vertebra), g - target image (input vertebra). The parameters of the flow are the same as for the compressible fluid with very viscosity.

Computed flow field provides information about translations of the nodes in both sections. After computation we obtain dislocation of nodes of the base grid onto new geometry (Fig. 26.).

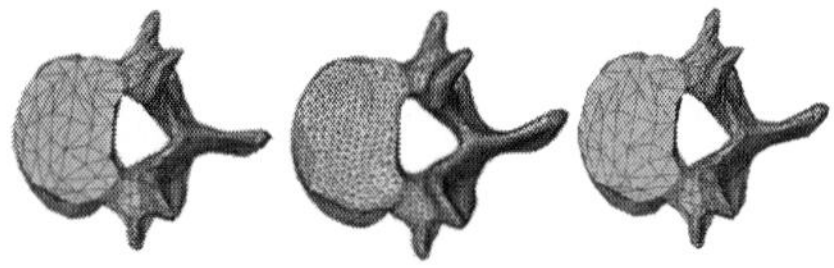

Fig. 26. Grid deformation (from the left): base object (base grid), new object inserted to database, base grid on geometry of the new objects.

4.2.3 Results of 3D PCA analysis – Femur bones

The database used in analysis contains 15 femur bones. Each bone has different geometry and is described by triangle surface grid (Fig. 27) with the same structure (14 thousands nodes, 30 thousands elements).

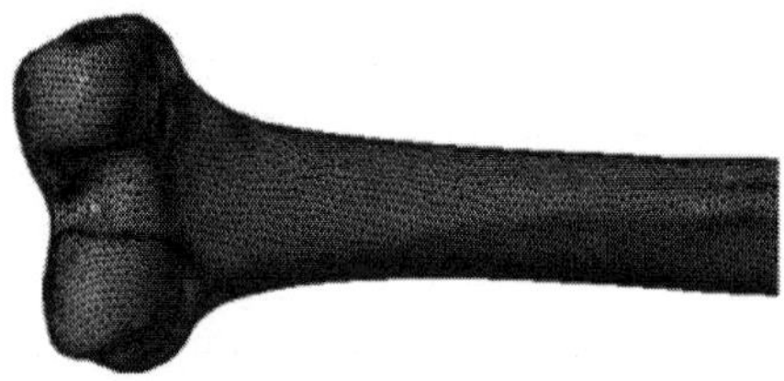

Fig. 27. Triangle surface grid of femur bone.

For this database the Principal Component Analysis was done. The result of this operation is the mean object, fifteen modes and coefficients.

The first fourteen modes include 100% of information about decomposed geometry (Table 4). Mode fifteen contain only a numerical noise and they are not used for further calculations.

Modes describing the features of the femur bones (Fig. 28). The first mode describes transformation of the length of the femur bone. Second mode represent position conversion of the head of the bone, third describe change the arc of the shaft (body). Next modes describing more complex deformations, e.g. fourth mod describe change the position of the greater trochanter and lesser trochanter, also thickness of the shaft (body).

In this experiment the value of average error for reconstructed geometry of the bone was equal 0,3mm (reconstruction done with using of 14 modes).

Study of the value of the coefficients, give us additional information about the analyzed bones. For presented database we can found, correlation between coefficient value of first mode and gender. Negative coefficient value "-" of first mode is connected with female bones (one exception bone nr 8), when positive coefficient value "+" describe male bones (Fig. 29.).

Number of the mode	Participation of the mode [%]	Total participation of the modes [%]
1	74.9212416	74.9212416
2	10.5438352	85.4650767
3	4.2699519	89.7350286
4	3.3128685	93.0478971
5	1.6659793	94.7138765
6	1.4234329	96.1373093
7	1.0359034	97.1732127
8	0.6781645	97.8513772
9	0.5866122	98.4379894
10	0.4796167	98.9176061
11	0.3301463	99.2477523
12	0.3080968	99.5558492
13	0.2516839	99.8075330
14	0.1924670	100.0000000
15	0.0000000	100.0000000

Table 4. Participation of the modes in decomposition.

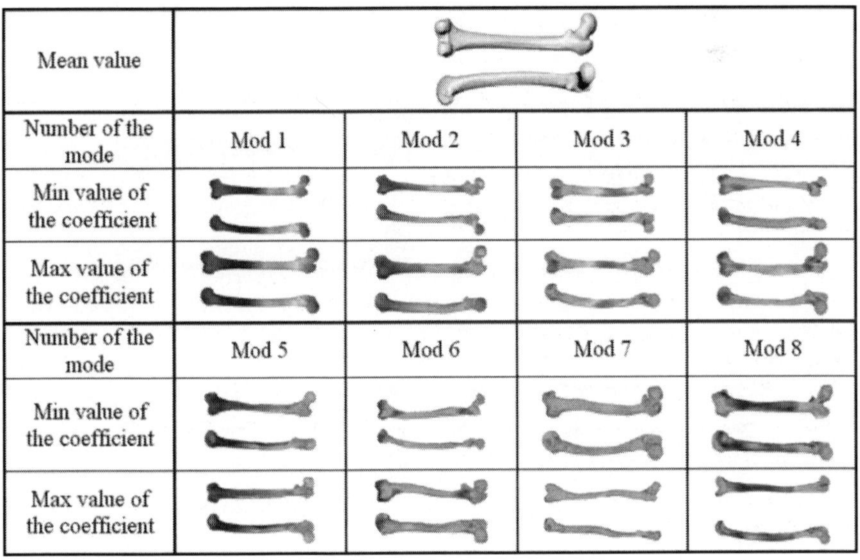

Fig. 28. 3D visualization of mean value and first eight modes of femur bones (for each bone the anterior and posterior view is shown).

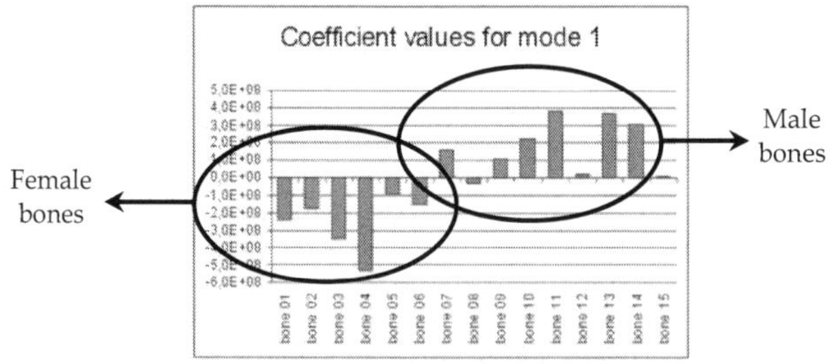

Fig. 29. Correlation between coefficient value of first mode and gender: the negative value "-" is correlated to female bone, positive value "+" is associated with male bones.

Other interesting feature of coefficients is individual set of coefficients values for each bone. This aspect is similar to "fingers prints". Because each bone have another geometry also they have individual set of coefficient values. On Figure 30 is presented graphs of coefficient values and visualization of the geometry for three different bones.

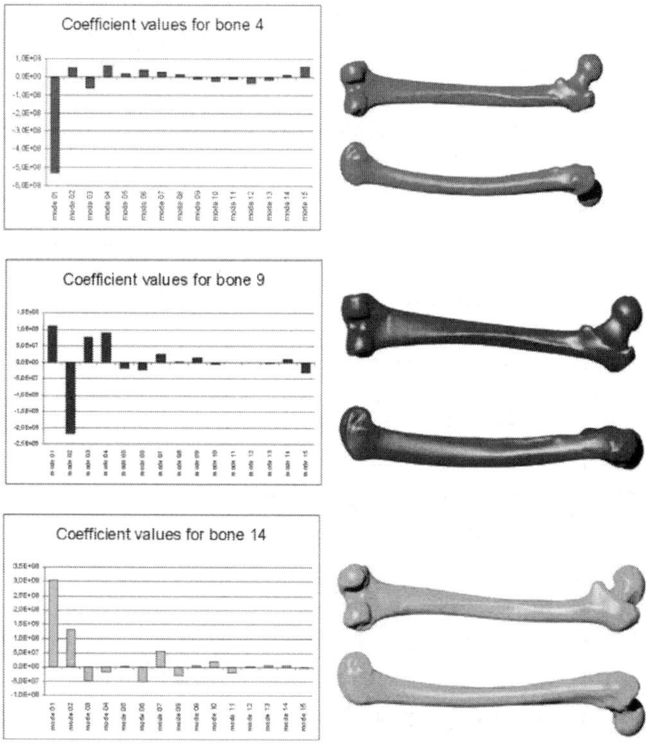

Fig. 30. Correlation between coefficient value and geometry of the bone for three different femur bones (all pictures of bones are made in the same scale).

4.3 Reconstruction method of 3D geometry of the bones basis on RTG images and empirical modes database

Another advantage of property of real 3D anthropometric database is possibility of using this information as the "knowledge base". Knowledge base is necessary for the reconstruction of 3D geometry, basing on few RTG images (e.g. two or three ,depends from complication of the object shape). Method developed by authors [Rychlik M., 2004, Rychlik M. at al., 2005] can be used instead of CT images processing. The result of the reconstruction is 3D virtual model which can be used for develop individual prosthesis. The high accuracy (comparison with CT and contact 3D scanners) and low costs, making this method more common.

4.3.1 Alghorithm of the reconstruction method

The Algorithm of the method is following (Fig. 31.). Searched three-dimensional object are represented by the set of RTG images (minimum two images from different directions). These RTG images are compared with DRR - Digitally Reconstructed Radiographs [Milickovic N. at al. 2000, Russacof D. B. 2003] from database.

Data base includes DRR images and set of the modes and coefficients. Modes and coefficients are received from Principal Component Analysis. After comparison of images, the most similar objects from database are selected. In the next step we manipulate the coefficients of modes as long as the minimization of the mean square deviation of the images RTG and DRR is accomplished. Finally we receive reconstructed 3D model in CAD system.

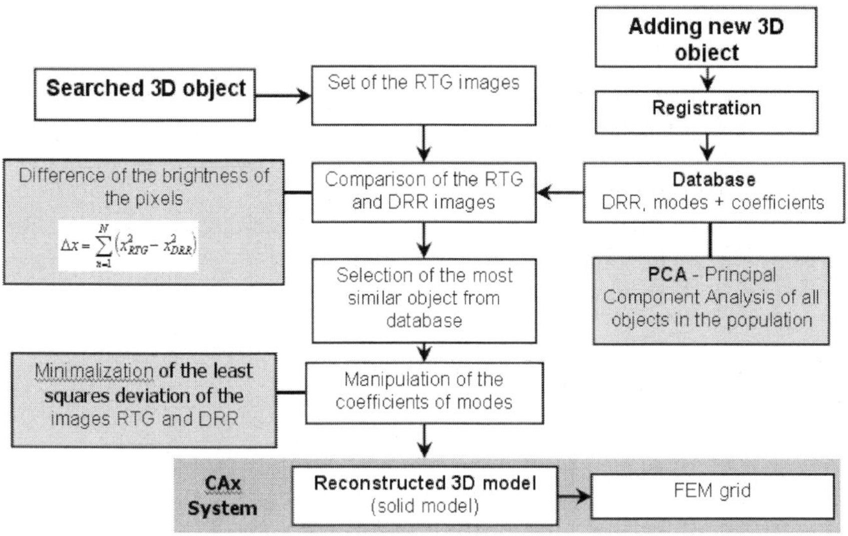

Fig. 31. Algorithm of the reconstruction method.

4.3.2 Input data – Artifical database

The database used in experiment contains 99 lumbar vertebra's (Fig. 32.). Each vertebra has different geometry, and is described by FEM grid with the same structure (616 nodes, 2000 elements).

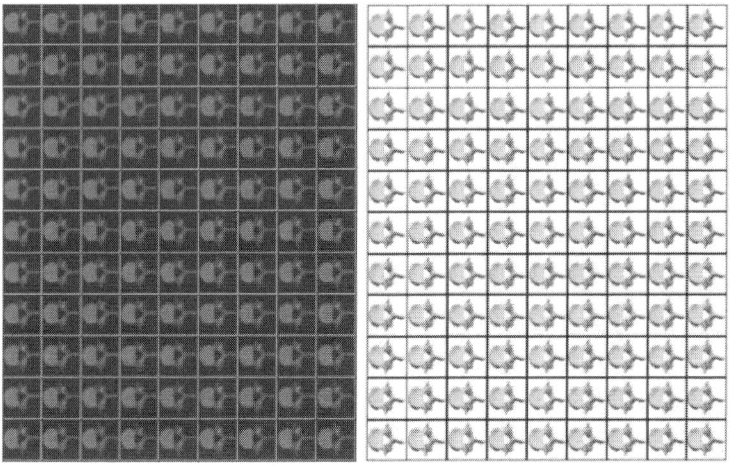

Fig. 32. Data base: DDR images (left side), 3D CAD models (right side).

4.3.3 Results of 3D PCA analysis – Vertebra bones

For this database the Principal Component Analysis was done. The result of this operation is the mean object, 11 modes and coefficients.

The first five modes include 96% of information about reconstructed geometry (Table 5.). Modes: twelfth and others contain very low information (this is only a numerical noise) and they aren't used for further reconstruction.

Modes describe the features of the vertebras (Fig. 33.). The first and fourth mode describe the deformation of the vertebral body, the second, third and seventh mode represent the deformation of the spinosus process. Other modes describe the deformation of the transverse process.

To verify this method the new vertebra has been made. It is deformed by three features (spinous process, vertebral body, transverse process) but has completely new values (there is no similar shape in data base).

In the next step we compare the DRR images of the searched and created vertebra and manipulate of the coefficients of modes. To compute the values of coefficients for all modes Jacobi criterion was used.

The final result of this experiment is the solid CAD model (Fig. 34.) and FEM grid.

Number of the mode	Participation of the mode [%]	Total participation of the modes [%]
1	60,7418270	60,7418270
2	18,7637347	79,5055617
3	8,0275130	87,5330747
4	7,5452177	95,0782924
5	1,1870943	96,2653867
6	0,9569025	97,2222892
7	0,6885226	97,9108118
8	0,5571059	98,4679177
9	0,5541704	99,0220881
10	0,5054029	99,5274910
11	0,4725086	99,9999996
12	0,0000002	99,9999998
13	0,0000001	99,9999999

Table 5. Participation of the modes in reconstruction.

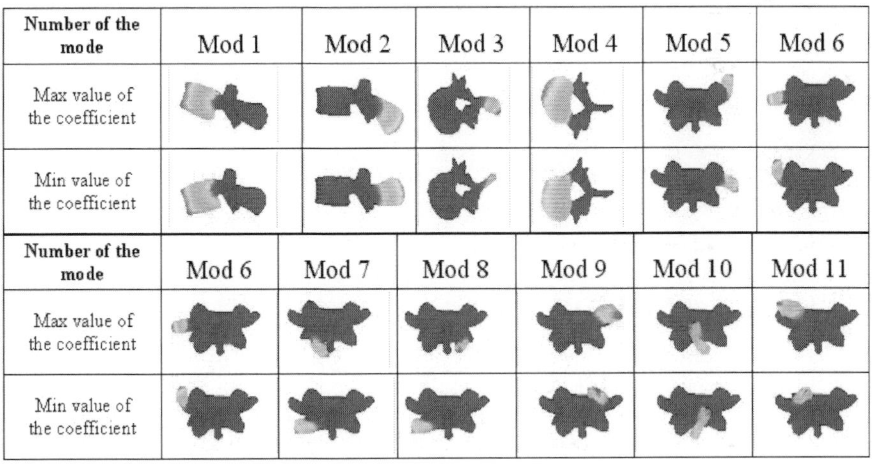

Fig. 33. Three dimensional visualization of 11 modes.

To verify the quality of the reconstruction, the anthropometric measurements [Berry J. L., 1987] of the reconstructed vertebra was done. Average inaccuracy of the reconstruction is about 0,25 mm (~1%). Volume differences between searched and reconstructed vertebra is about 0,11% and surface difference is 0,95%.

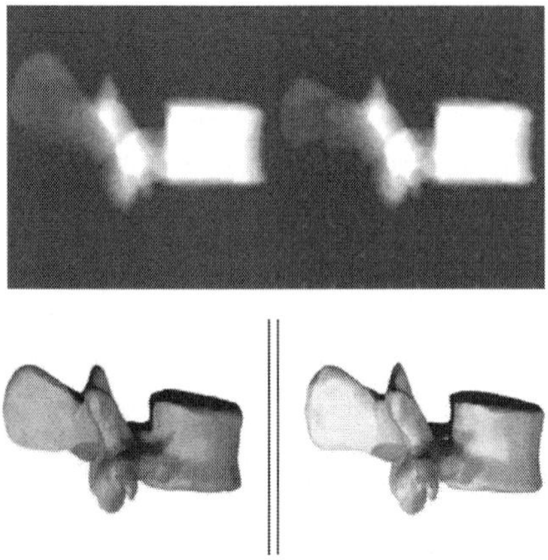

Fig. 34. Correlated images (from left): RTG image of searched object, DRR image of created (deformed) model, image of CAD solid model searched vertebra (left side) & reconstructed vertebra (right side).

5. Conclusions

Many modern methods and techniques known from classic mechanics and engineering solutions, they are applicable in many other disciplines of knowledge. One of such new "beneficent" is biological branch of knowledge. In presented research authors concentrate attention on present several applications of three-dimensional version of Principal Component Analysis in biological cases. However to describe geometry of 3D objects the numerous modal methods can be used; only empirical modes gives an optimal statistical database. Empirical modes, represent features of the objects composed in database. Characters of features are dependent from frequent occurrence in population.

The first presented application of 3D PCA is biometrics. Many security systems need ID key, which will be fast and guarantees high level of protection. The 3D PCA make possible using 3D faces as the access code (Faceprint). Each face has individual set of coefficient values - unique face code. That information (code) can be easily recorded onto electronic ID card - similar to 2D biometric data's. Presented method as the source of data-input, apply cheap non-contact measurement method and full 3D face information - instead of "control" points set (few nodal points in "golden triangle" area). The 3D geometry of the face (3D faceprint) is more complicated than "flat" image and by this way more proof onto fake, than 2D face recognition systems. Other advantage of this method is automatically receiving unauthorized attempt (face of unauthorized persons) without require specialist decipher. For results interpretation of verification procedure, any special equipment or knowledge is not necessary. Results of verification can be understanding for everybody (without special training) and used immediately as the image or 3D model, for further analysis, e.g.: in police departments or other 3D modeling.

Presented method was tested onto very specific group of data - faces of twins. Results of this analysis, was confirmed that even for very similar monozygotic twins faces (which can be very difficult for distinguish by human visual perception) the numerical ID - code of each face, was different and individual. Trends curves of coefficient values of modes have general the same trajectory but in local comparison still they are different. Them bigger difference between faces them larger distance between trend curves. For comparison of two faces of different twins the trend curves are completely different - analogical like for two different persons. The basic input information for PCA, not necessary must be limited only to geometry of the object, but can be enlarged by additional information's (e.g. thermal images) into multi-dimensional database. In presented paper the 2D infrared images of faces was added to the basic database. Also this data can be coded and used as a thermal faceprint. Big disadvantage of thermal images of face surface is strong influence of environment temperature. As the more stabile and independent from temperature of atmosphere, the system based on thermal images of face veins is suggested.

Second presented application of 3D PCA analysis is anthropometrics. 3D PCA make possible extraction of mean shape and geometrical features of biological objects set. Mean shape characterize all 3D body (not only few 2D dimensions, like it is, in traditional anthropometric database). Features are describing principal deformations of analyzed group of objects (bones). This method can be used to create of full three dimensional anthropometric database of the skeleton system. One of advantages of that three dimensional anthropometric database, is possibility of measured any necessary dimensions on the surface of the mean bone. Mean shape and geometrical features (knowledge about shape and trends of deformations) can be used for developing new, more useful types of prosthesis. Such 3D anthropometrics analysis also can be important in anthropology, gives us information about the changes that appear in the human skeletal structure in different populations or ages.

As a third application the method of reconstruction of three-dimensional shape of biological object was presented. The reconstructed geometry is compatible with CAD systems. Reconstruction algorithm, developed by authors, is based on the few 2D RTG images and knowledge about object geometry recorded in empirical database. Presented method use full volume information from RTG images and can be used not only for reconstruction of the biological objects.

Accuracy of the method is higher than reconstructions based on CT-imagining and comparable with 3D scanners (about 0,3 mm). Important characteristic of presented method is the automation of searching of the solution (elimination of landmarks) and that this method is non-invasive and non-destructive.

6. Future directions of research

Based onthe resultsof analysis presented above, in the following chapter authors propose further directions of researches. This work would have to expand possibilities of existing 3DPCA and to examine other methods of statistical analysis, such as: ICA-Independent Component Analysis.

For application of PCA in 3D biometric systems the unified system of data recording (included areas of measurements) must develop. Furthermore, the optimal data acquisition process should be clearly defined for obtain highest accuracy level of measurement during the shortest time and the maximum simplification of the measuring equipment. An important element that should be subjected to further testing is the issue of facial expressions of the subjects. This aspect strongly influence on the obtained results. Also study of the influence of other objects such as glasses, beard, hat, etc., on the results should be examined. Considering the three-dimensional biometric system can be interesting to increase the number of dimensions included in the analysis of the PCA. Such additional information may be infrared images. However in this case, user must remember about strong impact of the ambient temperature on the obtained results. One solution to this problem may be the use of thermal images containing the facial structure of blood vessels.

Development of the PCA method in the anthropometric application should include the development of precise and effective tool of registration process. This procedure should include the specific areas of individual bones and the anatomical elements of the human body. Very interesting results can provide a PCA analysis of other human organs. Also basic research on the structure of the external shape of human body would have produced very valuable results for the ergonomic environment.

Another direction of development of the above considerations is the method of three-dimensional reconstruction of the geometry of the object. Described method basis on the two-dimensional X-ray images and the 3D database generated by PCA analysis. For correct reconstruction is necessary to make set of measurements and analysis, contains: geometry measurements, PCA analysis and verification of reconstruction process performed on the of RTG images. Develop a comprehensive; coherent system for the reconstruction of geometry could allow the significantly spread the use of computer models in everyday medical practice.

7. Acknowledgment

The part of this work was supported under research grant no: N518 496039 from the Polish Ministry of Science 2010-2012.

8. References

Akhloufi, M, Bendada A., 2008,*Infrared Face Recognition Using Distance Transforms*, World Academy of Science, Engineering and Technology Nr 40, pp. 160-163.

Anderson, R. J., (2008), *Security Engineering: A Guide to Building Dependable Distributed Systems*, Wiley Publishing Inc., Indiana, USA ISBN-13: 9780470068526.

Anil K. J., Prabhakar S., Pankanti S., (2002), *On the Similarity of identical twin fingerprints*, The Journal of Patter Recognition Society Nr 35, pp. 2653 –2663.

Benameur S., Mignote M., Parent S., Labelle H., Skalli W., De Gusie J., (December 2001), *3D Biplanar Reconstruction of Scoliotic Vertebrae Using Statistical Models.* 20th IEEE International Conference on Computer Vision and Pattern Recognition, CVPR'01, volume II, pp. 577-582.

Berry J. L., Moran J. M., Berg W. S.,Steffee A. D., (1987), *A morphometric study of human lumbar and selected thoracic vertebrae,*Spine, Volume 12, Number 4.

Bro-Nielsen, M., Gramkow, C., (1996), *Fast fluid registration of medical images,* In: Proc. Visualization in Biomedical Computing (VBC'96), Springer Lecture Notes in Computer Science, vol. 1131, Hamburg

Holmes P., Lumley J. L., Berkooz G., (1996),*Turbulence, coherent, structures dynamical systems and symmetry,* Cambridge University Press.

Holmes, P., Lumley, J., L., Berkooz, G., (1998), *Turbulence, Coherent Structures, Dynamical Systems and Symmetry,* Cambridge University Press, Cambridge, New Edition.

Jain A.K., Ross A. and Pankanti S., (1999) , *A Prototype Hand Geometry-based Verification System,* Proceedings of 2nd International Conference on Audio- and Video-based Biometric Person Authentication (AVBPA), (Washington D.C.), pp.166-171.

Jantz, R.L. and P.H. Moore-Jansen, (1988), *A Data Base for Forensic Anthropology: Structure, Content and Analysis,* Report of Investigations no 47. Knoxville, TN: University of Tennessee.

Mainguet J-F. Biometrics, (2004), URL: http://pagesperso-orange.fr/fingerchip/biometrics/biometrics.htm

Milickovic N., Baltas D., Giannouli S., Lahanas M., Zamboglou N., (2000)*CT imaging based digitally reconstructed radiographs and its application in brachytherapy.* Phys. Med. Biol. 45, pp. 2787-2800.

Moore-Jansen, P.M., S.D. Ousley, and R.L. Jantz, (1994), *Data Collection Procedures for Forensic Skeletal Material.* Report of Investigations no 48. Knoxville, TN: University of Tennessee.

Morzynski M., Afanasiev K., Thiele F., (1999). *Solution of the eigenvalue problems resulting from global non-parallel flow stability analysis,* Computer Methods Applied in Mechanical Engineering.

Prokoski. F., (2000) *History, Current Status, and Future of Infrared Identification,* IEEE Workshop on Computer Vision behind the Visible Spectrum: Methods and Applications (CVBVS 2000), pp 5-14.

Russacof D. B., Rohlfing T., Rueckert D., Shahidi R., Kim D., (2003), *Maurer Calvin R. Fast calculation of digitally reconstructed radiographs using light fields,* Medical Imagining 2003, Image Processing, Proceedings SPIE Vol. 5032.

Rychlik M., (2004), Original title In Polish: *Metoda odtwarzania złożonych kształtów przestrzennych dla systemów CAD, przy zredukowanej ilości danych pomiarowych,* PhD work, Poznań University of Technology, Poznan Poland.

Rychlik M., Morzyński M., Stankiewicz W., (2005), *Applications of CFD and PCA methods for geometry reconstruction of 3D objects,* Proceedings of the 10th International Conference Mathematical Modeling and Analysis, Vilnius, pp 123-128. ISBN 9986-05-924-0.

Sanchez-Reillo R., Sanchez-Avila and Gonzales-Marcos A., (2000), *Biometric Identification Through Hand Geometry Measurements,* IEEE Transactions on Pattern Analysis and Machine Intelligence.

Schneider W., (2007), *Report of the Defense Science Board Task Force on Defense Biometrics,* Department of Defense United States of America, Washington D.C.

Syn, M., H-M., Prager, R., W., (1994), *Mesh models for three-dimensional ultrasound imagining,* CUED/F-INFENG/TR 210, Cambridge University Engineering Department, Cambridge.

Vitek C., (2005), *A comparison in osteological measurements of two populations from East Tennessee,* University of Tennessee at Chattanooga.

Vranic, D., Saupe, D., (2002), *Description of 3D-shape using a complex function of the sphere,* Department of Computer and Information Science, University of Konstanz.

Xiaoguang Lu, (2006), *3D Face Recognition across Pose and Expression,* PhD thesis, Michigan State University

5

Mathematical Modelling of Gene Regulatory Networks

Ana Tušek and Želimir Kurtanjek
Faculty of Food Technology and Biotechnology, University of Zagreb
Croatia

1. Introduction

Living cells can be observed as complex dynamical systems that are constantly remodelling themselves as response to changes in their environment (Zak et al., 2005). The cell metabolism includes number of reactions and products of reactions which interact forming a metabolic network. The aim of modern biology is to understand the structure and dynamic of those complex interactions.

Due to the fact that large amount of date about processes in living cells are being collected every day, it become necessary to use computers for data processing and analysis. Introducing computer technologies into biology new discipline has been develop, systems biology or computational biology. The aim of system biology is describing and understanding how parts of organism interact in one complex system; systems biology aims to develop mathematical model of biological systems by integrating experimental and theoretical techniques (Hecker et al., 2009, Albert, 2004). Systems biology studies biological systems by systematically perturbating them (biologically, genetically or chemically) monitoring the genes, proteins and informational pathway response (Strizh et al., 2007). According to Bruggeman & Westerholl, 2007 a complete systems biology approach requires (i) characterisation of organism molecular composition, (ii) components dynamics (spatial and temporal) and (iii) detail analysis of molecular response to internal and external stimuli.

Progress in molecular biology led to development of complete maps of genomes of many organisms; it is also possible to identify and classify proteins. Although the number of completely sequenced genomes is mounting rapidly, our knowledge of transcription regulation is limited to a few model organisms (Janga & Collado-Vides, 2007). The interactive regulation of genes, working together to create gene networks has been considered the origin of many functions of organism (Mochizuki, 2008). Classical molecular method (Northern blotting, reporter genes and DNA footprinting) have provided great insight into regulatory relationship between genes; advancement in genetic experimental technologies DNA microarray analysis provide an effective and efficient way to measure the gene expression levels of up to tens of thousands of genes simultaneously under many different conditions (Xu et al., 2007). The control of the gene transcription is an integrated mechanism involving the interaction of genes and proteins (Knott et al., 2010). Every gene has one or more activators and one or more inhibitors that are regulating the specific gene expression, depending on the situation in the cell and cell environment. The complex network of genes and there activators and/or inhibitors is defined as gene regulatory network. Gene regulatory networks can be very usefully for understanding the organisation within cells, because in gene regulatory networks information form the cell state and the outside environment are translated into correctly timed gene expression (Crombach & Hogeweg, 2008). Gene regulatory networks are usually described as network models where the dependencies between genes are presented by direct graph, in which nodes represent genes, proteins, enzymes or other chemical substances and edges led form a regulator to its target (edges represent transformation, eg. phosphorylation and dephosphorylation, or activation and deactivation)(Wilczynski & Furlog, 2010; Dilão & Muraro, 2010). Ideally, gene regulatory network display flow of information throughout embryogenesis (Hunman et al., 2009). To easily analyse those complex systems, mathematical models of gene regulatory networks have been developed. Mathematical models of gene regulatory networks include set of differential equations, graphical networks, stochastic functions and simulation models. Models can be used for making novel predictions and to plan future experiments.

In this chapter the theory of gene regulatory networks will be presented. The chapter will start with ideas how gene regulatory networks are constructed. There will be data on different types of gene regulatory networks and approaches for modeling those systems. This chapter will try to explain why is the modeling of complex regulatory networks important for genetic engineering and how can the mathematical analysis of gene regulatory networks be used for genetic engineering experiments planning and results interpretation.

2. Genes and genome

The hereditary nature of every living organism is defined by genome. Genome is formed of long sequences of DNA that provide information necessary to construct organism (Lewin, 2004). So genome can be divided into series of DNA sequences called genes. Each gene represents single protein (there is relationship between the base sequences of a gene and the amino acid sequence of the polypeptide whose synthesis directs the gene) (Berg, 2001). Genome of living organism can contain from less than 500 genes (for mycoplasma) to more than 40 000 genes (for human genome) (Table 1).

Phylum	Species	Genome (bp)
Algae	*Pyrenomas salina*	$6.6 \cdot 10^5$
Mycoplasma	*M. pneumoniae*	$1.0 \cdot 10^6$
Bacterium	*E. coli*	$4.2 \cdot 10^6$
Yeast	*S. cerevisiae*	$1.3 \cdot 10^7$
Slime mold	*D. discoideum*	$5.4 \cdot 10^7$
Nematode	*C. elegans*	$8.0 \cdot 10^7$
Insect	*D. melanogaster*	$1.4 \cdot 10^8$
Bird	*G. domesticus*	$1.2 \cdot 10^9$
Amphibian	*X. laevis*	$3.1 \cdot 10^9$
Mammal	*H. sapiens*	$3.3 \cdot 10^9$

Table 1. The genome size of some organisms (Lewin, 2004)

The number of genes in genome can be identified in several ways: (i) by defining open reading frames, (ii) by identifying all the mRNAs (transcriptome) or (iii) by identifying all the proteins (proteome). Due to the fact that some of the genes are presented in more then one copy or are related to one another, the number of different types of genes is less than total number of genes.

Over the past decade genome sequencing has generated large amount of new information. The main goal in sequencing is the identification of molecular and cellular function of all gene products. Interpretation of raw DNA sequences data includes identification and annotation of genes, proteins and metabolic and regulatory pathways (Médigue & Moszer, 2007). Accurate annotation of the human and genome of other organisms is essential for drug discovery (Rust et al., 2002). The mostly used annotation method is sequence homology recognition. According to Yakunin et al., 2004 apart sequence-based method, few others approaches can be used: (i) analysis of temporal, spatial and physiological proteins regulation, (ii) analysis of protein interactions, (iii) analysis of gene neighborhood, (iv) analysis of gene knockout phenotype, (v) analysis of the protein activities, (vi) analysis of post-translational modifications and (vii) protein structural analysis.

More information about components interaction allows multidimensional annotation; one dimensional annotation includes identification of genes in genome and description of functionality; two dimensional annotation specifies the cellular components and their interactions; three dimensional annotation of genome includes description of intracellular arrangement of chromosome and other cellular components, while four dimensional genome annotation could include changes in genome sequences due to the evolution (Reed et al., 2006). Genome annotation is usually preformed using one of the bioinformatics tools, GLIMMER, GlimmerM and GENSCAN (those programs include gene finding algorithm) or BLAST, FASTA and HAMER (sequence-homology search tools) (Reed et al., 2006).

2.1 Gene regulation

Taking in account central dogma of molecular biology developed by Francis Crick (transfer of sequence information between different biopolymers: RNA, DNA and proteins) there are three possible places of regulation of production of an active gene; first is the transcriptional regulation, second the translation regulation and the third post-translation or post-transcriptional regulation (Fig.1.). Regulation of gene expression is fundamental for the coordinate synthesis, assembly and localization of the macromolecular structures of cells (Halbeisen et al., 2007).

Regulation of gene expression at transcriptional level is evolutionary conserved mechanism in all cellular organisms. This process is mediated by physical interactions between transcription factors and *cis*-acting regulatory elements in promoter region of target genes (Janky et al., 2009). During transcription, mRNA is synthesized using mRNA polymerase. This process can be divided in four steps: (i) promoter recognition, (ii) chain initiation, (iii) mRNA chain elongation and (iii) chain termination and regulation can occur at each step.

Protein synthesis occurs during the translation process; mRNA is "translated" into specific polypeptide according to rules of tri nucleotide genetic code. This step of protein biosynthesis can also be divided into three parts: (i) initiation, (ii) elongation and (iii) termination. Each of these phases requires a specific group of translocation factors (Day & Tuite, 1998).

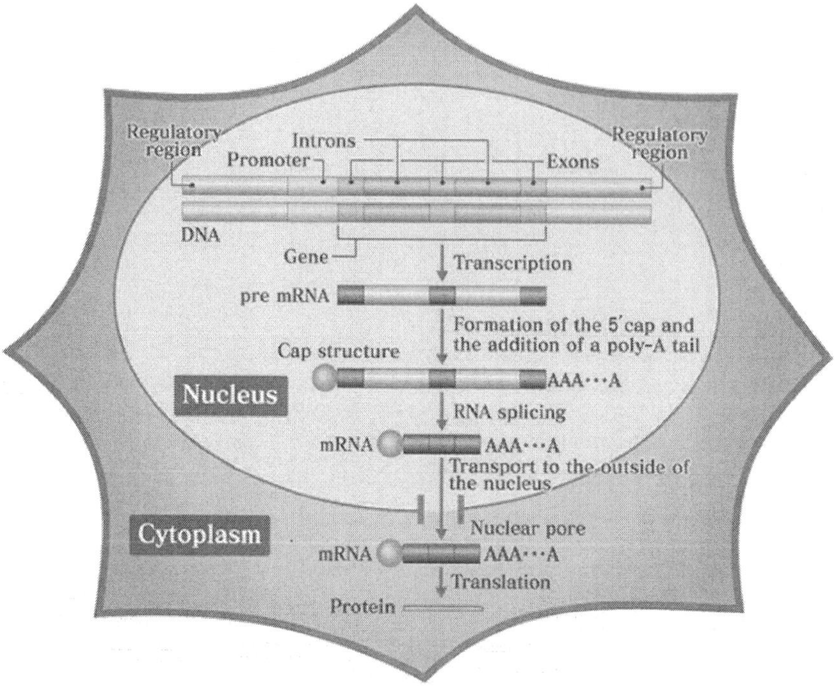

Fig. 1. Gene expression (http://csls-text.c.u-tokyo.ac.jp/active/04_03.html)

Translation initiation includes events that lead to positioning of 80S ribosome at the start codon of mRNA. Translation rates are primarily regulated at initiation level involving large number of initiation factors (Macdonald, 2001). The amount of mRNA available for translation can be changed at different steps of RNA maturation. Two families of proteins (the RNA binding proteins and RNA helicases) determinate the fate of pre-mRNAs and mRNA by regulating steps from transcription to translation (Mazzucotell et al., 2008). Translation control is critical in regulating wide range of process in cells form development, cell differentiation and proliferation to regulation of metabolic pathways. It is also important for protection of cell from external effects (Garcia-Sanz et al., 1998).

Transcription and translation regulation mechanisms are till now described in literature quite detail, but there is still only few data of post-transcriptional and post-translational regulation mechanism. Due to the fact that large number of RNA molecules is being synthesis in the cell, the precise post-transcriptional regulation is necessary to control the activity and location of produced RNA molecules. This mechanism is controlled by RNA-binging proteins (Halbeisen et al., 2007). Post-transcriptional regulations of gene expression occur at the levels of pre-messenger RNA (mRNA) processing (capping, splicing, and polyadenylation), mRNA stability, and mRNA translation (Floris et al., 2009). The last level of gene expression control is the post-translational regulation. This step is responsible for controlling the levels of protein activity. Post-translation protein modifications are important for clinical research. There are few hounded of described post-translation modification; the most common are phosphorylation, ubiquitination, glycosylation, *S*-nitrosylation, proteolysis and methylation (Egorina et al., 2008).

3. Gene regulatory networks

When talking about biochemical network they can be divided into three groups: (i) metabolic network-describing chemical transformations between metabolites, (ii) protein networks (signaling networks)-describing protein-protein interaction and (iii) gene networks- describing relationships between genes (Brazhnik et al., 2002, Schlitt & Brazma, 2005). Key differences between regulatory and metabolic networks are listed in the Table 2.

Network feature	Metabolic networks	Regulatory networks
Structure	Hazard stochiometry	Qualitative statements
Evolutionary conservation	Enzyme sequences highly conserved across species	Limited conversion of *cis* regulatory sites between closely related species
Malleability	Fixed structure in terms of the substrates that a particular enzymes can process	Adjustable structure, because of the possibility that mutations in the *cis* regulatory sites change binding specificity
Level of biochemical characterization	Fairly complete understanding of most subsystems in microbial organisms	Most subnetworks have not been well characterized even in microbial model organisms
Modelling approaches	Quantitative constraint-based models can be constructed at the genome-scale	Quantitative models can be currently constructed only on a small scale; qualitative discrete network models can be used to study large networks
Role of noise	Relatively small because of the high concentrations of metabolites involved in most reactions	Possibly significant in determining both structural features of the network and the overall response of the network to a stimulus

Table 2. Differences between regulatory and metabolic networks (Herrgård et al., 2004)

Gene regulatory networks regulate the expression of thousands of genes. It can be sad that gene regulatory networks are maps of the interactions between regulatory gene products and their *cis* regulatory elements (gene and gene products interact and form networks), as well between signaling ligand and their receptor. So, basic functional unit of gene regulatory network is promoter region of a gene or operon which contains *cis* regulatory binding site for transcription factors, The location of binding sites and affinity of transcription factors determinate the level of gene expression (Herrgård et al., 2004) (Fig. 2).

Gene regulatory maps display flow of regulatory information throughout embryogenesis (Hinman et al., 2009). Gene network analysis provides many important information:

1. gene network provides information to help annotate genome
2. it helps to uncover the biochemical network in a cell
3. it provides new idea to treat some diseases (Liu et al., 2006).

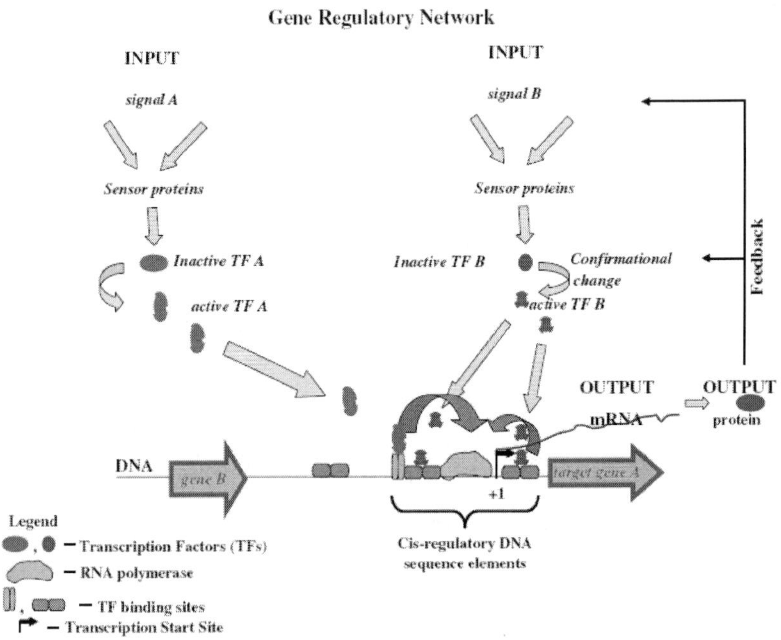

Fig. 2. Genomic view of gene regulatory network. From genomic perspective transcriptional regulation can be presented as an interplay between *cis*-regulatory elements and different transcription factors (Janga & Collado-Vides, 2007)

The activity of functional genes is influenced by few factors: transcriptional factors and cofactor that effects transcription, by degradation of proteins and transcripts and by post-translational modifications (Hecker et al., 2009). The idea of gene regulatory network is to describe dependence between molecules included in gene activity. Gene regulatory network is composed of nodes (representing genes proteins or metabolites) and edges (representing molecular interactions) (Hecker et al., 2009). Identification of gene regulatory networks is based on deterministic models of gene expression (Cinquemani et al., 2008).

The architecture of gene regulatory networks arise directly form DNA sequences of the genome and representation of gene regulatory networks must have specific emphasis on predicted DNA inputs and it has to be viewable at a number of different levels (Longabaugh et al., 2008). Identifying gene networks from large-scale dataset measurements is a difficult computational and experimental problem (Tegnér & Björkegren, 2006).

4. Mathematical modelling of gene regulatory network

As mentioned before, gene regulatory networks are becoming more and more usefully tool for analysis and understanding organization within cells and their dynamics (Crombach & Hogeweg, 2008). To better understand the complex process in gene regulatory networks, mathematical models of those systems have been developed. Mathematical models are very useful for predicting the effect of nonlinear interactions (Smolen et al., 2000) and can provide insight into systems understanding of regulation of processes in the cell (Zak et al., 2005). Gene regulatory networks are modelled as networks composed of nodes representing genes, proteins or metabolites and edges representing molecular interactions (protein-protein, DNA-protein or relationships between genes) (Hecker et al., 2009). The biggest problem in a field of mathematical modelling of gene regulatory networks is still in development of model based on experimental data because it is very difficult to defining the quality of available experimental data. There are many approaches for defining gene regulatory networks identification; in the most general manner we can defer unstructured and structured approach (Zak et al., 2005). In unstructured modelling approach there is assumption that every gene regulates every other gene. Using additional domain knowledge it is possible to develop structured model. Subcellular structure, nuclear connectivity and dynamical model structure have to be taken into consideration when developing structured model (Fig 3).

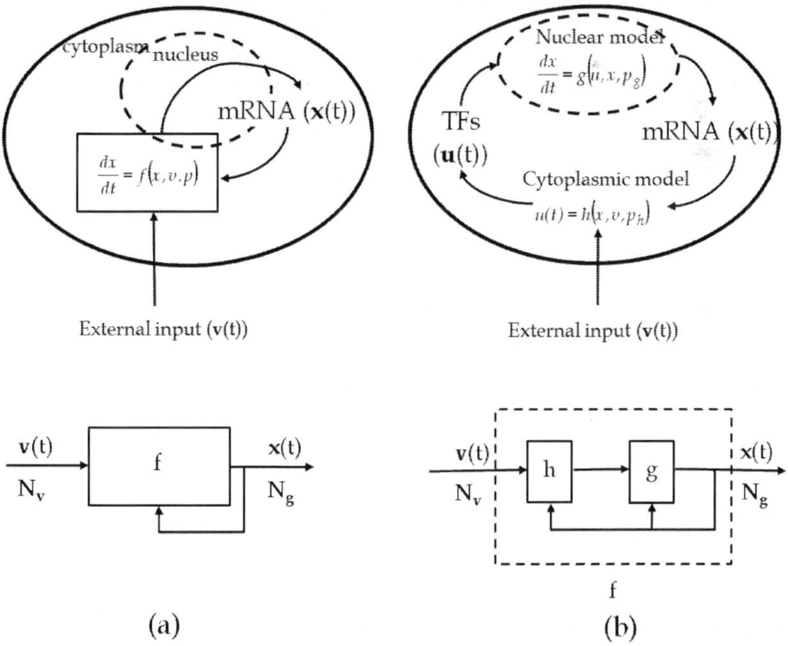

Fig. 3. (a) Unstructured and (b) structured gene regulatory network modelling (Zak et al., 2005)

Mathematical sciences can contribute to biology in field of models diversity. Different types of cell are developed as a consequence of the gene activity which is under control of gene regulatory network (Fig. 4) (Mochizuki, 2008).

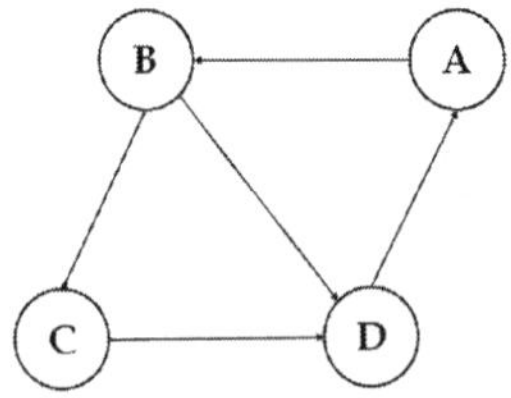

Fig. 4. Example of gene regulatory network (Mochizuki, 2008)

When developing model two facts have too be taken into account: (i) gene expression levels are regulated by the combined action of multiple gene products, (ii) the number of measurements is relatively small compared to the number of measured genes and measures noise has to be taken into account (van Someren et al., 2002). According to Schlitt & Brazma, 2005 gene networks models can be divided into four groups according to increasing level of detail in the models: (i) part lists, (ii) topology models, (iii) control logic models, (iv) dynamic models.

All mentioned approaches face the same two problems which make the automatic discovery of gene networks form experimental data far form trivial (van Someren et al., 2002). The first is statistical robustness and the second biological interpretation of the results (how to differ regulation form co-expression and indirect regulation form direct regulation) (Lulli & Romauch, 2009). When talking about statistical robustness the focus is the fact that high-dimensionality problem cusses the hypothetical models to be highly susceptible (number of microarray experiments is usually much smaller that number of genes included into network) (Chan et al., 2008).

4.1 Parts list

The first step in developing gene regulatory network is construction of a part list of the components included into network (Hu et al., 2010). High-throughput genome sequencing project have made available complete genomic lists of many organism (Alm & Arkin, 2003). Those lists include genes, transcriptional factors, promoters, binding sites and many other molecules important for functioning of gene network (Schlitt & Brazma, 2007).

4.2 Topology models

After defining the components of the gene networks, the next step of the modelling of the gene regulatory network is definition of the connections between nodes (definition of the edges). Development of network topology includes decision about genes are included into the networks, which acts as inhibitors or activator of transcription (Mendes et al., 2003). The different topology classes of networks (regular lattice, small-world, random networks…) are consequence of different ways how large sets of elements are connected (Gonçalves & Costa, 2008). Network growth model is present in Fig. 5. To quantitatively describe a network topology at minimum three metrics are employed:

1. clustering coefficients - for node i in a network with k_i edges connecting it to the nearest neighbours, the clustering coefficient is defined with Eq. 1.

$$C_i = \frac{2n}{k_i(k_i - 1)} \tag{1}$$

   were n represents the number of edges between nearest neighbours. C_i can have numerical values between 0 and 1. When C_i=0 node is linked to disconnected group, and when C_i=1 node is connected to interlinked group.
2. network diameter - is defined as the smallest number of the links by which starting from one node another node can be reached
3. degree distribution – is probability $P(k)$ that a node has k links (Lukashin et al., 2003).

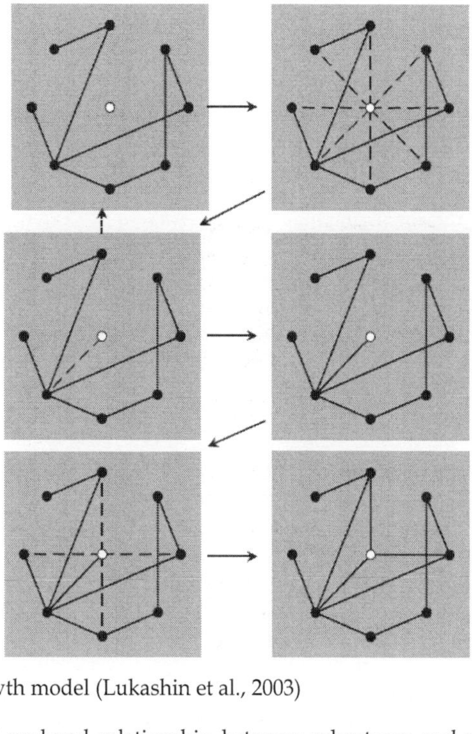

Fig. 5. Network growth model (Lukashin et al., 2003)

Ciliberti et al., 2007 analysed relationship between robustness and network topology for millions of networks with different topologies. Results showed that significantly different network architecture can show the same gene expression patterns. It was also noticed that some networks are highly robust to gene expression noise and mutations whereas some are quite fragile. Crombach & Hogeweg, 2008 analysed the evolution of gene regulatory networks. Their results showed that interplay between long term evolution process and short term gene regulation dynamics leads to increase in efficiency of crating adapted offspring.

4.3 Control logic models

After defining the network topology, the next step in development of gene regulatory network is analysis of the rules of the interaction between the network elements (Schlitt and Brazma, 2007). Transcriptional-regulatory systems is based on the presence of transcription factor binding sites of genes which are responsible for receiving temporal regulatory input signals; sequential logic model (SML) can be used for description of trans-activation and temporal mRNA expression profiles (Yeo et al., 2007). SML technique can ensure detail insight into gene regulation and it can ensure systematically analysis of the dynamic transcriptional inputs.

4.4 Dynamic models

The nodes in gene network population of genes, proteins and other regulatory molecules. There can be from few to few thousands of copies of those molecules in cell. Components of the gene regulatory networks can be changed in response to internal and external stimuli. It is important to include those interactions into network; this is possible using dynamic modelling approach. Dynamic modelling frameworks are usually classified along two axes: continuous versus discrete (describes the level of detail of node state) and deterministic versus stochastic (in view of uncertainties and variability of the transfer functions) (Albert, 2007). Dynamic models can also be divided into quantitative (base on system of ordinary differential equations) and qualitative models (piecewise linear differential system) (Chaouiya, 2007).

4.4.1 Boolean models

Boolean networks describe the state of genes with binary (ON/OFF) variables. Dynamic behaviour of each variable is governed by Boolean function (Albert, 2004). Although Boolean networks allow the analysis of the dynamics of the gene regulatory networks, they ignore the effect of genes at intermediate levels (Xu et al., 2007). Boolean networks have been intensely investigated as models for genetic control in cells. In those networks, each gene represents the node, and as mentioned before each node has two states ON (producing the protein) or OFF (there is no protein production). The biological basis for development of Boolean netwok as a model of gene regulatory network lies in the fact that during regulation of functional states the cell exhibits switch-like behaviour; this form of behaviour ensures the movement of cell from one state to another (Shmulevich et al., 2002). In the network there are links between nods (one node has impact on the other) (Pomerance et al., 2009). The Boolean networks have ability to contain very large number of nodes but are very crude in their approximation in biology (Karlsson & Hörnquist, 2007). In Boolean network form (Fig.6.), the genome is presented by set of binary variables, $g_1, g_2 \ldots g_N$. The expression of each gene changes with time according to Eq.2.:

$$g_n(t+1) = F_n\left(g_{n_1}(t), g_{n_2}(t) \ldots g_{n_{k_n}}(t)\right) \tag{2}$$

where F_n is Boolean function constructed according to the inhibition or activation nature of the regulators. According to Balleza et al, 2008 if $F(g_1,g_2)$ is the function of two regulators g_1 and g_2 than function F can be in one of the following forms: $F(1,1)=1$, $F(1,0)=1$, $F(0,1)=0$ and $F(0,0)=1$. Regulatory phrase for $F=1$ is activator and for $F=0$ inhibitor.

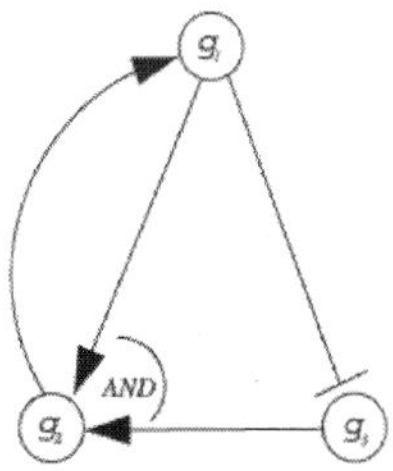

Fig. 6. Boolean network of three entities (Steggles et al., 2007)

Continuous models give more realistic description of the process, but development of those models requires large amounts of experimental data. As mentioned before in Boolean models at each time point the gene state depends on the state of the gene regulators at previous time step (Giacomantonio & Goodhill, 2010).

Some modification of traditional Boolean gene regulatory network models can be found in literature. One of them is temporal Boolean network. The difference between those two network models is in the fact temporal Boolean network allows the state of gene at time *t+1* depends on state of genes at times *t*, *t-1*,....., *t-(T-1)*(Silvescu & Honavar, 2001). Another approach is propped by Shulevich et al, 2002; probabilistic Boolean network. Probabilistic Boolean network includes properties of Boolean networks (rule-based dependence between genes), but due to the probabilistic nature this approach is suitable for systematic study of regulatory networks.

4.4.2 Petri net models

Petri net theory provides graphical notation with mathematical background. A Petri net is directed, bipartite and labelled graph which is build of four parts: (i) palces, denoted with circle representing biological compounds (metabolites), (ii) transitions, denoted with black rectangle, representing biochemical reactions between metabolites (iii) arcs, denoted with arrows and (iv) tokens denoted by black rectangle (Fig.7.) (Steggles et al., 2007).

As mentioned before, places represent resource of the system and can contain movable objects (tokens). Tokens represent quantitative unit of compounds. Transitions correspond to events that can change the state of the resources. Arcs (arcs label corresponds to stoichiometric number in reaction equation). Places represent resource of the system, and transitions correspond to events that can change the state of the resources. Arcs connect places to transitions (Chaouiya, 2007) and are allowed only between places and transitions and vice versa, never between places or between transitions (Koch et al., 2005).

According to Steggles et al., 2006, it is possible to develop gene regulatory network model based on Petri net starting from Boolean network. The idea was to use logic minimization to extract Boolean terms representing gene network and then to translate this into Petri net structure; the resulting Petri net model is capable to correctly capture dynamic behaviour of gene networks.

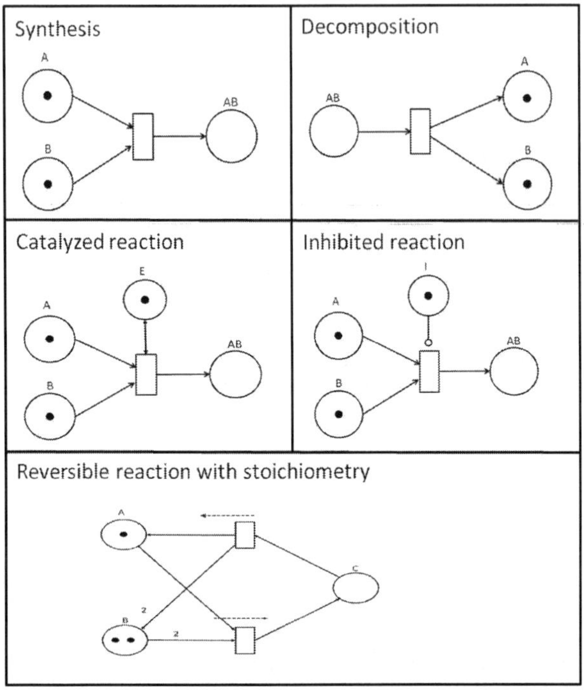

Fig. 7. Petri net modelling of different reactions (Chaouiya, 2007)

4.4.3 Difference and differential equation models

Using ordinary differential equations for representing gene regulatory networks concentrations of proteins, mRNAs and other molecules are presented as continuous time variables (Polynikis et al., 2009). Flexibility of ordinary deferential equations allows the description of complex relations between components of the net. Differential equations can describe complex dynamic behaviour like oscillations, cyclical patterns, multistationary and switch-like behaviour (Gebert et al., 2007). According to Hecker et al., 2009 the dynamic of gene regulatory networks can be described with (Eq.3.):

$$\frac{dx}{dt} = f(x,p,u,t) \tag{3}$$

were $x(t) = (x_1(t)......x_n(t))$ represents gene expression vector of genes for 1 to n, f is function that describes the rate of change of variable x. p presents model parameter set and u external perturbation signals. Transcription and translation can be model using ordinary differential equations (Eq. 4-5):

$$\frac{dr_i}{dt} = F\left(f_i^R(p_1), f_i^R(p_2)....f_i^R(p_n)\right) - \gamma_i r_i \tag{4}$$

$$\frac{\mathrm{d}p_i}{\mathrm{d}t} = f_i^P(r_i) - \delta_i p_i \tag{5}$$

the function $f_i^R(p_j)$ is usually non-linear and describes the dependence of mRNA concentration on protein concentration. According to Hecker et al., 2009 ordinary differential equations for description of gene regulatory network can be divided into:

1. linear differential equations can used for description of gene expression kinetics (Eq.6)

$$\frac{\mathrm{d}x_i}{\mathrm{d}t} = \sum_{j=1}^{N} w_{i,j} x_j + b_i u \tag{6}$$

Gebert et al., 2007 used developed model of pecewise linear differential equation for description of interaction between genes in regulatory networks; variables of the model were mRNA concentrations (Fig.8.).

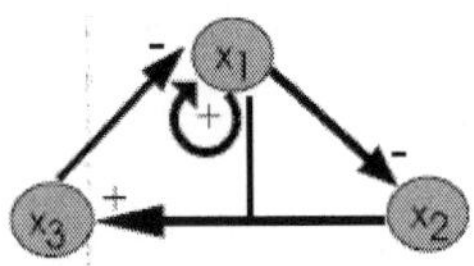

Fig. 8. Model of gene regulation (Gebert et al., 2007)

Model was based on assumption that regulation between genes can be described using piecewise linear differential equations (Eq 7-9).

$$\dot{x_1} = k_{1,1} h^+\left(x_1, \theta_{1,1}, m_{1,1}\right) + k_{1,3} h^+\left(x_3, \theta_{1,3}, m_{1,3}\right) - \gamma_1 x_1 \tag{7}$$

$$\dot{x_2} = k_{2,1} h^+\left(x_1, \theta_{2,1}, m_{2,1}\right) - \gamma_2 x_2 \tag{8}$$

$$\dot{x_3} = k_{3,1,2} h^+\left(x_1, \theta_{3,1}, m_{3,1}\right) h^+\left(x_2, \theta_{3,2}, m_{3,2}\right) - \gamma_3 x_3 \tag{9}$$

were γ represents the degradation rate of mRNA and k are rate constants.
Wu et al., 2004 proposed method to model gene expression dynamic from measured time-course data including linear equations. Developed dynamic equations described the relationships between internal state variables and observation variables.

2. non-linear differential equations are used for describing complex dynamic behaviours. Comparing to linear models, identification of the non-linear differential equation model is computationally more intensive and it requires more data (Quian & Wang, 2007). The numerical representation of non-linear ODE model of gene regulatory network (Eq.10):

$$\frac{\mathrm{d}x_i}{\mathrm{d}t} = f_i\left(x_1, x_2, \ldots, x_n\right) + v_i \qquad i = 1, 2, \ldots N \tag{10}$$

where f_i represents the non-linear function which can be determinated from experimental data, it can be polynomial (Eq.11):

$$f_i = \sum_{j=1}^{L_i} \left[\left(w_{ij} + \mu_{ij} \right) \Omega_{ij} \left(x_1, x_2, \ldots, x_n \right) \right] \qquad i = 1, 2, \ldots N \tag{11}$$

where L_i is the number of terms in f_i, w_{ij} represent parameters that need to be estimated and $\Omega_{ij}(x_1, x_2, \ldots x_N)$ is the component of the nonlinear function.
Quian and Wang, 2007 developed gene regulatory network model including evolutionary algorithm and filtering approach; noise was modelled using nonlinear ordinary differential equations. Simulation showed the usage of proposed model on experimental data for microarray experiments.

Using set of ordinary differential equations for description of gene network, the inference of genetic networks is often defined as a function optimization problem to minimize the defences between gene expression levels obtained numerically and levels measured in experiments (Kimura et al., 2009). The problems that occurs when working with differential equation model are that those models include many parameters which have to be estimated form experimental data or obtained from literature. It also has to be taken into consideration that for complex differential equations analytical solution and analysis of the equations can be very complex.

4.4.4 Stochastic modelling

All cellular events depend on probabilistic collisions between molecules. Due to the fact that number of events occurring in the cells is not large and events are dependent, it is not possible to use deterministic rate equations for description of the gene network (gene expression is stochastic process (Paulsson, 2005). There are many important stochastic phenomena during the life time of the cell, like random fluctuations that initiate transcription, spontaneous jumps in mRNA or protein concentrations (Rosenfeld, 2007). Study of stochastic properties in genetic systems involves formulation of molecular noise, formulation of approximation of these representations and development of computational algorithms capable for describing complexity of network dynamics (El Samad, et al., 2005).

According to Rosenfeld, 2007 for mathematical description of stochastic dynamics of gene regulatory networks two approaches can be used:

1. non-linear dynamics paradigm – treats the biochemical components included in gene expression regulation as continuous variables and describes their variations using non-linear differential equations
2. Markov process paradigm – due to the fact that some molecules included into gene expression regulation can occur in cell in very low concentrations they can not be treated as a continuous variables and their random fluctuations can be very high.

Stochastic modelling approach is mathematically represented with Eq.12:

$$p(x, t + \Delta t) = p(x, t + \Delta t) \cdot \left(1 - \sum_{j=1}^{m} \alpha_j \Delta t \right) + \sum_{j=1}^{m} \beta_j \Delta t \tag{12}$$

where x represents the amount of molecules (state variable), $p(x,t)$ probability distribution. Assuming that $\Delta t \to 0$, the equation for stochastic representation of gene regulatory network is developed Eq. 13:

$$\frac{\partial p(x,t)}{\partial t} = \sum_{j=1}^{m} \left(\beta_j - \alpha_j p(x,t)\right) \tag{13}$$

4.4.5 Finite state linear models

Methodology of finite state linear modelling (FSLM) was developed by Bramza & Schlitt, 2003; it combines discrete and continuous aspects of gene regulation in structured way. Model was developed on few assumptions: (i) gene activity is defined by state of transcription binding sites in promoter region, (ii) each binding site can be in one of the finite number of states, (iii) active gene produces substance with rate dependant on activity level, (iv) state of binding site depends on concentrations of transcription factors. The continuous parts of the model consist of the state of the proton concentrations. As mentioned before it also includes Boolean-type model gene regulation (each gene and each binding site can have only two sates; ON or OFF). Bramza & Schitt, 2003 used finite state linear model for construction of biological network of λ-phage (Fig.9.)

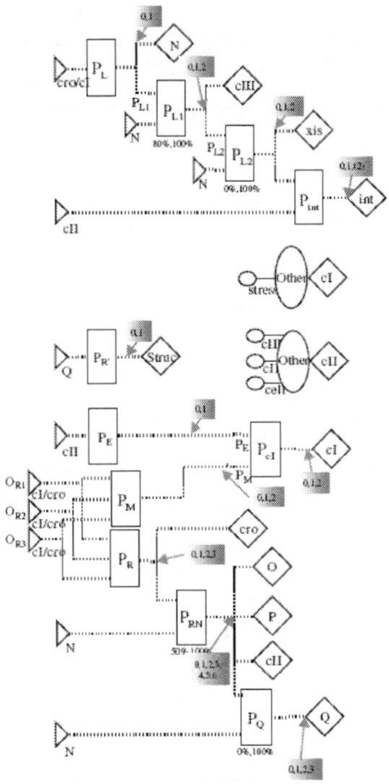

Fig. 9. Gene network of λ-phage (Bramza & Schitt, 2003)

Ruklisa et al., 2005 used previously described FSLM model for testing some theoretical properties of the model: (i) what kind of network dynamic could be modelled using this framework, (ii) is it possible to describe chaotic network dynamics and some others. A series of experiments were performed to estimate the regularity of behaviour of random networks; networks were simulated in 10000 steps and results show that FSLM models can be suitable for describing biological reality.

4.4.6 Hybrid models

Due to fact that boundaries between discreet and continuous model depend on the level of details included into the model there is an attempt to develop the models that could include both approaches (Schlitt & Bramza, 2007). Matsuno & Doi, 2000 proposed hybrid Petri net model for presentation of gene regulatory networks of λ-phage. Hybrid Petri net is an extension of Petri net that has continues and discrete elements and can be easily used for protein or mRNA concentration. Another approach to development of hybrid model is present by Crudu et al., 2009. They proposed unified framework for hybrid simplification of the Markov models of stochastic gene network dynamics. It was shown that those simplified models describe with good accuracy the stochastic properties of the gene networks and can be used for multi-scale biochemical systems.

5. Conclusion

Gene expression can be regulated on few levels. Gene regulatory networks are defined as collections of DNA segments in cells which interact with each other. Construction of gene regulatory networks is first step in biological analysis. It is very import to understand and explain the dynamic of gene regulatory networks. To explain and understand those complex biochemical systems different mathematical models have been developed. Techniques of mathematical modelling defer in level of details. Each modelling technique has its advantages and disadvantages and that has to be taken into consideration when developing mathematical model, because proposed model has to provide good insight into gene regulation process and be useful for prediction of some possible mutations or any other change.

6. Future direction section

When modelling gene regulatory networks the fact that model describes only some properties has to be taken into consideration. So there is always open question how real the developed model can be (Schlitt & Bramza, 2007). Using new molecular methods large amount of data can be collected ensuring the better insight into process in the cell. Including all this information in the model more detail model can be developed. When talking about mathematical modelling of gene regulatory networks the neural networks have been used lately for modelling (Lee & Yang, 2008; Xu et al., 2008). For example Knott et al., 2010 presented approach to model gene regulatory networks as non-liner system using artificial neural network. There is also idea in developing synthetic networks. All described approaches have one goal developing simple model which would describe the process in the cell; so the future direction of modelling of gene regulatory networks would be in funding the way how to reduce the complexly of biological systems and to preserve the model functionality.

7. Acknowledgment

This work was supported by Ministry of Science, Education and Sport of Republic of Croatia grant MZOŠ 0589.

8. References

Alm, E. & Arkin, A.P. (2003) Biological network. *Current Opinion in Structural Biology*, Vol. 13, No. 2, (April, 2003), pp. 193-202, ISSN 0959-440X

Albert, R. (2004) Boolean modelling of genetic regulatory networks. *Lecture Notes in Physics*, Vol.650, pp. 459-481, ISSN 0075-8450

Albert, R. (2007) Network inference, analysis, and modelling in systems biology. *The Plant Cell*, Vol. 19, (November 2007), pp.3327-3338, ISSN 1532-298X

Balleza, E.; Alvarez-Buylla, E.R., Chaos, A., Kauffman, S., Shmulevic, I. & Aldana, M. (2008) Critical dynamics in genetic regulatory networks: examples from four kingdoms. *Plos One*, Vol. 3, No. 6, (June 2008) pp. 1-10, ISSN 1932-6203

Berg, J.M.; Tymoczko, J.L., Stryer, L. & Clarke, N.D. (2001) Biochemistry, W.H. Freeman and Company, ISBN 0-7167-4954-8

Bramza, A. & Schlitt, T. (2003) Reverse engineering of gene regulatory networks: a finite state linear model. *Genome Biology*, Vol. 4, No. 6, (April 2003) pp. P5, ISSN 1465-6906

Brazhnik, P.; de la Fuente, A. & Mendes, P. (2002) Gene networks: how to put the function in genomics. *Trends in Biotechnology*, Vol. 20, No. 11, (November 2002) pp. 467-472, ISSN 0167-7799

Bruggeman, F.J. & Westerhoff, H.V. (2007) The nature of systems biology. *Trends in Microbiology*, Vol. 15, No. 1, (January, 2007), pp. 45-50, ISSN 0966-842X

Chan, Z.S.H.; Havaukkala, I., Jain, V., Hu, Y. & Kasabov, N. (2008) Soft computing methods to predict gene regulatory networks: An integrative approach on time-series gene expression data. *Applied Soft Computing*, Vol.8, pp. 1189-1199, ISSN 1568-4946.

Chaouiya, C. (2007) Petri net modelling of biological networks. *Briefing in Bioinformatics*, Vol.8, No.4, (July 2007), pp. 210-219, ISSN 1477-4054

Ciliberti, S.; Martin, O.C. & Wagner, A. (2007) Robustness can evolve gradually in complex regulatory gene networks with varying topology. *Plos Computational Biology*, Vol. 3, No. 2, (February 2007), pp. 0164-0173, ISSN 1553-734X

Cinquemani, E.; Milias-Argeitis, A., Summers, S. & Lygeros, J. (2008) Stochastic dynamics of genetic networks: modeling and parameter identification. *Bioinformatics*, Vol. 24, No. 23, pp. 2748-2754, ISSN 1471-2105

Crombach, A. & Hogeweg, P. (2008) Evolution of evolvability in gene regulatory networks. *Plos Computational Biology*, Vol.4, (July 2008), pp. 1-13, ISSN 1553-7358

Crudu, A.; Debusschu, A. & Radulesc, O. (2009) Hybrid stochastic simplifications for multiscale gene networks. *BMC Systems Biology*, Vol.3, pp. 89-114, ISSN 1752-0509.

Day, D.A. & Tuite, M.F. (1998) Post-transcriptional gene regulatory mechanisms in eukaryotes: an overview. *Journal of Endocrinology*, Vol. 157, pp.361-371, ISSN 1479-6805

Dilão, R. & Muraro, D. (2010) A software tool to model genetic regulatory networks. Applications to the modelling to threshold phenomena and of spatial patterning in *Drosophila*. *Plos One*, Vol. 5, No. 5 (May 2010), pp. e1074, ISSN 1932-6203

Egorina, E.M., Sovershaev, M.A. & Østerud, B. (2008) Regulation of tissue factor procoagulant activity by post-translational modifications. *Thrombosis Research*, Vol. 12, No. 6, pp. 831-837, ISSN 0049-3848

El Samad, H.; Khammash, M., Petzold, L. & Gillespie, D. (2005) Stochastic modelling of gene regulatory networks. *International Journal of Robust and Nonlinear Control,* Vol. 15, pp. 691-711, ISSN 1049-8923

Floris, M.; Mahgoub, H., Lanet, E., Robaglia, C. & Benoit, M. (2009) Post-transcriptional regulation of gene expression in plants during abiotic stress. *International Journal of Molecular Sciences,* Vol. 10, pp. 3168-3185, ISSN 1422-0067

Garcia-Sanz, J.A.; Mikulits, W., Livingstone, A., Lefkovits, I. & Müllner, E.W. (1998) Translational control: a general mechanism for gene regulation during T cell activation. *The Journal of the Federation of American Societies for Experimental Biology,* Vol. 12, No.3, (March 1998), pp.299-306, ISSN 1530-6860

Gebert, J.; Radde, N. & Weber, G.-W. (2007) Modelling gene regulatory networks with piecewise linear differential equations. *European Journal of Operational Research,* Vol. 181, pp. 1148-1165, ISSN 0377-2217

Halbeisen, R.E.; Galgano, A., Scherrer, T. & Gerber, A.P. (2007) Post-transcriptional gene regulation: From genome-wide studies to principles. *Cellular and Molecular Life Sciences,* Vol. 65, No. 5, (March 2008), pp. 798-813, ISSN 1420-9071

Hinman, V.F.; (2009) Evolution of gene regulatory network architectures: Examples of subcircuit conservation and plasticity between classes of echinoderms

Hecker, M.; Lambeck, S., Toepfer, S., van Someren, E. & Guthke, R. (2009) Gene regulatory network inference: Data integration in dynamic models-A review. *BioSystems,* Vol.69, No.1, (April 2009), pp. 86-103, ISSN 0303-2647

Herrgård, M.J.; Covert, M.W. & Palsson, B.Ø. (2004) Reconstruction of microbial transcriptional regulatory networks. *Current Opinion in Biotechnology,* Vol. 15, No.1, (February 2004), pp. 70-77, ISSN 0958-1669

Hu, J.; Wan, J., Hackler Jr., L., Zack, D.J. & Qian, J. (2010) Computational analysis of tissue-specific gene networks: application to murine retinal functional studies. *Bioinformaics,* Vol. 26, No.18, (September 2010), pp. 2289-2297, ISSN 1471-2105

Janga, S.C. & Collado-Vides, J. (2007) Structure and evolution of gene regulatory networks in microbial genome. *Research in Microbiology,* Vol.158, No.10 (December 2007), pp. 787-794, ISSN 0923-2508

Janky, R.; van Helden, J., Madan Babu, M. (2009) Investigating transcriptional regulation: from analysis of complex networks to discovery of *cis*-regulatory elements. *Methods,* Vol. 48, No. 3, (July 2009), pp. 277-286, ISSN 1046-2023

Karlsson, F. & Hörnquist, M. (2007) Order or chaos in Boolean gene networks depends on the mean fraction of canalizing functions. *Physica A: Statistical Mechanics and its Application,* Vol. 384, No.2 (October 2007), pp. 747-757, ISSN 0378-4371

Kimura, S.; Nakayama, S., Hatakeyama, M. (2009) Genetic network inference as a series of discrimination tasks. *Bioinformatics,* Vol. 25, No. 7 pp.918-925 ISSN 1471-2105

Knott, S.;Mostafavi, S. & Mousavi, P. (2010) A neural network based modelling and validation approach for identifying gene regulatory networks. *Neurocomputing,* Vol. 73, No. 13-15, (August, 2010), pp. 2419-2429, ISSN 0925-2312

Koch, I.; Junker, B.H. & Heiner, M. (2005) Application of Petri net theory for modelling and validation of the sucrose breakdown pathway in the potato tuber. *Bioinformatics,* Vol. 21, No. 7, pp. 1219-1226, ISSN 1471-2105

Lee, W.-P. & Yang, K.-C. (2008) A clustering-based approcah for interfernig rucerrent neural netwoks as gene regulatory networks. *Neurocomputing,* Vol. 71, No. 4-6, (January 2008), pp. 600- 610, ISSN 0925-2312

Lewin, B. (2004) Genes, Pearson Prentoce Hall, ISBN 0-13-123924-4

Liu, T.-F.; Sung, W.-K. & Mittal, A. (2006) Model gene network by semi-fixed Bayesian network. *Expert Systems with Application,* Vol.30, No.1, (January 2006), pp. 42-49, ISSN 0957-4174

Longabaugh, W.J.R.; Davidson, E.H. & Bolouri, H. (2009) Visualization, documentation, analysis, and communication of large-scale gene regulatory networks. *Biochimica et Biophysica Acta,* Vol. 1789, No. 4, (April 2009), pp. 363-374, ISSN 0006-3002

Lukashin, A.V.; Lukashev, M.E. & Fuchs, R. (2003) Topology of gene expression networks as revealed by data mining and modelling. *Bioinformatics,* Vol. 19, No. 15, (October 2003) pp. 1909-1916, ISSN 1471-2105

Lulli, G. & Romauch, M. (2009) A mathematical program to refine gene regulatory networks. *Discrete Applied Mathematics,* Vol. 157, pp. 2469-2482, ISSN 0166-218X

Macdonald, P. (2001) Diversity in translational regulation. *Current Opinion in Cell Biology,* Vol. 13, No.3, (June 2001), pp. 326-331, ISSN 0955-0674

Matsuno, H. & Doi, A. (2000) Hybrid Petri net representation of gene regulatory networks. *Biocomputing 2000, Proceeding of the Pacific Symposium,* pp. 338-349, ISBN 981-238-598-3, Hawaii, USA, January 23-27, 2000

Mazzucotelli, E.; (2008) Abiotic stress response in plants: When post-transcriptional and post-translational regulations control transcription. *Plant Science,* Vol. 174, No. 4, (April 2008), pp. 420-431, ISSN 0168-9452

Médigue, C. & Moszer, I. (2007) Annotation, comparison and databases for hundreds of bacterial genomes. *Research in Microbiology.* Vol. 158, No. 10 (December 2007), pp. 724-736, ISSN 0923-2508

Mendes, P.; Sha, W. & Ye, K. (2003) Artificial gene networks for objective comparison of analysis algorithms. *Bioinforamtics,*Vol.19, No.2, pp. 122-129, ISSN 1460-2059

Mochizuki, A. (2008) Structure of regulatory networks and diversity of gene expression patterns. *Journal of Theoretical Biology.* Vol. 250, No. 2 (January 2008), pp.307-321, ISSN 0022-5193

Paulsson, J. (2005) Models of stochastic gene expression. *Physics of Life Reviews,* Vol.2, No.2, (June 2005), pp. 157-175, ISSN 1571-0645

Polynikis, A.; Hogan, S.J. & di Bernardo, M. (2009) Comparing different ODE modelling approaches for gene regulatory networks. *Journal of Theoretical Biology,* Vol. 261, pp. 511-530, ISSN 0022-5193

Pomerance, A.; Ott, E., Girvan, M. & Losert, W. (2009) The effect of network topology on the stability of discrete state models of genetic control. *PNAS,* Vol. 106, No. 20, (May 2009), pp. 8209-8214, ISSN 1091-6490

Qian, L. & Wang, H. (2007) Inference of genetic regulatory networks by evolutionary algorithm and H_ filtering. *14th IEEESP Workshop on Statistical Signal Processing SSP 07,* pp. 21-25, ISBN 9781424411979

Reed, J.L.; Famili, I., Thiele, I. & Palsson, B.O. (2006) Towards multidimensional genome annotation. *Nature Reviews Genetics,* Vol.7, (February 2006), pp. 130-141, ISSN 1471-0056

Rosenfeld, S. (2007) Stochastic cooperativity in non-linear dynamics of gene regulatory networks. *Mathematical Biosciences,* Vol. 210, No. 1, (November 2007), pp. 121-142, ISSN 0025-5564

Ruklisa, D.; Bramza, A. & Viksna, J. (2005) Reconstruction of gene regulatory networks under finite state linear model. *Genome Informatics,* Vol. 16, No. 2, pp. 225-236, ISSN 0919-9454

Rust, A.G.; Mongin, E., Birney, E. (2002) Genome annotation techniques: new approaches and challenges. *Drug Discovery Today*, Vol. 7, No. 11, (May 2002), pp. s70-s76, ISSN 1359-6446

Silvescu, A. & Honavar, V. (2001) Temporal Boolean Network Models of Genetic Networks and their Inference from Gene Expression Time Series. *Complex Systems*, Vol. 13, pp. 61-78, ISSN 0891-2513

Schlitt, T. & Brazma, A. (2005) Modelling gene networks at different organisational levels. *FEBS Letters*, Vol.579, No.8, (March 2005), pp. 1859-1866, ISSN 0014-5793

Shmulevich, I., Doughtery, E.R., Kim, S. & Zhang, W. (2002) Probabilistic Boolean networks: a rule-based uncertainty model for gene regulatory networks. *Bioinformatics*, Vol. 18, No. 2, pp. 261-274, ISSN 1460-2059

van Someren, E.P.; Wessels, L.F.A., Backer, E. & Reinders, M.J.T. (2002) Genetic network modeling. *Pharmacogenomics*, Vol. 3, No. 4, pp.507-525, ISSN 1462-2416

Smolen, P.; Baxter, D.A. & Byrne, J.H. (2000) Mathematical modelling of gene networks. *Neuron*, Vol. 26, (June 2000), pp. 567-580, ISSN 0896-6273

Steggles, L.J.; Banks, R., Shaw, O. & Wipat, A. (2007) Qualitatively modelling and analysing genetic regulatory networks: a Petri net approach. *Bioinformatics*, Vol.23, No.3, (March 2007), pp. 336-343, ISSN 1460-2059

Steggles, L.J.; Banks, R. & Wipat, A. (2006) Modelling and analysing genetic networks: From Boolean networks to Petri nets. *Lecture Notes in Computer Sciences*, Vol.42, (October 2006), pp. 127-141, ISSN 0302-9743

Strizh, I.; Joutchkov, A., Tverdokhlebov, N. & Golitsyn, S. (2007) Systems biology and grid technologies: Challenges for understanding complex cell signaling networks. *Futire Generation Computer Sytems*, Vol.23, No.3 (March, 2007), pp. 428-434, ISSN 0167-739X

Tegnér, J. & Björkegren, J. (2007) Perturbations to uncover gene networks. *Trends in Genetics*, Vol. 23, No. 1, (January 2007), pp. 34-41, ISSN 0168-9525

Wilczynski, B. & Furlong, E.E.M. (2010) Challenges for modelling global gene regulatory networks during development: insight from *Drosophila*. *Developmental Biology*. Vol. 320, No. 2, (April 2010), pp. 161-169, ISSN 1471-213X

Wu, F.X.; Zhang, W.J. & Kusalik, A.J. (2004) Modeling gene expression from microarray expression data with state-space equations. *Biocomputing 2004, Proceeding of the Pacific Symposium*, pp. 581-592, ISBN 981-238-598-3, Hawaii, USA, January 6-10, 2004

Xu, R.; Venayagamoorthy, G.K. & Wunsch, D.C. (2007) Modelling of gene regulatory netwoks with hybrid differential evolution and particle swarm optimization. *Neural Networks*, Vol. 20, pp. 917-927, ISSN 0893-6080

Yakunin, A.F.; Yee, A.A., Savchenko, A., Edwards, A.M., Arrowsmith, C.H. (2004) Structural proteomics: a tool for genome annotation. *Current Opinion in Chemical Biology*, Vol. 8, No. 1 (February 2004), pp. 42-48, ISSN 1367-5931

Yeo, Z.X.; Wong, S.T.,Vel Arjunan, S.N. Piras, V., Tomita, M., Selvarajoo, K., Guiliani, A. & Tsuchiya, M. (2007) Sequential logic model deciphers dynamic transcriptional control of gene expressions. *Plos One*, Vol. 2, No. 8 (August 2007), pp. 1-18, ISSN 1932-6203

Zak, D.E.; Vadigepalli, R., Gonye, E.G., Doyle, F.J., Schwaber, J.S. & Ogunnaike, B.A. (2005) Unconventional systems analysis problem in molecular biology: a case study in gene regulatory network modelling. *Computational and Chemical Engineering*, Vol.29, No.3, (February 2005), pp. 547-563, ISSN 0098-1354

6

Modern Methods Used in the Complex Analysis of the Phonocardiography Signal

Nicolae Marius Roman[1] and Stefan Gergely[2]
[1]*Technical University, Cluj-Napoca,*
[2]*National Institute for Research and Development of Isotopic and Molecular Technologies, Cluj-Napoca, Romania*

1. Introduction

Sometimes we need an accurate or approximate representation of a quantity in a different form; either the quantity is given by an analytical expression or by the finite set of values. Using transformations, we usually measure the similarity of a given function with an entire class of functions depending on one or more parameters (such as the frequency in the Fourier transform) which may change continuously or discretely. The wavelet representation is given in the space-frequency domain, opposite to the Fourier analysis that gives only a frequency representation. Compact supports of wavelets provide a space, and their oscillatory nature provides a frequency representation of a transformed function. It is clear that such representation is essential for the non stationary signal. The wavelet representation of a function has the multiresolution property, which means that it is given on several resolution scales. Details defined on various refinement levels (fine meshes) are added to the rough approximation determined on a coarse mesh. The dimension of the data set that store information about the function is considerably decreased while the most important information is not lost. This is very important for a good compression that saves storage in a system memory. A data compression is fundamental for an efficient analyzing of a signal with an extremely high noise density and a large variety of shapes (Abbas K.Abbas & Rasha Bassam, 2009).

If a compression scheme is lossless it can be always recover the entire original message by uncompressing then a compressed message that has the same total entropy as the original, but in fewer bits.

Another problem that has to be solved during the filtering process is the so called boundary distortion. This appears at the end samples of the signal because there are left fewer samples than multiplying coefficients. The easiest way to resolve this issue is to introduce zeros at the end of the signal. This does not affect the entropy of the iteration even if the signal is not following the original pattern. All the filtering processes are done by using of the wavelet transform.

Wavelet functions are localized both in frequency and in time domain by shifting and scaling function without a projection over the entire transformed signal. Another important aspect is that in terms of number of calculations which are necessary for the Fourier transform. The Fourier transform requires a number of $O(n \cdot log_2(n))$ operations instead of only $O(n)$ mathematical operations for the wavelet transform.

2. The fast wavelet transform

The approximation at the m+1 scale is given by equation 1

$$S_{m+1,n} = \int_{-\infty}^{\infty} x(t)\Phi_{m+1,n}(t)dt \tag{1}$$

by replacing 1 we get:

$$S_{m+1,n} = \int_{-\infty}^{\infty} x(t)\cdot\left[\frac{1}{\sqrt{2}}\sum_k c_k \Phi_{m,2n+k}(t)\right]dt \tag{2}$$

For a much better illustration, by rearranging the terms it yields:

$$S_{m+1,n} = \frac{1}{\sqrt{2}}\sum_k c_k\left[\int_{-\infty}^{\infty} x(t)\Phi_{m,2n+k}(t)dt\right] \tag{3}$$

and finally the approximation coefficient $S_{m,2n+k}$ for each k we get:

$$S_{m+1,n} = \frac{1}{\sqrt{2}}\sum_k c_k S_{m,2n+k} = \frac{1}{\sqrt{2}}\sum_k c_{k-2n} S_{m,k} \tag{4}$$

In a similar manner we get the wavelet detail coefficients:

$$T_{m+1,n} = \frac{1}{\sqrt{2}}\sum_k b_k S_{m,2n+k} = \frac{1}{\sqrt{2}}\sum_k b_{k-2n} S_{m,k} \tag{5}$$

As a result the equations 4 and 5 are forming the multi-resolution decomposition algorithm used in our paper.

2.1 Choosing the optimal wavelet function for the analysis of PGC

Every application which requires the using of a wavelet transform requires the adaptation or finding of a certain type of wavelet function. The first criterion is defined by the correlation factor between the wavelet function and the analyzed signal. Unfortunately the shape of the correlated wavelet function is capable to indicate only the family of wavelet functions but gives no indication regarding the number of the wavelet coefficients. To compute the necessary coefficient numbers, we used the wavelet toolbox of the Matlab program. The PCG signal is decomposed accordingly the algorithm shown in figure 1:

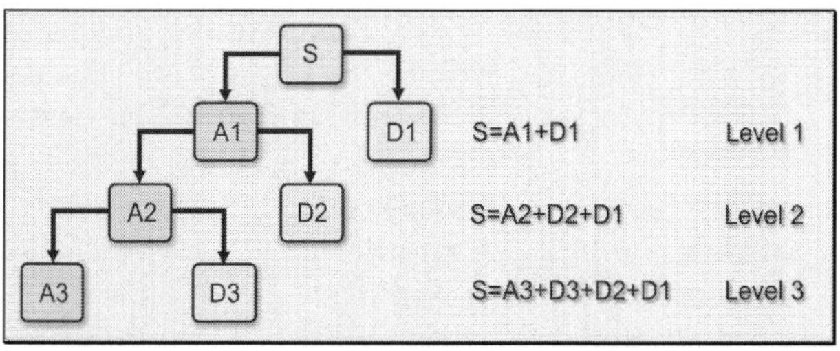

Fig. 1. Three level decomposition algorithm

A key criterion in determining the type of wavelet function consists in evaluation the overall reconstruction error, for the given type of signals that will appear in the application. So the evaluation must be made for signal reconstruction at the extreme in terms of spectral content. We imposed this condition for the decomposition algorithm to use a minimum number of coefficients, to optimize the convolution calculation time. Therefore the evaluation of the reconstruction error is done by using the functions from the Matlab toolbox which are shown in figure 2 (Gergely S., 2011).

```
load Normal;                   %Load file
s=Normal(1:32768);
[C,L]=wavedec(s,3,'db2');
A3=wrcoef('a',C,L,'db2',3)  %Computing the decomposition of level 3
D1=wrcoef('d',C,L,'db2',1);
D2=wrcoef('d',C,L,'db2',2);
D3=wrcoef('d',C,L,'db2',3);
sig=A3+D3+D2+D1;            %Reconstruction from signal parts
err=max(abs(s-sig));        %Error computation
```

Fig. 2. Evaluation of the reconstruction error

After computing the wavelet function we tested the validity of the selection by taking on all detail components of reconstructed signal and computing the reconstruction error. The goal was to find a maximum error therefore the maximum sensitivity of the wavelet function to the given input signal. The tables are presenting the overall computed errors which must be the lowest possible and the component extraction error which must indicate the highest sensitivity of the wavelet functions.

These two conditions are met by the Daubeschies db2 function. It seemed that this function did answer very well to the PCG signal which is a strongly polynomial type due the massive presence of arbitrary heart murmur signals. Due to the Matlab convention the db2 wavelet function is mathematically defined by four coefficients which are computed by using the orthogonally conditions along with a specially imposed condition which gives the smoothness of the Daubeschies functions

The Daubeschies functions family plays an important role in signal analysis because it is most often used to break down signals into sub-band components. Therefore the use of Db4 function requires the computation of the scaling coefficients. The scaling equation for a wavelet function having four coefficients is given by equation (6): (Gergely et al. 2011)

$$\Phi(t) = c_0\Phi(2t) + c_1\Phi(2t-1) + c_2\Phi(2t-2) + c_3\Phi(2t-3) \tag{6}$$

And the equation for the wavelet function is:

$$\psi(t) = c_0\psi(2t) - c_1\psi(2t-1) + c_2\psi(2t-2) - c_3\psi(2t-3) \tag{7}$$

Prof. Ingrid Daubeschies imposed a supplementary condition regarding the smoothness of the wavelet function which is given by equation 8:

$$\sum_{k=0}^{N_k-1} (-1)^k c_k k^m = 0 \tag{8}$$

For $m \in Z, m = 1,2,3,...,N_k / 2 - 1$. This means that the wavelet function can suppress or show up parts of the signal which are polynomial structure up to $N_k / 2 - 1$ grade, or better put out the signal parts that have a polynomial behavior. Finally by solving the system of equations shown in figure 3 it yields the solutions from table 1:

	c_0	c_1	c_2	c_3
$\Phi(t)$	$\frac{1+\sqrt{3}}{4}$ 0.6830	$\frac{3+\sqrt{3}}{4}$ 1.1830	$\frac{3-\sqrt{3}}{4}$ 0.3170	$\frac{1-\sqrt{3}}{4}$ -0.1830
$\Phi(-t)$	$\frac{1-\sqrt{3}}{4}$ -0.1830	$\frac{3-\sqrt{3}}{4}$ 0.3170	$\frac{3+\sqrt{3}}{4}$ 1.1830	$\frac{1+\sqrt{3}}{4}$ 0.6830

Table 1. Coefficients of the wavelet function

```
clear, syms c0 c1 c2 c3;

eq1='c0 +c1 +c2 +c3  = 2';
eq2='c0^2+c1^2+c2^2+c3^2 = 2';
eq3='c0 -c1 +c2 -c3  = 0';
eq4='  -c1+2*c2-3*c3  = 0';

[c0,c1,c2,c3] = solve(eq1,eq2,eq3,eq4,c0,c1,c2,c3);
disp('c0= '),disp(c0), disp( double(c0));
disp('c1= '),disp(c1), disp( double(c1));
disp('c2= '),disp(c2), disp( double(c2));
disp('c3= '),disp(c3), disp( double(c3));
```

Fig. 3. Equations system for solving the Daubeschies 4 coefficients

Therefore in the case of Daubeschies multiresolution algorithm we get:

$$S_{m+1,n} = \frac{1}{\sqrt{2}}\left(c_0 S_{m,2n} + c_1 S_{m,2n+1} + c_2 S_{m,2n+2} + c_3 S_{m,2n+3}\right) \tag{9}$$

By replacing with the computed coefficients, we get the final form:

$$S_{m+1,n} = 0.483 \cdot S_{m,2n} + 0.837 \cdot S_{m,2n+1} + 0.224 \cdot S_{m,2n+2} - 0.129 \cdot S_{m,2n+3} \tag{10}$$

In the same manner by replacing $b_k = (-1)^k c_{N_k-1-k}$ and also the computed coefficients in equation 5, it yields:

$$T_{m+1,n} = -0.129 \cdot S_{m,2n} - 0.224 \cdot S_{m,2n+1} + 0.837 \cdot S_{m,2n+2} - 0.483 \cdot S_{m,2n+3} \tag{11}$$

Equations 9 and 10 are used to compute the partial multiresolution decomposition up to level seven, which is used in the characterization of the PCG signals. The wavelet transform is done by using *Daubeschies 4* coefficients along with signal decimation by two. Another benefit of using the wavelet transform is due the filtering effect which reduces the bandwidth of the signal.

2.2 The time-frequency representation of PCG signals

A common situation which occurs in the analysis of the PCG signals is that the domains of signal frequency spectra are almost identical but the temporal distribution of spectral components is totally different. For this reason the frequency analysis requires a different approach to traditional methods. The main parameter that leads to differentiation of the two signals is the energy distribution in time domain, which is well evidenced by Parseval's relation given in equation 12:

$$\sum_{i=0}^{N-1} x[i]^2 = \frac{2}{N}\sum_{k=0}^{N/2} MagX[k]^2 \tag{12}$$

So the best approach is a non-stationary analysis of signal properties coupled with a time-frequency representation type. Wavelet representation is made in time-frequency domain opposed to Fourier analysis as only be effective in the frequency domain representation. The compact support offered by the wavelet transform allows the analysis by space and the oscillating character of a signal. This type of analysis is best suited for non-stationary signal type. Although apparently PCG signal is characterized by time periodicity of cardiac activity, the high frequency components of the signal spectrum are strongly marked by acoustic noise which is created by blood flow through vessels and cardiac valves. Wavelet representation of a function is characterized by multi-resolution property which means that it can be decomposed in several scales. By performing wavelet transform on a signal it results a considerably signal vector size decreases due to decimation by 2, at each level of transform. This is essential as a good signal compression to store transform in a low amount of available memory and having limited resources which is specific to the embedded type of microcomputers. The simulation software packages of the Matlab programming environment, offers a wide range of functions as a representation of time-frequency analysis but their export is generally possible only at the graphic level. The correct design of the time-frequency scalogram algorithm requires more detailed study of how the spectrum inversion occurs at the decimation by two of the wavelet high pass filter. Identifying the areas in which the frequency spectrum inversion occurs can be done by the representation of wavelet packet on several levels. In figure 4 it can be observed the inversion algorithm then takes place.

The time-frequency scalogram decomposition is actually a total multi-resolution analysis, so that the representation of time-frequency scalogram requires the correct reordering of the resulted spectrum fields. So it can be seen how the spectrum fields results from filtering G (high pass), following the decimation by 2 produces spectral inversion. Given the above observations, in figure 4 we can see another interesting phenomenon in the last decomposition, where the order of occurrence of the frequency domains follows a pattern similar to the Gray code (A.Jensen & A. la Cour-Harbo, 2001). Spectral range as natural frequency ordering is done by interpreting the initial results of permutations that are written in binary 000, 001, 011, 010, 110, 111, 101, 100 (the string of numbers marked in green).

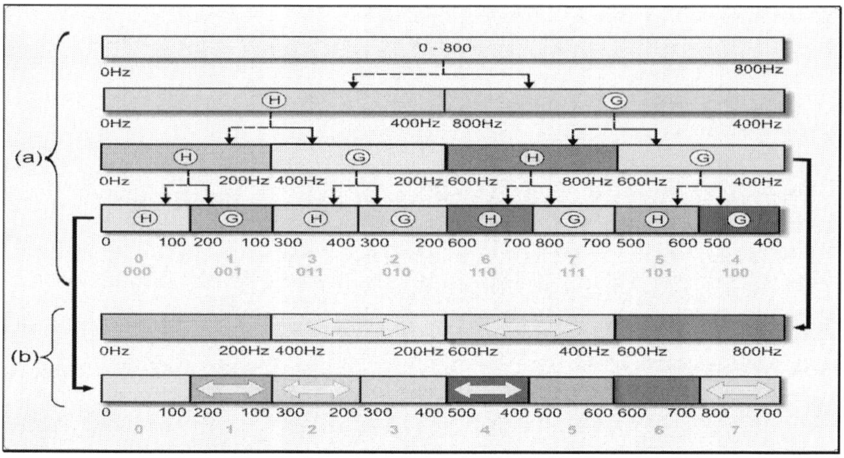

Fig. 4. (a) Wavelet packet order (b) natural order

An autonomous medical device witch is using a graphical color display, showing a time-frequency scalograme as a result of multiple wavelets transforms, is a very complex problem. To solve the implementation on a microcontroller, the specific problems associated with time-frequency representation have following steps:

a. Correct scaling of the calculated results of multi-resolution wavelet transforms on both x, y coordinates.
b. Calculation of the samples power average coefficient scaling.
c. Construction of time-frequency plane by allocating the appropriate memory addresses for each levels of decomposition.
d. Correction of the natural order of frequency representation. Due to decimation by 2 at each level of decomposition, the filtered frequency domain appears in the mirror.
e. Setting the calculated energy values to the equivalent RGB colors.
f. Converting data from the memory allocated time-frequency representation to a bxp type file. We assigned this type of graphics file to the DEM128160 display. The graphic conversion program between bmp files and bxp files were done by using the graphics library of the Embarcadero C + + program.

The time-frequency plane is used to describe the way in which the signal energy is distributed along the signal. The time-frequency scalogram is actually a full decomposition when analyzing multi-resolution, so that proper representation requires reordering the domain of the resulted spectrum. Spectral areas ordering by following the natural frequency, is done by interpreting the initial permutations results which are written in binary 000, 001, 011, 010, 110, 111, 101, 100. The new frequency order follows a Gray code pattern. It may be noted that Gray property type permutations is changing a single bit to change from one value to another. The computation of the time-frequency plane requires reiterating the wavelet transform routines for 254 times. The samples numbers of the original signal are decreasing to half after each transformation. Therefore the total amounts of required operations are 32768*7=229376 MAC instructions. At the level of the dsPIC30F6012 microcontroller the overall computing time is approximately 0.96 seconds. The displaying of the scalogram requires the construction of a special algorithm which is capable to calculate the addresses allocated to each pixel. The address of the first pixel is programmed for the upper left corner. This reference address position is convenient for standard graphics display and alphanumeric character set implementation.

In the case of the scalogram the standard display mode changes the addresses on the vertical axis by computing the interlaced Gray code addressing mode used to correct the spectral distribution. For a continuous representation throughout the full 62-800Hz spectral range, the algorithm displays only the spectral bands found in the decomposition of level 7. The displaying algorithm (Gergely et al.) of the time-frequency plane is shown in figure 5:

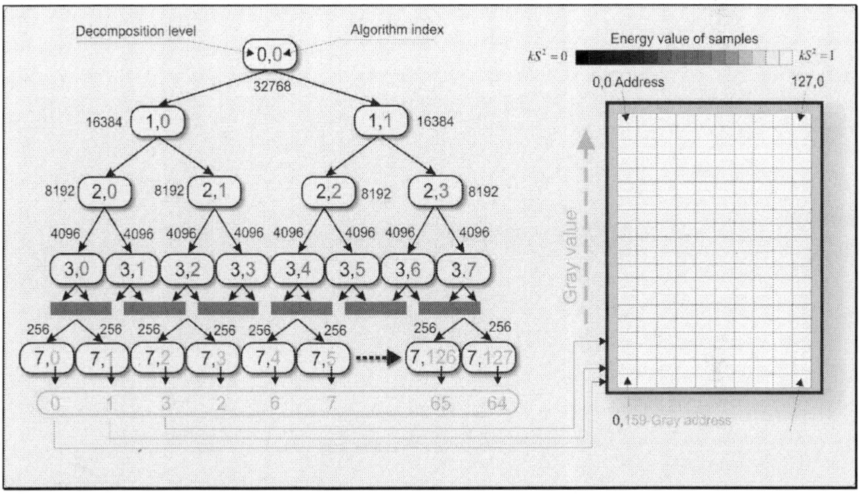

Fig. 5. Time-frequency plane algorithm

After the total decomposition the obtained frequency resolution is given by equation 13:

$$\Delta f = \frac{\Delta f_{Band}}{nr[INDEX_{dec}]} = \frac{800-62}{128} = 5.76Hz \tag{13}$$

Adding a further level of decomposition, increases the frequency resolution by increasing the number of bands, but also it occurs a lower temporal resolution by reducing the number of samples. This is a consequence of the principle that states that a time-frequency representation has an intrinsic limitation, as the product in time and frequency resolution is limited by Heisenberg's uncertainty principle which expresses the equation 14:

$$\Delta t \cdot \Delta f > \frac{1}{2} \tag{14}$$

Where Δt and Δf are given by equations 15 and 16:

$$\Delta t = \sqrt{\frac{\int t^2 |\psi(t)|^2 dt}{\int |\psi(t)|^2 dt}} \tag{15}$$

$$\Delta f = \sqrt{\frac{\int \omega^2 |\Psi(\omega)|^2 d\omega}{\int |\psi(\omega)|^2 d\omega}} \tag{16}$$

Where $\Psi(\omega)$ is the Fourier transform of base wavelet function $\psi(\omega)$

In figure 6 it is showed a few time-frequency scalograms obtained by using of the multi-resolution algorithm presented in figure 5.

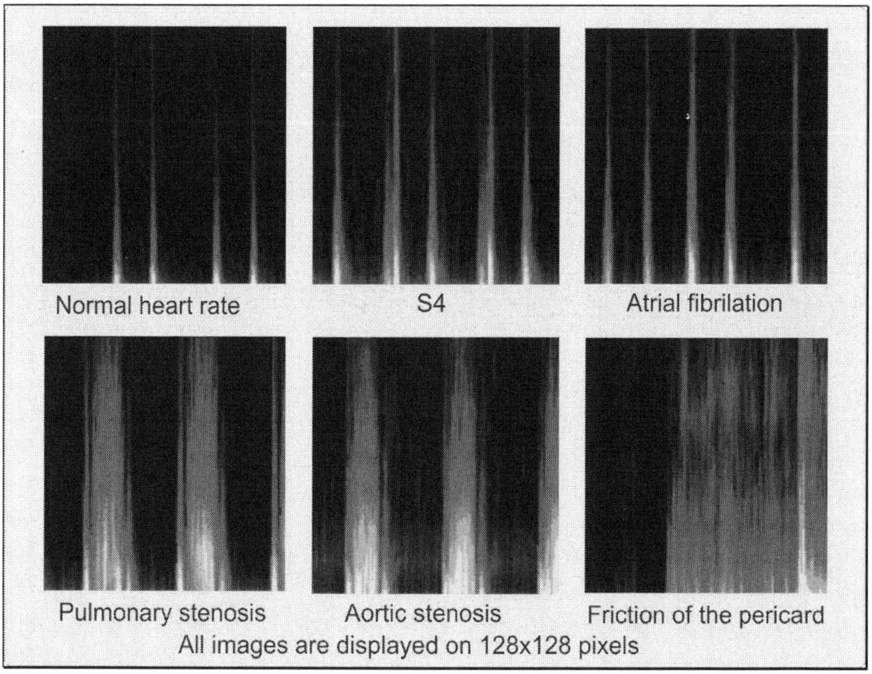

Fig. 6. Time-frequency scalograms of the acquired PCG signals

2.3 The Shannon multirate entropy in computing of the Euclidian distance of the PCG pathology

In information theory, entropy is a measure of the uncertainty associated with a random variable. In this context, the term usually refers to the Shannon entropy, which quantifies the expected value of the information contained in a message, usually in units such as bits.

Equivalently, the Shannon entropy is a measure of the average information content one is missing when one does not know the value of the random variable. In the wavelet transform theory the Shannon entropy is the measure for a cost function as how much decomposition has to be made to attain a full decomposition. After the signal decomposition, the level iterations contain a specific narrow signature reflected in the information content in a specific frequency band. At the end of the decomposition the signal is characterized by a number of Shannon's entropy coefficients. The first step in the characterization of the PCG signals is to compute the multi-resolution decomposition of the signal by using of the wavelet transform. The level at which the decomposition stops is given by the optimization is the number of calculations and the content of information of on levels below a certain threshold where it no longer pays a further decomposition. The multi-resolution wavelet decomposition shown in figure 7 presents a PCG signal with pathology. These representations are the result of simulations made under the National Instruments - LabWindows CVI platform without using any embedded software packages for the wavelet transform.

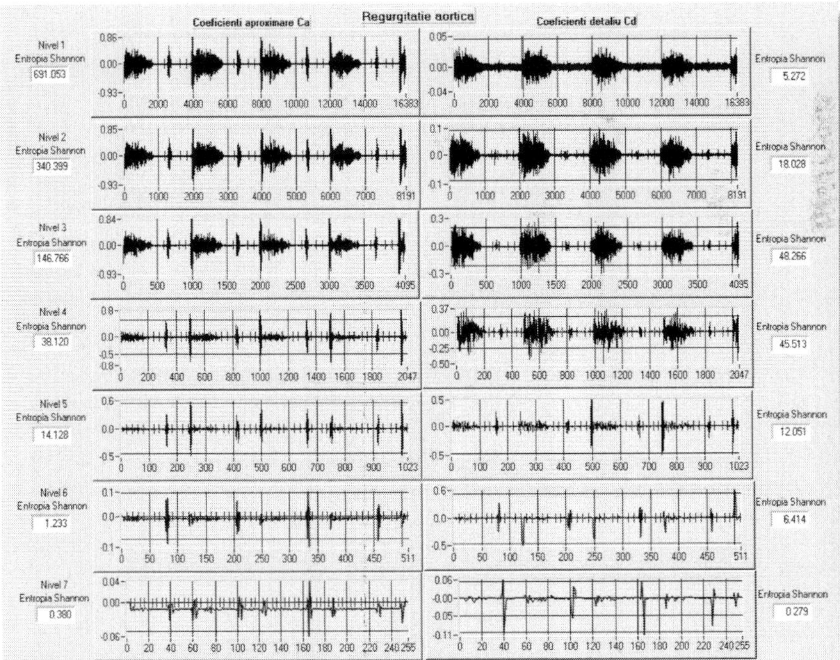

Fig. 7. Shannon entropy of PCG signal decomposition

Equation 17 (Gergely S., 2011) represents the matrix of a PCG signal which is decomposed on up to L levels and containing N samples for the original signal.

$$W_L(N) = \begin{vmatrix} c_{11} & c_{12} & c_{13} & c_{14} & \cdots & c_{1N} \\ c_{21} & c_{22} & c_{23} & \cdots & c_{2N/2} & 0 \\ c_{31} & c_{32} & \cdots & c_{3N/4} & 0 & 0 \\ c_{41} & c_{42} & \cdots & c_{4N/8} & 0 & 0 \\ \cdots & \cdots & \cdots & \cdots & \cdots & \cdots \\ c_{L,1} & c_{L,2} & \cdots & c_{L,N-2^L} & 0 & 0 \end{vmatrix} \tag{17}$$

Such a signal can be represented and stored using only 14 coefficients by replacing each line in the matrix with 2 coefficients obtained by computing the Shannon entropy of each individual level of decomposition. These two coefficients are taken from the above figure. By simulation of the calculation algorithms directly in C language, it was significantly reduced the time required to implement the DSP programs. For this reason, the code generation for the DSP microcontroller was used in another C compiler but with the same source code optimized for a different level of precision. Quantization errors which are inherent in floating point calculations do not alter the results because all evaluations were made by identifying only the minimum values of Euclidian distance. The Euclidian distance is computed by using equation 18:

$$d(p_{ij}, q_{ij}) = \sqrt{\sum_{i=1}^{m} \sum_{j=1}^{n} (q_{ij} - p_{ij})^2} \tag{18}$$

The signal coefficients are stored in the SD memory card in specific vectors (address) which represent the comparison reference for the recognizing process of the specific pathology. By using the Shannon entropy coefficients there is not necessary to store the entire pathology signals. These coefficients represent the compressed form of the pathology signals. The pathology signals have therefore specific spectral fingerprints which are used to compute the Euclidian distance between the stored reference vectors and the currently analyzed signal. By using the wavelet transform in the analyzing of *PCG* signals it is possible to compress and to preserve all time-frequency characteristics of the signals. On the other hand either time domain or frequency domain analysis does not fully describe the nature of non-stationary signal. A pathological *PCG* signal is dominated by the high frequency components along with the low frequency *S* type pulses. The statistical characterization method is usable only for a primary signal classification. A precise *PCG* signal characterization done with the intention of pathology recognizing, is possible only if a reference signal is in fact compared with the fully or partially acquired signal. The frequency content in the multilevel wavelet transform may well be evaluated by the information content of each level defined by the Shannon entropy which is presented in the following equation:

$$S = -\sum_{i=0}^{N} x_i^2 \log(x_i^2) \tag{19}$$

The estimation of the signals envelope as a final characterization is a difficult task that involves intensive computing resources. Therefore the algorithm was designed to be implemented on a device using *DSP* engine for the signal processing.

2.4 Correlation of the PCG signals

The correlation algorithm is using only the approximation coefficients of the wavelet transform. So that the question is which decomposition level is to be used for the signal correlation algorithm? The envelope of the signal must contain as much as possible amount of samples to get a specific pathology characterization. The property of the multilevel wavelet transform is that, each computed approximation coefficients do contain both the approximation and detail coefficients of the next level. The envelope of the PCG signal is computed by using the third level of signal decomposition which is shown in figure 8:

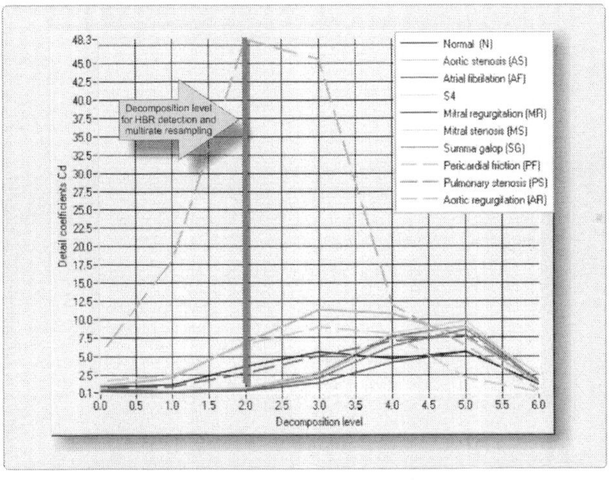

Fig. 8. Decomposition levels of the PCG signals

After all the issue is to test the correlation between the acquired signal and all reference signals that are stored in the *SD* card. Our studies showed that the heart beat rate does not affect the overall spectral density of the *PCG* signal. The Shannon sampling theorem has been extended to allow for sampling times which are not uniformly spaced (Gergely S., 2011; Fliege N.J., 1994). Several slightly different versions of the non-uniform sampling theorem have arisen. The differences lie in the spaces of functions being considered and the different classes of sampling times which are permitted. The theorem essentially says that a band-limited signal $x(t)$ is uniquely determined by knowledge of its samples $\{an = x(tn)\}$ as long as the sampling times $\{tn\}$ occur at a rate which is on average higher than the *Nyquist* rate. By compressing or expanding the signal the envelope remains shift able and also the resulted frequency variations are not important. The frequency content is previously analyzed by the using of the

Shannon entropy which classifies the *PCG* signal at each wavelet decomposition level. The complex overall algorithm is shown in figure:

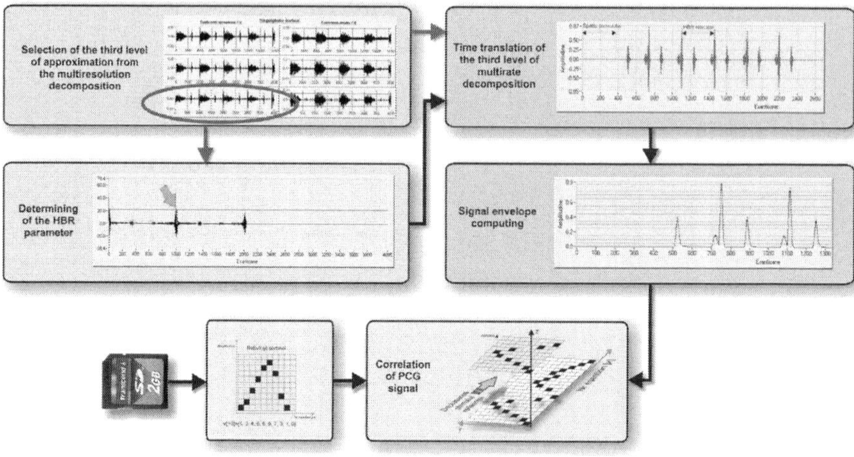

Fig. 9. PCG signal correlation algorithm

The above presented algorithm is capable to analyze the extremely complex structure of the PCG signal which is characterized by a signal envelope which is amplitude modulated and in the same time it is frequency modulated having specific and distributed "carrier" frequencies. The frequency band of the original PCG signal is limited extremely sharp by using a 512 coefficients FIR filter which follows the input anti-alias analog filter. The useful frequency band of the PCG signal is situated between 62-800 Hz.

The main difficulty in doing the correlation task is that, the acquired signal is never at the same *HBR* (Heart Beat Rate) like the reference signals; as a result the time shift will corrupt the peak value of the cross-correlation. All signal envelopes references are recorded at a known *HBR*, information which is stored in the file of each signal. In signal processing, auto-correlation is a measure of similarity of two waveforms as a function of a time-lag applied to one of them. This is also known as a sliding dot product or inner-product. It is commonly used to search a long duration signal for a shorter, known feature. The auto-correlation (Broersen Piet M.T., 2006). of the third level decomposition is done by using the equation:

$$R_{xx}(j) = \sum_{i} x_i x_{i-j} \tag{20}$$

The reason for which we have used the third level of decomposition instead of the original signal is because of the necessity to reduce the number of computation operations. By using the third level of decomposition, the overall computations are reduced by a factor of 64 due to the squaring of the samplings reduction which is at a factor of 8. The using of the cross-correlation is the only practical method to extract a certain sequence from a noisy PCG signal which is dominated by the murmur of the heart (Abdallah et al.,1988).. The resulted auto-correlation is shown in figure 10:

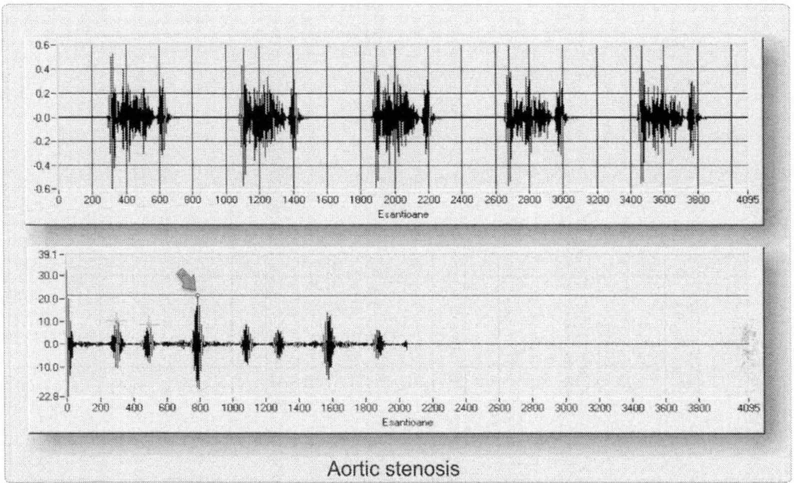

Fig. 10. Auto-correlation of the third level decomposed PCG signal

After the computing of the autocorrelation the HBR parameter is obtained with the equation 21:

$$HBR(beats/\min) = \text{int}\left(\frac{60 \cdot nW_3}{n[index] \cdot T_{sampling}} \right) \tag{21}$$

The correct cross-correlation is complete after the re-sampling of the acquired signal in accordance to the reference signal *HBR*. After re-sampling, the signal is interpreted as having the same original sampling rate. The necessary re-sampling rate is given by the ratio between the HBR parameter of the analyzed signal and the HBR parameter of the reference:

$$\frac{Sr \uparrow x(tn)}{Rr \downarrow x(tn)} = \frac{L}{M} = R_{Ratio} \tag{22}$$

Where L is the interpolation factor which means that between two consecutive signal samples there are inserted a number of L-1 zeros. M is the decimation factor which is always constantly equal with 100. Extensive simulations have proved that the algorithm is permissive to an R_{RAtio} from 0.43 to 0.99. The reference signal is always converted to a HBR equal to 100 before it is stored in the pathology data base. As a consequence the above algorithm has the drawback of using a lot of memory space in the systems memory.

The sensitive part of the overall algorithm is the interpolator used in the multirate sampling module. It turned out that the final correlation operation is obviously sensitive to the unmatched envelope. The issue is the lag over the real envelope of the computed values in case of a under filtering or a diminishing and distorted wave form in case of an over filtering. Therefore it was necessary to calculate the interpolation filter. The first step of using a linear interpolator has the ability of good low frequency attenuation but on the other hand the high frequency components of the envelope signal are slightly distorted. Finally we have preferred a FIR filter. The usually used two filters for the re-sampling process is reduced to a single filter which is chosen by using equation 23; (Fliege N.J., 1994)

$$\theta_c = \min\left(\frac{\pi}{L}, \frac{\pi}{M}\right) \tag{23}$$

At the third level of signal decomposition the new sampling rate is interpreted as 1000 Hz

The frequency domain which must be covered by the filters is shown in figure 11:

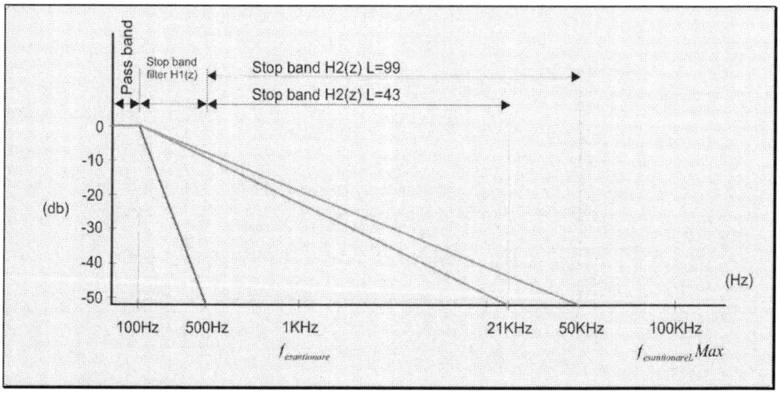

Fig. 11. Frquency domain of the multirate sampling filter

Therefore the imposed conditions to the re-sampling filter are:

1. Pass band 0÷100Hz
2. First stop band 100÷500Hz
3. Second pass band 0÷100Hz
4. Second stop band 500Hz÷50KHz
5. Pass band ripple 0.02db
6. Stop band attenuation 53db
7. Used window: Hamming

Below are presented the equations used to compute the interpolation filter:

The impulse response of the low pass filter is given by equation 24:

$$h(n) = \begin{cases} \frac{\Omega_c}{\pi} & n = 0 \\ \frac{\sin(\Omega_c n)}{n\pi} & \text{for } n \neq 0 \text{ , } -M \leq n \leq M \end{cases} \tag{24}$$

The filter coefficients are weighted with the Hamming window:

$$w_{Ham}(n) = 0.54 + 0.46\cos\left(\frac{n\pi}{M}\right) \quad \text{where } -M \leq n \leq M \tag{25}$$

$$h_w(n) = h(n) \cdot w_{Ham}(n) \tag{26}$$

The number of filtering coefficients is computed with equation 6.8

$$\Delta f = \frac{f_{STOP} - f_{PASS}}{f_{sampling}} \tag{27}$$

$$N = \frac{3.3}{\Delta f_{sampling}} \tag{28}$$

The cutting frequency does not depend on the interpolation factor L and is given by:

$$f_t = \frac{f_{PASS} + f_{STOP}}{2} = 300Hz \tag{29}$$

For HBR between 43 - 99

$$R_{Ratio} = \frac{HBR_{aquired}}{HBR_{ref}} \tag{30}$$

Where HBR_{ref} =100

It yields for L interpolation factor between 43 to 99 a number of 355 to 817 coefficients.

For the above mentioned R_{Ratio} interval we got a number of coefficients between 355 and 817. The result of the re-sampling process is shown in the figure 12. These values aren't large in comparison to the permanently used 512 coefficients in the overall band pass filter. All these coefficients are stored in the program memory of the DSP microcontroller.

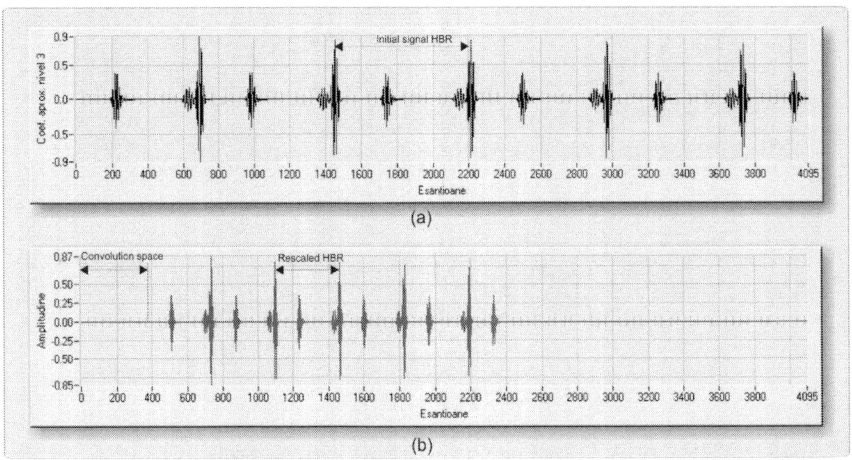

Fig. 12. Time compression of the PCG signal by using the third level of decomposition

2.5 Computing of the PCG signals envelope

Hilbert transform is a process which is capable to extract the precise envelope of a given signal. Generating a signal in the complex domain and out of phase by 90 degrees from the real signal provides a series of numerical processing such as quadrature modulation and demodulation of signals, and the implementation of automatic gain control systems. Time and frequency representation shows how the Hilbert transform cosine signal spectral component rotates with -j and the negative component by +j. An important property of the Hilbert transform is that it is a theoretical system with frequency response magnitude one and phase equal to 90 degrees for all frequencies. This means that a signal passing through a Hilbert system will be weighted by $\sqrt{2}$ the amplitude and phase will be modified by ¼ the period T. If a real signal $x_r(t)$ is modulated in amplitude, then the modulated signal envelope is that it contains the useful information. So the instantaneous envelope E(t) becomes:

$$E(t) = |x_c(t)| = \sqrt{x_r(t)^2 + x_i(t)^2} \tag{31}$$

The above equation is the envelope of the modulator signal and is used to calculate also the PCG signal envelope. Traditional signal demodulation of amplitude modulated signal consists of previously rectifying the signal by squaring and applying a smoothing low pass filter for the carrier frequency. This type of demodulation has been tested for PCG signal envelope but a comparison shows that the voltage ripple obtained by Hilbert transform is clearly in favor. The filter ripple for both methods is shown in figure 13:

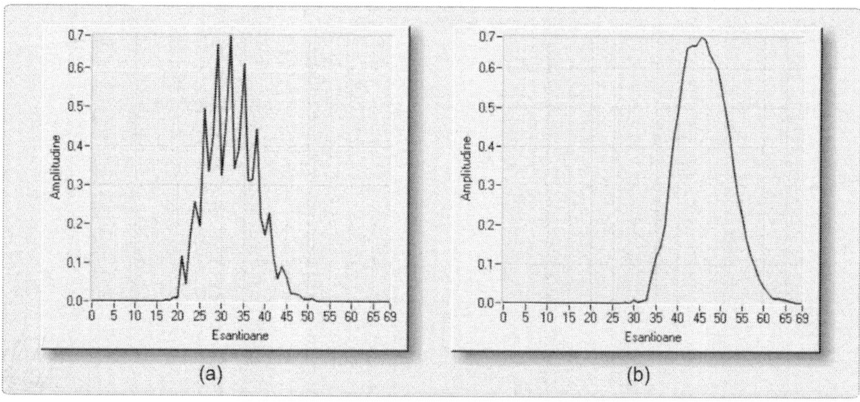

Fig. 13. Voltage ripple (a) Squaring method (b) Hilbert transform

In terms of the number of calculations required, the Hilbert transform method is faster because it involves the using of a filter with a lower number of coefficients.

Implementation of Hilbert transform involves the calculating of the impulse response of a system considered linear. So that for arbitrary signal:

$$h(t)=\frac{1}{2\pi}\int_{-\omega_s/2}^{\omega_s/2}H(\omega)e^{j\omega t}d\omega=\frac{1}{2\pi}\int_{-\omega_s/2}^{0}je^{j\omega t}d\omega+\frac{1}{2\pi}\int_{0}^{\omega_s/2}-e^{j\omega t}d\omega \tag{32}$$

$$=\frac{1}{2\pi t}\left(e^{j0}-e^{-j\omega_s t/2}-e^{-j\omega_s t/2}+e^{j0}\right)=\frac{1}{\pi t}\left[1-\cos(\omega_s/2)\right] \tag{33}$$

For a discrete signal the above result has to be adapted, therefore the final form is given by equation 34:

$$h(n)=\frac{f_s}{\pi n}\left[1-\cos(\pi n)\right] \tag{34}$$

For $n\neq 0,\ and\ \left[h(n)=0, pentru\ n=0\right]$ where

n is the time domain index,
f_s is the sampling rate in samples/second

The impulse response of the Hilbert transform is shown in figure 14:

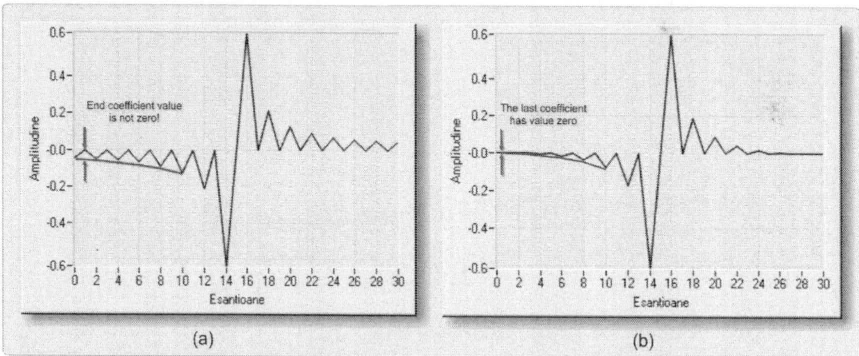

Fig. 14. (a) Impulse response of the Hilbert transform (b) using of a Blackman window

It is possible to use a signal envelope in the evaluation process of the PCG signal because the algorithm does not care about the frequency spectrum of the original signal. The frequency spectrum of the signal was previously evaluated in a probabilistic manner by the Shannon entropy. The Hilbert transform is software implemented by computing the filtering coefficients using the finite impulse response of the transform.

Therefore the FIR coefficients are computed by replacing the n index in the above equation. Choosing an odd number of coefficients is an essential criterion because of the center tap of the signal phase condition. To improve the low frequency response of the Hilbert transform we used a supplementary Blackman window. The Hilbert transform implementation is shown in figure 15:

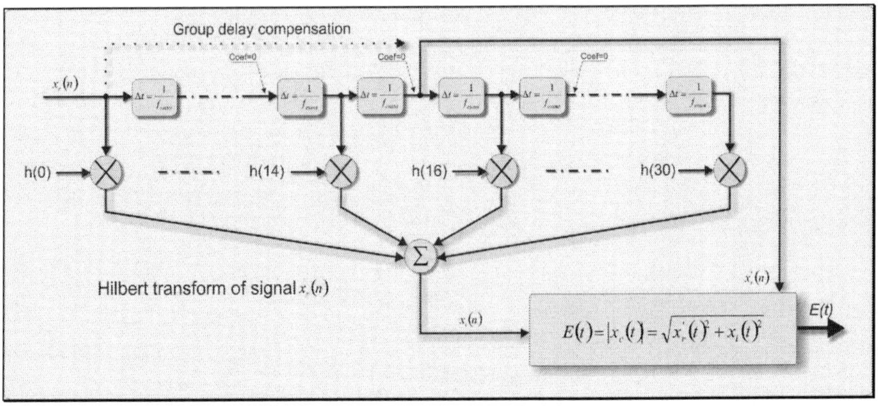

Fig. 15. Software implementation of the Hilbert transforms

The results by using the Hilbert transform are shown in figure 16. It can be observed the almost perfect envelope of a signal having a complex frequency spectrum below the detected envelope. The Hilbert transform does not influence the peak value of the signal which is an important feature of the envelope extraction procedure.

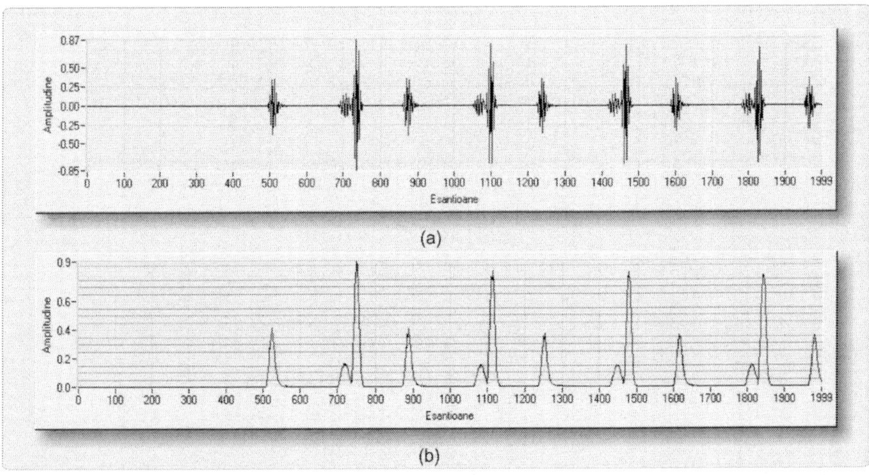

Fig. 16. Envelope detection of the PCG signal

Due to the complex structure of the PCG signal which is characterized by the presence of a large number of distributed peak values, it was necessary to introduce supplementary information regarding the amplitude of the signal. During the researches we applied a new method to analyze the PCG signal by introducing an additional coordinate to the signal vector which is visible in picture 17. The idea is that we switched to two-dimensional analysis similar to pattern recognition located in an image (Andrew K.Chan & Steve J.Liu, 1998). Thus the points defined in terms of measured values X0Y are introducing a second dimension of the signal and can thus be interpreted as an image. Reducing the number of calculations required to scale the amplitude vector x[t] for a number of dots (pixels).This type of resulted image can be processed by using advanced image processing methods. On a closer analysis, there is an important feature which allows to limit one of the coordinates of the vector w[y][x]. It can be observed that both signals involved in the algorithm are scaled to the same number of values on the Y coordinate, which provides a significantly higher computing speed. This was imposed because the simple convolution of the reference signal with the analyzed signal in order to get the pathology correlation is not efficient. The solution to the problem was to convert the one dimensional signal vector to a two-dimensional vector which at the end represents a graphical image of the PCG signal (Anke Meyer-Base, 2004). The conversion starts with the dividing of the sample amplitude to a given number of desired vertical pixels. If the value is in the computed domain it will be replaced by the value of 1, or if the value is outside of the domain it becomes zero. The signal conversion process is shown in figure 17.

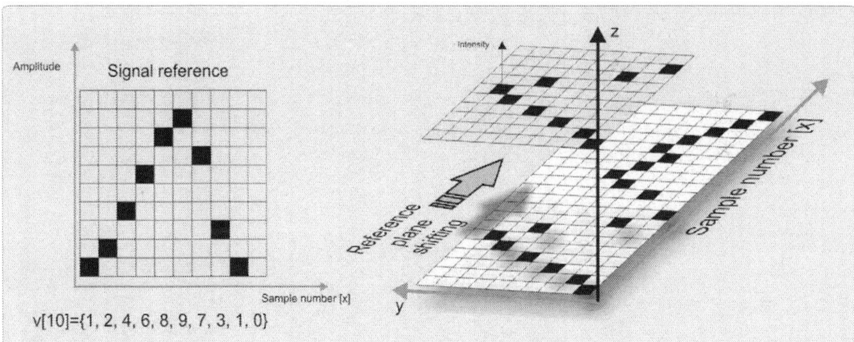

Fig. 17. Two-dimensional conversion of the PCG signal

By extending the method it is possible to give a different magnitude to different image segments by inserting different values instead of ones. As a result the image performs as a picture having a new z coordinate. The modified method makes possible the transformation from absolute pathology detection to a probable type of detection which is useful for primary pathology classification. This way the PCG signal image of the envelope is processed by using conventional image processing algorithms.

The extraction of the PCG signal references is done using a custom designed program which is fully interactive and provides the necessary support for the archiving of the results. All extracted reference vectors are stored in the SD card of a hand held device. The amount of necessary memory to store a reference image does not exceed 2KB. Some reference images are shown in figure 18:

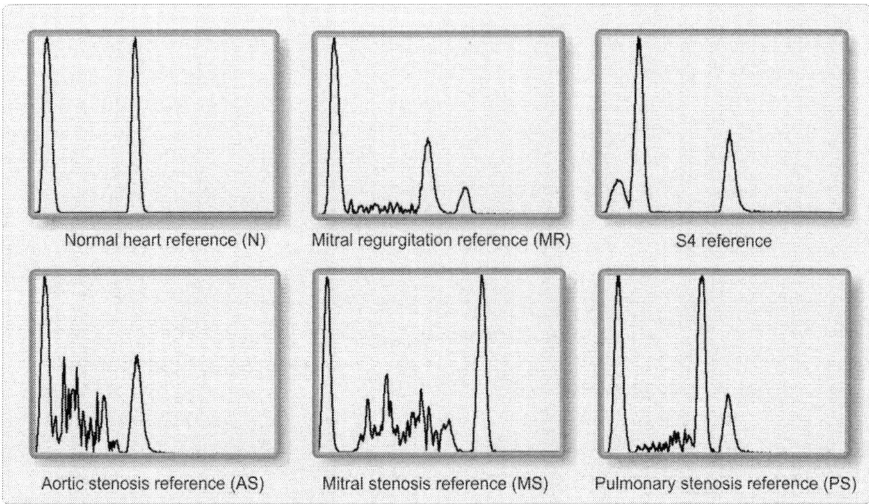

Fig. 18. PCG signals reference images

Pathology reference images were extracted from the real signals and shows how easy it can be identified with the pathology of origin. The obtained signals does resemble with the well known EKG signals. All noises under the signals envelope were eliminated for a better pathology exploration. By computing the Euclidian distance in order to evaluate the correlation between these reference signals and the analyzed signals, finally we got a nearly perfect match which is shown in figure 19:

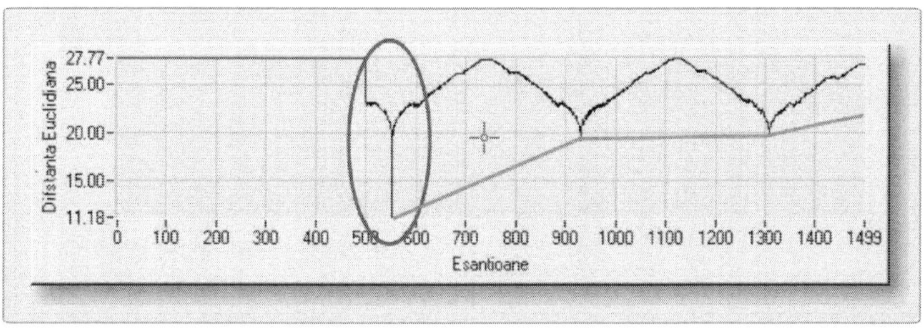

Fig. 19. Perfect correlations of two PCG signals

The construction of the above shown algorithm is achieved through a very simple calculation routine that consists only of a few lines of program. Reference signals were rescaled to 1Volt for a total of 50 points. The x axis number of points remains unchanged against the original signal and dynamically allocated between 100 and maximum 350 points. Under these conditions the reference image is represented in a matrix of 50x350 points. To test the recognition algorithm, the routine uses computer generated pixels of the image without intensity parameter Z (pixel has value 1) and no interpolation therefore a minimum number of points. The lowest number of points (42) is contained by the reference of normal heart rhythm. Analogous to the procedure for the reference signal, it applies the same above procedure for the analyzed signal. As a pattern recognition method, we have used the computation of the Euclidian distance between the analyzed signal and the stored references.

3. Construction of a PCG signal analyzer device

The equipment's operating system (Gergely S., 2011) is programmed to handle internal data flow between its component microcontrollers, communication with the outside through the USB port and graphics system. An important component of the program management module for distributing data is between the two microcontrollers. The operating system was designed to allow on board test routines running for the speed performance evaluation of the development system. The hardware system connects to a PC via USB2 interface which is managed by its own program, designed specifically for this application. The host program was implemented in LabWindows CVI which is capable to load into RAM or SD card any routine to emulate the original data in the DSP microcontroller. The resulting data are then transmitted back to the PC for evaluation. This was required because between the programs which are running on your PC and development board are differences in the computing precision. While DSP microcontroller does run routines with the precision given by organizing the data in Q1.15 format, all written routines in LabWindows CVI for the initial simulation are in double precision. The hardware uses a dsPIC30F6012 microcontroller with built-in DSP unit and a PIC18F4550 microcontroller equipped with built-in USB (Gergely S., 2011; Axelson Jan, 2006) full speed mode.

The hardware set of elements which are entering in the composition of the DSP module are specialized for rapid calculation of the amount of products. This equation is fundamental in digital signal processing and mathematical point of view is based on the convolution operation. The development is designed so that it carries out all processes signal analysis using equation 35:

$$S = \sum_{i=0}^{N-1} a_i b_i \tag{35}$$

Recursive FIR filter implementation can be done easily by using modulo addressing type programming which after computing the values; it provides the return address used for the filter coefficients. Hilbert transform calculation assumes a similar algorithm but to simplify modulo addressing type, due to the small amount of Hilbert coefficients the zero values are inserted in the looping list.

The DSP microcontroller has two direct hardware implemented instructions to compute the Euclidian distance with or without accumulation (ED and EDAC). The minimum value for the distance measured to all references represents the match with the analyzed signal. The data stored on the SD card is downloaded via the USB.

The experiments were made using the internal 12 bit ADC converter. The final objective was to construct an algorithm capable of discriminate between certain pathological situations. The measured frequency band of the phonocardiography signal is between 62Hz to 800Hz. The chosen sampling frequency is a standard 8 KHz. As a result the sampling frequency is much higher than the required Nyquist criterion. This way the aliases are pushed far from the used frequency band. The over-sampling is the best way to design a low order anti-alias analog filter for the input. After the acquisition process the signal is normalized to an amplitude of ±1V or in other words is converted to the Q15 binary signed fraction representation which means 0x7FFF (32767) to 0x8000 (-32768). This way any multiplying with the normalized filtering coefficients does not exceed the value of 1. Obviously because the ADC has only 12 bits the over range risk is less likely.

During the acquisition of the PCG signal the samples are previously filtered with a 512 taps FIR band pass filter to cut under 60db the low frequency noises generated by the patient moving along with the operators hand moving. The presence of the FIR filter is crucial due to the necessity of a band limited signal required by the wavelet transform. The DSP engine is well suitable for the fast computing of the required convolution between the acquired signal and the filtering coefficients. This is a similar process to any FIR or IIR filter which is a familiar in digital signal processing (Emmanuel C. Ifeachor & Barrie W. Jervis, 2002). The wavelet filter uses the hardware implemented MAC (Multiply Accumulate) instruction. Usually by design the FIR filter coefficients are symmetrical, having one or two middle values identical. In the case of the wavelet filter a special attention requires the correct order of indexing the filtered signal coefficients, because of the non-symmetrical coefficient values. In case of a wrong order or array flipping, the process of the convolution ends with a cross-correlation with unexpected output values. This is happening because the two DSP processes are mathematically related. Thus the memory address of the hardware DSP circular buffer of the coefficient data memory space has to be initiated properly. The wavelet filtering process starts with the saving of the stored data to a SD memory card, card preferable FAT formatted for direct file writing-reading. Each filtering iteration is done first for the approximation coefficients and secondly for the detail coefficients. After the iteration is done the sample number is half of the original signal or the previous approximation coefficients. The results are stored back to the memory card and this way the DSP processes may possibly be tested through the systems USB connectivity by an external PC. The overall necessary processing time for a scale index equal with 7 but only on the wavelet tree is equal to 12.5s, including al the read and write time to the SD memory card. In case of using a large static RAM instead of a SD memory card the overall time goes down to 25ms. The system is equipped with a color LCD display therefore is capable of displaying the signals coefficient scalogram in a complex time-frequency representation. The Daubeschies 4 coefficients are used in a similar manner to compute the wavelet transforms, but the circular buffer is addressed in a way that the resulted signal coefficients are decimated by two.

For a much shorter name using, the two microcontrollers are called "north" and "south". These two units are controlled by an operating system which is embedded in the south microcontroller. The south microcontroller is slower but it has the USB communication module. This module makes possible the firmware update via the USB port or a fast data exchange between the device and the host PC program. The structure of the operating system is presented in figure 20:

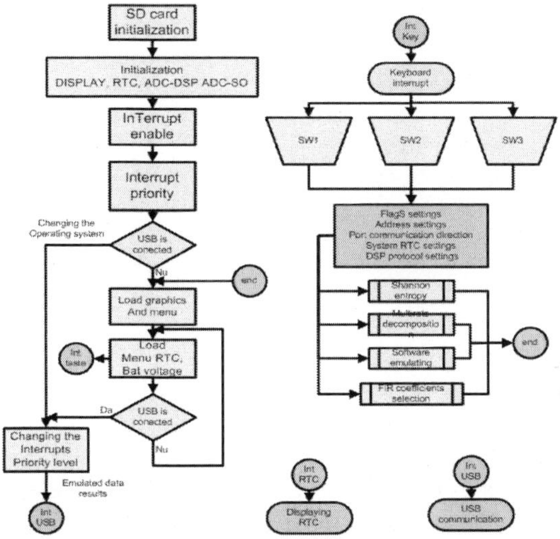

Fig. 20. The structure of the operating system

The above mentioned operating system is an ideal structure which makes possible a separate development of the DSP computing routines. At the end the final program structure can be embedded in one single DSP microcontroller. In that case the system requires an external USB hardware. All resulted data and graphics are displayed on a 1.8″ color LCD. This 128x160 pixels display is sufficient for a small portable unit but if the user wishes all graphical data may be transferred to a host PC for a much better image resolution. The display uses a Himax HX8345-A controller which has to be programmed through the 18 bit parallel port. It turned out that the initial high color depth is useless in the application; therefore this was downgraded to 65536 color levels by reducing the bit number of the parallel port. The hardware bus configuration is shown in figure 21:

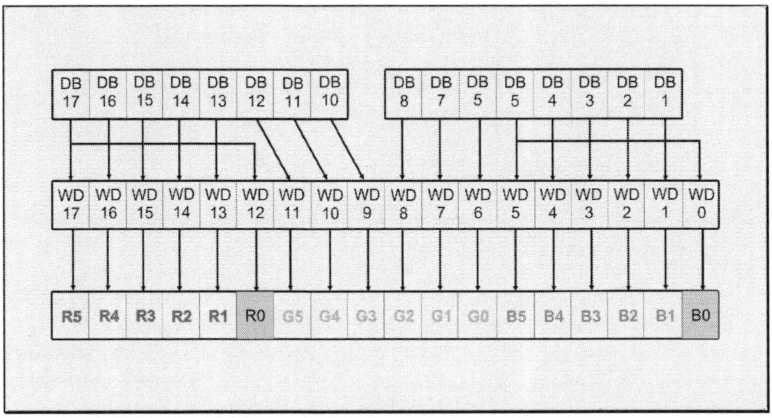

Fig. 21. Configuration of the reallocated parallel port

For data displaying it was built a custom designed character set which is structured on 13xW pixels where the W parameter may vary from 4 to 8. By using a dynamically allocated character width, the displayed text does have a much realistic appearance. The device uses also some graphics which uses a BMP structure. The conversion of the images from 18 bit to 16 bit RGB565, required the design of a auxiliary conversion program which makes also possible the transferring of the raw bmp pictures to the SD card of the device. For intermediary data storage the device is using a 4Mb static RAM addressed in a 16 bit structure. The memory can be addressed by both microcontrollers but the data flow is managed by the south master microcontroller. In order to avoid bus conflicts the system uses two buffered data transceivers. The south microcontroller can address the RAM only indirectly because of the 19 bit port which is generated by the DSP north microcontroller. The structure of how the RAM is accessed is shown in figure 22:

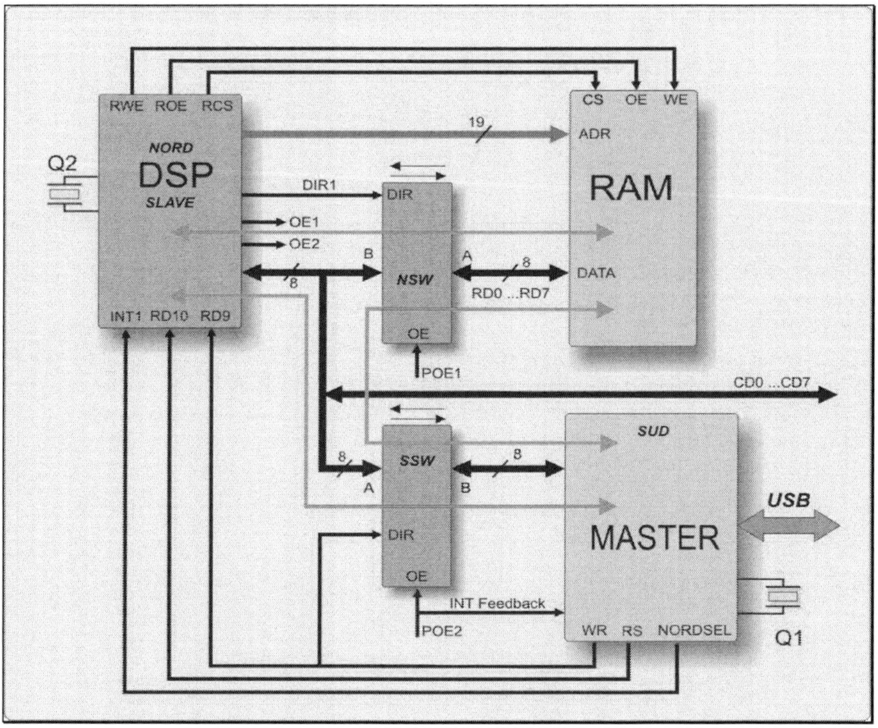

Fig. 22. RAM accessing protocol

As it can be seen in the above picture, the DSP microcontroller may well access RAM directly, but entering into this routine is subject to the interrupt generated by the master microcontroller. Meaning the data is controlled by setting the direction of the data access switches SSW and NSW. For optimal control of data flow and to avoid transfer conflicts, the master microcontroller will set that directly or indirectly the access to RAM, by the DSP microcontroller through SW-NSW. To increase the transmission speed we preferred the use of a parallel transmission protocol instead of the SPI transmission. Of course this mode of transmission does increase complexity of the designed hardware. NORDSEL signal selects DSP microcontroller which answers after interruption by turning on SSW that generates parallel port command words transfer by activating RS. If the sent command to the DSP is to acquire an acquisition, than it can communicate directly to RAM. After transmission, the DSP microcontroller sends an interrupt to the south POE2 confirmation signal. The answer will be change south direction by activating the DSP to send other commands. Data transfer between the south microcontroller and the RAM memory is done indirectly by DSP microcontroller.

Data obtained during the execution of signal processing routines and all graphical elements are stored on a SD memory card or MMC card. In this way the available system memory is practically unlimited given the fact that the 32-bit addressing way allows access to 4GB of memory. The memory card can have access to FAT16 or as access to physical memory sectors. Because the FAT protocol is a copyright of Microsoft Corporation, yet we preferred to access the SD card memory as physical memory. Of course in this way, only the host PC can access the card by using a proprietary memory structure. The advantage of this mode of operation is having a full control of stored data without the possibility of unauthorized copying of the content. Bringing the SD card in active state and data transferring to memory is done according to a predetermined by the manufacturer protocol, which includes a series of command words. Also the speed of accessing the SPI communication protocol is critically dependent on the state in which the SD card is accessed. A series of data related to memory capacity, internal organization and memory speed are programmed in a sometimes inaccessible memory area, which is equivalent to hard disks MBR. The organization by predefined memory sector structure is similar to a hard disk. The major difference from a hard disk access speed is very limited on some models. The Best SD cards reach a speed of 20MB/sec but the slower may be under 250Kb/sec. For this reason the SD memory card is the slowest element in the operating system which was taking into account at the design of software routines. The SD card memory of the designed prototype is organized as shown in figure 23:

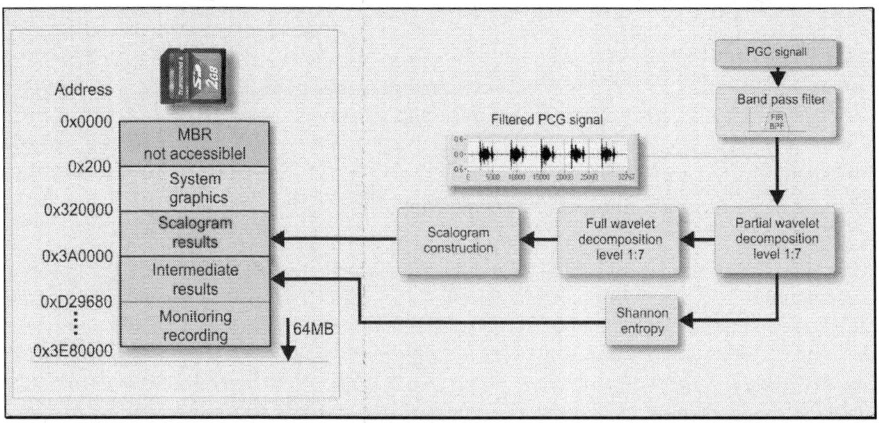

Fig. 23. Data structure of the SD card memory

SPI interface is based on a different protocol, not using the native mode of communication used by the SD card. This interface allows the use in advantageous terms on a SD card SPI port type that is found as a peripheral module in all modern microcontrollers. The communication protocol of an SD card consists of two types of data. Initialization and normal operation involves sending a first set of codes in the form of control bytes followed by receiving a response. That way the established communication type between a SD card and a host microcontroller becomes bidirectional. The control data packet which is transmitted between the SD card and microcontroller has a fixed length of 6 bytes as shown in figure 24.

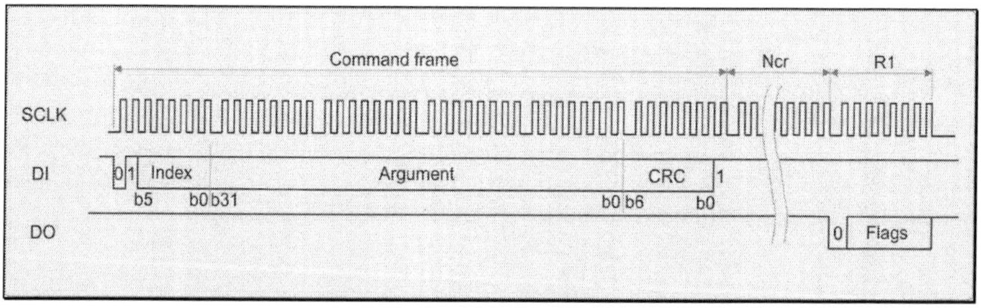

Fig. 24. Data packets in SPI transmission mode

After sending a control packet to the card, the microcontroller will receive a response R1, R2 or R3; because data transfer is ensured by generating a clock signal, the host must always send a false 0xFF byte type to keep the communication channel active. The allocated response time after sending a command packet (NCR) of the SD card has a length of 0-8 bytes. Ultimately the CRC field is optional to check the validity of data and becomes critical only when using high-speed transmission between host and SD card. To ensure compatibility with SD cards having limited capacity, the application design does not use CRC field because the transmission rate was reduced to a rate of 250Kb. Normally, this rate of transmission can use a minimum speed 400Kb. The necessary condition for the activation of the SD card is to exceed the power supply voltage value of 2 volts then that CS and DI is set to high level for at least 170 SCLK transmitted clock periods. Immediately after activating the card, it can receive native commands. After activating the card it will receive automatically a soft reset. This sets the SPI port system clock to 100 KHz and it is send CMD0 with CS at low level for entry into reset mode. After entry into SPI mode the host will switch off the SD card verification CRC. After acceptance of commands CMD0 the card goes in idle mode. Switching to Idle mode takes up to 400ms while the card is not accessible to the host microcontroller.

The hardware of the device is divided in two parts which are separated by the independent microcontrollers. The DSP microcontroller uses an 80MHz clock frequency which makes possible a real time FIR filtering of the input signal by using of 512 coefficients in about 18μs for every sample. Obviously, that the FIR filtering is used following the anti-alias filtering of the input signal. The supplementary FIR filtering is necessary to avoid the occurrence of frequency artifacts during the wavelet filtering. The hardware structure of the device is shown in figure 25:

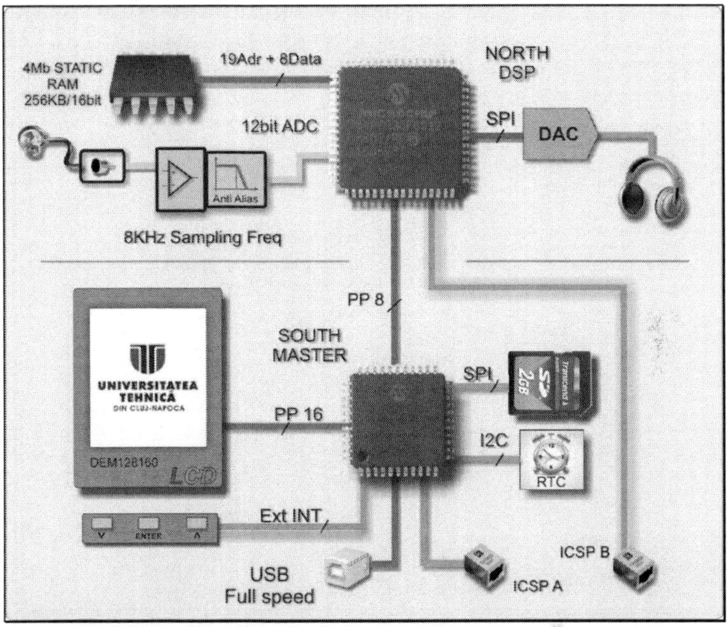

Fig. 25. Hardware structure of the PCG signal analyzer

The preconditioning of the PCG signal is completed by using a 6th order Sallen-Key filter which has to cut all unwanted frequency harmonics below 72db at the half of the sampling frequency. That way the 12bit analog-digital converter is acquiring a clean non-aliased signal. The frequency response of the combined anti-alias and FIR filter is presented in figure 26. It can be observed the outstandingly sharp, band-pass characteristic of the overall filter.

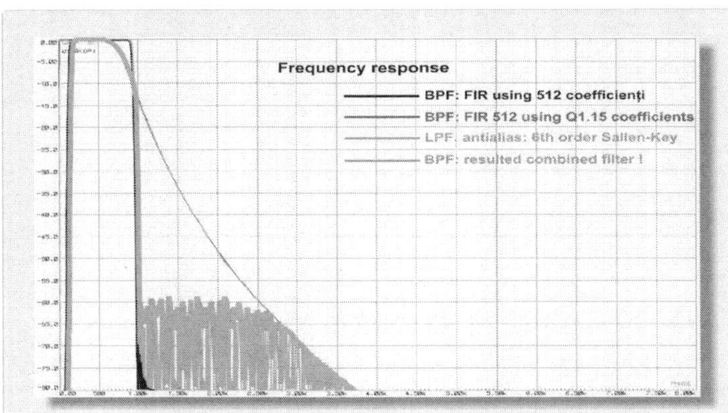

Fig. 26. Frequency response of the signal preconditioning module

The device is equipped also with a digital-analog converter which converts in real time the acquired and filtered signal into sound through a headphone amplifier. Therefore the device is capable to offer to the physician the possibility of standard auscultation along with recording and storing the data.

The input FIR filter can be chosen to obtain the emulated "Bell", "Diaphragm" or "Band-pass" characteristics of a standard stethoscope. The working device is shown in figure 27:

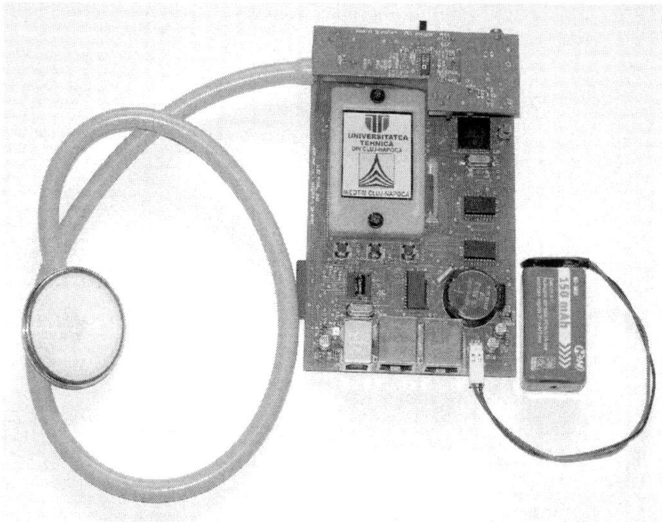

Fig. 27. The working prototype of the PCG signal analyser

The device uses a friendly menu equiped with sufficient graphical elements. This feature is important because it helps the medical staff for a quick use of the device without the need of a instruction manual by using a clear explanatory demo.

For the same purpose the interface uses a keyboard of only three keys which meaning are automatically configured. After boot-up the system displays a waiting image, the time (RTC) and the voltage of the power supply. For the moment by selecting the main menu, the system displays the working menu which makes possible the selection of the implemented program routines.

In order to testing the desired program routines, the operating system allows the independent data downloading from a host PC. Flashing of the menu can be made for any desired application by changing text messages from the operating system program. At this stage until the final release point of the processing algorithms, the DSP microcontroller executes routines calculation in external assistance of the computer.

The activation of selected computer routine transfers in RAM and SD card data to be processed. After selecting the routine, the operating system checks if USB is listed by the computer. If the USB connection is active operating system commands from the computer expects. The first calculation routines were programmed in DSP microcontroller through direct compilation of C language into machine code. This was imposed primarily by the lack of a compiler able to handle directly the microcontroller DSP module, which imposed direct writing routines in assembly language DSP. The immediate consequence was increasing difficulty in debugging programs. So we preferred the original C language debugging even if this greatly increases processing time. At this moment the system is capable to compute autonomously the time-frequency scalogram and the Shannon entropy of the acquired PCG signal. Currently we are working at the implementation of the correlation algorithm which requires first of all, the construction of a pathology data base. The displayed results of a time-frequency scalogram are shown in figure 28:

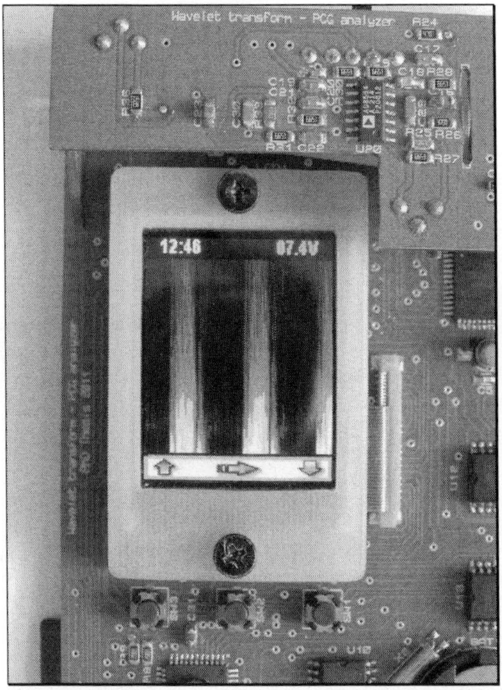

Fig. 28. Time-frequency scalogram of the „Aortic stenosis" pathology

The "System Settings" menu includes setting of the sampling frequency. Changing the sampling rate requires the recalculation of the input anti-alias filter and the use of another board for the analog circuit. The operating menu can be reconfigured easily by changing the menu text in each command line of which belongs to a menu page. The programming menu is made so that it can implement a large number of pages of which limitation is imposed only by the memory capacity of the hosting microcontroller.

By rewriting part of the operating system it can be designed a menu option which automatically is loaded from the SD card, depending on the application. In conclusion the same operating system can manage multiple applications which are completely customizable.

4. Conclusion

Smart use of digital processing tools helps in a new approach as concerning the classical cardiac auscultation, the innovative techniques with the ultimate goal of improvement in prevention and cardiology care. Early identification of cardiac pathologies is closely related to the physician's capacity to perceive and correctly interpret the heart sounds. By using a medical electronic device for PCG signal analysis, it can be increased the rate to identify heart abnormalities, compared with classical method of auscultation. The absolute novelty of the work consists of providing a series of original algorithms that can be used to accurately identify cardiac pathologies. This opens a new road in the PCG signal analysis said to be almost unapproachable. So far, most noninvasive type tests are extracted from the ECG signal. Transformation of PCG signal into a signal with a precise and predictable envelope classified after a pattern archive, together with a known spectral behavior makes possible a full characterization of cardiac pathology obviously within the limits set by a cardiologist professional.

Algorithms presented in this paper refer to those which can be implemented immediately in embedded analysis software. Development of new algorithms for analysis is directly linked to the hardware capabilities of the systems that are to implement, therefore the project started to show weakness when we decided to implement the convolution algorithm of the computed PCG images. The immediate problem that arose was insufficient RAM for the large number of two-dimensional vectors which had to be temporarily stored. Temporary solution was to transfer the algorithm towards the development system by computing the interpolation routine segments with intermediate storage of data on SD memory card. High memory access time of the SD card increases the calculation times to impractical values. So at this moment, the prototype system is capable at this development stage only for the Shannon entropy calculations which are necessary for the display of signal's time-frequency scalogram. The introduction of the additional intelligent decision-making algorithms to the operating system presented in the paper can be a powerful tool for characterization of cardiac pathologies by acquiring the PCG signal. Although this new medical imaging device suffers from a low spatial and temporal resolution; it could be proved to be a good choice for low-cost and mobility strategy in cardiac imaging, rather than the expensive ultrasound imaging devices. The classical auscultation technique benefits from a great quality improvement by using a device which is capable to offer a time-frequency representation.

5. Future directions

The expected research direction is to be guided to improve the image quality on a larger display and increase the number of wavelet decomposing levels to avoid the necessary interpolations used in present. In terms of hardware we can go two ways of solving the lack of resources. The first way is redesigning part of the current development system to increase the RAM capacity, or alternatively to satisfy also the condition of low energy demand which consist of a total redesign by migrating to the Texas Instruments microprocessors. The change of the microprocessor version implies full rewrite of the operating system. TMS320C5000 series microprocessors are low cost with fixed-point DSP capabilities and having a very low consumption in terms of supply using a voltage of 1.8

volts and an integrated memory of 320KB/16biți. The move to Texas Instruments microprocessors is supported also by an additional argument; the TI components do have accreditation for standard medical use. Development of electronic equipment is linked to building a database of reference PCG signal images for a large variety of pathologies. The cross-correlation algorithm is although under construction but the proved interest for this device among the cardiologists, makes us confident for the utility of the newly designed features.

6. Acknowledgements

We wish to thank in this way Mr. Robert Owen, responsible for the European academic program initiated by the Texas Instruments company for the donation of development systems which are necessary to continue the research on this project.

7. References

A. Jensen & A. la Cour-Harbo (2001). *Ripples in mathematics, The discrete wavelet transform*, Springer, ISBN: 3-540-41662-5

Abbas K.Abbas & Rasha Bassam (2009). *Phonocardiography signal processing*, MCP, ISBN: 9781598299762

Abdallah et al. (1988). *Arterial stenosis murmurs: an analysis of flow and pressure fields*, Journal Acoust. Soc Am. 83(1): 318-34

Addison S. Paul (2002). *The illustrated wavelet transform handbook*, IOP, ISBN: 0-7503-0692-0

Andreas Antoniu (2006). *Digital signal processing: signals systems and filters*, McGraw-Hill, ISBN: 0-07-145424-1

Andrew K.Chan & Steve J.Liu (1998). *Wavelet toolware*, ISBN 0121745953

Anke Meyer-Base (2004). *Pattern recognition for medical imaging*, Elsevier, ISBN:0-12-493290-8

Axelson Jan (2006). *USB Mass storage*, ISBN-13: 978-1-931448-05-5

Bachman George, Lawrenc Narici & Edward Beckenstein (2000) *Fourier and wavelet analysis*, Springer, ISBN:0-387-98899-8

Broersen Piet M.T. (2006). *Automatic Autocorrelation and Spectral Analysis*, Springer, ISBN-10: 1-84628-328-0

Bu-Chin (2008). *Radar image processing*, Wiley&Sons, ISBN: 978-0-470-18092-1

Emmanuel C. Ifeachor & Barrie W. Jervis (2002). *Digital signal processing; A practical approach sec.ed.*, ISBN 0201-59619-9

Fliege N.J. (1994). *Multirate digital signal processing; multirate systems, filter banks, wavelets*, ISBN: 0-471-93976-5

Gergely S, Roman M.N. & Ciupa R.V. (2011). *Portable PCG signal analyzer*, International Conference on Advancements of Medicine and Health Care through Technology IFMBE Proceedings, Volume 36, Part 2, 140-143, DOI: 10.1007/978-3-642-22586-4_29

Gergely S, Roman M.N., Fort C. (2011). *Multirate sampling in PCG signal correlation*, International Conference on Advancements of Medicine and Health Care through Technology IFMBE Proceedings,Volume 36, Part 3, 198-201, DOI: 10.1007/978-3-642-22586-4_43

Gergely S., M.N. Roman & R.V.Ciupa (2011). *Wavelet transform using DSP microcontroller*, 5th European IFMBE Conference, IFMBE Proceedings 37, pp. 117–120, Budapest, ISBN 978-3-642-23507-8, ISSN 1680-0737

Gergely S. PhD. Thesis (2011). *Research and implementation of medical electronic equipment, to use in cardiology*, Technical University of Cluj-Napoca, Romania

7

Osteocytes Characterization Using Synchrotron Radiation CT and Finite Element Analysis

Zully Ritter[1], Andreas Staude[2], Steffen Prohaska[3] and Dieter Felsenberg[1]

[1]*Charité Universitätsmedizin Berlin*

[2]*Federal Institute for Materials Research and Testing, BAM*

[3]*Zuse Institute Berlin, ZIB*

Germany

1. Introduction

Since a correlation between osteocyte number and their morphology with bone aging or its response to pharmacological treatment appears to exist, a methodology to characterize osteocytes from bone biopsies becomes important. In this chapter, the usage of synchrotron measurements, algorithms for image analysis (Amira, ZIB), and the finite element method using parallelized computational resources for topological analysis of osteocytes is explained and discussed. Different routines normally applied for material characterization of network-like structures (skeletonization) have been adapted to visualize osteocytes along bone cement lines at high resolution (2.174 μm). The different steps concerning to counting osteocytes and analyzing the mechanical behavior of bones are illustrated with an example.

The methods were developed to answer some scientific questions such as: Does bone osteocyte distribution, number and volume differ between healthy and osteoporotic bone? How much does the osteocytes' morphology and topology contribute to load transmission capacity in bones? Which parameters are useful to characterize bones and their changes due to aging? Which strategies can be used to maintain a balance of osteocyte number and connectivity in order to balance for minimizing bone aging effects?

Usage of the combined methodologies from CT up to numerical analysis (fem) are presented in this chapter in an easy, feasible and repeatable way allowing osteocytes characterization, whose topology is an indicator of bone adaption under different mechanical or pharmacological conditions. The interdisciplinary work between Charité Universitätsmedizin Berlin (Center for Muscle and Bone Research), BAM (federal Institute for Materials Research and Testing) and Zuse Institute Berlin (ZIB) was essential for quantifying and characterizing osteocytes at different age stages. The required techniques, advantages and disadvantages of the combined methods as well as the expected results are discussed in the chapter.

1.1 Scientific background

Osteocytes are differentiated bone cells from osteoblasts, which are embedded into osteons and connected in between by means of their processes. There is evidence that osteocytes are not only responsible for sensing mechanical stimuli but also for transmitting the amplified signal to the bone surface (You *et al.* 2001; Cowin 2002; Whitfield 2003; Han *et al.* 2004; Anderson *et al.* 2008; Jacobs *et al.* 2010; Cheung *et al.* 2011). In normal conditions, the sensed mechanical stimulus is transduced in biochemical and bioelectrical signals captured for the osteoblast and osteoclast thus starting bone formation and bone resorption activities. At a macro level, the bone geometry and density is continuously adapted to guarantee bone mechanical functionality under physiological loads. It is known that bone adaption follows the Wolf's and Roux's rules for allowing maximal strength by optimized bone mass.

A misbalance in this process (osteocytes-mechanosignal transmission-osteoblastic and osteoclastic activities) will generate changes in the bone geometry and density distribution such as observed in bone diseases. In the elderly, a misbalance between an accelerated osteoclastic activity and an incapacity of osteoblasts to form new bone results in a progressive reduction of the trabecular bone structures, an increment in the cortical porosity and a reduction of the cortical thickness. At a micro-level, bone is a composite material formed by hydroxylapatite and collagen. Other alterations in the signal pathway from osteocytes to osteoblasts and/or osteoclasts are related with induced changes in the hydroxylapatite crystals by increased secretion of Ca. Thereby the hydroxylapatite crystal number increases and the collagen content decrease and a glass-like bone structure is formed (osteogenesis imperfecta) (Boyde *et al.* 1999; Roschger *et al.* 2008; Dong *et al.* 2010). Similarly, an overproduction of collagen fibrils results in a hyper elastic bone material with a gummy-like mechanical behavior (osteomalacia) (Feng *et al.* 2006). In all cases, osteocytes generated signals appear to be associated with these bone diseases. Osteoporosis is one of the most frequent bone diseases affecting the elderly population, whose number will probably sharply increase in the future, thus we will concentrate firstly in the analysis and comparison of osteocytes from osteoporotic in comparison with healthy bone biopsies. The method explained here is of course applicable independently of the bone biopsies or disease type, including bone samples after pharmacological interventions.

As the signal coming from the osteocytes will stimulate both bone formation and bone resorption, many pharmacological interventions try to effect the receptors for these signals: osteoblast and osteoclast, more than acting directly on the osteocytes. Additionally, it is known that bone resorption velocities are in general higher as required for bone formation (Huiskes 2000; Liu 2001; Nabavi *et al.* 2001; Huang *et al.* 2010). The pharmacy industry develops therefore principally antiresorptive drugs, which will reduce or inhibit osteoclastogenesis. The most used antiresorptive drugs are bisphosphonates, estrogen receptor modulators (SERMs), calcitonin, parathyroid hormone (PTH), cathepsin K inhibitors, Denosumab and strontium ranelate. This last drug might not only have an antiresorptive effect but is also able to stimulate osteoblastic activities. However, it is not clear how much the hydroxylapatite crystal is morphologically changed by replacement of Ca atoms through Sr atoms. Thus it is unclear how much the densitometric measurements are affected. Osteocytes characterization from bone biopsies of patient treated with strontium ranelate will help to illustrate how osteocytes (and consequently osteoblastic and osteoclastic activities) are affected after alteration of the hydroxylapatite bone crystal.

Bone adaption or its pathological changes in time are nowadays monitored by densitometric and *in vivo* CT or similar radiological measurements. After measurement evaluation, the density bone distribution is calculated by comparison of measured absorptiometry coefficients with those from phantom measurements of materials of known density values. Cortical bone density and trabecular bone density can thus be determined. After segmentation structural bone parameters such as BV/TV and cortical thickness are calculated. There are additional structural and geometrical parameters (e.g. trabecular thickness, trabecular separation, cortical porosity) that are derived from mathematical relations of the density parameters combined with the geometrical contours or bone segmentation.

Osteoporosis implies a fracture risk whose asymptomatic development is not seriously considered by the affected population. CT-techniques allow analysis of bone structure, geometry and density in time (*in vivo*) or its detailed analysis in nanometer scales by analysis of *in vitro* CT measurements. Actually clinical CTs possess a resolution of 150 µm.

Some indicators calculated after reconstruction and evaluation of bones are widely accepted to show bone adaption and to estimate its fracture risk. Such parameters are however normally given as a mean value over the measured volume. Although these parameters are a good indicator of bone morphology, in some cases they are insufficient to show how bone is responding under a pharmacological treatment or newly adapted conditions. Osteocytes are not only directly responsible for starting bone remodeling regions, but their number, sizes and distribution in comparable bone volumes shows how bone has changed by a disease or by medication that alter bone mineralization such as strontium ranelate or bisphosphonates. We have concentrated on developing a methodology for osteocytes characterization using available commercial platforms and adapted algorithms. Radiological and tridimensional visualization allows understanding how a pathological condition or an alteration of the normal bone conditions is related to the osteocytes morphology and their distribution.

2. Related work

Evidences of osteocytes (monkeys) ultrastructural changes under microgravity (Rodionova *et al.* 2002)

Tensile strains regulate stem cell osteogenesis (Kearney *et al.* 2010)

Maintenance of subject specific cell mechanosensitivity for prevention of osteoporosis (Mulvihill *et al.* 2008)

Osteon diameter is related with the strain environment distribution (van Oers *et al.* 2008)

Osteocytes apoptosis induce angiogenesis (Cheung *et al.* 2011)

Osteonal geometry reconstruction and BMU activity analysis by using SR-CT (osteocytes are aligned around osteon cavities) (Cooper *et al.* 2011)

Specific location of osteon type structures correlate with its mechanical environment (external loads) (Beraudi *et al.* 2010)

It appears that osteocytes are physiologically adapted to "sense" its mechanical environment by means of its primary cilium (Whitfield 2003)

Visualizing osteocytes canaliculi network (limited VOI) able to show 2 osteocytes (lacunae) (Schneider *et al.* 2011)

It appears that osteocytes networks mimic the orientation of the surrounding extracellular bone matrix(Kerschnitzki *et al.* 2011)

3. Methodology

Osteocytes characterization has been made possible by combining radiological, image and numerical analysis. We have employed: laboratory micro-CT and Synchrotron radiation CT (SR-CT) (Rack *et al.* 2008) for radiological *in vitro* measurements, Amira (ZIB) (Stalling 2005) for image analysis and the finite element method (Abaqus) for estimating and comparing compressive stiffness from healthy and osteoporotic bone biopsies after SR-CT measurements. Additional algorithms were implemented in Matlab. Before describing the method in detail general considerations for sample preparation will be discussed.

3.1 General considerations

The first step is the bone sample preparation. Bone samples are normally fixed in methyl methacrylate or in ethanol for tissue conservation. In our study, the biopsies were maintained fixed in 70% ethanol and 30% water for allowing posterior histological analysis (e.g. von Kossa staining) when required. If subsequent analyses are not planned, biopsies embedded in methyl methacrylate guarantee CT measurements free from movement artifacts. Some studies have shown that derived bone structural analysis from biopsies first fixed in ethanol with those after methyl methacrylate do not present significant differences (Perilli *et al.* 2007). An ethanol fixation allows adapting the container to the requirements of the CT acquisition. In case of using an ethanol fixation, the samples should be acclimated to the ambient room temperature previous to SR-CT measurements, in order to avoid micro-movements during the measurement.

The method from CT measurement up to FE Analysis includes the following steps:

- Task 1: Bone biopsies extraction
- Task 2: Laboratory μCT measurements *in vitro* (minimal resolution: 20 μm)
- Task 3: 3D projections reconstruction
- Task 4: Standard bone structure and density parameters calculation (e.g. BT/TV, Trabecular Number (Tb.N), Trabecular Separation (Tb.Sp))
- Task 5: Selecting bone biopsies for SR-CT (based on compared parameters in task 5 (e.g. samples with a BV/TV variation > 60%)
- Task 6: Preparation of tailored bone containers for SR-CT measurements
- Task 7: Repeating Task 3 to Task 5
- Task 8: Image analysis including 3D stereoscopy (Amira)
- Task 9: Analysis of osteocytes topology (number and volume) by adapting skeletonization techniques
- Task 10: Comparison of obtained results in Task 9
- Task 11: Finite element mesh generation (script in Matlab interface Amira-Abaqus (for Amira version previous to 2010)
- Task 12: FEA and generation of comparative histograms from mechanical parameters (von Mises, minimum principal strains)
- Task 13: Comparison of obtained results in Task 12

3.2 Detailed methodology description

3.2.1 Task 1: Bone biopsies extraction

In our example study an analysis of the jaw was performed. For comparison and results interpretation, the regions of interest selected for study need to be biomechanically comparable. In our case, bone samples were extracted from region 36. For analysis of osteocytes morphological changes after prostheses implantation, it is recommendable not only to compare biopsies from the same regions of healthy subjects but with biopsies taken from the contralateral bone side of the same subject. The implantation of prostheses implies drastic induced changes in the mechanical bone environment, thus significant differences on osteocytes morphology could be erroneously measured by comparing with healthy subjects. On the other hand, considering that bone biopsies are an invasive procedure, an alternative would be to extract the biopsies at least one year after implantation, time in which bone adaption velocity achieves normal balanced levels again. After extraction, bone samples were maintained under routinely used conditions of constant -20°C temperature.

Since osteocytes characterization is basically performed by means of SR-CT measurements, a highly specialized technique, it is recommendable to pre-select the best biopsies that could show typical patterns for the bone disease or bone topic under study. We recommend, therefore, a previous image analysis using a typical CT laboratory such as outlined in task 2.

3.2.2 Task 2: Laboratory μCT measurements *in vitro* (minimal resolution: 20 μm)

SR-CT is a specialized CT measurement, which is time consuming and requires knowledge and good planning. Therefore, to obtain better results, the regions to be analyzed with this technique need to be firstly pre-selected after analysis and comparison of the bone structure and density parameters coming from, for example, laboratory CT measurements. In most of the cases, biopsies have typical dimensions of 2 mm in diameter and 10 mm in length. Cone-beam CTs with a resolution between 15 and 20 μm will be sufficient to determine bone structure and density. A high-energy X-Ray source will allow good contrast and reduced noise, thus improving measurement quality. For our study, we used 20 μm and a cone beam CT using 100 kV and 30 μAmpere. Flat and dark exposures were taken before and after the measurement, averaged, and used for correcting the projections.

3.2.3 Task 3: 3D reconstructions

After projection filtering, maximal and minimal values of the gray values corresponding to the attenuation coefficients of the bone are obtained. In general it is not recommendable to perform additional Gauss filtering to reduce the noise. This will results in loosing important information concerning the bone trabecular structure. Instead, a good segmentation is preferred. Analysis of the histograms of the gray value distribution from in the best case a random selection including 50% of the samples from each group or at least one sample from each group under study (here osteoporotic vs. healthy bone) allows the determination of the threshold values required for segmentation. The valleys formed between each peak-value in the histograms indicate the appropriate threshold values to be used. Advanced image analysis software such as Amira (ZIB) possesses tools (e.g. magic wand) for improving the segmented bone/material regions. This threshold needs to remain constant until finalizing the study, since calculation of bone structure, geometrical and density parameters depend on it. The BV/TV is the most accurately determinable structure parameter. Using the contours at the perimeter in each transversal segmented projection and filling the total area inside, the total volume containing the biopsy will be determined (BV). After determination of the bone volume from the segmented region, the tissue volume (TV) value will be determined. Thus the BV/TV ratio can be calculated. Once the BV/TV has been calculated for all biopsy samples and after comparison between the groups under study, it is recommendable to select biopsies with a difference larger than 60% in the BV/TV ratio between groups (here healthy vs. osteoporotic bone biopsies from the same jaw region (e.g. for our sample 36).

In a similar way as described above, 3D segmentation after SR-CT measurements can be performed.

3.2.4 Task 4: Standard bone structure and density parameters calculation (e.g. BT/TV, Trabecular Number (Tb.N), Trabecular Separation (Tb.Sp))

Commercial CTs scanners are able to perform an automatic evaluation of BV/TV and other structural and geometrical parameters. The most relevant structural bone parameters are Tb.N, Tb.Sp, cortical thickness (Ct.Th.), cortical perimeter (Ct.Pt), and from the density parameters group, cortical (Dcomp) and trabecular density (Dtrab). Frequently other parameters are reported (e.g. density at the center of the bone section: Dmeta, or immediately near to the cortical bone (Dinn) but these are mathematically derived from the Dcomp und Dtrab in combination with their geometrical location. In similar form, series of structural parameters can be mathematically obtained from BV/TV in combination with superimposed geometrical forms (e.g. spheres or ellipses). A linear relation of the measured attenuation coefficient distribution to the bone volume allows assignment of density values for each voxel.

3.2.5 Task 5: Selecting bone biopsies for SR-CT (based on compared parameters in task 5 (e.g. samples with a BV/TV variation > 60%)

As explained above, the BV/TV ratio is easy to calculate, without employment of external software. A non-automatic calculation allows following the process and to improve segmentation if required. The BV/TV will be calculated from standard laboratory CT-measurements (at least 20 μm). After that and for synchrotron radiation measurements, specimens with a difference of 60% in the BV/TV value between groups (e.g. osteoporotic vs. healthy) will be chosen for osteocytes morphology characterization.

3.2.6 Task 6: Preparation of tailored bone containers for SR-CT measurements

Containers with dimensions as close as possible to the biopsy dimension need to be selected. In our study, the containers were tailored +10% of the biopsy diameter. At such scales, it is recommendable first to fill the container partially with the ethanol solution (if applicable) to avoid air bubbles formation under the biopsy, to introduce the bone sample, and to continue up to complete filling. High temperature variations need to be avoided for suppressing possible additional movement artifacts.

3.2.7 Task 7: Repeating Task 3 to Task 5 (from SR-CT-measurements up to 3D volume reconstruction)

For SR-CT measurements with a pixel size of 2.174 μm of the total biopsy (height ca. 1 cm), two stacks each one with 2500 slices are required. Due to the high variability of the beam, flat exposures are collected every 100 projections.

For each data set the rotational axis can numerically determined. From this, the tilt angle and displacement are calculated for eliminating double contours, also allowing correction of each slice separately. An important aspect is to control the existence of ring artifacts, which in the case of our data is mainly caused by damages of and pollutions of the scintillator. If the location of the defect region is known, the attenuation coefficient corresponding to the region can be averaged from the neighbors and corrected computationally during the reconstruction process. The flatfield corrected projection data are filtered with a 3x3 median filter and reconstructed using a standard filtered back-projection algorithm with only a ramp filter. Thus the spatial resolution is degraded less than when using a smoothing filter (e.g. Shepp-Logan) and the high frequency noise is suppressed sufficiently.

3.2.8 Task 8: Image analysis including 3D stereoscopy

After segmentation and assignment of gray value ranges to each specific material, here bone and osteocytes, the first characterization parameter related to osteocytes characterization, that is their localization, will be obtained. For analysis of osteocytes trajectories, it is highly recommendable to use 3D stereoscopic views of the generated osteocyte surfaces embedded on the bone tissue. 3D-stereoscopy allows a detailed description of the trajectory especially in the trabecular bone volumes, in which the classical circular lamellae around the osteons are not visualized. By superposition of the orthoslices and using a minor contrast canal on the reconstructed volume, the osteocytes trajectories and patterns can clearly be identified; in this form, their relation to the cement lines location becomes understandable.

3.2.9 Task 9 - 10: Analysis of osteocytes topology (number and volume) by adapting skeletonization techniques

Once the projections from the SR-CT measurements containing the gray values have been reconstructed for each stack, this will be positioned and merged to obtain the total CT-biopsy measurement. A review of the orthoslices can be made for checking ring artifacts. For segmentation in Amira, a "label voxel" tool can be used for supplying the limit threshold values of the gray scales to separate each material type, or grade of mineralization in the bone label. In our study, the different grades of mineralization on the bone volume were not segmented separately. Air/Exterior, bone, osteons and osteocytes were segmented. As osteons canals, osteocytes (lacunae) and the exterior/air regions will have similar attenuation coefficients, making it difficult to determine an appropriate threshold value for osteocytes segmentation, it will be simple and semiautomatic to enable the options "voxel accuracy" and "bubbles" in Amira (ZIB) using the "label-voxel" toolbox. Thus the osteons will be segmented (separated using the magic wand). This tool causes all connected voxels with same material properties to be selected, separating osteons from osteocytes. The remaining bubble voxels could be adjudicated to "osteocyte" material. Optimal results depend on the grade of contrast and reduced noise of the original CT measurement. As mentioned above, at this scale, it is not recommendable to use Gauss filters or similar. Instead a good segmentation could be used. After segmentation, the number of the voxels for each material region (bone, osteons and osteocytes) and its total volume is determined (material statistics in Amira). Thus the relations total volume (biopsy volume)/tissue (bone) volume and total volume (bone)/tissue (osteocytes) volume are determinate.

Osteocytes number calculation. The osteocytes number can be calculated after skeletonization (Fouard *et al.* 2006) of the segmented biopsy, in which only the osteocytes are kept. Thus, the other materials should be selected and deleted only for this step (of course after saving the original Amira mesh containing all material regions). A skeleton is a schematic representation of a solid after extraction of geometrical and topological simplified shape features, thus facilitating its analysis on the extracted schema. In biomechanics this tool is commonly used for analysis of the nerve or the circular systems (e.g. diameter and length distribution of the vessel is obtained). The distant transformation map concept introduced by H. Blum calculates the closest boundary (vertices) for each point in the represented object. In the case of the osteocytes, this results in a center point inside the surface (bubble) at each osteocyte (Fig. 9). For large osteocytes, a two vertices joined by one line will be generated. Looking at the skeletonization results, the total number of vertices and lines corresponding to the segmented osteocytes are reported. The osteocytes number (N) is calculated subtracting the number of vertices (v) from the number of lines (l). This simple method was tested and validated by automatic counting compared with a manual counting of osteocytes in a reduce volume of the biopsy.

3.2.10 Task 11: Finite element mesh generation

After segmentation and previous to osteocytes counting procedure, a surface for each material is obtained. For mesh generation the semi-automatic tool from Amira ("tetragen") was employed. The triangular surface is then converted to solid tetrahedrons. Requisite for successful 3D meshing are that the triangulated surface fills the criterions of non-intersection, surface closeness, aspect ratio and non-wrong conserved orientation. Once the surface is ready, the tetrahedral mesh is automatically generated using an advancing front algorithm implemented in Amira. Prior to mesh generation, it is recommendable to check the number of expected finite elements. If the represented geometry is not affected, improvements in the mesh generation could be allowed. Finally, the mesh topology (coordinates and elements connectivity) can be written in an ASCII format, readable for the most common FE solvers (Abaqus, Ansys, etc.).

3.2.11 Task 12: FEA and generation of comparative histograms from mechanical parameters (von Mises, minimum principal strains)

In our study, the mesh topology was imported in Abaqus. Using Abaqus-CAE the boundary conditions, material properties and mechanical material behavior will be imposed in the solid model of the bone volume with the osteocytes. A compression test was simulated by encastring the nodes (all six degrees of freedom = 0) at the basis of the mesh and a distributed load on the top of the model. For comparison with other studies, the material properties were taken from literature (Boutroy *et al.* 2008; Rincon-Kohli *et al.* 2009; Varga *et al.* 2011; Vilayphiou *et al.* 2011). The materials were modeled to be isotropic and homogeneous and to possess a linear elastic behavior. The Abaqus solver was used to calculate the strain and strength tensors. After analysis, reports (ASCIÍ format) containing the magnitude of each mechanical parameter amount others (e.g. minimum principal strains and von Mises stress distribution) were exported for post-processing analysis. The magnitudes were averaged at the centroid of each element. Lists containing the element number and corresponding strength/strain values were represented in histograms in pre-selected thresholds. Logarithms representations of such distributions will conduce to wrong results interpretation. Thus, a natural scale of percental number of elements at each interval is preferred.

3.2.12 Task 13: Comparison of obtained results in Task 12

Traditionally, the power of the finite element analysis is to show zones of high stress or strains concentration, which are indicators of regions susceptible to mechanical failure, thus allowing redesigning by re-dimensioning or improving the strength or mechanical properties of the materials. For the analysis of biological tissues, it is not only important to visualize these zones of high stresses but to compare the effect of pharmacological interventions on the bone or the effect of artificial implants and to quantify these effects on bone tissues even at short times. Histogram distributions of stress and strains in pre-defined thresholds are used for this. Explicitly in the case of osteocytes, the zones of stress concentration were visualized and histograms were elaborated for analysis and comparison of the effect of the size, number and location on bone strength for osteoporotic and healthy biopsies of the jaw. For histograms, interpretation of the translational displacement and the picks of the histograms were analyzed. Translational displacement differences between groups (osteoporotic vs. healthy bone biopsies) are indicator of the compressive bone stiffness. If the histogram curve tends to be localized to the left (Y axis), a high percentage of finite elements possesses low stress values, thus indicating that the bone are more mechanically stable. On the other hand, the differences of the height of the histogram (Gauss distribution) are an indicator of stress concentration, thus under same mechanical boundary conditions, a sample experiencing highest magnitudes of stresses (highest pick) is less able to resist and to transmit external acting physiological loads, which imply highest damage tendency under physiological load (bad mechanical bone quality). The histogram generation and their comparisons can be performed by writing a simple Matlab subroutine or amongst others using the Python programming language.

4. Practical example (results)

Biopsies from osteoporotic and healthy bones were analyzed. The results from each of the task described above will be presented.

4.1 Task 1: Bone biopsies extraction

No special techniques were employed for bone biopsy extraction and no post-traumatic events were registered.

4.2 Task 2 - 6: Laboratory µCT measurements and 3D reconstruction *in vitro*

In an initial step, 20 healthy and 20 osteoporotic bone biopsies were scanned using an isotropic resolution of 20 µm. Three-dimensional volume reconstructions and image analyses performed using Amira (ZIB) are shown in the Fig. 1. A voxel based density distribution color map (red-orange: from low to middle density values and from yellow to white: highest density values) was used to identify new bone from old one, as well as the differently mineralized bone regions. After analysis of the histogram distributions of the gray values obtained from the CT-measurements (segmentation), the BV/TV ratios were calculated using the procedure explained above. Exemplarily, the calculated values are reported at the bottom of the figures 1 and 2. As observed, the highest calculated BV/TV differences were registered for the biopsy fr2 (from the healthy group at the center in Fig. 1) with a BV/TV= 0.3426 and for the biopsy fr7 (from the osteoporotic group at the right in Fig. 2), thus these two biopsies were selected for

SR-CT measurements to find out if the number of osteocytes, their volume, and their distribution along the cement lines are correlated with aging.

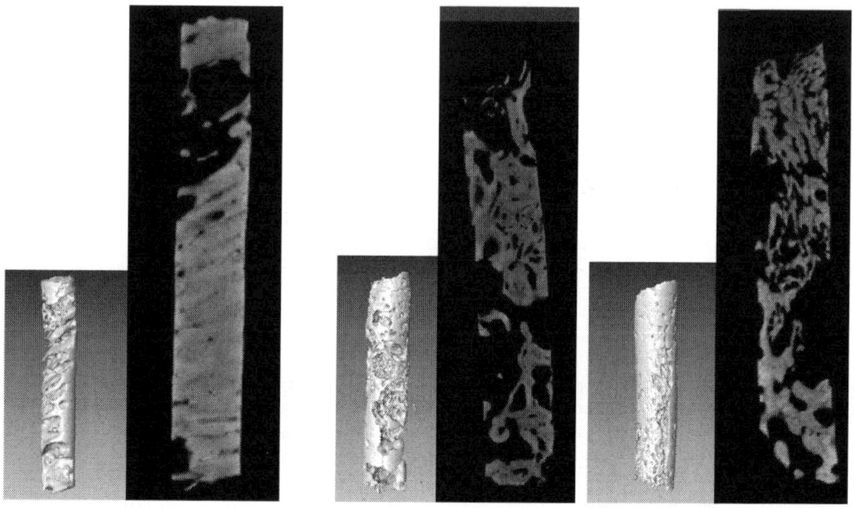

Fig. 1. Healthy bone biopsies from the jaw: 3D reconstructions and BV/TV determination after μCT laboratory measurements (20 μm isotropic resolution).

4.3 Task 8: SR-CT image analysis including 3D stereoscopy

4.3.1 Task 8.1: Image analysis

As explained above, after SR-CT measurements (ca. 5000 slices @2.174 μm isotropic resolution), the volumes were visualized using Amira (ZIB) as shown in the Figure 3. It appears that the osteocytes are more frequent in the healthy biopsy and that they are shorter compared with the osteoporotic one. Outside of osteons the osteocytes are localized along the cement lines. Additionally they seem to be more frequent in the high mineralized regions (more lightening voxels) as shown in the selected axial and orthogonal slices of the Fig. 3. In the Fig. 4, a view of the 3D volume reconstructions (osteoporotic and healthy) and a detail from the osteoporotic bone biopsy (fr7) through a slice using an inverse color map shows that near the bone surface osteocytes are minor in number and the bone appears to be less mineralized. Confirming the initial observations, osteocytes are mainly localized along to the cement lines and are less spaced inside the highly mineralized regions. Osteocytes distribution (red) embedded in the bone matrix for the healthy bone biopsy (section) are shown in the Fig. 5.

BSch-M4, fr4_20 BH5, fr5_20 KG7, fr7_20

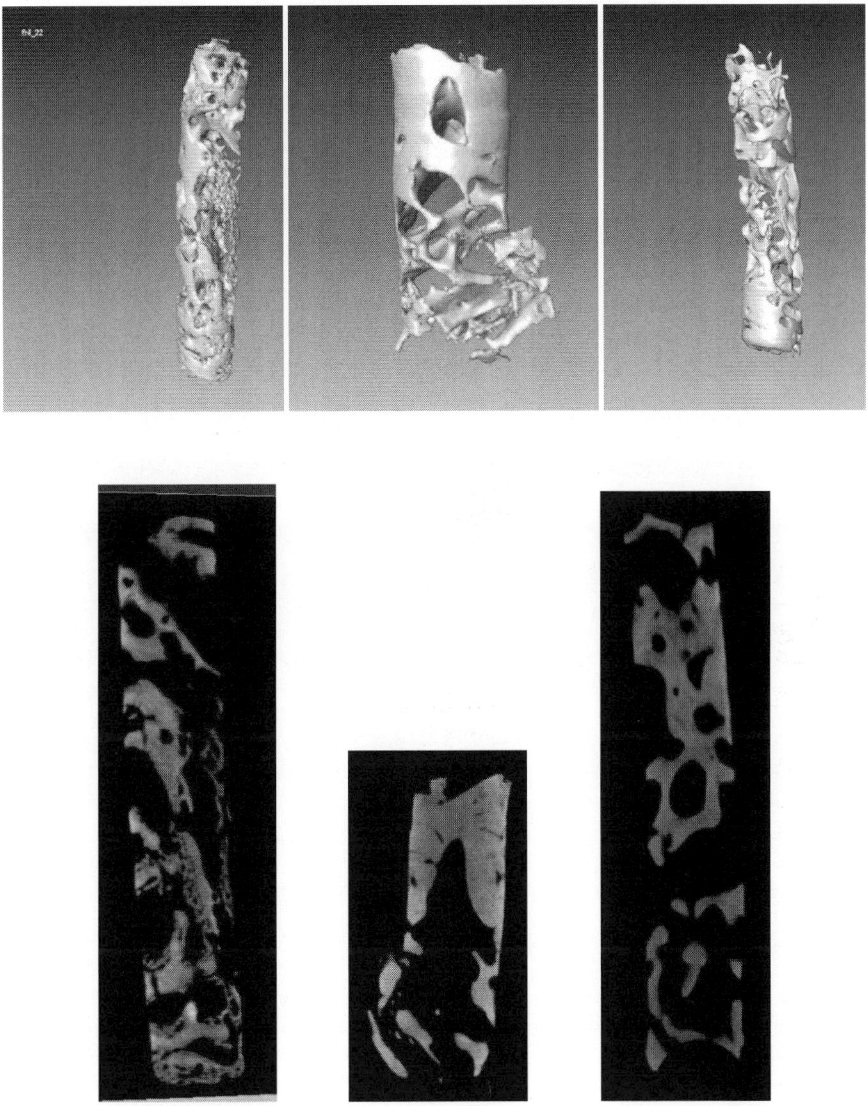

BV/TV = 0.2203 BV/TV = 0.237 BT/TV=0.1791

Fig. 2. Osteoporotic bone biopsies from the jaw: 3D reconstructions and BV/TV determination after μCT laboratory measurements (20 μm isotropic resolution).

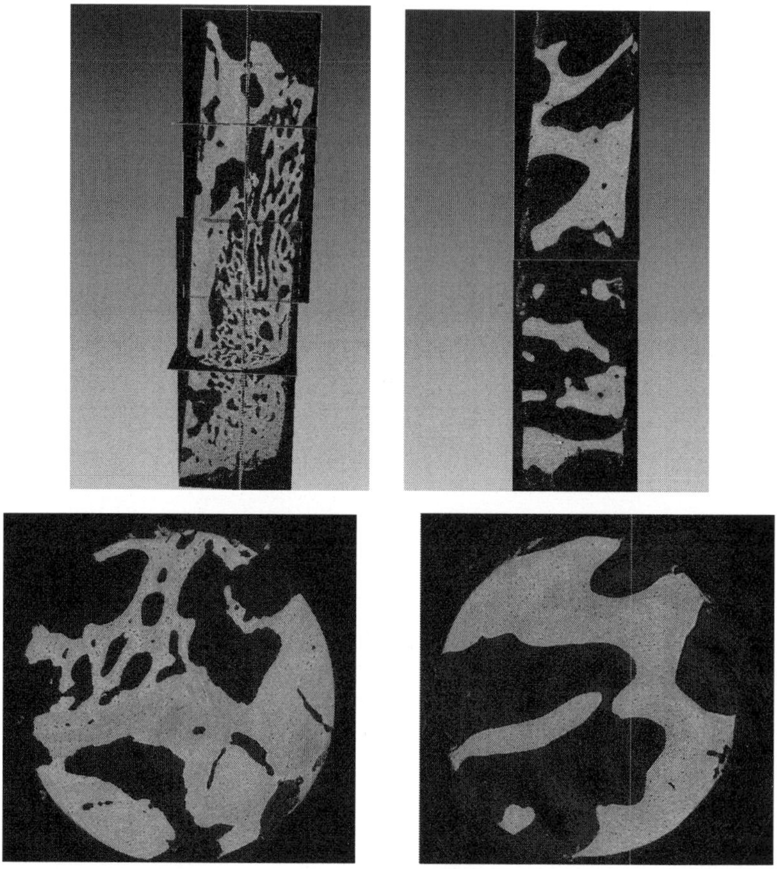

Fig. 3. Axial and orthogonal cuts showing the different grades of mineralization and osteocytes location for a healthy (fr2) and an osteoporotic (fr7) bone biopsy of the jaw region36 after SR-CT measurements @ 2.174 μm (BESSY).

4.3.2 Task 8.2: 3D stereoscopy (Amira ZIB)

Due to the high resolution of the scans, especially for the healthy biopsies in which a large number of osteocytes were visualized, it can be difficult to follow the osteocytes trajectory after surface rendering. We found that using stereoscopic views of the segmented and subsequently rendered volumes of osteocytes facilitates understanding osteocytes morphology. It appears that osteocytes presented an elliptical-like surface and that its major radius is mainly aligned with the longitudinal axis of the biopsies, which represents, in the case of the analyzed regions, the loading axis. Stereoscopic views are essential to understanding how osteocytes are really distributed inside the bone volume (exemplary shown for the osteoporotic bone biopsy; osteocytes colored in yellow (Fig. 6)), and their trajectory is clearly identifiable (Fig. 7).

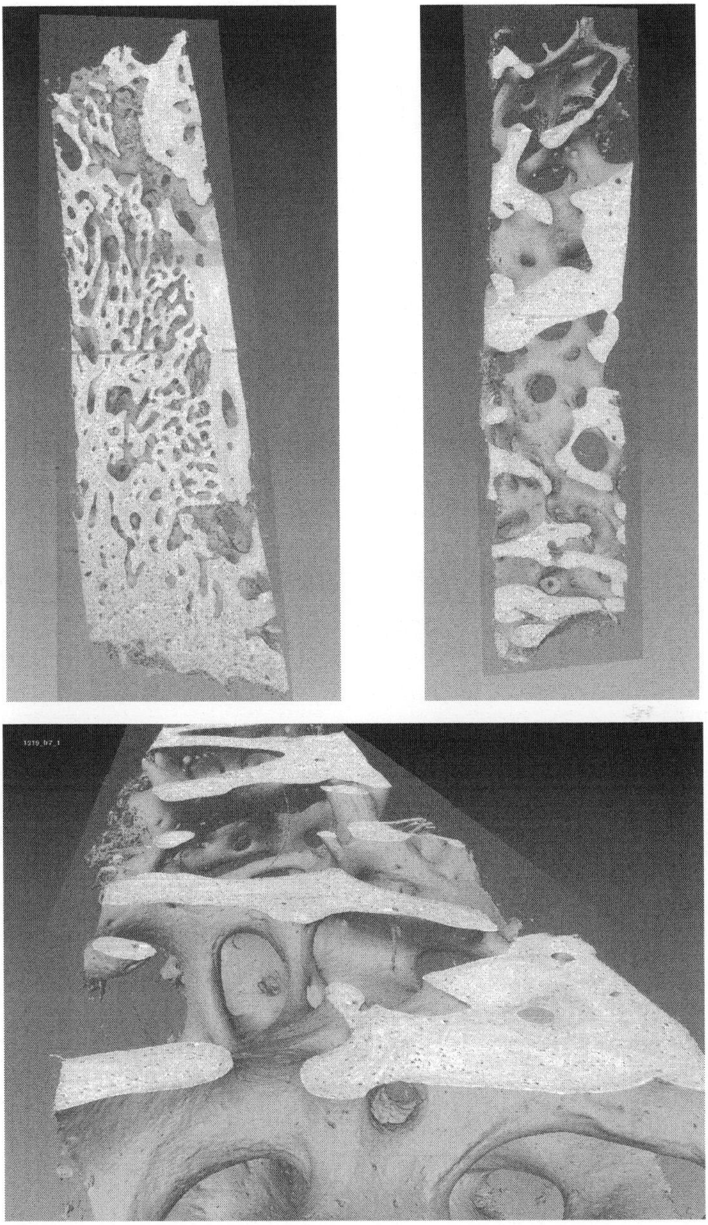

Fig. 4. 3D Reconstruction of a healthy (left) and an osteoporotic (right) bone biopsy after SR-CT measurements (2.174 μm). In slice (inverse color map) different mineralized regions and osteocytes are shown (bottom: detail).

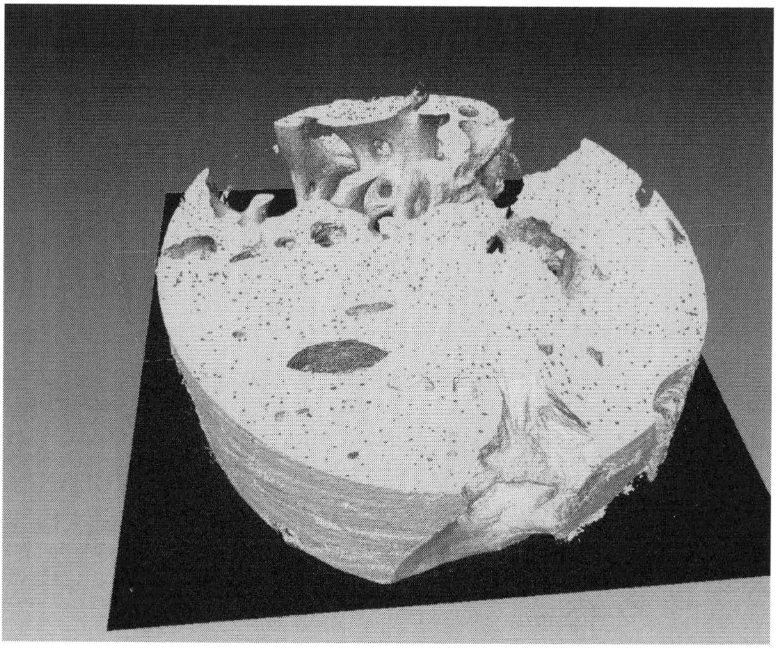

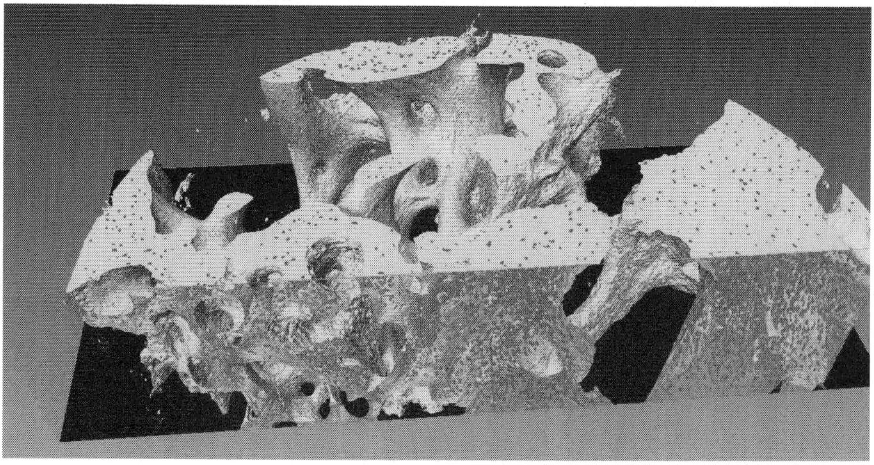

Fig. 5. 3D Volume rendering of a healthy bone biopsy (section) after SR-CT measurements @2.174 µm (BESSY), showing osteocytes (in red) embedded in the bone matrix (Amira ZIB, bottom: cut).

In both samples the osteocytes were localized mainly on the low mineralized regions (qualitatively) or enlarge of the cement lines as show exemplary in a cut of the projections from the healthy bone biopsy (Fig. 8).

The size of the osteocytes was higher in the osteoporotic biopsies. After qualitatively analysis the center points representing each osteocyte were quantified and compared as show in the next section.

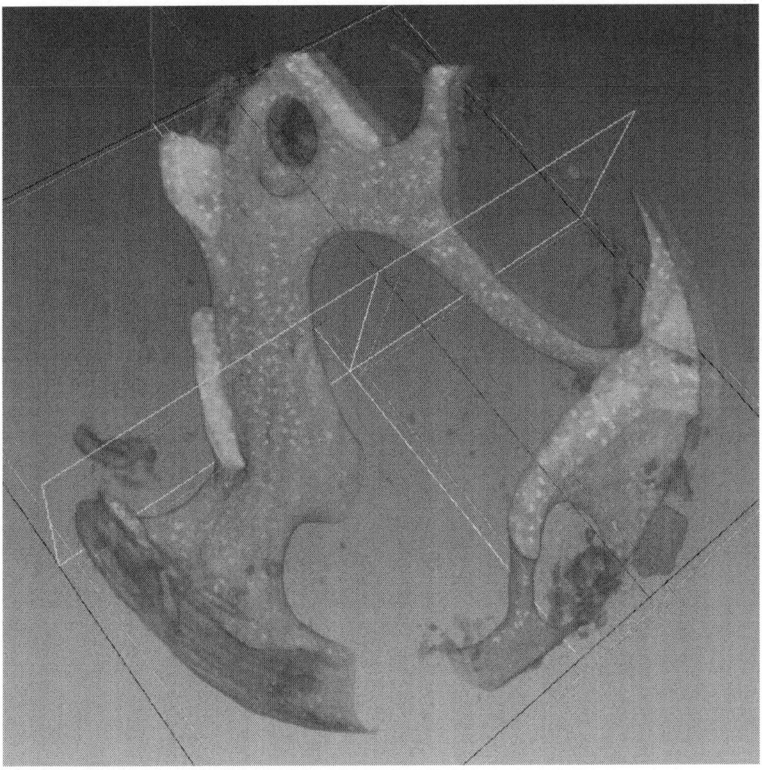

Fig. 6. Example of a stereoscopic 3D view for the osteoporotic biopsy section showing the osteocytes in yellow aligned in the load direction.

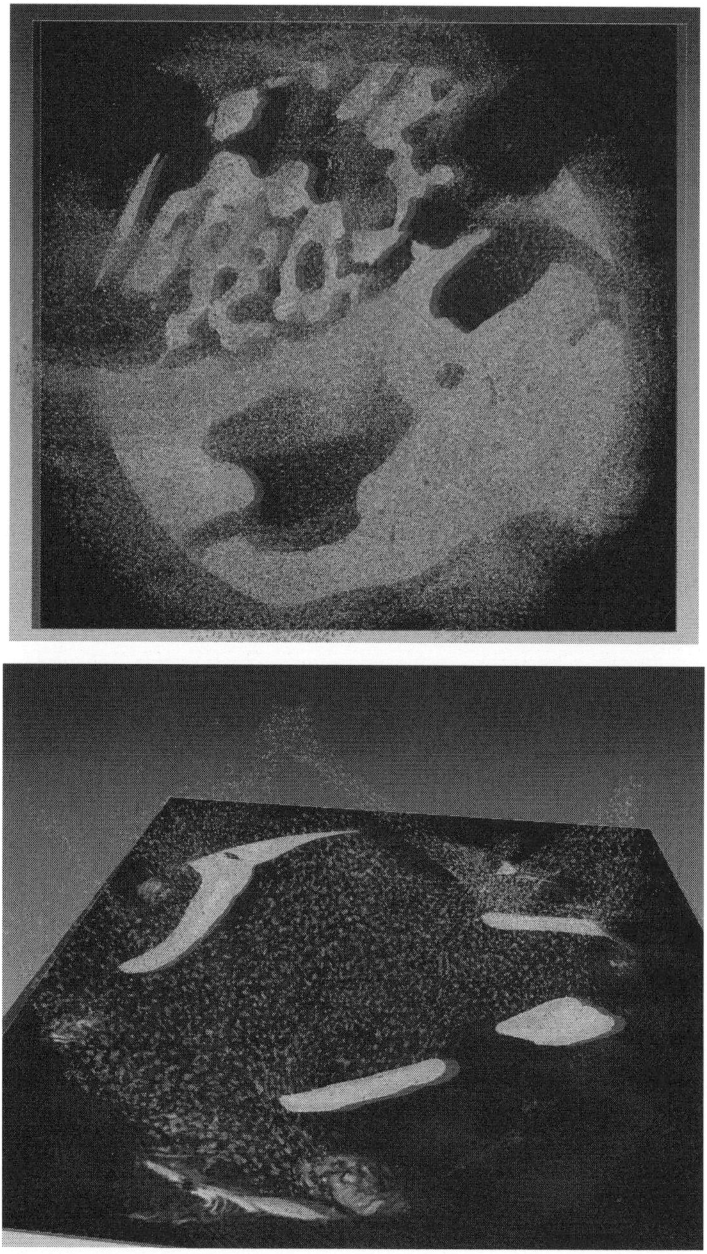

Fig. 7. Stereoscopic view of osteocytes path distribution in a healthy (top) and an osteoporotic (bottom) bone biopsy section.

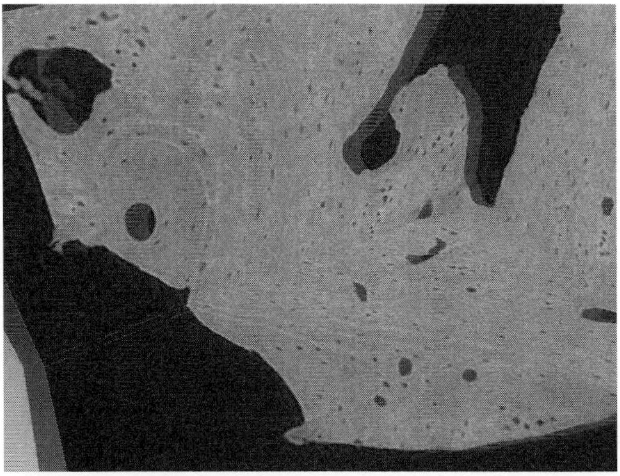

Fig. 8. Stereoscopic view of the projection from the healthy bone biopsy showing the osteocytes aligned along to the cement lines (SR-CT measurements @2.174 μm).

4.4 Task 9 - 10: Analysis of osteocytes topology

After using the skeletonization tool from the voxel topology as described in 4.2.9, the osteocyte number was determined, which was larger in a healthy bone biopsy. To confirm these findings two additional biopsies from the jaw with identical regions, one from an osteoporotic and one from a healthy bone, were analyzed following the same protocol. After comparing osteocytes number quantification (Fig. 10), it was found that osteoporotic bone could have up to of 85.4% (mean comparisons) less osteocytes in the jaw in the same region (36). As healthy bone possesses higher bone mass, the osteocytes number related to the analyzed bone volume (identical biopsy section) as well as the osteocytes volume related to the bone volume were additionally quantified, compared, and shown in Figs. 11 and 12 respectively.

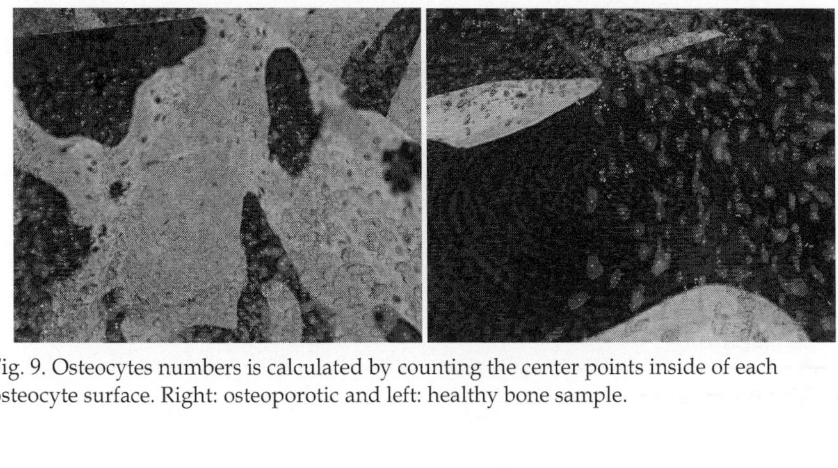

Fig. 9. Osteocytes numbers is calculated by counting the center points inside of each osteocyte surface. Right: osteoporotic and left: healthy bone sample.

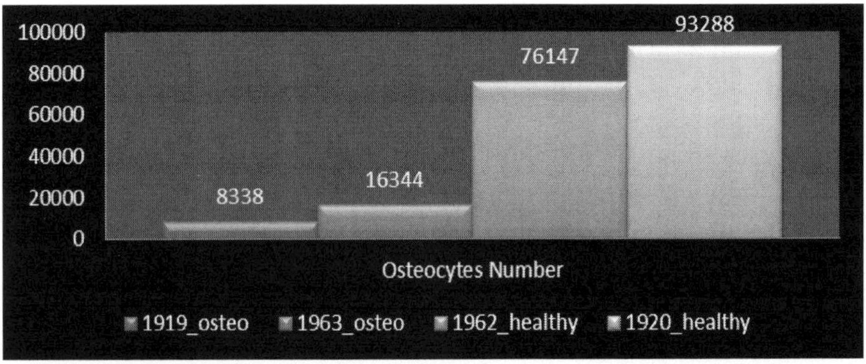

Fig. 10. Osteocytes number for healthy and osteoporotic bone biopsies of the jaw (section).

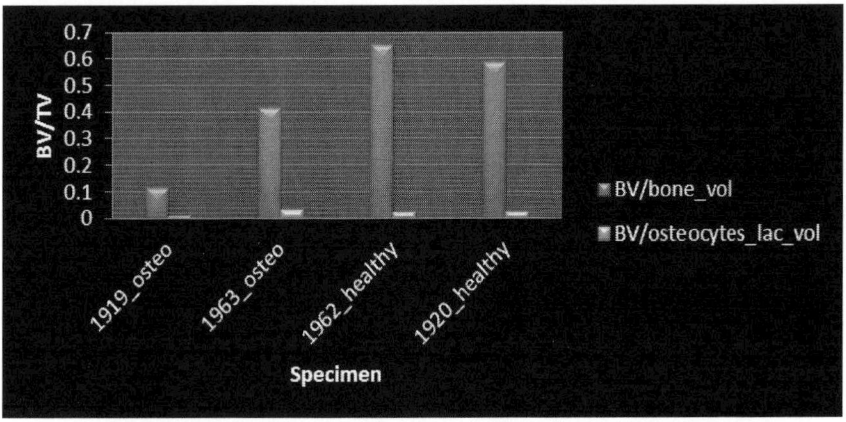

Fig. 11. BV/TV relations.

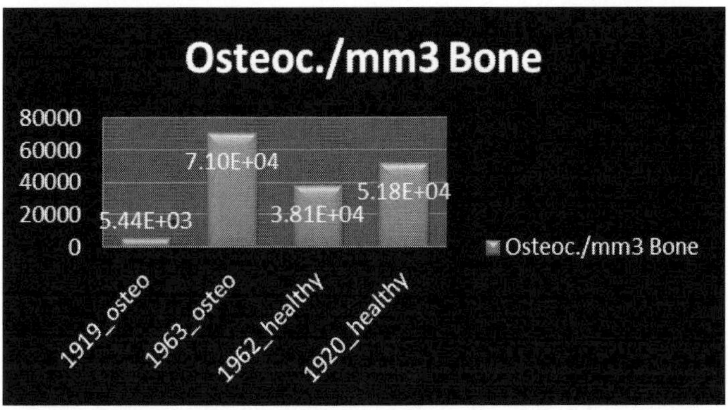

Fig. 12. Osteocytes number related to the bone volume.

4.5 Task 11 - 13: Finite element analysis

Due to the high computational costs, only a section from the healthy and bone biopsies from equivalent anatomical regions were analyzed. After meshing following the protocol described in 4.2.10, boundary conditions and material properties were imposed in the FE models (Fig. 13 and 14).

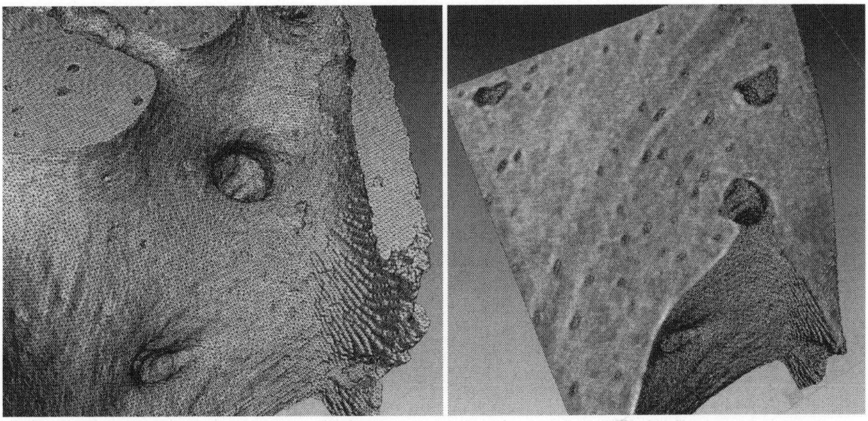

Fig. 13. FEM from a bone biopsy (left) and a zoomed section (right) with a cutting plane showing the projection in a false color map and the meshed osteocytes inside in red.

For osteocytes an elastic Young modulus of 1% of the elastic modulus of bone was given. Due to the fact that with the used resolution it was not possible to visualize the canaliculi, non-hydrostatic properties were chosen for the osteocytes. Thus for the same reason and in order to keep simplicity, the bone was not modeled as biphasic but as homogenous, isotropic and linear elastic. To compare with other studies, in which *in vivo* analysis of human μFE-models has been analyzed, material properties and boundary conditions (load magnitude and application) were taken from literature. Thus, an E-modulus of 17 GPa, a Poisson ratio (γ) of 0.3 and 1.7 GPa and γ = 0.45 for bone and osteocytes were used respectively. As explained above the differently mineralized regions were not segmented and consequently meshed together. Similarly for comparison with other analyses, a compression load of 1000 N was applied ramp-like and linear in the step. The step has a total time of 100 seconds, and reports of the results were set to be printed each 25 seconds. This allows visualization of the first regions that achieve maximal stress and strains tensors (Fig. 15). After analysis of the results, under the same conditions the load transmission capacity in the osteoporotic bone was reduced up to approx. 23% compared with the healthy biopsy after interpreting von Mises stress and minimum principal strain distribution. It appears that the size of osteocytes is more important than their number. Of course these findings need to be confirmed by analyzing more bone samples not only for the same region but other anatomical regions from healthy subjects and osteoporotic patients.

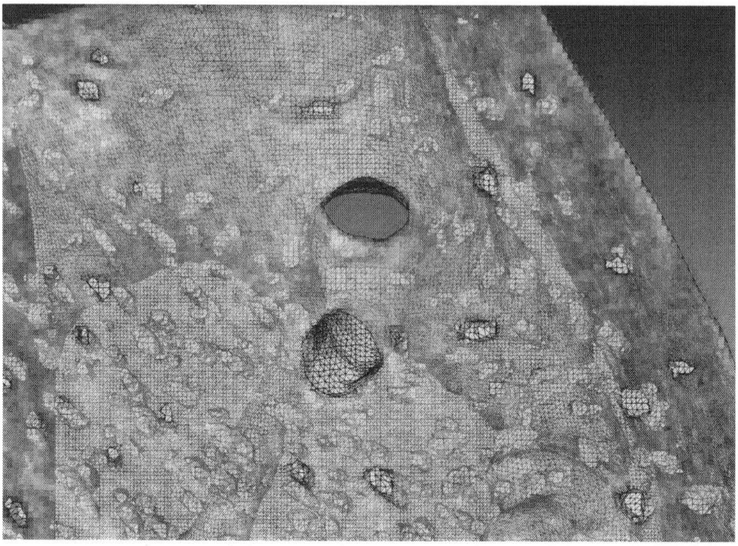

Fig. 14. Detail (through-view) of the FE-Mesh of the bone and osteocytes embedded in the bone matrix.

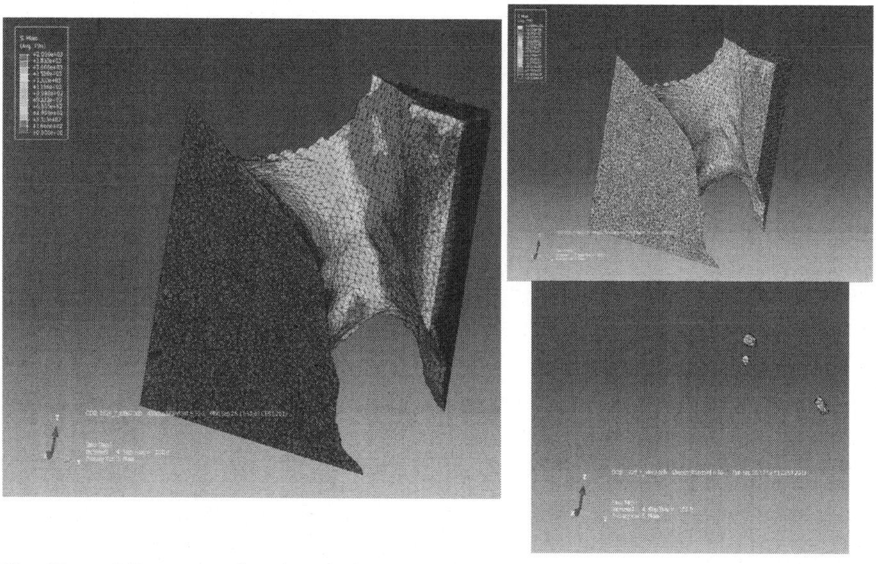

Fig. 15. von Mises stress distribution for a bone section and selected osteocytes with high stress values.

5. Specific scientific relevance and innovative aspects of osteocytes characterization

CT-Techniques and image analysis already allow bone structure, geometry and density evaluation over time (*in vivo*) or its detailed analysis at the nanometer scale (*in vitro*). However, it appears to be more challenging to describe how bones respond to pharmacological treatment or new mechanical conditions. Considering that osteocytes are not only directly responsible for starting bone remodeling regions, but that their number, size and distribution in comparable bone volumes shows how bone changed due to diseases or medications (e.g. as strontium ranelate or bisphosphonates, which alter bone mineralization), we have therefore developed a methodology for osteocytes characterization. For the first time, the complete method from laboratory CT (using a standard resolution of 20 µm), SR-CT (voxel size 2.174 µm) up to their finite element analysis was carried out.

Considering the actual developments in software and hardware, it has become possible not only to measure and reconstruct the bone biopsies using both 20 µm (laboratory CT) but also for the first time the total volume biopsy (2.2 mm diameter and 1cm length) using 2.174 µm isotropic resolution. It was important to visualize osteocytes distribution in their whole length and to verify the positioning of the osteocytes inside the total bone volume of the biopsy. The evaluation of bone biopsies (e.g. intact vs. unhealthy such as shown in this chapter, or after pharmacological treatments) will be a relevant and in the future important indicator for bone quality evaluation.

6. Potential users of the methodology and results

Once the relation between osteocytes and bone healthiness is understood, the methods described in this chapter will be used for the design of technologies to intervene in the mechanobiological process directed for the osteocytes. Patient specific pharmacological interventions or training conditions will be designed for it.

The method described here uses commercially available computational software and hardware and can easily be reproduced for visualization of the osteocytes lacunae and their processes distribution (to visualize this last a higher SR-CT resolution will be needed). In general, healthy bone matrix or its alterations due to genetics, aging or reduction in the bone mechanical stimuli could be studied and analyzed using this method.

In the future, the analysis of environment conditions and necessities of each patient will be carried out. After SR-CT measurements, its analysis requires advanced computational tools. Although the method described here is easy and reliable, it will not be readily available for all interested parties. Biopsies are an invasive technique. Maybe in the future and due to the continuous development in CTs technologies, reduced volume of bone samples will be sufficient for analysis but conserving the requirements of sufficient bone mass with a considerable number of osteocytes that allows comparisons and understanding bone diseases or bone response after usage of designed pharmacological interventions. However it remains speculative to suppose a minimal bone volume size to understand how osteocytes are acting. For future studies, it could be interesting for better understanding of osteocytes' morphology and their role on bone behavior to analyze bone samples from regions with high turn-over metabolic process, thus to analyze osteocytes morphology and their interconnectivity. We propose the methodology described here as standard method, hence comparison between results from different studies will provide valuable knowledge on osteocytes nature.

7. Discussion

7.1 On the method

Considering that non necrotic bone tissue was present in the biopsies, it is assumed that in each osteocyte lacunae resides a living, active osteocyte with identical and normal functionality. Thus, the comparison of osteocytes morphology from bone samples, as e.g. osteoporotic and healthy analyzed and reported here, are valid providing information about relations between bone mechanics response and osteocytes morphology.

An obvious requirement is the measurement quality. For laboratory CT measurements, it is not critical because after reconstruction, it is possible to repeat the measurement in an adequate time. But, at least for the synchrotron measurements at BESSY, it was critical to repeat a SR-CT measurement, due to considerable time requirements for measuring and projections reconstruction and an inflexible time schedule. Thus, the selection of the biopsies and their preparations are not trivial at all.

One of the principal advantages of CT is its non-destructive nature, implying that measurements not only at different CT resolutions of the same samples and regions are possible, but it can also be combined with other techniques (e.g. atomic force microscope for studying the interaction with proteins). After comparisons of measured parameters at different scales, quantitative relations between density, bone structural parameters and number of osteocytes can be derived.

Combined CT techniques for measurement and reconstruction, image analysis and the finite element method are adequate to study and analyze osteocytes morphology and their relation with bone stiffness.

7.2 On the findings

As confirmed in this study the relation BV/TV is a good indicator of the bone quality. Considering that as observed in the laboratory μCT measurements (20 healthy and 20 osteoporotic bone biopsies) and observed in detail in the SR-CT measurements, in most cases the highest mineralized regions are localized at the center of each geometrical bone structure. Thus the possible effects on the ratios determination due to partial volume effects are counterbalanced independently from the scale used for scanning (of course for 20 μm and less).

After analysis of the first two biopsies selected for SR-CT measurements, the number of osteocytes for the healthy bone biopsy was clearly larger than for the osteoporotic bone sample, as expected, and although a major number of biopsies need to be analyzed this finding was confirmed after measurements of two additional samples. But an interesting fact was that osteocytes size appears to be smaller in the healthy bone biopsies.

8. Conclusion and future direction

Our findings showed a clear alignment of the osteocytes along the cement lines. Interestingly at the regions near the bone surface with reduced mineralization grade osteocytes were mainly aligned along the close to high mineralized region. Apparently, not only osteocytes number is reduced with aging but their size increases and become sparely distributed in comparison with the healthy bone samples from the human mandible.

Automatic tetrahedron mesh generation using the "tetragen" tool from Amira worked adequately for meshing the biopsies with a resolution of 20 μm, but meshing biopsies with osteocytes embedded on the bone matrix from the SR-CT samples consumes an enormous amount of time, due to necessary adjustments for avoiding intersections and conserving model closeness.

It is important to consider that this study has been initiated in 2008 (first scans with 20 μm) and remains an on-going study for performing the rest of SR-CT measurements, and for quantifying osteocytes/grade of mineralization. It was given importance to visualize osteocytes (lacunae) in the complete bone volume biopsy, and although the method has been established, new questions occurred: How is the grade of connectivity between osteocytes? Are there changes in the number and direction of the osteocytes dendrites for the osteoporotic and healthy bone biopsies? Is it possible that osteocytes for the osteoporotic bone samples are large but that all osteocytes possesses more or less the same number of processes (canaliculi), such that the number of canaliculi will become an specific characteristic of this bone cells? Or will due to aging a general mal-functioning of the osteocytes occur, such that only a reduced number of processes will be expected? In this last case, the pathway of the mechanical stimuli to osteoblastic and osteoclastic bone cell will be interrupted, and bone formation will never be initiated for regions with unconnected osteocytes and new bone will not be formed, similarly bone resorption required for initiating bone repair will be stopped.

8.1 Future direction

To finalize with such speculations, new measurements of the same 4 biopsies measured at BESSY with 2.174 μm (results report in this chapter) have been performed using a resolution of approx. 0.2 μm. We expect to see the canaliculi network, to perform 3D volume visualization and their quantitative analysis, following the established protocol presented here.

Additionally and since in osteoporotic bones osteocytes size appears to be larger as for healthy, additional analysis on the sample group included in this study will be performed for confirming or neglecting this finding. If the initial finding is true, it could be important to analyze if the grade of mineralization and number, size and distribution of osteocytes are related. SR-CT is able to show different degrees of mineralization. These analyses will be then realized at short time by including additional steps using the skeletonization tool after segmentation of the different mineralized regions in Amira, allowing their quantification and comparison.

There are some reports about the morphology and connectivity between osteocytes. However it is not clear how they are distributed in relation to the different grades of mineralization. The SR-CT measurements using 0.2 μm spatial resolution will clarify this point.

Although not shown in this chapter, as the analysis has not been completed, we observe some micro- fissures whose pattern extended in 3D through complete biopsy, which we will be analyzed.

Visualization of osteocytes in their natural environment facilitates interpretation of the findings. Thus one can understand their role in the bone architecture by means of their morphological characterization.

9. Acknowledgments

Only the interaction and team work between different disciplines, and groups has allowed visualization and analysis using good established tools such as the finite element method and to incorporate new developments from Amira and the BAM procedures for measurements and reconstructions.

10. References

Anderson, C. T., Castillo, A. B., Brugmann, S. A., Helms, J. A., Jacobs, C. R. and Stearns, T. Primary cilia: cellular sensors for the skeleton. *Anat Rec (Hoboken)* Vol.291,(9), 2008, pp:1074-8.

Beraudi, A., Stea, S., Bordini, B., Baleani, M. and Viceconti, M. Osteon classification in human fibular shaft by circularly polarized light. *Cells Tissues Organs* Vol.191,(3), 2010, pp:260-8.

Boutroy, S., Van Rietbergen, B., Sornay-Rendu, E., Munoz, F., Bouxsein, M. L. and Delmas, P. D. Finite element analysis based on in vivo HR-pQCT images of the distal radius is associated with wrist fracture in postmenopausal women. *J Bone Miner Res* Vol.23,(3), 2008, pp:392-9.

Boyde, A., Travers, R., Glorieux, F. H. and Jones, S. J. The mineralization density of iliac crest bone from children with osteogenesis imperfecta. *Calcif Tissue Int* Vol.64,(3), 1999, pp:185-90.

Cheung, W. Y., Liu, C., Tonelli-Zasarsky, R. M., Simmons, C. A. and You, L. Osteocyte apoptosis is mechanically regulated and induces angiogenesis in vitro. *J Orthop Res* Vol.29,(4), 2011, pp:523-30.

Cooper, D. M., Erickson, B., Peele, A. G., Hannah, K., Thomas, C. D. and Clement, J. G. Visualization of 3D osteon morphology by synchrotron radiation micro-CT. *J Anat,* 2011.

Cowin, S. C. Mechanosensation and fluid transport in living bone. *J Musculoskelet Neuronal Interact* Vol.2,(3), 2002, pp:256-60.

Dong, X. N., Zoghi, M., Ran, Q. and Wang, X. Collagen mutation causes changes of the microdamage morphology in bone of an OI mouse model. *Bone* Vol.47,(6), 2010, pp:1071-5.

Feng, J. Q., Ward, L. M., Liu, S., Lu, Y., Xie, Y., Yuan, B., Yu, X., Rauch, F., Davis, S. I., Zhang, S., Rios, H., Drezner, M. K., Quarles, L. D., Bonewald, L. F. and White, K. E. Loss of DMP1 causes rickets and osteomalacia and identifies a role for osteocytes in mineral metabolism. *Nat Genet* Vol.38,(11), 2006, pp:1310-5.

Fouard, C., Malandain, G., Prohaska, S. and Westerhoff, M. Blockwise processing applied to brain microvascular network study. *IEEE Trans Med Imaging* Vol.25,(10), 2006, pp:1319-28.

Han, Y., Cowin, S. C., Schaffler, M. B. and Weinbaum, S. Mechanotransduction and strain amplification in osteocyte cell processes. *Proc Natl Acad Sci U S A* Vol.101,(47), 2004, pp:16689-94.

Huang, C. and Ogawa, R. Mechanotransduction in bone repair and regeneration. *Faseb J* Vol.24,(10), 2010, pp:3625-32.

Huiskes, R. If bone is the answer, then what is the question? *J Anat* Vol.197,(Pt 2), 2000, pp:145-156.

Jacobs, C. R., Temiyasathit, S. and Castillo, A. B. Osteocyte mechanobiology and pericellular mechanics. *Annu Rev Biomed Eng* Vol.12, 2010, pp:369-400.

Kearney, E. M., Farrell, E., Prendergast, P. J. and Campbell, V. A. Tensile strain as a regulator of mesenchymal stem cell osteogenesis. *Ann Biomed Eng* Vol.38,(5), 2010, pp:1767-79.

Kerschnitzki, M., Wagermaier, W., Roschger, P., Seto, J., Shahar, R., Duda, G. N., Mundlos, S. and Fratzl, P. The organization of the osteocyte network mirrors the extracellular matrix orientation in bone. *J Struct Biol* Vol.173,(2), 2011, pp:303-11.

Liu, X. Y. Effects of microgravity on Ca mineral crystallization and implication for osteoporosis in space. *Applied Physics Letters* Vol.79,(21), 2001, pp:3539-41.

Mulvihill, B. M. and Prendergast, P. J. An algorithm for bone mechanoresponsiveness: implementation to study the effect of patient-specific cell mechanosensitivity on trabecular bone loss. *Comput Methods Biomech Biomed Engin* Vol.11,(5), 2008, pp:443-51.

Nabavi, N., Khandani, A., Camirand, A. and Harrison, R. E. Effects of microgravity on osteoclast bone resorption and osteoblast cytoskeletal organization and adhesion. *Bone*, 2001.

Perilli, E., Baruffaldi, F., Visentin, M., Bordini, B., Traina, F., Cappello, A. and Viceconti, M. MicroCT examination of human bone specimens: effects of polymethylmethacrylate embedding on structural parameters. *J Microsc.* Vol.225,(Pt 2), 2007, pp:192-200.

Rack, A., Zabler, S., Mueller, B. R., Riesemeier, H., Weidemann, G., Lange, A., Goebbels, J., Hentschel, M. and Goerner, W. High resolution synchrotron-based radiography and tomography using hard X-rays at the BAMline (BESSY II). *Nuclear Instruments and Methods in Physics Research Section A* Vol.586,(2), 2008, pp:327-344.

Rincon-Kohli, L. and Zysset, P. K. Multi-axial mechanical properties of human trabecular bone. *Biomech Model Mechanobiol* Vol.8,(3), 2009, pp:195-208.

Rodionova, N. V., Oganov, V. S. and Zolotova, N. V. Ultrastructural changes in osteocytes in microgravity conditions. *Adv Space Res* Vol.30,(4), 2002, pp:765-70.

Roschger, P., Paschalis, E. P., Fratzl, P. and Klaushofer, K. Bone mineralization density distribution in health and disease. *Bone* Vol.42,(3), 2008, pp:456-66.

Schneider, P., Meier, M., Wepf, R. and Muller, R. Serial FIB/SEM imaging for quantitative 3D assessment of the osteocyte lacuno-canalicular network. *Bone* Vol.49,(2), 2011, pp:304-11.

Stalling, D., Westerhoff, M., and Hege, H.-C. (2005). Amira: a highly interactive system for visual data analysis. *The Visualization Handbook*. C. D. Hansen, and Johnson, Christopher R., Elsevier: 749-767.

van Oers, R. F., Ruimerman, R., van Rietbergen, B., Hilbers, P. A. and Huiskes, R. Relating osteon diameter to strain. *Bone* Vol.43,(3), 2008, pp:476-82.

Varga, P., Pahr, D. H., Baumbach, S. and Zysset, P. K. HR-pQCT based FE analysis of the most distal radius section provides an improved prediction of Colles' fracture load in vitro. *Bone* Vol.47,(5), 2011, pp:982-8.

Vilayphiou, N., Boutroy, S., Szulc, P., Van Rietbergen, B., Munoz, F., Delmas, P. D. and Chapurlat, R. Finite element analysis performed on radius and tibia HR-pQCT images and fragility fractures at all sites in men. *J Bone Miner Res*, 2011.

Whitfield, J. F. Primary cilium--is it an osteocyte's strain-sensing flowmeter? *J Cell Biochem* Vol.89,(2), 2003, pp:233-7.

You, L., Cowin, S. C., Schaffler, M. B. and Weinbaum, S. A model for strain amplification in the actin cytoskeleton of osteocytes due to fluid drag on pericellular matrix. *J Biomech* Vol.34,(11), 2001, pp:1375-86.

8

Specific Absorption Rate Analysis of Heterogeneous Head Models with EEG Electrodes/Leads at 7T MRI

Leonardo M. Angelone[1,2] and Giorgio Bonmassar[2]

[1]*Division of Physics, Office of Science and Engineering Laboratories, Center for Devices and Radiological Health, U.S. Food and Drug Administration, Silver Spring, MD*

[2]*Athinoula A. Martinos Center for Biomedical Imaging, Department of Radiology, Massachusetts General Hospital, Harvard Medical School, Charlestown, MA USA*

1. Introduction

In this chapter we explore the use of anatomically accurate head models for radio frequency (RF) dosimetry and design of electroencephalography (EEG) electrode and leads. The study is conducted at 300 MHz, which is the frequency used to elicit the proton-based Magnetic Resonance Imaging (MRI) signal at 7 Tesla (7T). The use of electrically heterogeneous vs. homogeneous numerical models is explored in terms of investigation of antenna-effect for EEG leads. While the results in the homogeneous model can be validated with direct measurements in phantoms, the experimental validation of numerical simulations with electrically heterogeneous head models would require the use of a multi-structure physical phantom, much more cumbersome and expensive to build. This study aimed to evaluate whether the use of a more complex heterogeneous head model would provide additional information when looking at energy absorbed by a human head wearing EEG electrodes/leads and exposed to a 300 MHz RF field.

MRI-based high-resolution homogeneous and heterogeneous head models were implemented for this study. The electromagnetic (EM) interactions between EEG electrodes/leads on the human head and the incident RF field used to elicit the MRI signal were investigated in terms of electromagnetic field, induced currents in the leads, and specific absorption rate (SAR) in a human head. Both perfectly conductive and resistive EEG leads were studied.

Non-significant differences in whole-head SAR (i.e. less than 5%) and a 30% difference in peak-10g-averaged SAR values were observed with the homogeneous vs. heterogeneous models. The difference for peak-1g-averaged SAR estimated with the homogeneous vs. heterogeneous model was up to 100%. The presence of an insulating layer between EEG electrode and skin resulted in a change of 10% of peak-10g-averaged SAR and 280% for peak 1g-averaged SAR. Results of this study suggest that a homogeneous model could be used to estimate the changes on whole-head and 10g-averaged SAR due to the antenna effect of EEG leads at 7 T MRI. Precise modeling of the electrically conductive interface between electrode and head surface is also fundamental.

Simultaneous EEG and MRI/fMRI recordings are frequently performed in clinical research as they provide fundamental information on the physiological and hemodynamic activity of the brain [Allen 2000, Benar 2003, Comi 2005, Kobayashi 2005, Liebenthal 2003, Matsuda 2002, Mirsattari 2004, Mulert 2005, Purdon 2009]. While clinical application for this technology (e.g. epilepsy) are mainly limited to MRI fields up to 1.5 T [Stern 2006], the possibility of increased spatial resolution and signal to noise ratio for brain structural and functional information drives an increasing number of research groups toward the use of high field MRI, namely 3T [Goldman 2000, Iannetti 2005, Purdon 2009, Scarff 2004] and even 7T [Mullinger 2008, Vasios 2006].

EEG recordings at high-field MRI present several technological challenges, including signal and safety issues. The EEG electrodes/leads can affect the MRI signal [Bonmassar 2001], and the MRI can add noise into the EEG signal [Allen 2000, Lemieux 1997]. The safety issues present are intrinsic to high-field MRI [Ibrahim 2007] as well as due to interaction between static, gradient and RF field with EEG electrodes and leads on the human head [Schenk 2000, Shellock 2011].

Safety issues for simultaneous EEG and high-field MRI recordings are typically categorized as: force and torque on device due to static and spatial gradient fields [Schenk 2000], peripheral nerve stimulation due to gradient-switching [Shellock 2011], and potential issues due to induced currents and related adverse thermal effects associated with energy dissipation inside the head [IEC 2002, FDA 2003].Because of the low magnetic permeability of the human body [Polk 1986], RF heating from magnetic energy dissipated inside the human head is typically disregarded and only the electric component of the incident field is considered when calculating RF heating. The electric energy fed into the RF coil of the MRI systems is partly radiated into the empty space and partly dissipated with the EEG leads and the head. If the energy dissipated inside the head is not properly balanced by the thermoregulatory system, potential adverse thermal effects can occur [Adair 1986]. The quantity used to quantify the amount of power dissipated in the human body is the SAR, measured in W/kg [NCRP 1981].

A full evaluation of RF-induced heating requires the calculation of electric field in each point of the volume of interest. The electric coupling can be analyzed in terms of both a) Faraday-induced non-conservative coupling and b) conservative capacitive coupling:

$$\vec{E} = -j\omega\vec{A} - \nabla V \tag{1}$$

Faraday's induced currents ("eddy currents"), represented by the non-conservative term of eq. (1) $j\omega\vec{A}$, are generated by coupling between the MRI gradient and/or RF field and conductive loops within EEG leads, inside the human head, and/or between EEG leads and human head [Dempsey 2001]. Capacitive coupling - represented by the conservative term of eq. (1) ∇V, occurs when the dimensions of the load (i.e., head with leads) are comparable with the incident wavelength, and the time-varying electric component is "picked up" by the load, acting as scattering antennas [Armenean 2004, Balanis 2005, Dempsey 2001, Yeung 2002]. Hence, there is a difference of potential (∇V in eq. 1) due to charge accumulation that contributes to the conservative component of the electric field.

For MRI fields up to 1.5 T the EM wavelength (e.g., 4.7m in empty space at 64 MHz/1.5T) is much longer than dimensions of the head and the capacitive coupling can be disregarded ("quasi-static approximation") [Bottomley 1978]. Consequently, previous studies evaluating RF heating for EEG leads and MRI systems up to 1.5T have mainly focused on faraday-induced eddy currents [Lemieux 1997]. Based on these studies, some solutions have been proposed to overcome the issue of the induced currents along EEG leads, such as twisted pair configuration [Godlman 2002], or the use of current-limiting resistors [Lemieux 1997].

At high field MRI (3 T or higher) however, this approximation is no longer valid (e.g., RF wavelength at 300 MHz/7T in empty space is 1m) and a full-wave characterization of the incident RF field [Ibrahim 2007] is necessary. The full-wave model requires the analysis of the complete Maxwell equations; given the complexity of the geometries considered, numerical solutions have been implemented [Collins 2005, Gandhi 1999, Jin 1997, Kainz 2003, Trakic 2007, Van der Berg 2007]. Among the different algorithms used, the Finite Difference Time Domain [Kunz 1993, Taflove 2005] is often the method of choice.

The "antenna-effect" defines the physical phenomenon for which a conductive lead immersed in an EM field scatters the incident field, becoming a transmitting-antenna [Balanis 2005]. This mechanism creates two different issues: 1) a mismatch of conductivity at the interface between a lead and the skin, with charge accumulation ("capacitive" effect) and enhancement of electric field in the area underneath the electrode [Guy 1975]; 2) a perturbation of the EM field compared to the one generated by the RF coil only, with related changes of SAR in the head.

The currents induced along the EEG leads in an RF field depend on the geometry of the leads, the characteristics of the incident EM field, and the material properties of the lead. The efficiency of the leads as antennas, hence their effect into the incident EM field, is higher for lead dimensions comparable with the wavelength of the incident field. Given the typical length of EEG leads (~50-100 cm) the EM fields generated by rapid gradient switching have wavelengths too long to generate a significant antenna behavior for the EEG leads [Dempsey 2001]. Conversely, the antenna effect of the leads will be significant at the RF frequencies used for imaging. The RF current induced in the leads depend on the relative position of the leads with respect to the incident RF field, being maximal with leads parallel to the RF field and null with the leads perpendicular to the RF field [Balanis 2005].

Given the geometrical complexity of the problem considered, computational EM can help to further understand the interaction between variably-resistive EEG leads and the human body. Whole-body averaged, partial body, and whole-head averaged SAR [IEC 2002, FDA 2003] are the values of reference used in the MRI systems to control the maximum RF transmitted power allowed during an MRI examination. A spatial resolution of $2\times2\times2.5\text{mm}^3$ to model the human head is considered accurate when evaluating whole-head SAR in MRI [Collins 2003]. However, in the specific case of a human head with conductive leads during MRI, the interactions between leads and the RF-field are expected to generate local peaks of electric field and SAR near the electrodes [Guy 1975]. In this case, the use of the whole-head SAR as an exclusive dosimetric parameter for safety profile is inaccurate and the estimation of local 1g- or 10g-averaged SAR is more appropriate [Angelone 2010, Nitz 2005]. In this study, the hypothesis that $2\times2\times2.5\text{mm}^3$ is sufficient for SAR computation was rejected, and a MRI-based head model with $1\times1\times1\text{mm}^3$ isotropic spatial resolution was implemented [Angelone 2008, Makris 2008]. A similar model has been used to study the effect of purely metallic EEG leads [Angelone 2004], to evaluate the use of high resistive leads with numerical simulations on a homogeneous model [MRI 2006], and to evaluate the effect of EEG electrodes/leads in the human head exposed to RF sources of mobile-phone [Angelone

2010]. In this chapter we investigate the effect of using electrically heterogeneous vs. homogeneous human head models.

2. Methods

Numerical head model: Anatomical segmentation and classification at radio-frequency by electrical properties. MRI data - One healthy 37-year-old, right-handed adult male volunteer participated in this study. Informed consent was obtained in accordance with Massachusetts General Hospital policies. High-resolution anatomical MRI data were acquired with a quadrature birdcage transmit/receive head coil on a 1.5 T scanner (General Electric, Milwaukee, WI). Data were collected with a T1-weighted 3D-SPGR sequence (TR/TE = 24/8 ms) with 124 slices, 1.3 mm thick (matrix size 256×192, FOV 256 mm). The volume data was resampled to isotropic voxels with dimensions of 1x1x1 mm^3. Segmentation was then applied to this dataset volume.

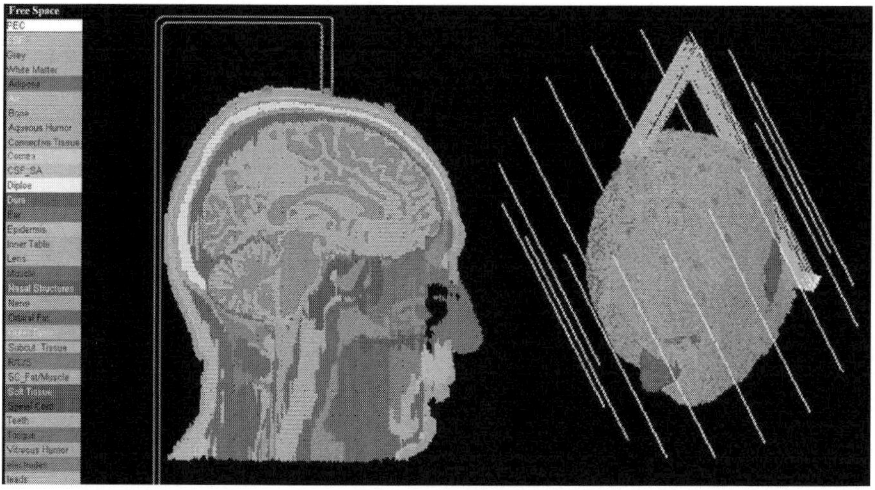

Fig. 1. High resolution head model with 32 electrodes/leads and RF coil. The 3D view shows the head model with EEG leads centered in a 16-wire RF coil.

Anatomical segmentation - Twenty-five non-brain anatomical structures (**Figure 1**) were manually segmented from the MRI data by an expert anatomist [Makris 2008]. Three brain structures (Cerebro Spinal Fluid, Grey and White matter) were additionally segmented with an automatic segmentation algorithm [Dale 1999, Segonne 2004] and coregistered with the non-brain structures. The final head model consisted of a total of 28 anatomical structures (**Table 1**). The total number of Yee cells [Yee 1966] was 4,642,730. The head dimensions were 170 mm in width, 217 mm in depth, and 238 mm in height.

	Anatomical Structures	Heterogeneous Density (kg/m^3)	Heterogeneous 300 MHz (d) σ (S/m)	Heterogeneous 300 MHz (d) ε_r	Homogeneous Density (kg/m^3)	Homogeneous 300 MHz (d) σ (S/m)	Homogeneous 300 MHz (d) ε_r
BRAIN	Grey Matter	1030(a)	0.69	60.00	1040	0.80	59
BRAIN	White Matter	1030(a)	0.41	43.77			
BRAIN	Cerebro Spinal Fluid	1010(a)	2.22	72.73			
NON-BRAIN	Adipose	920(a)	0.07	11.74			
NON-BRAIN	Air (Resp./Diges./Sinus)	1.3(b)	0.00	1.00			
NON-BRAIN	Bone (Facial)	1850(b)	0.08	13.43			
NON-BRAIN	Connective Tissue	1100(a)	0.55	46.77			
NON-BRAIN	Cornea	1076(c)	1.15	61.37			
NON-BRAIN	Diploe / Bone Marrow	1080(b)	0.21	23.16			
NON-BRAIN	Dura	1030(a)	0.80	47.95			
NON-BRAIN	Ear / Pinna	1100(a)	0.55	46.77			
NON-BRAIN	Eye Humor (Aqueous)	1010(a,c)	1.51	69.01			
NON-BRAIN	Eye Humor (Vitreous)	1010(a,c)	1.51	69.01			
NON-BRAIN	Eye Lens	1100(c)	0.64	48.95			
NON-BRAIN	Epidermis/Dermis	1100(a)	0.64	49.82			
NON-BRAIN	Inner Table	1850(b)	0.08	13.43			
NON-BRAIN	Muscle	1040(d)	0.79	58.97			
NON-BRAIN	Nasal-Structures	1100(a)	0.55	46.77			
NON-BRAIN	Nerve	1040(a)	0.41	36.90			
NON-BRAIN	Orbital Fat	920(a)	0.07	11.74			
NON-BRAIN	Outer Table	1850(b)	0.08	13.43			
NON-BRAIN	Retina/Choroid/Sclera	1170(a)	0.97	58.90			
NON-BRAIN	Spinal Cord	1040(a)	0.41	36.90			
NON-BRAIN	Soft Tissue	1100(a)	0.55	46.77			
NON-BRAIN	Subcutaneous Tissue	1100(a)	0.55	46.77			
NON-BRAIN	Subcutaneous Fat	920(a)	0.07	11.74			
NON-BRAIN	Teeth	1850(b)	0.08	13.43			
NON-BRAIN	Tongue	1040(d)	0.79	58.97			

Table 1. Anatomical structures and electrical properties of high-resolution heterogeneous head model at 300 MHz. The electrical properties were constant for all the anatomical structures in the homogeneous model. (a) [Li 2006]; (b) [Collins 2004], (c) [DeMarco 2003], (d) [FCC website] based on [Gabriel 1996].

Classification of anatomical structures at radio-frequency by their electrical properties - The classification of anatomical structures in terms of electrical properties is necessary to precisely compute the EM field and SAR in the human head during an MRI experiment. The electrical properties of anatomical structures, such as electrical conductivity and permittivity, vary depending on their structural composition. Specifically, the electrical properties of the models used in this study were considered as [Vorst 2006]: a) linear with electric field, b) isotropic, c) dispersive, and d) heterogeneous in space. Under these conditions, complex permittivity (ε^*) is defined as:

$$\begin{aligned} \varepsilon^*(\omega) &= \varepsilon_r(\omega) - j\varepsilon''(\omega) \\ &= \varepsilon_r(\omega) - j\frac{\sigma_{tot}(\omega)}{\omega\varepsilon_0} = \varepsilon_r(\omega) - j\left(\frac{\sigma_i(\omega)}{\omega\varepsilon_0} + \varepsilon_d(\omega)\right) \end{aligned} \quad (2)$$

where $\varepsilon_r(\omega)$ is the frequency-dependent relative permittivity of the material, ε_0 is the permittivity of free space (equal to $8.854 \cdot 10^{-12}$ F m^{-1}), ω is the angular frequency of the field ($\omega = 2\pi f$, with *f* frequency in Hz); $\varepsilon''(\omega)$ is the frequency-dependent loss factor, with $\sigma_{tot}(\omega)$ the total conductivity, that includes a frequency-independent ionic conductivity ($\sigma_i(\omega)$) and the frequency-dependent losses due to dielectric polarization ($\varepsilon_d(\omega)$). The frequency used in this study was 300 MHz which is approximately the RF frequency needed to elicit proton MRI signal at 7 T.

In the EEG leads, typically built with metals or non-biological materials, the loss component is due to free electrons only:

$$\varepsilon''(\omega) = \frac{\sigma_{tot}(\omega)}{\omega\varepsilon_0} = \frac{\sigma_i(\omega)}{\omega\varepsilon_0} \quad (3)$$

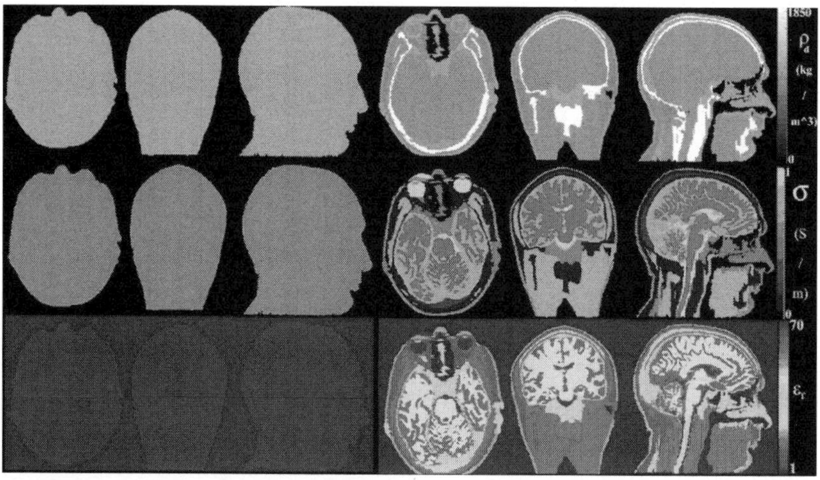

Fig. 2. Biophysical properties for homogeneous and heterogeneous model at 300 MHz. The high-spatial resolution of the model allowed distinguishing contiguous structures with different electrical properties, such as bone-marrow vs. outer table, skin vs. fat.

The anatomical classification, mass density and electrical properties at 300 MHz are shown in **Table 1** and mapped in **Figure 2**. Two different electrical models - a homogeneous and a heterogeneous one - were implemented. For the homogeneous case, the same physical properties were assigned to all the anatomical structures, i.e., conductivity $\sigma_{\text{tot}} = 0.8\,\text{S}/\text{m}$, relative permittivity $\varepsilon_{\text{r}} = 59$, and density $\rho_{\text{d}} = 1040\,\text{kg}/\text{m}^3$, corresponding to the average properties of muscle at 300 MHz [FCC Website]. For the heterogeneous model, each anatomical structure was assigned more specific electrical properties, based on the data of the comprehensive study by Gabriel et al. [Gabriel 1996a, 1996b, 1996c] (**Table 1**). The values of mass density were derived from literature [Collins 2004, DeMarco 2003, Gabriel 1996, FCC website, Li 2006]. An average value of conductivity and permittivity was assigned to the anatomical structures without a direct equivalence in the database (i.e., "Subcutaneous Tissue", "Connective Tissue", and "Soft tissue") [Makris 2008].

Numerical Model of EEG electrodes and Leads - The layout of thirty-two EEG electrodes on a 2D mask was designed using Circuit Maker (Altium Inc, San Diego, CA) and imported into Matlab (Mathworks, Natick, MA). The mask was co-registered with the axial slice of largest diameter on the head model. The EEG electrodes and leads of the mask were projected and placed on the surface of the head model ("epidermis" tissue, see **Figure 1**) [Angelone 2006]. The EEG electrodes were modeled as small cylinders (radius: 7 mm, thickness: 3 mm) and were positioned in direct contact with the skin as for the expanded 10-20 montage [Regan 1989]. The leads were modeled as metallic leads ($\rho_{el/leads} = \rho_{copper} = 1.67 \cdot 10^{-8}\ \Omega\, m$), and were bundled above the Cz electrode [Regan 1989],oriented vertically, and curved downward as shown in **Figure 1**. The complete model (i.e., head with 32 EEG electrodes/leads) was then imported into the XFDTD software (Remcomi Inc., State College, PA). EEG leads were shortened on one side, to simulate the short circuit created by the low-pass filter in the input stage of the EEG recording system [Purdon 2008], and connected on the other side to the head surface.

Numerical Model of RF Coil - The RF source was based on a volume RF coil [Jin 1997, Collins 2001]. The coil was modeled with 16 perfect electrically conductive rods of 295 mm in length and disposed around the head with circular symmetry (diameter 260mm) (**Figure 1**). The RF source was simulated as a circular excitation driving the current generators placed on the centers of the rods with 1A peak-to-peak amplitude and a 22.5° phase-shift between any two adjacent generators.

FDTD simulations - Numerical simulations were performed using commercially available software XFDTD, based on the Finite-Difference-Time-Domain (FDTD) algorithm. Numerical simulations were performed at a frequency of 300 MHz. A total of seven perfectly matching layers were used for boundary conditions [Berenger 1994]. The total volume, including the free space around the model, was 297×353×303 mm^3; the time step used to meet the Courant condition for numerical stability [Taflove 2005] was 1.92 ps, and the total number of time steps was 25,000. Simulations provided the magnitude of electromagnetic field and induced currents for each voxel, as well as whole-head averaged SAR, 1g- and 10 g-averaged SAR [IEC 2002, FDA 2003].

3. Results

Model without EEG electrodes/leads - **Figure 3** shows the magnetic flux density $\|\vec{B}\|$, and **Figure 4** the electric field $\|\vec{E}\|$ and induced currents $\|\vec{J}\|$ computed with homogeneous and heterogeneous head model. The load of the head on the RF coil (i.e. the impedance seen by each of the 16 sources) was similar (± 10%) in both models, in line with physical RF coil tuning on the bench with anatomically accurate phantoms or human head [Ibrahim 2005]. The characteristic Central Brightening Effect at 7T [Collins 2005] was present in both models. The superposition of electromagnetic fields determined a complex pattern of electric field inside the head and local peaks of electric field at the boundaries between skin and air as well as inside the head. The effect of the tissue conductivity focused the currents in the most conductive structures (e.g., Cerebro Spinal Fluid and eye region).

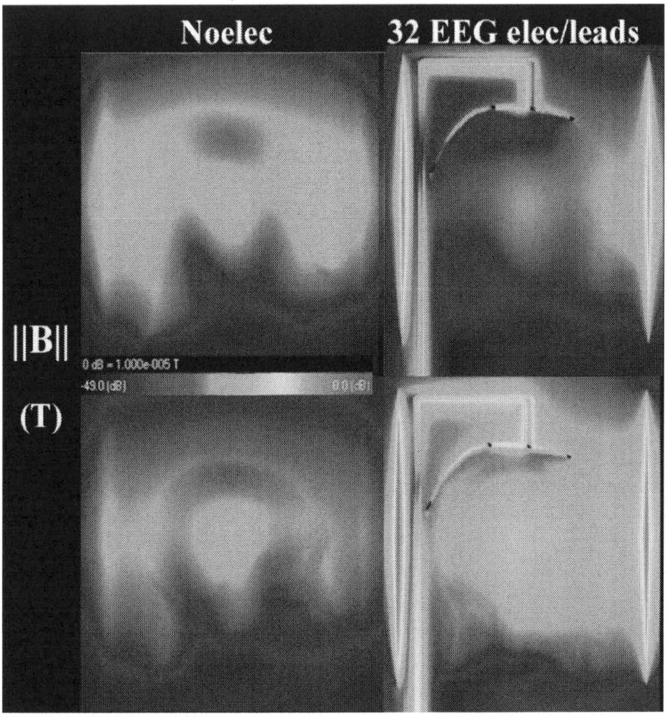

Fig. 3. Amplitude of magnetic flux density $\left\|\vec{B}\right\|$ computed with homogeneous and heterogeneous head model without ("Noelec") and with EEG electrodes/leads. The characteristic Central Brightening Effect at 7T [Collins 2005] was present in both models.

Head plus metallic leads - **Figure 4** shows the effect of metallic leads with the head. The superposition of the electric field radiated from the RF coil and field scattered by the leads resulted in an increase of the field near the leads and on the skin, and in a reduction of the field at the center of the head ("shielding effect of the EEG leads") [Hamblin 2007]. There was a peak of induced currents on the skin, near the leads. Because of the EEG-leads acting as antennas, the coil load and the magnetic field inside the head were different compared to the control case of no leads.

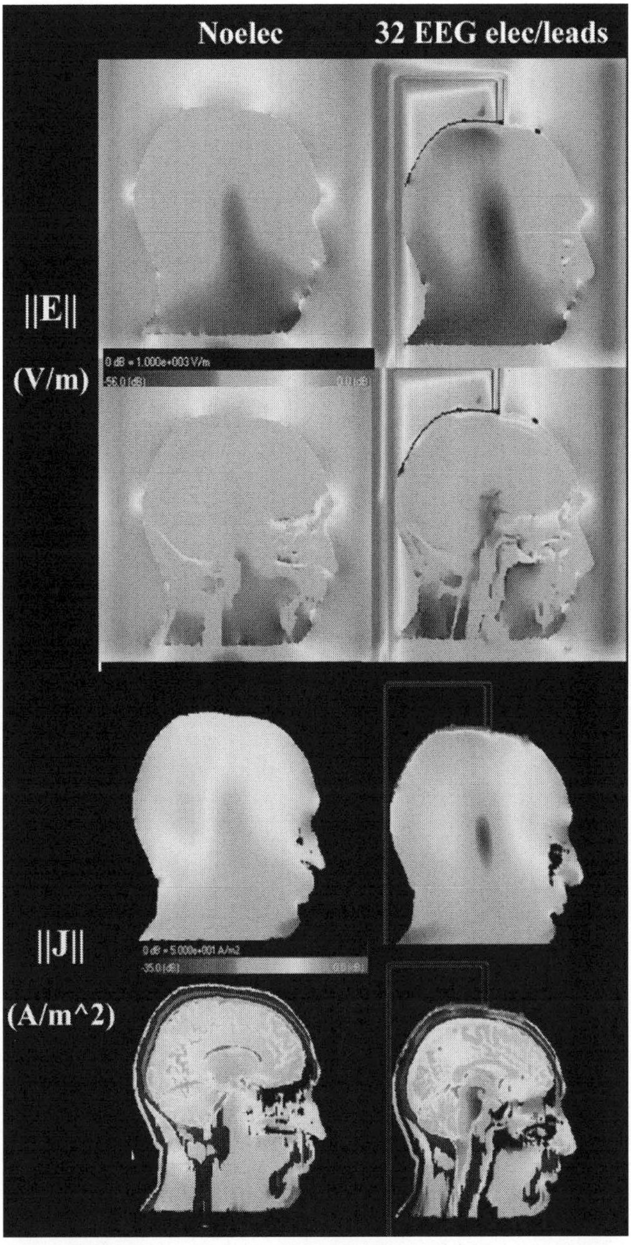

Fig. 4. Amplitude of electric field $\|\vec{E}\|$ and induced currents $\|\vec{J}\|$ computed with homogeneous and heterogeneous head model, without ("Noelec") and with EEG electrodes/leads.

SAR - The whole-head SAR computed with the two models (with/without leads) was similar (i.e., 3% difference, see **Table 2**). No significant difference (<5%) in whole-head SAR was observed for the case with perfectly conductive EEG leads. The heterogeneity of the structures and the local differences of electrical properties affected the 1g-averaged SAR, with up to two-fold difference for the peak 1g-averaged SAR (**Figure 5**) in the control case without leads (1^{st}vs. 3rd column, **Table 2**), and a 30% difference with EEG leads (2^{nd}vs. 4th column, **Table 2**). Smaller differences with homogeneous vs. heterogeneous model were observed in the computation of 10-g averaged SAR, with a 15% difference without leads and 20% difference with EEG leads (**Table 2**).

300 MHz	Homogeneous		Heterogeneus	
	noelec	32elec-copper	noelec	32elec-copper
Max SAR [W/kg]	1.1	33.9	2.3	38.8
Peak 1g avg. SAR [W/kg]	0.48	1.37	0.92	1.05
Peak 10g avg. SAR [W/kg]	0.29	0.32	0.33	0.40
Whole Head [W/kg]	0.10	0.09	0.10	0.09
Input power [W]	4.1	3.3	4.5	3.6
Power dissipated in head[W]	2.0	1.4	2.4	1.8
Radiated power [W]	2.1	1.8	2.1	1.9
Efficiency	52%	56%	47%	51%

Table 2. Results for simulations with homogeneous and heterogeneous model, without and with copper EEG leads.

4. Discussion

While the results in the homogeneous model can be validated with direct measurements in phantoms, the validation of numerical simulations with heterogeneous head models require a multi-structure phantom, which would be much more cumbersome and expensive to build. This study aimed to evaluate whether the use of a more complex heterogeneous model would provide additional information when looking at SAR changes due to EEG electrodes/leads in a human head exposed to a 300 MHz RF field.

For this purpose, the study was based on a high-resolution head model segmented by an expert anatomist from MRI data of an adult healthy subject (**Figure 1**). In the control-case of a head model without EEG electrodes/leads, thei EM field was slightly asymmetric [Amjas 2005, Sled 1998]. The EM fields and induced currents were also different between the homogeneous and heterogeneous models [Amjad 2005].

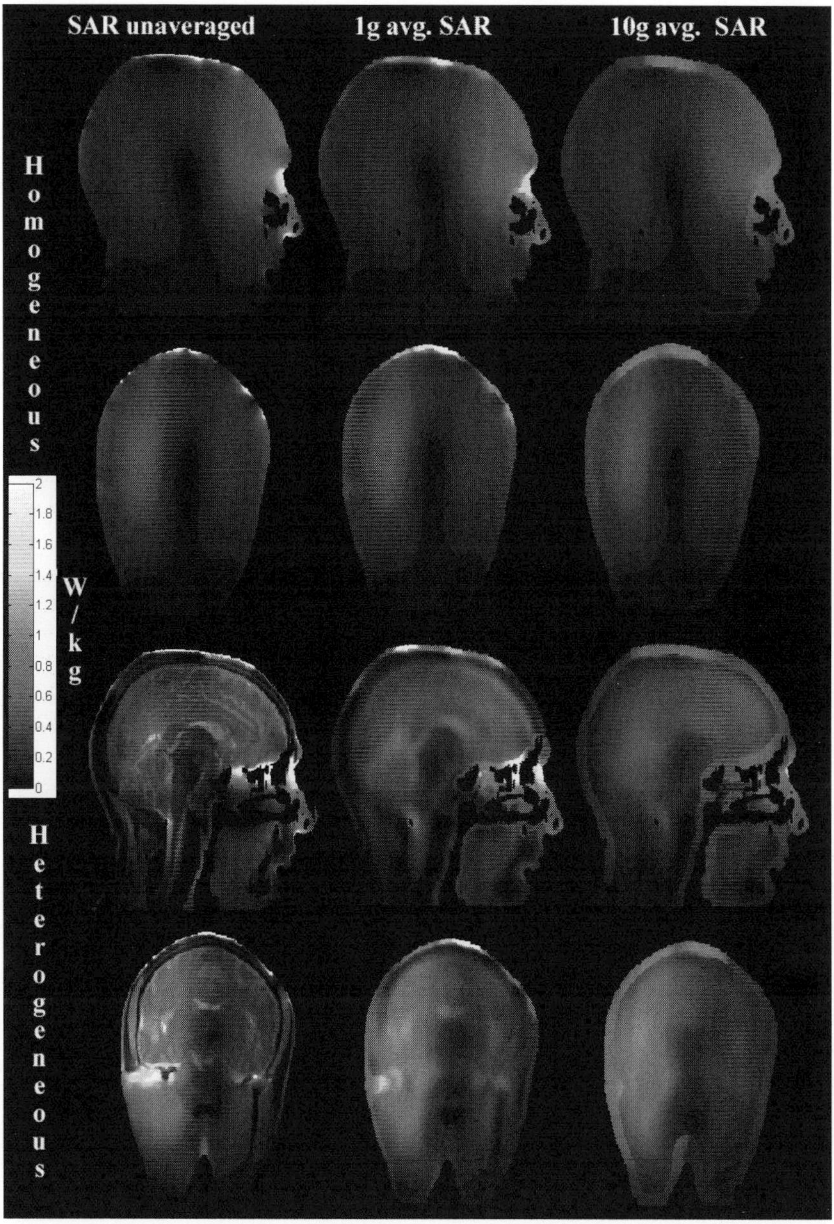

Fig. 5. Specific Absorption Rate (SAR) computed with an electrically homogeneous (top) and electrically heterogeneous (bottom head) model. Sagittal and coronal maps for SAR unaveraged, 1g-averaged and 10g-averaged SAR are shown.

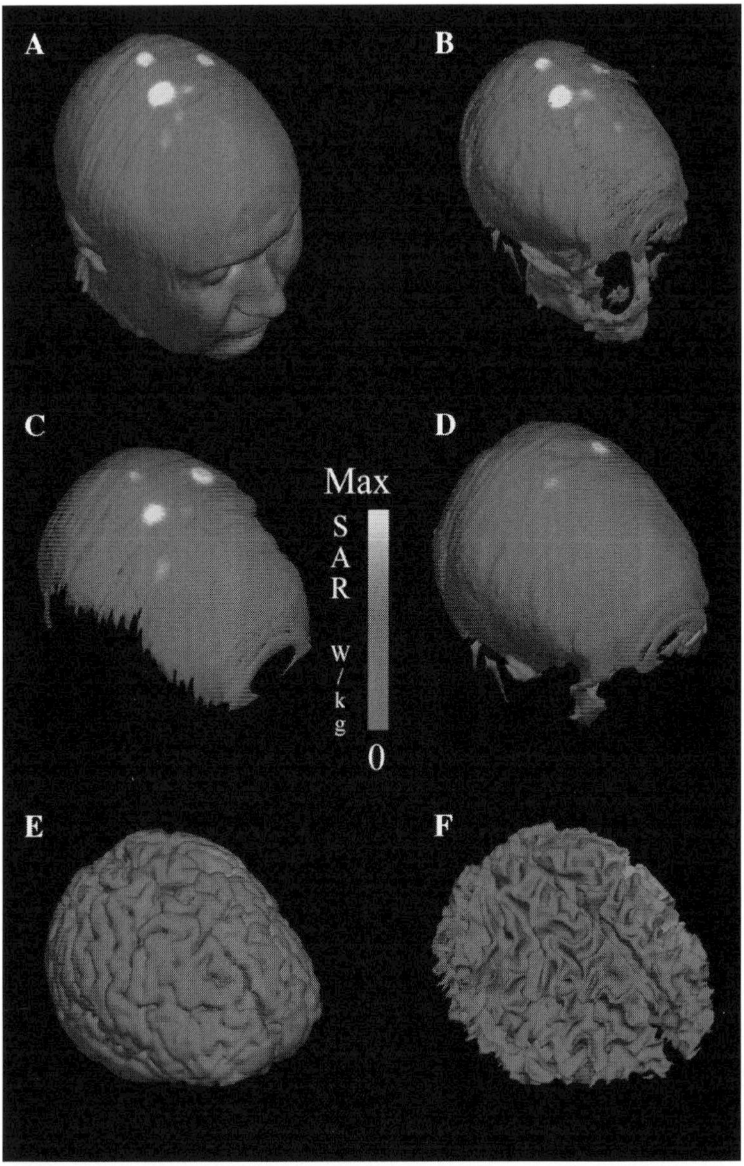

Fig. 6. 3D view of SAR (W/Kg) with copper leads on epidermis and bone structures (outer table, inner table, bone, teeth). The high-resolution of the model allowed for precise anatomical definition of thin structures, such the epidermis, where the contact with copper EEG leads induces local electric field and SAR enhancement. Max SAR = 10 W/kg. Values normalized to 1 W of Input Power.

SAR estimation with homogeneous and heterogeneous model- No significant differences were observed for whole-head SAR computed with or without EEG leads for both the homogeneous and heterogeneous models, suggesting that whole-head SAR may be an excessively smoothing parameter for RF dosimetry with EEG leads. The small difference in peak SAR estimated with homogeneous or heterogeneous model for the case with metallic EEG leads was likely due to the specific location of the peak SAR (i.e., few mm underneath the electrodes); the volume of interest in the heterogeneous model included only two structures, epidermis and subcutaneous tissue, with electrical properties similar to the one used for the homogeneous model. On the other hand, because of the spatially-limited characteristics of SAR changes it is important to properly model the variably-conductive interfaces between EEG electrodes, epidermis, and subcutaneous tissues, both in terms of anatomical structures and electrical properties. As a further test, we have compared the results obtained with the homogeneous model with metallic leads with a model where the external layer (i.e., the epidermis) was substituted with perfectly insulating material ($\sigma = 0\ S/m$). Whole-head and 10g-averaged SAR were not affected by the dramatic change in conductivity at the interface, but there was a 280% change in computed 1g-averaged SAR.

The use of a heterogeneous head model may allow for improved SAR computation and visualization for heterogeneous structures with different electrical properties, such as skin, fat, muscle or bone marrow (**Figure 2**). However, the use of an anatomically fine-grained head model may add potential errors when modeling the internal structures of the head [Gajsek 2002]. Due to the difficulties in matching exactly all the anatomical definitions to existing literature, some of the anatomical structures were assigned the same electrical properties; 16 different electrical properties were used to characterize the anatomical structures (**Figure 2**). Further work may be performed to improve the electrical characterization of the numerical head model and to validate using direct measurements with corresponding physical models.

Effect of geometry - This study focused on evaluating the effect of head electrical heterogeneity as well as lead resistivity on SAR. The geometrical model was constant with respect to other physical variables (**Figure 1**) which may affect SAR: number of electrodes, length and orientation of the leads, position of the head inside the RF coil, and RF source geometry, as well as size and shape of the head model. In clinical applications, these variables will be affected by various external constraints, such as length of the imager used for the MRI recording, position of EEG system inside the MRI room, and geometry of RF coil used to obtain the best Signal to Noise Ratio (SNR). For example, EEG leads may be connected to a pre-amplifier placed either on the back of the imager (EEG leads from the top of the head oriented farther away from the head) or in the front of the scanner (EEG leads placed along the head and exiting from the neck down); in this case the minimal physical length of the leads will depend on the placement of the pre-amplifier. We have modeled 32 electrodes and leads, a configuration currently used in many laboratories for EEG-MRI recordings. The results of this study cannot be directly extrapolated to different number of electrodes, because the presence of more leads may increase the interaction with the EM field, with resulting SAR in the head that could be higher or lower, depending on the geometry, the shielding effect of the EEG leads [Hamblin 2007] and the frequency considered [Angelone 2004].

Antenna effect - The typical length of EEG leads is in the order of ~ 50-100cm, which is comparable with the wavelength of the RF field at 300 MHz (i.e., 1 m in empty space). The interactions of the EEG leads and RF coils will induce changes in the EM field inside the head (i.e., "shielding effect" of the EEG leads) [Hamblin 2007] and local SAR enhancement at the interface between electrodes and skin [Armenean 2004, Yeung 2002]. Low resistivity EEG leads ($\rho_{lead} < \rho_{\min} \approx 0.0001\,\Omega\,m$) behave as lossless antenna [Balanis 2005] and will have maximum induced currents along the leads. The high discontinuity of resistivity between lead and surrounding medium ($\rho_{lead} = 1.67 \cdot 10^{-8}\Omega\,m$ vs. $\rho_{skin} = 1/\sigma_{skin}\,1.56\,\Omega\,m$ for the skin/epidermis, **Table 1**) determines an electric field enhancement at the interface between leads and head surface (i.e., epidermis). This observation is in line with theoretical models [Guy 1975] and physical evidence of reports of burns due to "antenna-effect" of leads [Dempsey 2001].

5. Conclusions

The aim of this study was to investigate the possible effect of using complex heterogeneous head models when investigating SAR in a human head wearing EEG electrodes/leads while exposed to RF field of high-field MRI. MRI-based high-resolution homogeneous and heterogeneous head models with 32 EEG electrodes/leads were implemented. Electromagnetic simulations based on FDTD algorithm were performed. Non-significant differences in whole-head SAR (i.e. less than 5%) and a 30% difference in peak 10g-averaged SAR values were observed with the homogeneous vs. heterogeneous models. The presence of an insulating layer between EEG electrode and skin resulted in a three-fold change in computed 1g-averaged SAR. Results of this study suggest that when whole-head, 10g-averaged, and 1g-averaged SAR in a human head wearing EEG electrodes/leads are computed with a homogeneous rather than electrically heterogeneous model this can result in a difference of up to 30%. In all cases, a precise modeling of the electrically conductive interface between electrode and head surface is fundamental to avoid a significant underestimation of the local SAR.

Future directions – The systematic analysis presented in this chapter improved the scientific understanding of the complex interactions between radiofrequency electromagnetic field and a human head with EEG leads. Such a numerical framework can be used to support the design and development of novel leads for multimodal recording at ultra high-field MRI. Future work may be directed toward investigating the effect of the specific head model used, in terms of inter-subject variability and in the presence of anatomical pathologies. Moreover, further improvement of the electrical model, namely the electrical properties associated with each anatomical structure, can be obtained by taking advantage of MRI-based direct measurements, i.e., electrical properties tomography (EPT). Finally, while the specific absorption rate is the current parameter used for RF dosimetry, the use of temperature is a more biologically significant quantity, and future work may be directed toward a better evaluation of the changes in temperature – rather than only SAR – in the body. The experimental validation with properly matching geometries between numerical and physical models will most likely be the final fundamental step toward a complete dosimetric evaluation.

6. Acknowledgments

We would like to thank Dr. Nikos Makris, Jonathan Kaiser, and the Center for Morphometric Analysis at Massachusetts General Hospital for their help for this study. We also would like to thank Drs. CK Chou, Bu Sik Park, and Jana Delfino for the useful insights.

The mention of commercial products, their sources, or their use in connection with material reported herein is not to be construed as either an actual or implied endorsement of such products by the Department of Health and Human Services. This research was carried out in whole or in part at the Athinoula A. Martinos Center for Biomedical Imaging at the Massachusetts General Hospital, using resources provided by the *Center for Functional Neuroimaging Technologies, P41RR14075,* a P41 Regional Resource supported by the Biomedical Technology Program of the National Center for Research Resources (NCRR), National Institutes of Health. This work was also supported in part by the National Institute of Biomedical Imaging and Bioengineering (R01EB006385) (GB), and by the National Eye Institute (R21EY020961-01) (GB).

7. References

Adair E.R., and Berglund L.G. On the thermoregulatory consequences of NMR imaging. Magn Reson Imaging, 1986. 4(4): p. 321-33.

Allen P.J., Josephs O., and Turner R. A method for removing imaging artifact from continuous EEG recorded during functional MRI. Neuroimage, 2000. 12(2): p. 230-9.

Amjad A., Kamondetdacha R., Kildishev A., Park S.M., and Nyenhuis J. Power deposition inside a phantom for testing of MRI heating. IEEE Trans on Magnetics, 2005. 41(10): p. 4185-4187.

Angelone L.M., Potthast A., Segonne F., Iwaki S., Belliveau J., and Bonmassar G. Metallic electrodes and leads in simultaneous EEG-MRI: specific absorption rate (SAR) simulation studies. Bioelectromagnetics, 2004. 25(4): p. 285-295.

Angelone L.M., Vasios C.E., Wiggins G., Purdon P.L., and Bonmassar G. On the effect of resistive EEG electrodes and leads during 7 T MRI: simulation and temperature measurement studies. Magn Reson Imaging, 2006. 24(6): p. 801-12

Armenean C., Perrin E., Armenean M., Beuf O., Pilleul F., and Saint-Jalmes H. RF-induced temperature elevation along metallic wires in clinical magnetic resonance imaging: influence of diameter and length. Magn Reson Med, 2004. 52(5): p. 1200-6.

Balanis, C.A., Antenna theory : analysis and design. 3rd ed. 2005, Hoboken, NJ: John Wiley. xvii, 1117 p.

Benar C., Aghakhani Y., Wang Y., Izenberg A., Al-Asmi A., Dubeau F., and Gotman J. Quality of EEG in simultaneous EEG-fMRI for epilepsy. Clin Neurophysiol, 2003. 114(3): p. 569-80.

Berenger J.P. A perfectly matched layer for the absorption of electromagnetic waves. Computational Physics, 1994. 114: p. 185-200.

Bonmassar G., Hadjikhani N., Ives J.R., Hinton D., and Belliveau J.W. Influence of EEG electrodes on the BOLD fMRI signal. Hum Brain Mapp, 2001. 14(2): p. 108-15.

Bottomley P.A. and Andrew E.R. RF magnetic field penetration, phase shift and power dissipation in biological tissue: Implications for NMR imaging. Phys. Med. Biol., 1978. 23: p. 630–643.

Collins C.M., and Smith M.B. Spatial resolution of numerical models of man and calculated specific absorption rate using the FDTD method: a study at 64 MHz in a magnetic resonance imaging coil. J Magn Reson Imaging, 2003. 18(3): p. 383-8.

Collins C.M., Liu W., Wang J., Gruetter R., Vaughan J.T., Ugurbil K., and Smith M.B. Temperature and SAR calculations for a human head within volume and surface coils at 64 and 300 MHz. J Magn Reson Imaging, 2004. 19(5): p. 650-6.

Collins C.M., Liu W., Schreiber W., Yang Q.X., and Smith M.B., Central brightening due to constructive interference with, without, and despite dielectric resonance. J Magn Reson Imaging, 2005. 21(2): p. 192-6.

Comi E., Annovazzi P., Silva A.M., Cursi M., Blasi V., Cadioli M., Inuggi A., Falini A., Comi G., and Leocani L. Visual evoked potentials may be recorded simultaneously with fMRI scanning: A validation study. Hum Brain Mapp, 2005. 24(4): p. 291-298.

Dale A.M., Fischl B., and Sereno M.I. Cortical surface-based analysis. I. Segmentation and surface reconstruction. Neuroimage, 1999. 9(2): p. 179-94.

DeMarco S.C., Lazzi G., Liu W., Weiland J.D., and Humayun M.S. Computed SAR and thermal elevation in a 0.25-mm 2-D model of the human eye and head in response to an implanted retinal stimulator - part I: models and methods. Antennas and Propagation, IEEE Transactions on, 2003. 51(9): p. 2274-2285.

Dempsey M.F., Condon B., and Hadley D.M. Investigation of the factors responsible for burns during MRI. J Magn Reson Imaging, 2001. 13(4): p. 627-31.

Federal Communication Commission http://www.fcc.gov/fcc-bin/dielec.sh

Food and Drug Administration (FDA) Center for Devices and Radiological Health. *Criteria for Significant Risk Investigations of Magnetic Resonance Diagnostic Devices*. 2003.

Gandhi O.P., and Chen X.B. Specific absorption rates and induced current densities for an anatomy-based model of the human for exposure to time-varying magnetic fields of MRI. Magn Reson Med, 1999. 41(4): p. 816-23.

Gabriel C., Gabriel S., and Corthout E. The dielectric properties of biological tissues: I. Literature survey. Phys. Med. Biol., 1996. 41: p. 2231–2249.

Gabriel C., Gabriel S., and Corthout E. The dielectric properties of biological tissues: II. Measurements in the frequency range 10 Hz to 20 GHz. Phys. Med. Biol., 1996. 41: p. 2251–2269.

Gabriel C., Gabriel S., and Corthout E. The dielectric properties of biological tissues: III. Parametric models for the dielectric spectrum of tissues. Phys. Med. Biol., 1996. 41: p. 2271–2293.

Gajsek P., Walters T.J., Hurt W.D., Ziriax J.M., Nelson D.A., and Mason P.A. Empirical validation of SAR values predicted by FDTD modeling. Bioelectromagnetics, 2002. 23(1): p. 37-48.

Goldman R.I., Stern J.M., Engel J. Jr., and Cohen M.S. Simultaneous EEG and fMRI of the alpha rhythm. Neuroreport, 2002. 13(18): p. 2487-92.

Guy A. W. Biophysics - Energy Absorption and Distribution, vol. AGARD Lectures Series 78, p. 4-1 to 4-14, 1974.

Hamblin D.L., Anderson V., McIntosh R.L., McKenzie R.J., Wood A.W., Iskra S., and Croft R.J. EEG electrode caps can reduce SAR induced in the head by GSM900 mobile phones. IEEE Trans Biomed Eng, 2007. 54(5): p. 914-920.

Iannetti G.D., Niazy R.K., Wise R.G., Jezzard P., Brooks J.C., Zambreanu L., Vennart W., Matthews P.M., and Tracey I. Simultaneous recording of laser-evoked brain potentials and continuous, high-field functional magnetic resonance imaging in humans. Neuroimage, 2005. 28(3): p. 708-19.

Ibrahim T.S., Kangarlu A., and Chakeress D.W. Design and performance issues of RF coils utilized in ultra high field MRI: experimental and numerical evaluations. IEEE Trans Biomed Eng, 2005. 52(7): p. 1278-84.

Ibrahim T.S., Mitchell C., Abraham R., and Schmalbrock P. In-depth study of the electromagnetics of ultrahigh-field MRI. NMR Biomed, 2007. 20(1): p. 58-68.

IEC, International Standard, medical equipment - part 2-33: Particular requirements for the safety of the magnetic resonance equipment for medical diagnosis, 2nd revision. 2002, International Electrotechnical Commission 601-2-33: Geneva. p. 29-31.

Jin J., and Chen J. On the SAR and field inhomogeneity of birdcage coils loaded with the human head. Magn Reson Med, 1997. 38(6): p. 953-63.

Kainz W., Chan D.D., Casamento J.P., and Bassen H.I. Calculation of induced current densities and specific absorption rates (SAR) for pregnant women exposed to hand-held metal detectors. Phys Med Biol, 2003. 48(15): p. 2551-60.

Kobayashi, E., Bagshaw A.P., Jansen A., Andermann F., Andermann E., Gotman J., and Dubeau F. Intrinsic epileptogenicity in polymicrogyric cortex suggested by EEG-fMRI BOLD responses. Neurology, 2005. 64(7): p. 1263-6.

Kunz K.S., and Luebbers R.J. The finite difference time domain method for electromagnetics. 1993, Boca Raton: CRC Press. 448 p.

Lemieux L., Allen P.J., Franconi F., Symms M.R., and Fish D.R. Recording of EEG during fMRI experiments: patient safety. Magn Reson Med, 1997. 38(6): p. 943-52.

Li Q.X., and Gandhi O.P. Thermal Implications of the New Relaxed IEEE RF Safety Standard for Head Exposures to Cellular Telephones at 835 and 1900 MHz. IEEE Trans Microwave Theory and Technique, 2006. 54(7): p. 3146-3154.

Liebenthal E., Ellingson M.L., Spanaki M.V., Prieto T.E., Ropella K.M., and Binder J.R. Simultaneous ERP and fMRI of the auditory cortex in a passive oddball paradigm. Neuroimage, 2003. 19(4): p. 1395-404.

Makris N, Angelone L, Tulloch S, Sorg S, Kaiser J, Kennedy D, Bonmassar G. MRI-based anatomical model of the human head for specific absorption rate mapping. Med Biol Eng Comput. 2008. 46(12): p. 1239-1251.

Matsuda T., Matsuura M., Ohkubo T., Ohkubo H., Atsumi Y., Tamaki M., Takahashi K., Matsushima E., and Kojima T. Influence of arousal level for functional magnetic resonance imaging (fMRI) study: simultaneous recording of fMRI and electroencephalogram. Psychiatry Clin Neurosci, 2002. 56(3): p. 289-90.

Mirsattari S.M., Lee D.H., Jones D., Bihari F., and Ives J.R. MRI compatible EEG electrode system for routine use in the epilepsy monitoring unit and intensive care unit. Clin Neurophysiol, 2004. 115(9): p. 2175-80.

Mulert C., Jager L., Propp S., Karch S., Stormann S., Pogarell O., Moller H.J., Juckel G., and Hegerl U. Sound level dependence of the primary auditory cortex: Simultaneous measurement with 61-channel EEG and fMRI. Neuroimage, 2005. 28(1): p. 49-58.

Mullinger K., Debener S., Coxon R., and Bowtell R. Effects of simultaneous EEG recording on MRI data quality at 1.5, 3 and 7 Tesla. Int J Psychophysiol. 2008 Mar;67(3): p. 178-88.

National Council Radiation Protection and Measurements (NCRP). Radiofrequency electromagnetic fields: properties, quantities and units, biophysical interaction, and measurement. 1981, Bethesda, MD.

Nitz W.R., Brinker G., Diehl D., and Frese G. Specific absorption rate as a poor indicator of magnetic resonance-related implant heating. Invest Radiol, 2005. 40(12): p. 773-6.

Polk C. and Postow E. CRC handbook of biological effects of electromagnetic fields. 1986, Boca Raton, Fla.: CRC Press. 503 p.

Purdon PL, Millan H, Fuller PL, Bonmassar G. An open-source hardware and software system for acquisition and real-time processing of electrophysiology during high field MRI. J Neurosci Methods. 2008 Nov 15;175(2): p.165-86.

Purdon PL, Pierce ET, Bonmassar G, Walsh J, Harrell PG, Kwo J, Deschler D, Barlow M, Merhar RC, Lamus C, Mullaly CM, Sullivan M, Maginnis S, Skoniecki D, Higgins HA, Brown EN. Simultaneous electroencephalography and functional magnetic resonance imaging of general anesthesia. Ann N Y Acad Sci. 2009 Mar;1157: p.61-70.

Regan D. Human brain electrophysiology: Evoked potentials and evoked magnetic fields in science and medicine. 1989, New York: Elsevier, 415 p.

Scarff C.J., Reynolds A., Goodyear B.G., Ponton C.W., Dort J.C., and Eggermont J.J. Simultaneous 3-T fMRI and high-density recording of human auditory evoked potentials. Neuroimage, 2004. 23(3): p. 1129-42.

Schenck J. Safety of strong, static magnetic fields. J Magn Reson Imaging, 2000. 12(1): p. 2-19.

Segonne F., Dale A.M., Busa E., Glessner M., Salat D., Hahn H.K., and Fischl B. A hybrid approach to the skull stripping problem in MRI. Neuroimage. 2004 Jul; 22(3): p. 1060-75.

Shellock F.G. Reference Manual for Magnetic Resonance Safety, Implants, and Devices: 2011. Biomedical Research Publishing Company, 650 p.

Sled J. G., and Pike G. B. Standing-wave and RF penetration artifacts caused by elliptic geometry: an electrodynamic analysis of MRI.1998, IEEE Trans. Med. Imaging, vol. 17, p. 653-662

Stern J.M., Simultaneous electroencephalography and functional magnetic resonance imaging applied to epilepsy. Epilepsy Behav, 2006. 8(4): p. 683-92.

Taflove A., and Hagness S. C. Computational Electrodynamics: The Finite-Difference Time-Domain Method, 3rd ed. 2005, Artech House, Norwood, MA.

Trakic, A., F. Liu, H.S. Lopez, H. Wang, and S. Crozier, Longitudinal gradient coil optimization in the presence of transient eddy currents. Magn Reson Med, 2007. 57(6): p. 1119-30.

Van den Berg C.A., van den Bergen B., Van de Kamer J.B., Raaymakers B.W., Kroeze H., Bartels L.W., and Lagendijk J.J. Simultaneous B1 + homogenization and specific absorption rate hotspot suppression using a magnetic resonance phased array transmit coil. Magn Reson Med, 2007. 57(3): p. 577-86.

Vasios C.E., Angelone L.M., Purdon P.L., Ahveninen J., Belliveau J.W., and Bonmassar G. EEG/(f)MRI measurements at 7 Tesla using a new EEG cap ("InkCap"). Neuroimage, 2006. 33(4): p. 1082-92.

Vorst A.v., Rosen A., and Kotsuka Y. RF/microwave interaction with biological tissues. 2006, John Wiley & Sons, IEEE, Hoboken, N.J.: xiii, 330 p.

Yee K.S. Numerical Solution of Initial Boundary Value Problems Involving Maxwell's Equations in Isotropic Media. IEEE Transactions on Antennas and Propagation, 1966. 14(3): p. 302-307.

Yeung C.J., Susil R.C., and Atalar E. RF heating due to conductive wires during MRI depends on the phase distribution of the transmit field. Magn Reson Med, 2002. 48(6): p. 1096-8.

9

Simulating Idiopathic Parkinson's Disease by *In Vitro* and Computational Models

Tjitske Heida[1], Jan Stegenga[1], Marcel Lourens[2], Hil Meijer[2], Stephan van Gils[2], Nikolai Lazarov[3] and Enrico Marani[1]
[1]*Department of Biomedical Signals and Systems, University of Twente*
[2]*Department of Applied Analysis and Mathematical Physics, University of Twente*
[3]*Department of Anatomy and Histology, Medical University Sofia*
[1,2]*The Netherlands*
[3]*Bulgaria*

1. Introduction

1.1 Short history

The motor disorder of Parkinson's disease (PD) results from injury of the basal ganglia (BG). Understanding of the pathophysiology came late, especially with regard to the involvement of the substantia nigra. The description of 'shaking palsy' or 'paralysis agitans' (Parkinson, 1817) did not bring forward the recognition of its pathological origin. Lewy (1912, 1913) put emphasis on the globus pallidus and putamen. Von Economo's emphasis (1917) on the substantia nigra (SN) in encephalitis lethargica, with analogous clinical appearance, prompted others to pay attention to this nucleus. Tetriakoff (1919) was the first to describe SN involvement in paralysis agitans. Hassler (1937, 1938, 1939), by studying the normal cytoarchitecture of the SN, discovered a differential damage in the pars compacta using the collection of Cecile and Oscar Vogt. Moreover, he described the damage in the locus coeruleus. It was Friede, already in 1953 (1953, 1966), using histochemical techniques, who proposed a relation with catecholaminergic systems. Although the SN-catecholamine doctrine was regularly scrutinized in the early days of catecholamine research (see e.g. Mettler, 1964), it has not been overthrown up till now.

1.2 Idiopathic Parkinson's disease

Parkinson's disease is nowadays subdivided in idiopathic Parkinson's disease and Parkinson plus syndromes (see Usunoff et al., 2002). Parkinson plus syndromes counts for 15% of all Parkinsonism, although in large autopsy series the percentage augmented to 20-25% (Hughes et al., 1992), thus leaving idiopathic Parkinson's disease as the most frequently occurring form (Jellinger, 1987). Nevertheless contested (see e.g. Gibb, 1988; Kingsburry et al., 1999), the suggestion that the vulnerability of SN neurons is related to the neuromelanin/tyrosine hydroxylase content is favored in idiopathic Parkinsonism (Hirsch et al. 1988). Idiopathic Parkinson's disease is characterized by neuromelanin-containing cell loss and by the presence of Lewy inclusion bodies in surviving neurons in the SN and other areas (for an overview see Usunoff et al., 2002). "Lewy bodies in the SN are considered the pathological hallmark of Parkinson's disease, which means that if they cannot be found, the diagnosis is not Parkinson's disease" (Usunoff et al., 2002). The conclusion that idiopathic Parkinson's disease involves degeneration of pigmented neurons of the brain stem is inevitable (Greenfield & Bosanquet, 1953). This conclusion is also based on the distribution of Lewy bodies in other brainstem areas. However, within the human SN not all subareas degenerate (for an overview see Usunoff et al., 2002). Since topography is present in the human SN, circuits of these sparse unharmed areas do survive.

1.3 Models of idiopathic Parkinson's disease

Animal research profoundly increased by the detection of MPTP. In 1982, a young male, age 29, in northern California, used a new synthetic heroin, which brought him and his also addicted brother and several others, profound and unremitting Parkinsonism (Langston et al. 1999). In this case Meperidine (Demerol, Pethidine) was used. MPPP, the 'Designer heroin' (1-methyl-4-phenyl-4-propionoxypiperidine) contained not only MPPP but also 2.5 to 2.9% of MPTP (1-methyl-4-phenyl-1,2,3,6-tetrahydropyridine) by weight, a byproduct in the synthesis of MPPP. Biotransformation produces from MPTP the 1-methyl-4-phenylpyridinium ion (MPP^+), which is taken up by the dopamine transporter of the SN neurons, where it blocks the mitochondrial respiratory chain (see Langston et al., 1999 and references herein). An experimental monkey model was developed (see Vitale et al., 2009, for ethical criticism on this monkey model). MPTP was quickly shown experimentally to selectively destroy nerve cells in the SN after systemic administration. The resulting striatal dopamine depletion explained most, if not all of the clinical features of Parkinson's disease (for an extensive summary see Langston et al., 1983; Langston et al., 1999, and a report of an earlier case by Davis et al., 1979). MPTP works in dogs, cats and pigs, but is less effective in rats and guinea pigs, while the MPTP effect is strain dependent in mice. The overview of monkey MPTP results (Israel and Bergman, 2008) shows that these studies demonstrated the importance of the inactivation of the STN, inducing Parkinson symptoms and that the onset of synchronized bursts and high frequency oscillations interfered with normal function of the spatio-temporal function of the basal ganglia.

"However, although an experimental animal model is present and enormous efforts have been carried out to detect the cause of Parkinsonism, what initiates the disease is still unknown. Moreover, human studies have an ethical drawback and a case as described above is seldom found in literature. Therefore, experimental results from animals, often not possible to translate to the human situation, especially rat and mouse results, is what scientists have to relay on. Consequently model studies, using systemic, neuroanatomically developed, models, are of the utmost importance in the study of Parkinson's disease and are significant in their contribution to the understanding of Deep Brain Stimulation (DBS), nowadays mainly carried out in the subthalamic nucleus (STN)" (Heida et al., 2008; see also Toulouse & Sullivan, 2008).

It is, therefore, the gathering and the correct transformation of experimental animal results into newly developed PD models that determine the success of such a model in the contribution to the understanding of idiopathic Parkinson's disease. This review paper will first give an overview of the (classic) connection scheme of the basal ganglia-corticothalamic circuit. Then we will concentrate on rat SN and STN experimental results as obtained in our group. On the one hand anatomical data of the afferent and efferent connections of the SN and STN are presented, while on the other hand electrophysiological data of the neuronal activity patterns as observed in dissociated STN cell cultures and brain slices is discussed. Finally, a selection of computational models developed in our Applied Analysis and Mathematical Physics, and Biomedical Signals and Systems groups, related to different aspects of idiopathic Parkinson's disease are summarized. One of the aims of these computational models is to understand the mechanism of DBS. This review relies also on earlier publications, congress abstracts and presented posters (Cagnan et al., 2009; Heida et al., 2008, 2009, 2010a,b,c,d; Lourens et al., 2009, 2011; Marani et al., 2008, 2010; Meijer et al., in press; Moroney et al., 2008; Stegenga et al., 2009, 2010a,b,c).

2. Which connections are involved in idiopathic Parkinson's disease?

2.1 Classic connectivity diagram of the corticothalamic-basal ganglia network

The major pathways within the basal ganglia-thalamocortical circuit, which are known to be involved in the execution of voluntary movement, are illustrated in Figure 1 (see Gerfen & Wilson, 1996; and Groenewegen & Van Dongen, 2008). Albin et al. (1989) and De Long (1990) first proposed these pathways through the basal ganglia (BG). Two major connections link the BG input nucleus (striatum) to the output nuclei (globus pallidus interna (GPi)/substantia nigra pars reticulata (SNr)), namely the 'direct' and 'indirect' pathways. The critical balance between these two pathways determines normal motor behavior. The BG output nuclei have a high rate of spontaneous discharge, and thus exert a tonic, GABA-mediated, inhibitory effect on their target nuclei in the thalamus. The inhibitory outflow is differentially modulated by the direct and indirect pathways, which have opposing effects on the BG output nuclei, and thus on the thalamic targets of these nuclei.

The 'direct' pathway arises from inhibitory striatal efferents that contain both GABA and substance P and projects directly to the output nuclei. It is transiently activated by increased phasic excitatory input from the SNc (substantia nigra pars compacta) to the striatum. Activation of the direct pathway briefly suppresses the tonically active inhibitory neurons of the output nuclei, disinhibiting the thalamus, and thus increasing thalamocortical activity. The 'indirect' pathway begins with inhibitory striatal efferents that contain both GABA and enkephalin. These striatal neurons project to the GPe (globus pallidus externus). The GPe projects to the STN, via a purely GABAergic pathway, which finally projects to the output nuclei via an excitatory, glutamatergic projection. There is also a direct projection from the GPe to the output nuclei. The indirect pathway is phasically activated by decreased inhibitory input from the SNc to the striatum, causing an increase in striatal output along its pathway. Normally the high spontaneous discharge rate of GPe neurons exerts a tonic inhibitory influence on the STN. Activation of the 'indirect' pathway tends to suppress the activity of GPe neurons, disinhibiting the STN, and increasing the excitatory drive on the output nuclei. The decreased GPe activity also directly disinhibits the output nuclei. The resulting increase in activity of the output nuclei inhibits the thalamus further, decreasing thalamocortical activity. Activation of the direct pathway thus *facilitates* movement, whereas activation of the indirect pathway *inhibits* movement (see McIntyre and Hahn, 2010, for an extended overview).

The cortico-STN-GPi 'hyperdirect' pathway (Nambu et al., 2000, 2002; Nambu, 2005; Brown, 2003; BarGad et al., 2003; Squire et al., 2003) conveys powerful excitatory effects from the motor-related cortical areas to the globus pallidus, bypassing the striatum. The hyperdirect pathway is therefore an alternative direct cortical link to the BG, possibly as important to motor control as the direct pathway, which is typically considered to be the main cortical relay in the BG.

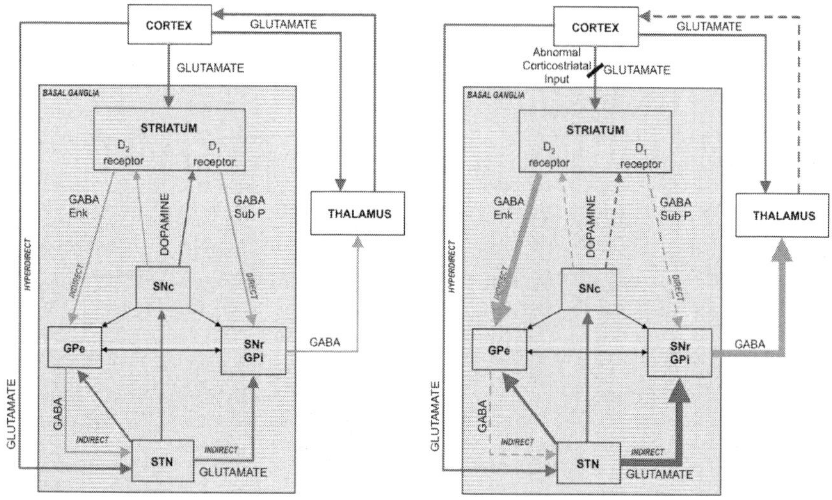

Fig. 1. Connection diagram of the basal ganglia-thalamocortical motor circuit. The relative connection strengths are indicated for Left: the normal healthy brain, and Right: the parkinsonian brain. Blue lines indicate inhibitory pathways; red lines indicate excitatory pathways. GPi: globus pallidus internus; GPe: globus pallidus externus; SNc: substantia nigra pars compacta; SNr: substantia nigra pars reticulata; STN: subthalamic nucleus; GABA: gamma amino butyric acid.

Nigrostriatal dopamine projections exert contrasting effects on the direct and indirect pathways (see Figure 1). Striatal neurons projecting in the direct pathway have D1 dopamine type receptors (D_1 and D_5) which cause excitatory post-synaptic potentials, thereby producing a net excitatory effect on striatal neurons of the direct pathway. Those projecting in the indirect pathway have D2 type receptors (D_2, D_3 and D_4), which cause inhibitory post-synaptic potentials, thereby producing a net inhibitory effect on striatal neurons of the indirect pathway. The facilitation of transmission along the direct pathway and suppression of transmission along the indirect pathway leads to the same effect - reducing inhibition of the thalamocortical neurons and thus facilitating movements initiated in the cortex. Thus, the overall influence of dopamine within the striatum may be to reinforce the activation of the particular basal ganglia-thalamocortical circuit which has been initiated by the cortex (Gerfen, 1992; Gerfen & Wilson, 1996; see also Hurley & Jenner, 2006). Due to the differential effects of dopamine on the D1 and D2 dopamine receptors of the striatum, a loss of striatal dopamine results in a reduction in transmission through the direct pathway and an increase in transmission through the indirect pathway, causing an imbalance between the two pathways.

The depletion of striatal dopamine changes neuronal firing rates in basal ganglia nuclei. Increased firing rates are found in the striatum, GPi and STN and a minimally decreased discharge in the GPe. A summary of tonic firing rates of BG nuclei in the normal and parkinsonian situation can be found in Heida et al. (2008). However, the pattern of discharge of basal ganglia neurons is thought to be equally as important as the rate of discharge in the execution of smooth movements. Several alterations in the discharge pattern have been observed in neurons of the BG in PD subjects. These alterations include a tendency of neurons to discharge in bursts, increased correlation and synchronisation of discharge between neighbouring neurons, rhythmic and oscillatory behaviour (Brown, 2003). Coherence between STN and GPi activity has been confirmed at tremor frequencies (3-10 Hz) (Brown et al., 2001). These oscillatory patterns are projected to GPi's thalamic projection site, the nucleus ventralis anterior thalami, and the cortex. In addition, STN and GPi demonstrate a tendency to synchronization at 11-30 Hz, which is likely to be driven from the motor areas of the cortex (Brown, 2003). In this circuit, the thalamus is in a key position as it receives the convergent afferent input from the GPi, the cortex, and the peripheral system, which it then projects back to the cortex, including motor areas (Smith et al., 1998).

2.2 Pedunculopontine and cholinergic connections

Gait is related to the pedunculopontine nucleus (Piallat et al., 2009), and therefore this nucleus plays an important role in gait and balance disorders that are common in Parkinson's disease. Topographically a pars compacta and a pars dissipatus of the PPN is discerned (Jacobsohn, 1909; Olszewski and Baxter, 1954). The pars dissipatus is supposed to contain glutamatergic neurons. Both parts contain cholinergic neurons. In humans the pars compacta exists of 90% cholinergic cells and the pars dissipatus of 25-75% (Mesulam et al., 1989). It should be noted, that intra-striatal pathways and PPN connections towards the SNc are mainly cholinergic. Cholinergic systems are also degenerated in Parkinson's disease. Nevertheless, next to a dopamine receptor balance a dopamine-acetylcholine balance also plays a role and "a cholinergic overactivity has been used to explain the improvement of some motor signs such as tremor, reported after muscarinic receptor blockade" (Calabresi et al., 2006), although a more cooperative role is supported for acetylcholine and dopamine in human cognitive performance. Cholinergic drugs do also have an improving effect on cognitive behavior in Parkinson's patients (Calabresi et al., 2006).

Physiological studies subdivided PPN neurons in three types (I, II and III) identified on the basis of their electrophysiological membrane properties obtained by intracellular recording. Type I neurons are characterized by low threshold calcium spikes (LTS), which give rise to a burst of fast action potentials after the offset of a hyperpolarizing current. The neurons also fire bursts of spikes when a depolarized stimulus is given during hyperpolarization. According to Takakusaki and Kitai (1997) Type I neurons are glutamatergic. Type II neurons do not burst. Instead they fire single action potentials with large after-hyperpolarizations in response to injections of depolarizing current. This type is thus suited to generate a relatively slow tonic repetitive firing pattern. About 50% of Type II neurons are cholinergic. Type III neurons miss characteristics of Type I and Type II PPN neurons, thus lacking low-threshold spikes. The PPN neuron receives pallidal information, gathers information from the STN-SN network with strong SN influence, also from the cortex, from the limbic system and hypothalamus, from the cerebellum and from the brainstem and can transmit it towards nearly all nuclei of the thalamus (both the cholinergic and non-cholinergic ones), and weakly towards the cortex and basal ganglia (Usunoff et al., 2003).

PPN plays a role in the control of muscle tone by means of its excitatory projections to the muscle tone inhibitory system in the brainstem. The PPN is also thought to produce the main influence on the parafascicular thalamic nucleus in cases of SN degeneration; the parafascicular nucleus being involved in motor control (Yan et al., 2008). In Parkinson's disease the increased inhibitory basal ganglia output, together with a decrease in cortical excitation of the PPN, may increase the level of muscle tone causing rigidity (Takusaki et al., 2004).

2.3 Subthalamic nucleus connections

The STN projection neurons are glutamatergic, excitatory, and heavily innervated by widely branching axons of the substantia nigra (SN), the internal pallidal segment (GPi), followed by the external pallidal segment (GPe) and the pedunculopontine tegmental nucleus (PPN). The most well-known afferent connections of the STN arise in the GPe. The STN is also innervated by glutamatergic corticosubthalamic axons. A substantial, bilateral cholinergic/glutamatergic projection arises in the PPN, while the thalamic centromedian-parafascicular complex also innervates the STN (see Table I). Finally, serotoninergic fibers from the raphe nuclei terminate profusely within the STN. The nigrosubthalamic connection was demonstrated by axonal transport techniques, and transmitter immunocytochemistry. The nigrosubthalamic connection arises from the dopaminergic (DA) neurons of the SN pars compacta (SNc). In addition, a moderate projection was described from the parvalbumin immunoreactive, presumably GABAergic neurons of the SN pars reticulata (SNr) to the STN. The nigrosubthalamic connection has always been described as ipsilateral, but rat tracer studies now oppose this view (see below and Marani et al., 2008). STN-pallidal fibers arborize more widely and terminate on more proximal neuronal elements of the pallidum than striato-pallidal fibers. Thus, the striatal and STN inputs to GPi form a pattern of fast, widespread, divergent excitation from the STN, and a slower, focused, convergent inhibition from the striatum (Squire et al., 2003). Furthermore, cortico-STN neurons and cortico-striatal neurons belong to distinct populations. Thus, signals through the hyperdirect pathway may broadly inhibit motor programs; then signals through the direct pathway may adjust the selected motor program according to the situation (the 'center-surround' model of Nambu, 2005). STN neurons can discharge continuously and repetitively at low frequencies (10-30 Hz) and can fire with bursts of high frequency spikes. STN neurons are physiologically subdivided in non-plateau neurons (neurons that react with low threshold spikes) and plateau generating neurons (those that can react with bursts, low threshold spikes or plateau potentials). The neuron has to be in a hyperpolarized state, for depolarizing or hyperpolarizing current pulses to induce plateau behavior (Beurrier et al., 1999). The tonic discharges are sodium-dependent, while its hyperpolarizing phases are calcium dependent. Bursts are calcium-dependent phenomena.

3. Rat experimental results: Anatomy and electrophysiology

3.1 Anatomy: Outline of SN connections in the rat

The afferent and efferent connections of the rat SN, studied with degenerative and tracer techniques, are restricted to the cortex, brainstem and cerebellum (the cerebellum and its connections are not treated in this review). All thalamic connections are SN efferent, except for the parafascicular thalamic nucleus. The afferent SN connections of this nucleus are ipsilateral. All efferents of the SN to the other thalamic nuclei are also ipsilateral, with the exception of the connections to medial dorsal-, ventral medial- and central lateral thalamic nucleus, which are both ipsi- and contralateral, like those of the pedunculopontine nuclei and superior and inferior colliculus connections. Ipsi- and contralateral afferents to the SN are found for the hypothalamus, laterodorsal tegmental nucleus and the parabrachial nuclei. All other connections, including cortex, caudate-putamen and pallidum connections are afferent and/or efferent and always ipsilateral. It means that SN influence is mainly ipsilateral and only a few pathways can also steer the contralateral side of certain thalamic nuclei, lateral habenular nucleus, superior and inferior colliculus, periaquaductal gray, and the pedunculopontine nucleus (see Table I and Marani et al., 2008).

Afferents to substantia nigra							**Efferents from substantia nigra**					
SNr		SNc		SNl			SNr		SNc		SNl	
ipsi	con	ipsi	con	ipsi	con		ipsi	con	ipsi	con	ipsi	con
x		x		x		Cortex	x		x		x	
x		x		x		Caudate-Putamen	x		x		x	
x		x				Pallidum	x		x			
x		x				Accumbens			x			
						Hippocampus			x			
		x		x		Amygdala			x		x	
						Lateral dorsal thalamic nucleus	x					
						Medial dorsal thalamic nucleus	x	x	x			
						Ventral medial thalamic nucleus	x	x	x			
						Central medial thalamic nucleus	x		x			
						Central lateral thalamic nucleus	x			x		
x		x		x		Parafascicular thalamic nucleus	x			x		
						Paracentral thalamic nucleus	x					
						Lateral posterior thalamic nucleus	x					
x		x		x		Lateral habenular nucleus			x	x		
						Dorsal lateral geniculate nucleus	x		x		x	

SNr		SNc		SNl			SNr		SNc		SNl	
ipsi	con	ipsi	con	ipsi	con		ipsi	con	ipsi	con	ipsi	con
						Zona incerta	x					
x		x		x		Subthalamic nucleus			x			
x	x	x	x	x	x	Hypothalamus	x		x		x	
						Superior colliculus	x	x				
						Red nucleus	x					
x		x				Entopeduncular nucleus						
						Inferior colliculus					x	x
						Periaqueductal gray			x	x		
x		x				Raphe dorsalis			x			
						Cuneiform nucleus	x					
						Mesencephalic reticular nucleus	x		x			
		x	x			Pedunculopontine tegmental nucleus	x	x	x			
x	x	x	x	x	x	Laterodorsal tegmental nucleus	x					
x	x	x	x	x	x	Parabrachial nuclei	x		x			
						Locus coeruleus	x		x		x	
						Parvocellular pontine reticular nucleus	x		x			
			x			Cerebellum		x		x		x

Table 1. Overview of afferent and efferent connections of the SN. SNr: substantia nigra pars reticularis; SNc: substantia nigra pars compacta; SNl: substantia nigra pars lateralis; ispi: ipsilateral; con: contralateral; x: existing connection.

3.1.1 Nigro-subthalamic connections in the rat

The outline of the nigro-subthalamic connections is shown by large injection sites with the anterograde BDA (biotinylated dextran amine) tracer that was injected into the lateral SNr (reticulata) and SNc (compacta). The axons running towards the brainstem and the mounting axons to the forebrain take at first a medial way towards the prerubral area. Few nigro-thalamic axons course dorsally towards the tegmentum. Most of the axons directed to the brainstem and forebrain progress immediately dorsal to SN, and some axons pass lateromedially of the SNc. Few axons bend ventromedially and travel along the border between SNr and the cerebral peduncle. Reaching the caudal pole of the STN, the labeled axons pierce into the nucleus through its lateral wedge, but also into its ventral border and enter also from the medially running bundle, dorsal to the STN. Within the STN, especially in the lateral half of the nucleus, along with passing fibers oriented mediolaterally, a large amount of terminal labeling is present. In the medial part of the STN mainly discrete bursts of labeled endings are noted. Midline crossing of SN axons occurs at several places. The most substantial component of crossed axons runs in the mesencephalic tegmentum ventral to the periaqueductal gray (PAG). Such bundles are found through the entire rostrocaudal extent of the mesencephalon. Some fibers in the rostral mesencephalon in fact come into the STN through its dorsal border. The midline is also crossed in the commissure of the superior colliculus and in the posterior commissure. The efferent SN axons cross the midline (crossed nigro-thalamic axons) rostral to the SN, and the last component of crossing axons runs in the supraoptic decussation, immediately above the optic tract. Some of these axons take a dorsomedial course towards the contralateral STN. In the contralateral STN a lower amount of labeled axons are noted. Nevertheless, they form very distinct mediolaterally extended patches. Most of these discrete fields of terminal labeling are in the central and lateral portions of the STN, but also medially some terminal 'whorls' are seen.

These results provide data for the existence of a substantial nigrosubthalamic connection in the rat, which emits also a moderate component to the contralateral STN (Figure 2). Ipsilaterally the efferent SN axons terminate in large, profuse terminal fields, whilst contralaterally they terminate in discrete, sharply circumscribed patches. Although the crossed nigrosubthalamic connection is moderate, exactly by its topical distribution, its 'point to point' connection is especially evident. The medial SNc projects to the contralateral medial STN, and the lateral SNc also projects mainly to the lateral half of the contralateral STN (see Marani et al., 2008).

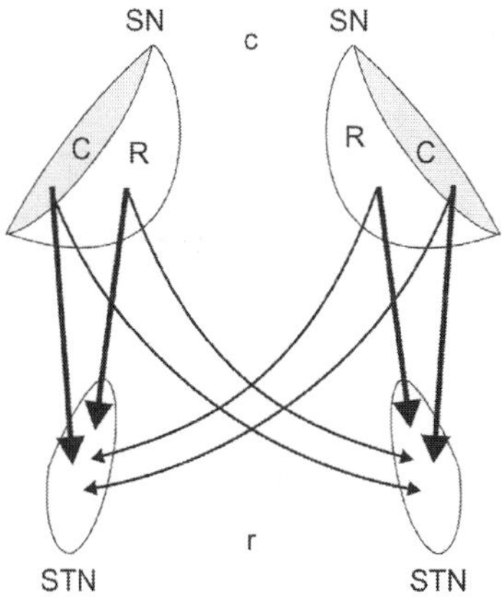

Fig. 2. Ipsilateral and contralateral nigro-subthalamic connections. SN: substantia nigra; STN: subthalamic nucleus; C: SN pars compacta; R: SN pars reticulata; c: caudal; r: rostral.

3.1.2 Nigro-trigeminal connections in the rat

It is generally accepted that also in the rat, the SN is involved in oral movements and oro-facial dyskinesias. Until now, is has been believed that the SN influences the trigeminal motoneurons via a multisynaptic pathway (see Usunoff et al., 1997; Lazarov, 2002). Histopathological changes in this rat model's substantia nigra have been demonstrated in tardive dyskinesias (Andreassen et al., 2003). Direct stimulation by STN DBS improves oro-facial dyskinesia in a rat model (Creed et al., 2010). Therefore, a renewed interest in the rat nigro-trigeminal pathway arose.

Specifically, the large BDA injection in the lateral SNc and parts of the adjacent SNr and SNl (lateral) resulted in anterograde labeling throughout the Me5 (mesencephalic trigeminal nucleus, see Usunoff et al., 1997) with a strong ipsilateral predominance, but contralateral labeling was also present. The results for SNc are summarized in Figure 3. Surrounding the injection site many intensely labeled neurons were present. Terminal labeling was observed among the perikarya of pseudo-unipolar neurons in the ipsilateral Me5c (caudal). At this sectional plane, virtually all pseudo-unipolar neurons were at least partially surrounded by varicose fibers, contacting their cell surface. The intensity of anterograde labeling in the Me5r (rostral) decreased almost bilaterally. Moderate terminal labeling was present around but not on pseudo-unipolar neuronal somata, both in the caudal and rostral Me5, on the contralateral side.

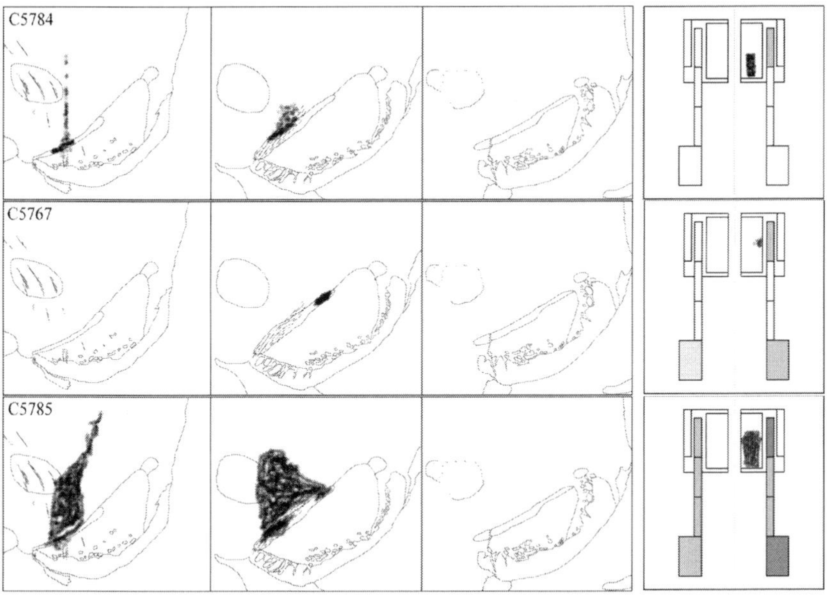

Fig. 3. Overview of the injection sites of three transversal slices of the SNc. The column at the right schematically shows the ipsi- and contralateral labeling in Me5, which is subdivided in a head and three tail areas. Anterograde labeling and injections (summed throughout the nucleus) are indicated in a map of the SN, with SNc, SNr and SNl, and Me5. Darker gray levels indicate a higher intensity of the labeling in Me5.

Selective injections into the medial SNc and lateral SNc produced labeled axons that were followed exclusively to the ipsilateral Me5c while the contralateral Me5c and Me5r on both sides displayed few labeled fibers (Figure 3). Terminal labeling was present in an extensive network in the ipsilateral Me5c, diminishing slightly from medial to lateral. Most of the terminal labeling surrounded the pseudo-unipolar mesencephalic trigeminal neurons. Some perikarya clearly displayed terminal and passing boutons covering their cell exterior. Throughout the neuropil of Me5c a meshwork of fine labeled fibers with varicosities was also present after injection into the lateral SNc. Single pseudo-unipolar neurons containing boutons en passant and boutons termineaux clearly visible on their surface were noted. The terminal labeling extended medially to the Me5c, to include the area of smaller cells in the locus coeruleus. A minute injection focus selectively infiltrated the SNl. In the Me5 area only few varicose fibers and their terminals reached the ipsilateral Me5c, while the rostral portion of this nucleus showed a slightly larger number of labeled fibers. In this case, no anterograde terminal labeling was observed in Me5 contralaterally.

The results of this study provide strong evidence that the SN also directly innervates the proprioceptive trigeminal neurons and thus, both the motor and sensory neurons controlling jaw muscles involved in mastication. Since pseudo-unipolar mesencephalic trigeminal nucleus neurons send axons to the pontine and spinal trigeminal nuclei, it appears that the entire trigeminal nuclear complex (see Usunoff et al., 1997) is profoundly influenced by the SN. Therefore, it can be inferred that inputs from SN possibly modify, modulate or interact with outputs from all these nuclei to control the masticatory behavior (see Marani et al., 2010).

3.2 Electrophysiology: Rat brain slices and dissociated STN cell cultures

We describe two approaches which can be followed to investigate the neuronal properties and network activity patterns *in-vitro*. Both use multi-electrode arrays (MEA's, Figure 4) to measure the extracellular membrane potential of neurons located close to the MEA's 60 electrodes. The first method we describe makes use of acute slices of rat brain, in which some of the structure remains intact but which can only be used for a short time (less than 8 hours). The second is to put neurons from a particular area in culture on top of the MEA, which loses all spatial structure, but can be used for months.

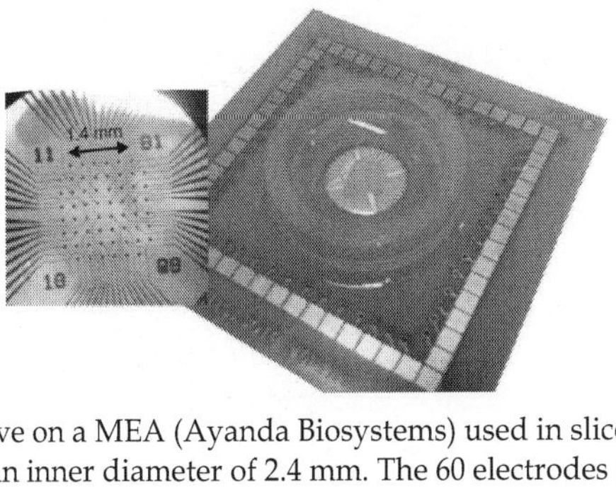

Fig. 4. View from above on a MEA (Ayanda Biosystems) used in slice research. The round culture chamber has an inner diameter of 2.4 mm. The 60 electrodes are spaced 200 µm apart in an 8 by 8 grid (the inset shows the electrodes covered by a slice). The electrodes are conically shaped, with the tips protruding 50-70 µm from the glass surface.

Horizontal slices of the STN-containing midbrain produced from rats, aged between 16-52 days, were placed such that the electrode matrix of the MEA was underneath the STN. Signals of spontaneous STN activity recorded in continuously perfused and carboxygenated artificial cerebro-spinal fluid (ACSF) were amplified, bandpass filtered (10 Hz-10 kHz) and digitized using a measurement system of MCS (MultiChannelSystems GmbH, Reutlingen, Germany). After software filtering (50-350 Hz), threshold crossings exceeding 5 times standard deviation were stored. Results show average firing rates of four neurons firing at mean frequencies of 0.1, 0.1, 0.06 and 1.2 Hz, respectively (Figure 5). In this example, the most active fourth neuron is the only neuron localized within (the motor cortex innervated area of) the STN. Neurons 2 and 4 were classified as 'bursty', neuron 1 was termed 'random' and neuron 3 was labeled 'regular' (for definitions of random, regular and bursty see Kaneoke and Vitek, 1996). On further inspection, many spikes were part of *doublets* (two spikes in close succession), while bursts of longer duration were rare. Such bursting STN activity was noted in many rat slices and the method used was able to discriminate several spiking patterns (Figure 6). Here, properties of random, regular and bursty spikes were allocated to the electrodes with their position within STN. Network connections may be detected by cross correlation analysis of spontaneous activity (Le Feber et al., 2007) or post-stimulus histograms (see Stegenga et al., 2010b). Moreover, the extranuclear network can also be studied (Figure 7, right panel).

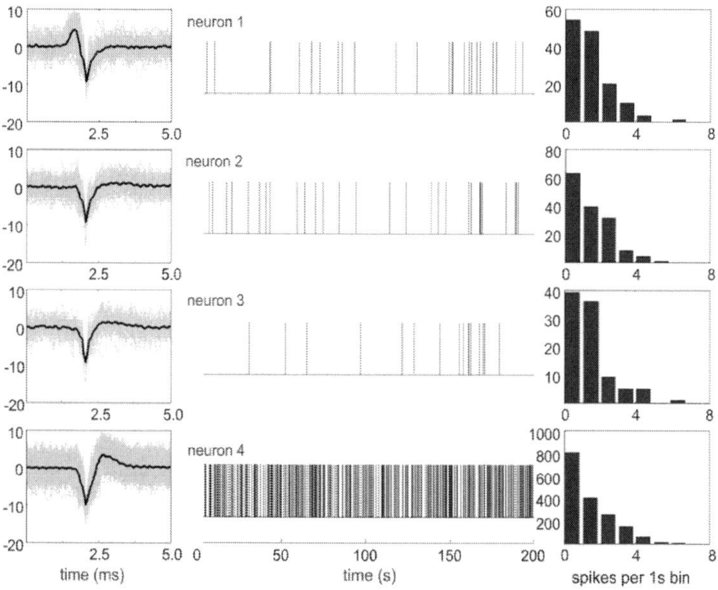

Fig. 5. Action potential waveforms and spike train analysis of 4 simultaneously recorded neurons in a horizontal slice of the rat brain including STN. Left: aligned action potential waveforms. Middle: spike trains of the 4 neurons. Right: density histograms of the spike trains, i.e. the number of occurrences that an interval of 1 s contained a certain number of spikes . The histograms were compared to a Poisson distribution for classification. Neuron 1: 'random'; neuron 3: 'regular'; neuron 2 and 4: 'bursty'.

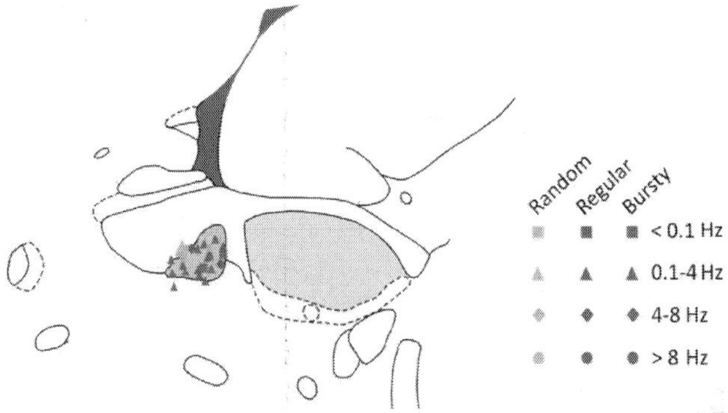

Fig. 6. Localization of activity in horizontal slices of STN (-8.1 mm from Bregma, figure 187 in Paxinos & Watson, 2007) classified according to mean frequency and spike train properties. STN neurons predominantly displayed low mean firing frequencies (<4 Hz) while spike trains were generally 'bursty'.

The addition of dopamine to acute slice preparations shows its effect on the firing rate and patterns of STN neurons, but also on SN neurons, depending on the placing of the MEA. Increasing concentrations of dopamine added to slices shows an increase in the spontaneous activity of the STN neurons, while a decrease of the spontaneous activity in SN was noted for a short period, before the increase started. Based on an analogous approach as done for intra-nuclear connections, mapping of extra-nuclear connections is also possible, here between STN and SN (Figure 7).

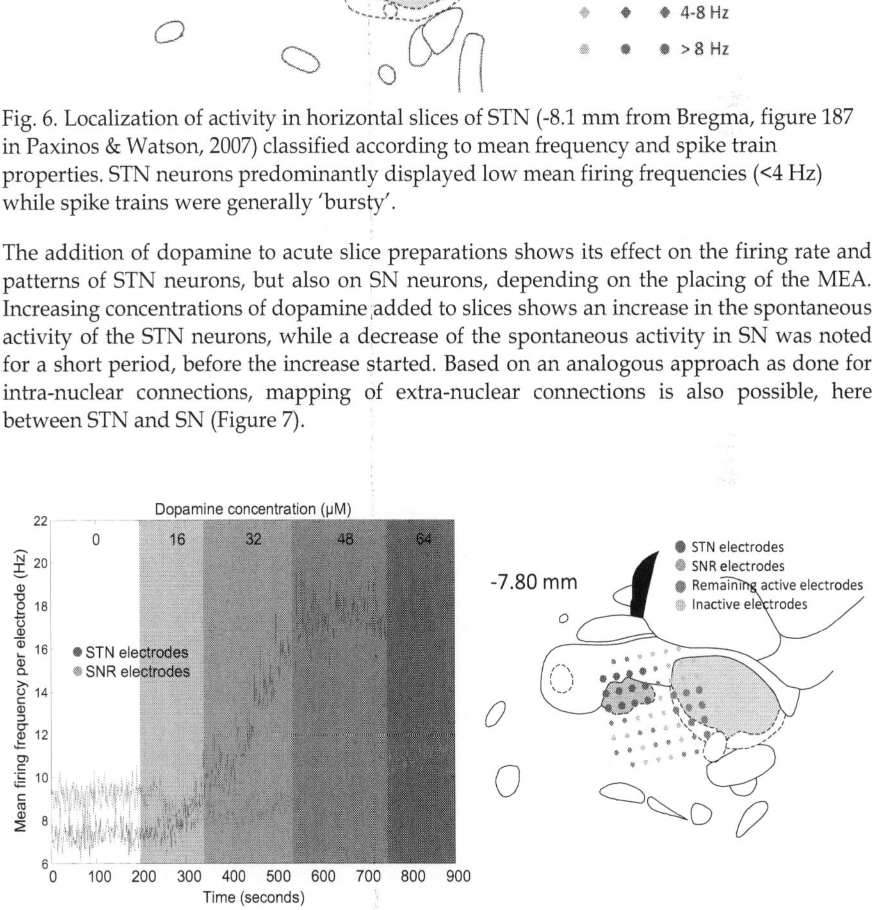

Fig. 7. Response of neurons located in STN and SN to dopamine application. Left: mean firing rate of 12 electrodes located in STN (blue) and 9 electrodes located in SN (green). The dopamine concentration was increased from 0 to 64 μM in steps of 16 μM (shaded gray background). Right: corresponding figure (188, Paxinos & Watson, 2007) with the position of the MEA electrodes included.

The rat neuroanatomical studies show a refined connection pattern between SN, Me5 and STN, which is new and hardly incorporated into models. Moreover rat dissociated STN neurons in culture and rat horizontal brain slices, containing the STN, provide the possibility to study artificial and original STN networks (in part), respectively. Herewith the mechanisms underlying bursting and oscillation of the rat STN neurons can be investigated, since the reaction of whole intranuclear, but also extranuclear networks can be studied together with single neuron reactions on artificial modulation of activity or by ablation of connections or by adding agonists and antagonists of neurotransmitters or receptors.

3.2.1 Mimicking the cholinergic PPN-STN connection in dissociated cultures

The pedunculopontine nucleus (PPN) is used as a new therapeutic target for DBS in patients suffering from Parkinson's disease with severe gait and postural impairment (Plaha & Gill, 2005). DBS of the PPN is only effective, if carried out at low frequencies (~20 Hz), while STN-DBS requires high frequencies (~130 Hz) to be successful. This is hardly comprehended. The projections from the PPN are reciprocal both towards the SN and the STN (see Usunoff, 2003). This nucleus contains cholinergic neurons (mainly Ch5 in the rat), that project onto the STN. There exists a direct relation between the severity of Parkinson's disease and the loss of cholinergic neurons in the PPN (Rinne et al., 2008), which provided the incentive to look into cholinergic effects on STN neurons.

To this end, rat STN areas from one day old rat pups were dissociated and cultured on the coated glass surface of a MEA similar to the example shown in Figure 4, in chemically defined, serum free, medium. Acetylcholine (ACh) was added in steps of 10 μM and extracelluar action potential activity of a maximum of 60 neurons was recorded. Addition of ACh reduced the spontaneous activity immediately and substantially for 50-100 seconds (Figure 8).

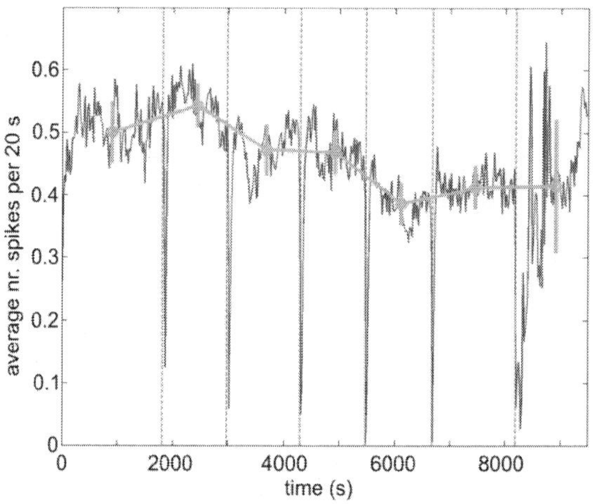

Fig. 8. Normalized spike activity in dissociated STN cultures after administration of ACh. Each red striped line marks the time at which the concentration ACh was increased by 10 μM. At the last line ACh was washed out. The action-potential activity of all recorded neurons was averaged and binned in 20 s bins. The green dots show the average activity for the different concentrations of ACh.

The total spike activity after the entire period of 1.5 hours (the period starting at the moment the first 10 μM was added till the moment ACh was washed out) was reduced by almost 25%. If synchronized bursting activity was present in the cultures, this activity was not reduced by addition of ACh. This suggests that cholinergic PPN input in the STN has a decreasing effect on the spontaneous activity of the STN. Loss of cholinergic input, on its turn, increases STN spontaneous activity (see Heida et al., 2008).

It should be noted that the symptoms of Parkinson's disease are a result of alterations in the network activity of the motor cortex, the thalamus and the basal ganglia. The alterations ultimately originate from a shortage of dopamine as a consequence of degeneration of (a.o.) the dopaminergic cells in the substantia nigra pars compacta. However, compensatory mechanisms effectively combat the effect of dopamine-shortage until roughly 80% of dopaminergic SNc cells have died. At any stage, we study not only the disease, but also the mechanisms nature uses to combat its effects (and maintain function). To model the disease and possible interventions (L-DOPA; DBS), fundamental research about the electrophysiology of all of the involved nuclei is needed.

Experiments with acute slices can provide us with detailed data, but only with respect to one moment in time and only by damaging a large part of the network that is involved in PD. The short-term effect of chemicals (drugs) and electrical stimulation (DBS) can be studied in tremendous detail and may lead to a better understanding of particularly the latter (and ultimately to better interventions). The progress made in MEA technology and slice preparation allows even more complex systems to be studied. For mice and rats, the maximum thickness of slices (~400 um) is enough to preserve much of the connectivity of the basal ganglia. The preservation of connections between distant nuclei (motor cortex, thalamus, substantia nigra) may well be possible, even though they may not be within a single slice. For now, these techniques allow us to check the models that have been created to study basal ganglia (dys)function such as the reciprocal coupling between STN and globus pallidus, which is claimed to result in bursting activity at low concentrations of dopamine. We can also test whether there is feedback from STN to the SN, thus ameliorating the effect of shortage of dopamine, but possibly speeding up PD progression (Blandini et al., 2000). We have already observed a marked increase in firing rate in both STN and SN with rising dopamine concentration. We expect that compensatory mechanisms (i.e. adaptation) will counter large changes in firing rate on the longer term, possibly by changing the firing patterns (i.e. neuronal and synaptic properties). Medication by L-DOPA may have the same effect in PD patients; enabling neurons to fire in patterns that, at least, do not interfere with normal function. The question of which patterns do not interfere with normal function, may be answered by simulating DBS in-vitro, since the effects of DBS are visible almost instantly.

For longitudinal studies, cultures of dissociated neurons, or even (non-dissociated) co-cultures can be used. Even though these will create networks that differ from those in the intact brain, they can be used to study basic mechanisms and how they evolve over longer periods of time. Here, more fundamental questions about neuronal adaptation to various inputs and chemical additions can be answered. From cultures of cortical neurons we know that basic properties of these networks (e.g. percentage of excitatory/inhibitory connections) develop in a similar way compared to in-vivo counterparts. This even allows the study of age-related effects.

4. Computational models of PD and DBS treatment

Computational studies are useful in investigating how pathological conditions and DBS induced activity may find their way through the basal ganglia-thalamocortical circuit. High-frequency stimulation leads to somatic inhibition of neurons that are close to the electrical field while simultaneously afferent and efferent axons may be excited. Both cellular and network effects may contribute to the overall clinical effects of DBS. McIntyre and Hahn (2010) claim that: "changes in the underlying dynamics of the stimulated brain networks may represent the core mechanisms of DBS and that those basic dynamical changes can be achieved via activation, inhibition, or lesion". Stimulation does not necessarily has to restore the network to a pre-pathological/normal state, but should allow improvement in Parkinson's symptoms.

Normally a parametric approach based on investigations of the biological system and network or molecular/channel characteristics, is preferred. Since not all systems are studied in detail, a non-parametric based model may be used, in which only input and output are considered, leaving the system a black box. Due to the extreme data gathering on Parkinson's disease non-parametric approaches are uncommon and the models brought forward can be classified as parametric. Here we will concentrate on the models for the thalamocortical relay neuron and the PPN neuron, thus directing towards an efferent thalamo-projecting model and an efferent spinal-projecting model.

4.1 Model of the thalamic relay neuron

The output of the basal ganglia network is directed towards the thalamic nuclei (Figure 1), which influences the motor cortex and its output is relayed via the pyramidal tract towards the secondary motor neurons. In two recent studies we have investigated how DBS can affect the functioning of the thalamus as a relay station (Cagnan et al., 2009; Meijer et al., 2011). Although this is a simplication, it is presumed that this relay should retransmit incoming information from cortex and sensory systems back to cortex. This extends earlier work by Rubin and Terman who showed that the mechanism of DBS may be regularizing the output of thalamus (Rubin & Terman, 2004). They demonstrated that under pathological conditions STN-GPe networks can show a pacemaker rhythm at tremor frequency (Terman et al., 2002). These phasic signals from basal ganglia may impair the transmission of thalamocortical information. When replacing the pathological oscillations by regular DBS input thalamocortical relay may be restored (Rubin & Terman, 2004; Guo et al., 2008).

We started to model a simpler situation by first focussing on rest tremor. A GPi-spike train obtained from a human PD patient during DBS surgery with characteristic patterns of rest tremor was used to generate GPi input to the thalamus. Without relay of cortical input (rest situation), the thalamic model response consisted of rebounds at the same tremor frequency (Figure 9).

By including excitatory input the combined effects of relay, PD and DBS could be examined. The pathological input was partially replaced by DBS pulses reflecting a limited volume of tissue being activated by the stimulation. For DBS there are two common targets: STN and GPi.

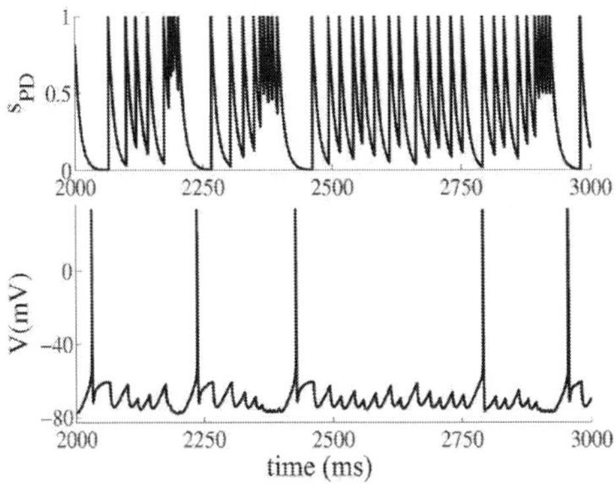

Fig. 9. Top: The model synaptic input reflects the burstiness of the activity of the measured GPi neuron. Bottom: The thalamic relay cell exhibits post-inhibitory rebound action potentials, i.e., during the pause after the GPi burst an action potential is generated.

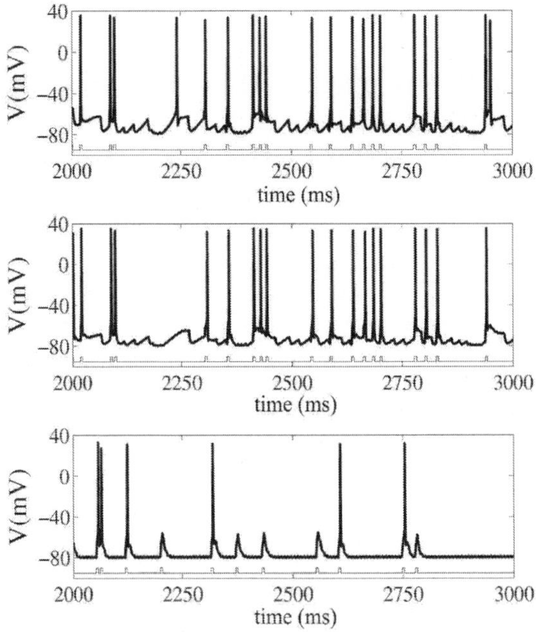

Fig. 10. The effect of overwriting the pathological GPi input by increasing DBS amplitude. The upper traces represent the membrane voltage (V) of the TC cell. The precise timing of the excitatory input (mean rate 16.5 Hz) is displayed beneath each voltage trace. Top: If the stimulation amplitude is too weak, rebounds and an incorrect signal relay occur. Middle: With moderate DBS amplitude, rebounds are quenched and relay is correct. Bottom: With high DBS amplitude, relay of sensory information is impaired.

Stimulation of the STN may recruit efferent fibers that excite GPi. In both cases it is therefore plausible that DBS leads to additional downstream GPi output. At the thalamus, the input from the basal ganglia comes from the GPi and is therefore inhibitory. A key property of thalamic relay cells is their low-threshold T-type calcium current. When the thalamic relay cell is inhibited long enough, it fires rebound action potentials (Janssen & Llinàs, 1984). The effect of such phasic pathological inhibition is that the thalamic output activity does not reflect the original input. This stems from two sources of errors. Long periods of inhibition diminish the responsiveness of the TC cell and rebound spikes are mixed with successful relays.

In the model we found that this extra inhibition can jam the transmission of pathological oscillations around the loop. Additionally we investigated the frequency dependence of this therapeutic regime and showed that in the model it persists to frequencies as low as 60 Hz, although the plateau starts at 100 Hz. In Cagnan et al. (2009) we considered a similar setup but considered the frequency content of the output. In particular, we showed that DBS can diminish the power at pathological frequencies in the spectrum of the thalamic output. Finally, we also found that if the frequency of the relay input is sufficiently high, and the variance low enough, this can also block the transmission of pathological low-frequency oscillations. This may be interpreted as a suppression of rest tremor.

4.2 Model of the PPN neuron

Due to its location in the brainstem and its function in locomotion and postural control, the pedunculopontine nucleus (PPN) has been suggested as a target for DBS to improve gait and postural instability. The glutamatergic PPN neurons are reciprocally connected with the basal ganglia and these neurons provide the descending PPN output to the spinal cord. Therefore, PPN has a pivot role in regulation of the basal ganglia and spinal cord, and providing indirect pathway for the basal ganglia to regulate the initiation of gait (Pahapill & Lozano, 2000; Hamani et al., 2007).

In Lourens et al. (2011) we have developed a computational conductance based model for the glutamatergic PPN type I to investigate the response of the PPN cell to various basal ganglia inputs. The specific characteristics of PPN currents are described by Takakusaki and Kitai (1997). A persistent sodium current is responsible for subthreshold membrane oscillations in PPN type I neurons, which underlies spontaneous repetitive firing. Moreover the LTS property is mediated by the T-type calcium current. The model is based on neurophysiological data of the thalamocortical relay neuron, and the pre-Bötzinger neuron. The PPN Type I is modelled as a single compartment model using the Hodgkin-Huxley formalism, except for the calcium current which is described by the Goldman-Hodgkin-Katz ion current equation. We used the basal ganglia model as proposed by Rubin and Terman (2004) to generate input to the PPN type I model. Moreover, we include the projection from the PPN back to the basal ganglia.

The model of an isolated type I PPN neuron shows the experimental behaviour as described in literature (Takakusaki & Kitai, 1997). The PPN neuron model shows spontaneous firing at 8 Hz, and bursting behaviour after the release of a hyperpolarizing input. In the network model, including 8 cells of STN, GPe and GPi and 1 PPN cell, we found that under PD conditions the firing rate of the PPN cell decreases and its firing pattern regularizes. In addition, we investigated the effect of DBS in PPN and STN on the behaviour of the PPN-basal ganglia network and on the relay property of the PPN cell. DBS is modeled as a train of positive current pulses, injected directly into the target cells. PPN-DBS is applied with high amplitude (100 μA cm^{-2}) at 40 Hz and STN-DBS is applied at 130 Hz with an amplitude of 400 μA cm^{-2}; both stimuli have a pulse width of 0.15 ms. For the relay property it turns out that combined high-frequency stimulation of STN and low frequency stimulation of PPN hardly improves the effect of exclusive STN stimulation. PPN-DBS eliminates the pathological firing pattern of STN and GPe cells, whereas STN-DBS and combined STN- and PPN-DBS eliminate the pathological firing pattern only from STN cells, see Figure 11.

5. Discussion

In general there is a wide gap between experimental animal results, especially with respect to neuroanatomical data, and computational modeling. In order to be able to investigate the anatomical and functional properties of afferent and efferent connections between the different nuclei of the basal ganglia, similar studies need to be performed as described for the substantia nigra. These studies, though very time-consuming, are essential to decide which pathways play important roles in normal functioning and therefore need to be included in modeling studies. In addition, it should be known what neuroanatomical changes take place resulting from the neurodegeneration associated with Parkinson's disease and how they affect network behavior. For instance, the direct effects of DBS on motor control are of interest, but since DBS has a low threshold to side effects, additional non-motor pathways are expected to be involved. Including these pathways in network models may shed light on the extent and effect of stimulation. Similarly, as PPN stimulation may have a beneficial influence on gait and balance, different pathways are important regarding the different motor symptoms of Parkinson's disease.

The classic diagram of the basal ganglia as presented in Figure 1 not only leaves out a number of connections that are discussed in this review, it also is based on average firing rates while currently it is known that firing patterns change under parkinsonian conditions. The irregular firing characteristics within the nuclei of the basal ganglia are transformed into a more synchronous and bursting activity pattern. Functionality of neuronal networks is dependent of neurotransmitters and their receptors, together with the channels present in the cell membrane. Studies on the properties and localization of the receptors and channels are therefore a prerequisite for adequate modeling. However, the enormous amount of receptors and channel types, and their variability in distribution makes it virtually impossible to describe neuronal function for all basal ganglia nuclei (see e.g. the eloquent studies on GABA in the basal ganglia; Tepper et al., 2007).

Dissociated neural cultures as well as brain slices positioned on multi electrode arrays open the possibility to study basal ganglia nuclear functional action and interaction, i.e. the overall result of all cell membrane activities of a neuron or group of neurons. By the addition of neurotransmitters, their agonists or antagonists, PD basal ganglia activity can be mimicked in-vitro. It is expected that this alternative route of studying PD will bring up the most needed extra information to support fine-tuning of neuron and neuronal network models and will as a consequence incorporate the more subtle connections nowadays described in neuroanatomical studies.

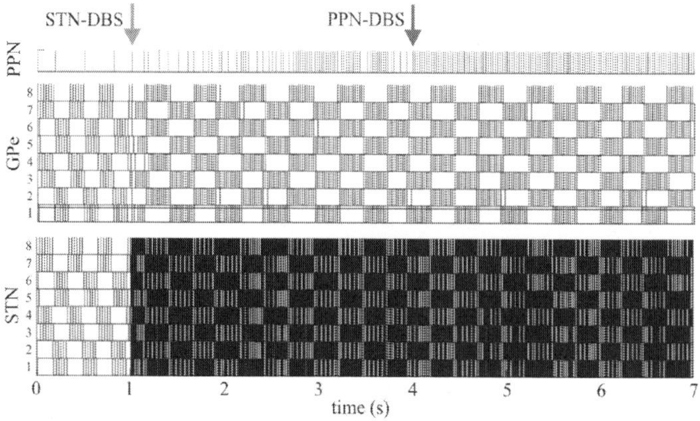

A)

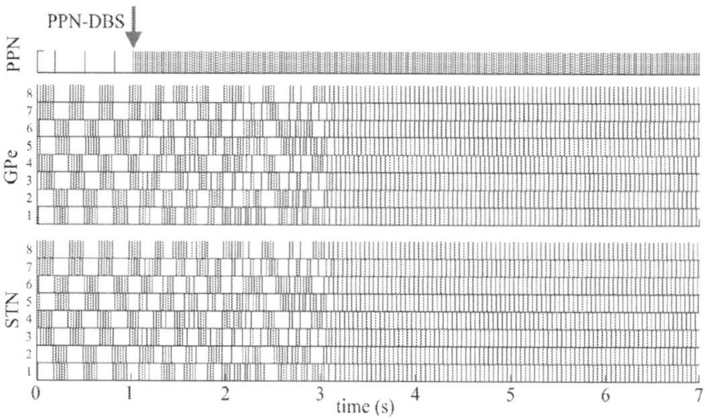

B)

Fig. 11. Effect of PPN-DBS and STN-DBS on the activity of GPe and STN cells. Stimulation starts at 1 s and 4 s, as indicated by the arrows. With STN-DBS stimulation clusters remain and the time period of the clusters gets longer in GPe, while STN cells are locked to the STN-DBS frequency. Addition of PPN-DBS shows no change (A). With only PPN-DBS (B) the STN and GPe clusters are disrupted after some transients.

Essential in modeling is to formulate reduced models that still capture essential properties of the dynamics but are able to include even these subtle connections. Models need verification by experiments to demonstrate that the model has reality value. With the increasing amount of in-vitro and in-vivo experimental data computational models may become applicable in human research and health care problems. The therapeutic stimulation parameters for DBS (polarity, pulse amplitude, pulse width, frequency) will in the near future rely more on the predictions made by model simulations (Cutsuridis et al., 2011).

6. Future direction

"Despite numerous diverse- and at times frankly bizarre- etiologic speculations over a considerable period of time, the cause or causes of Parkinson's disease remain unknown" (Stern, 1996). This statement still holds and therefore the efforts in Parkinson´s research are focused on investigating ´what goes wrong in the parkinsonian brain, and how can we reverse this pathological behaviour´. Medication and deep brain stimulation are meant to restore direct causes of the disease symptoms: compensating the loss of dopamine, and desynchronizing the pathological oscillations, respectively. A lot of attention is drawn to the basal ganglia and the causes and effects of its dysfunction. Individual neuronal receptor studies on basal ganglia or SNc cells hardly can give the overall outcome of the typical neuronal dysfunction. Dissociated neuronal cultures and brain slices presumably will be more successful.

Due to the neuronal plasticity of the brain, several mechanisms are involved in functional compensation for the progressive loss of dopamine. PD symptoms do not become clinically manifest until neuronal death exceeds a critical threshold: about 70–80% of striatal nerve terminals and 50–60% of SNc dopamine neurons (Bezard et al., 2003). While initially it was suggested that the preclinical state reflected the ability of the affected neuronal system to actively compensate for the loss of dopamine (Bezard et al., 2003), we now know that compensatory mechanisms outside that basal ganglia exist. Although the basal ganglia may be in a parkinsonian state, these mechanisms may prevent the appearance of symptoms. The overactivation of lateral premotor areas as found from PET and fMRI studies may express compensation processes (Samuel et al. 1997; Berardelli et al. 2001; Bezard et al., 2003). The cerebellothalamocortical circuit is proposed to play an important role in these processes since the cerebellum has strong connections with the lateral premotor areas. It is concerned with externally triggered movement, which may explain the beneficial effect PD patients experience from external cues in guiding movements. In contrast, the cerebellothalamic circuit was also hypothesized to play a role in tremor generation (Helmich et al., 2011). A prerequisite for the development of novel therapeutic methods in-vitro and computational models of Parkinson's disease is to include those circuits that are involved in compensating for the parkinsonian symptoms, based on cellular and connective studies.

7. References

Albin, R.L., Aldrige, J.W. & Young AB et al. (1989) The functional anatomy of basal ganglia disorders. *Trends Neurosci* 12, pp. 366-375

Andreassen, O.A., Ferrante, R.J., Aamo, T.O., Beal, M.F. & Jørgenson, H.A. (2003) Oral dyskineisas and histopathological alterations in substantia nigra after long-term haloperidol treatment of old rats. *Neuroscience* 122, pp. 717–725

Bar-Gad, I., Morris, G. & Bergman, H. (2003) Information processing, dimensionality reduction and reinforcement learning in the basal ganglia. *Progr Neurobiol* 71, pp. 439-473

Benabid, A.L., Pollak, P., Gervason, C., Hoffman, D., Gao, D.M., Hommel, M., Perret, J.E. & Rougemont, J.D. (1991) Long-term suppression of tremor by chronic stimulation of the ventral intermediate thalamic nucleus. *Lancet* 337, pp. 403–406

Berardelli, A., Rothwell, J.C., Thompson, P.D. and Hallett, M. (2001) Pathophysiology of bradykinesia in Parkinson's disease. *Brain* 124, pp. 2131-2146

Bezard, E., Gross, C.E. and Brotchie, J.M. (2003) *Trends Neurosci* 26, 215-221

Blandini, F., Nappi, G., Tassorelli, C. & Martignoni, E. (2000) Functional changes of the basal ganglia circuitry in Parkinson's disease. Prog Neurobiol 62, pp. 63-88

Brown, P., Oliviero, A., Mazzone, P., Insola, A., Tonali, P. & Di Lazzaro, V. (2001) Dopamine dependency of oscillations between subthalamic nucleus and pallidum in Parkinson's disease. *J Neurosci* 21, pp. 1033-1038

Brown, P. (2003) Oscillatory nature of human basal ganglia activity: relationship to the pathophysiology of Parkinson's disease. *Mov Disord* 18, pp. 357-363

Bullock, D. & Grossberg, S. (1988) Neural dynamics of planned arm movements: Emergent invariants and speed-accuracy properties during trajectory formation. *Psycholo Rev* 95, pp. 49–90

Beurrier, C., Congar, P., Bioulac, B. & Hammond, C. (1999) Subthalamic nucleus neurons switch from single spike activity to burst-firing mode. *J Neurosci* 19, pp. 599-609

Calabresi, P., Picconi, B., Parnetti, L. & Di Fillipo, M. (2006) A convergent model for cognitive dysfunctions in Parkinson's disease: the critical dopamine-acetylcholine synaptic balance. *Lancet Neurol* 5, pp. 974-983

Cagnan, H., Meijer, H.E., Van Gils, S.A., Krupa, M., Heida, T., Rudolph, M., Wadman, W.J. & Martens, H.C.F. (2009) Frequency-selectivity of a thalamocortical relay neuron during Parkinson's disease and deep brain stimulation: a computational study. *Eur J Neurosci* 30, pp. 1306-1317

Creed, M., Hamani, C., Nobrega, J.N. (2010) Deep brain stimulation of the subthalamic or entopenducular nucleus attenuates vacuous chewing movements in rodent model of tardive dyskinesia. *Eur Neuropsychopharmacol* doi:10.1016/j.euroneuro.2010.06.012

Cutsuridis, V., Heida, T., Duch, W. and Doya K. (2011) Editorial: Neurocomputational models of brain disorders. *Neural Networks* 24(6), pp. 513-514

Davis, G.C., Williams, A.C., Markey, S.P., et al. (1979) Chronic parkinsonism secondary to intravenous injection of meperidine analogues. *Psychiatry Res* 1, pp. 249- 254

DeLong, M.R. (1990) Primate models of movement disorders of basal ganglia origin. *Trends Neurosci* 13, pp. 281-285

Destexhe, A., Neubig, M., Ulrich, D. & Huguenard, J. (1998) Dendritic low threshold calcium currents in thalamic relay cells. *J Neurosci* 18, 3574–3588

Friede, R. (1953) Ueber die mutmassliche Bedeutung des Melanins in der Substantia nigra. *Arch exp Pathol Pharmak* 118, pp. 285-289

Friede, R.L. (1966) *Topographic Brain Chemistry*. Academic Press, New York

Gerfen, C.R. (1992) The neostriatal mosaic: multiple levels of compartimental organization. Trends Neurosci 15, pp.133-139

Gerfen, C.R. & Wilson, C.J. (1996) The basal ganglia Chapter II In: *Integrated systems of the CNS, Part III of Handbook of chemical anatomy* vol 12, Eds. Swanson, L.W. et al., Elsevier, Amsterdam

Gibb, W.R.G. (1988) The neuropathology of parkinsonian disorders. In: *Parkinson's Disease and Movement Disorders*, Eds. Jankovic, J., Tolosa, E. Urban & Schwarzenberg, Baltimore, 205-223

Gillies, A. & Willshaw, D. (2004) Models of the subthalamic nucelus: the importance of intranuclear connectivity. *Med Eng Phys* 26, pp.723-732

Greenfield, J.G. & Bosanquet, F.D. (1953) The brain stem lesions in parkinsonism. *J Neurol Neurosurg Psychiat* 16, pp. 213-226

Groenewegen, H.J. & van Dongen, Y.C. (2008) Role of the Basal Ganglia. In: *Parkinsonism and related disorders*, Eds. Wolters, E.C., Van Laar, T., Berendse, H.W., VU University Press, Amsterdam

Guo, Y., Rubin, J.E., McIntyre, C.C., Vitek, J.L. & Terman, D. (2008) Thalamocortical relay fidelity varies across subthalamic nucleus deep brain stimulation protocols in a Data-drivencomputational model. *J Neurophysiol* 99, pp. 1477-1492

Hamani, C., Stone, S., Laxton, A., & Lozano, A.M. (2007). The pedunculopontine nucleus and movement disorders: Anatomy and the role for deep brain stimulation. *Parkinsonism Related Disord*, 13, pp. s276–s280

Hassler, R. (1937) Zur Normalanatomie der Substantia nigra. *J Psychol Neurol* 48, pp. 1-55

Hassler, R. (1938) Zur Pathologie der Paralysis agitans und des postencephalitischen Parkinsonismus. *J Psychol Neurol* 48, pp. 387-476

Hassler, R. (1939) Zur pathologischen Anatomie des senilen und des parrkinsonistischen Tremor. *J Psychol Neurol* 49, pp. 193-230

Heida, T., Marani, E. & Usunoff, K.G. (2008) The subthalamic nucleus. II Modelling and simulation of activity. *Adv Anat Embryol Cell Biol* 199

Heida, T. & Beaujean, N. (2009) Parkinsonian pattern transduction by GPi. In: Annual symposium of the IEEE-EMBS Benelux Chapter, 9-10 Nov 2009, Enschede, The Netherlands. 70. *Annual Symposium of the IEEE/EMBS Benelux Chapter* 4th Annual Symposium of the IEEE/EMBS Benelux Chapter. University of Twente. ISBN 978-90-365-2933-4

Heida, T., Moroney, R., Usunoff, K.G. & Marani, E. (2010a) Deep Brain Stimulation Modeling and Simulation in Parkinson's disease. In: *Biomedical Diagnostics and Clinical Technologies: Applying High-Performance Cluster and Grid Computing*, Eds. Pereira, M. & Freire, M., ISBN 1605662801, DOI: 10.4018/978-1-60566-280-0

Heida, T. & Marani, E. (2010b) Dissociated neurons from an extended rat subthalamic area - spontaneous activity and acetylcholine addition. In: *XII Mediterranean Conference on Medical and Biological Engineering and Computing*, 27-30 May, Chalkidiki, Greece. pp. 180-183. *IFMBE Proceedings* (29). Springer Verlag. ISSN 1680-0737 ISBN 978-3-642-13038-0

Heida, T. & Marani, E. (2010c) The human subthalamic nucleus - knowledge for the understanding of Parkinson's disease. In: *XII Mediterranean Conference on Medical and Biological Engineering and Computing*, 27-30 May, Chalkidiki, Greece. pp. 176-179. IFMBE Proceedings (29). Springer Verlag. ISSN 1680-0737 ISBN 978-3-642-13038-0

Heida, T. & Wentink, E.C. (2010d) Rest and action tremor in Parkinson's disease: effects of Deep Brain Stimulation. In: *XII Mediterranean Conference on Medical and Biological*

Engineering and Computing, 27-30 May, Chalkidiki, Greece. International Federation for Medical and Biological Engineering

Helmich, R.C., Janssen M.J.R., Oyen, W.J.G., Bloem, B.R. and Toni, I. (2011) Pallidal dysfunction drives a cerebellothalamic circuit into Parkinson tremor. *Ann Neurol* 69, pp. 269-281

Hirsch, E., Graybiel, A.M. & Agid, Y.A. (1988) Melanized dopaminergic neurons are differentially susceptible to degeneration in Parkinson's disease. *Nature* 1988; 334, pp. 345-348

Huguenard, J.R. & McCormick, D.A. (1992) Simulation of the currents involved in rhythmic oscillations in thalamic relay neurons. *J Neurophysiol* 68, pp. 1373–1383

Hughes, A.J., Daniel, S.E., Kilford, L. & Lees, A.J. (1992) Accuracy of clinical diagnosis of idiopathic Parkinson's disease, a clinico-pathological study of 100 cases. *J Neurol Neurosurg Psychiat*, 55, pp. 181-184

Hurley, M.J. & Jenner, P. (2006) What has been learned from study of dopamine receptors in Parkinson's disease? *Pharmacol Therap* 111, pp. 715-728

Israel, Z. & Bergman, H. (2008) Pathophysiology of the basal ganglia and movement disorders. From animal models to human clinical applications. *Neurosci Biobehavior Rev* 32, pp.367-377

Jacobsohn, L. (1909) *Ueber die Kerne des menschlichen Hirnstamms*. Ver Koenigl Akad Wissensch. Berlin

Jahnsen, H. & Llinàs, R. (1984) Electrophysiological properties of guinea-pig thalamic neurones: an in vitro study. *J Physiol* 349, pp. 205.226

Jellinger, K. (1987c) Quantitative changes in some subcortical nuclei in aging. Alzheimer's disease and Parkinson's disease. *Neurobiol Aging*, 8, pp. 540-544

Kaneoke, Y., & J.L. Vitek (1996) Burst and oscillation as disparate neuronal properties. *J Neurosci Methods* 68(2), pp. 211-223

Kingsbury, A.E., Marsden, C.D. & Foster, O.J. (1999) The vulnerability of nigral neurons to Parkinson's disease is unrelated to their intrinsic capacity for dopamine synthesis: an in situ hybridization study. *Mov Disord*, 14, pp. 206-218

Lakke, E.A. (1997) The projections to the spinal cord of the rat during development; a time-table of descent. *Adv Anat Embryol Cell Biol* 135, pp. 1-143

Langston, J.W., Ballard, P., Tetrud, J. & Irwin, I. (1983) Chronic parkinsonism in humans due to a product of meperidine-analog synthesis. *Science* 219, pp. 979-980

Langston, J.W., Forno, L.S., Tetrud, J., Reeves, A.G., Kaplan, J.A. & Karluk, D. (1999) Evidence of active nerve cell degeneration in the substantia nigra of humans years after 1-Methyl-4-phenyl- 1,2,3,6- tertahydropyridine exposure. *Ann Neurol* 46, pp. 598- 605

Lazarov, N.E. (2002) Comparative analysis of the chemical neuroanatomy of the mammalian trigeminal ganglion and mesencephalic trigeminal nucleus. *Prog Neurobiol* 66, pp. 19-59

Le Feber, J., Rutten, W.L.C., Stegenga, J., Wolters, P.S., Ramakers, G.J.A. & Van Pelt, J. (2007) Conditional firing probabilities in cultured neuronal networks: A stable underlying structure in widely varying spontaneous activity patterns. *J Neural Eng* 4, pp.54-67

Lewy, F.H. (1912) Paralysis agitans. I. Pathologische Anatomie. In: *Handbuch der Neurologie*, Ed. Lewandowsky, M.H., Bd 3. Springer, Berlin, 920-933

Lewy, F.H. (1913) Zur pathologischen Anatomie der Paralysis agitans. *Deutsch Zeitschr Nervenheilk* 50, pp. 50-55

Lourens, M.A.J., Meijer, H.G.E., Heida, T. & Van Gils, S.A. (2009) The pedunculopontine nucleus as alternative target for deep brain stimulation. In: *Proceedings of the 4th Annual symposium of the IEEE-EMBS Benelux Chapter*, 9-10 Nov 2009, Enschede, The Netherlands. 27. Annual Symposium of the IEEE/EMBS Benelux Chapter 4th Annual Symposium of the IEEE/EMBS Benelux Chapter. Twente University Press. ISBN 978-90-365-2933-4

Lourens, M., Meijer, H., Heida, T., Marani, E. & Van Gils, S. (2011). The pedunculopontine nucleus as an additional target for deep brain stimulation. *Neural Networks*, 24(6), pp. 617–630

Marani, E., Heida, T., Lakke, E.A.J.F. & Usunoff, K.G. (2008) The subthalamic nucleus. I Development, cytology, topography and connections. Adv Anat Embryol Cell Biol 198, pp. 117

Marani, E., Lazarov, N.E., Heida, T. & Usunoff, K.G. (2010) Nigro-subthalamic and nigro-trigeminal projections in the rat. In: *XII Mediterranean Conference on Medical and Biological Engineering and Computing*, 27-30 May, Chalkidiki, Greece. pp. 184-187. IFMBE Proceedings (29). Springer Verlag. ISSN 1680-0737 ISBN 978-3-642-13038-0

McCormick, D.A. & Huguenard, J.R. (1992) A model of the electrophysiological properties of thalamocortical relay neurons. *J Neurophysiol* 68, pp. 1384–1400

McIntyre, C.C., Grill, W.M., Sherman, D.L. & Thakor, N.V. (2004) Cellular effects of deep brain stimulation: model-based analysis of activation and inhibition. *J Neurophysiol* 91, pp. 1457–1469

McIntyre, C.C. & Hahn, J.P. (2010) Network perspectives on the mechanisms of deep brain stimulation. *Neurobiol Disease* 38, pp. 329-337

Meijer, H.G.E., Krupa, M., Cagnan, H., Lourens, M.A.J., Heida, T., Martens, H.C.F., Bour, L.J. & Van Gils, S.A. (2011) From parkinsonian thalamic activity to restoring thalamic relay using deep brain stimulation: new insights from computational modeling. *J Neural Eng*, 8, DOI:10.1088/1741-2560/8/6/066005

Mesulam, M.M., Geula, C., Bothwell, M.A. & Hersh, L.B (1989) Human reticular formation: cholinergic neurons of the pedunculopontine and laterodorsal tegmental nuclei and some cytochemical comparisons to forebrain cholinergic neurons. *J Comp Neurol* 283, pp. 611-633

Mettler, F.A. (1964) Substantia nigra and parkinsonism. *Arch Neurol* 11, pp. 529-542

Modolo, J. & Beuter, A. (2009) Linking brain dynamics, neural mechanisms, and deep brain stimulation in Parkinson's disease: An integrated perspective. *Med Engineer Physics* 31, pp. 615-623

Moroney, R., Heida, T. & Geelen, J. (2008) Increased bradykinesia in Parkinson's disease with increased movement complexity: elbow flexion–extension movements. *J Comput Neurosci* 25, pp. 501-519 DOI: 10.1007/s10827-008-0091-9

Nambu, A., Tokuno, H., Hamada, I., Kita, H., Imanishi, M., Akazawa, T., Ikeuchi, Y. & Hasegawa, N. (2000) Excitatory cortical inputs to pallidal neurons via the subthalamic nucleus in the monkey. *J Neurophysiol* 84, pp. 289-300

Nambu, A., Tokuno, H. & Takada, M. (2002) Functional significance of the cortico-subthalamo-pallidal 'hyperdirect' pathway. *Neuroscience Research* 43, 111-117

Nambu, A. (2005) A new approach to understand the pathophysiology of Parkinson's disease. *J Neurol* 252 suppl. 4, pp. IV/1-IV/4

Olszewski, J. & Baxter, D. (1954) *Cytoarchitecture of the human brain stem.* Karger Basel, 1-195

Otsuka, T., Abe, T., Tsukagawa, T. & Song, W.-J. (2004) Conductance based model of the voltage-dependent generation of plateau potential in the subthalamic neurons. *J Neurophysiol* 2, pp. 255-264

Pahapill, P.A. and Lozano, A.M. (2000). The pedunculopontine nucleus and parkinson's disease. *Brain*, 123, pp. 1767–1783

Parkinson, J. (1955) *An essay on the shaking palsy* (1817). In: Macdonald Critchley, Ed. Parkinson, J. (1755-1824) Macmillan, London

Paxinos, G. & Watson, C. (2007) *The rat brain in stereotactic coordinates.* Academic Press London

Piallat, B., Chabardes, S., Torres, N., Vraix, V., Goetz, L., Seigneuret, E., Bardinet, E., Ferraye, M., Debu, B., Krack, P., Yelnik, J., Pollak, P. & Benabid, A.L. (2009) Gait is associated with an increase in tonic firing of the sub-cuneiform nucleus neurons. *Neuroscience* 158, pp. 1201-1205

Plaha, P. & Gill, S.S. (2005) Bilateral deep brain stimulation of the pedunculopontine nucleus for parkinsons disease. *Neuroreport* 16, pp. 1883–1887

Rinne, J.O., Ma, S.Y., Lee, M.S., Collan, Y. & Röyttä, M. (2008) Loss of cholinergic neurons in the pedunculopontine nucleus in Parkinson's disease is related to disability of the patients. *Park Rel Disord* 14, pp. 553-557

Rubin, J.E., Terman, D. (2004) High-frequency stimulation of the subthalamic nucleus eliminates pathological thalamic rhythmicity in a computer model. *J Comp Neurosci* 16, pp. 211-235

Samuel, M., Ceballos-Baumann, A.O., Blin, J., Uema, T., Boecker, H., Passingham, R.E. and Brooks D.J. (1997) Evidence for lateral premotor and parietal overactivity in Parkinson's disease during sequential and bimanual movements: a PET study. Brain 120, pp. 963-976

Smith, Y., Bevan, M.D., Shink, E. & Bolam, J.P. (1998) Microcircuitry of the direct and indirect pathways of the basal ganglia. *Neuroscience* 86, pp. 353-387

Spann, B.M., Grofova, I. (1992) Cholinergic and non-cholinergic neurons in the rat pedunculopontine tegmental nucleus. *Anat Embryol* 186, pp. 215-227

Squire, L.R., Bloom, F.E., McConnell, S.K., Roberts, J.L., Spitzer, N.C. & Zigmond, M.J. (2003) Fundamental Neuroscience, 2nd edition, Academic Press. *The Basal Ganglia*, pp. 815-839

Stegenga, J. & Heida, T. (2009) Measuring activity of the subthalamic nucleus in acute slices using multi electrode arrays. In: *Annual symposium of the IEEE-EMBS Benelux*

Chapter, 9-10 november 2009, Enschede, The Netherlands. pp. 26-26. University of Twente. ISBN 978-90-365-2933-4

Stegenga, J., Le Feber, J., Marani, E. & Rutten, W.L.C. (2010a). Phase-dependent effects of stimuli locked to oscillatory activity in cultured cortical networks. *Biophysical Journal* 98, pp. 2452-2458

Stegenga, J. & Heida, T. (2010b) Oscillations in subthalamic nucleus measured by multi electrode arrays. In: *XII Mediterranean Conference on Medical and Biological Engineering and Computing*, 27-30 May 2010, Chalkidiki, Greece. pp. 784-787. IFMBE Proceedings (29). International Federation for Medical and Biological Engineering. ISSN 1433-9277 ISBN 978-960-99365-0-7

Stegenga, J., Van Wezel, R.J.A. & Heida, T. (2010c) Network Activity Patterns in the Subthalamic Nucleus of the Rat. In: *Conference proceedings of the 7th International Meeting on Substrate-Integrated Microelectrode Arrays*, 29 June - 2 July 2010, Reutlingen, Germany. pp. 49-50. FischBach Druck GmbH

Stern, G. (1996) Parkinson's disease: The apoptosis hypothesis. *Adv Neurol* 69, pp. 101-107

Takakusaki, K., Kitai, S.T. (1997) Ionic mechanisms involved in the spontaneous firing of tegmental pedunculopontine nucleus neurons of the rat. *Neuroscience* 78, pp. 771–794

Takakusaki, K., Saitoh, K., Harada, H. & Kashiwayanagi, M. (2004) Role of basal ganglia brainstem pathways in the control of motor behaviors. *Neurosci Res* 50, pp. 137–151

Tepper, J., Acrombie, E. & Bolam, J. (2007) GABA and the basal ganglia. *Prog Brain Res* 160, pp. 1-360

Terman, D., Rubin, J.E., Yew, A.C., Wilson, C.J. (2002) Activity patterns in a model for subthalamopallidal network of the basal ganglia. *J Neurosci* 2, pp. 2963-2976

Toulouse, A. & Sullivan, A.M. (2008) Progress in Parkinson's disease- Where do we stand? *Progr Neurobiol* 85, pp. 376-392

Tretiakoff, C. (1919) Contribution a l'etude de l'anatomie pathologique du locus niger de Soemmering avec quelques deductions relatives a la pathogenie des troubles du tonus musculaire et de la maladie du Parkinson. *Thesis No 293*, Jouve et Cie, Paris

Usunoff, K.G., Itzev, D.E., Ovtscharoff, W.A. & Marani, E. (2002) Neuromelanin in the Human Brain: A review and atlas of pigmented cells in the substantia nigra: *Rev Arch Physiol Biochem* 110, pp. 257-369

Usunoff, K.G., Itzev, D.E., Lolov, S.R. & Wree, A. (2003) Pedunculopontine tegmental nucleus. Part I. Cytoarchitecture, neurotransmitters, development and connections. *Biomedical Rev* 14, pp. 95-120

Usunoff, K.G., Marani, E. & Schoen, H.R. (1997) The trigeminal system in Man. *Adv Anat Embryol Cell Biol* 136, pp. 126

Vitale, A., Manciocco & A., Alleva, E. (2009) The 3R principle and the use of non-human primates in the study of neurodegenerative diseases: The case of Parkinson's disease. *Neurosci Biobehavior Rev* 33, pp. 33-47

Von Economo, C.J. (1917) Neue Beitrage zur Encephalitis lethargica. *Neurol Zbl* 36, pp. 866-878

Yan, W., Zang, Q.J., Liu, J., Wang, T., Wang, S., Liu, X., Chen, L. & Gui, Z.H. (2008) The neural activity of the parafascicular nucleus is conversely regulated by nigrostriatal pathway and pedunculopontine nucleus in rat. *Brain Res* 1240, pp. 204-212

10

Vascular Stent Design Optimisation Using Numerical Modelling Techniques

Houman Zahedmanesh, Paul A. Cahill and Caitríona Lally
Dublin City University
Ireland

1. Introduction

Since their first introduction in 1985 by Palmaz et al. (1985), balloon-mounted vascular stents have revolutionised the treatment of atherosclerosis, and in particular coronary artery disease. Vascular stents were developed to restore blood flow in stenosed arteries of the body, thereby preventing ischemia and myocardial infarction in peripheral and coronary arteries, respectively. A modification to these first stents by Schatz et al. (1987) led to the development of the first commercially successful stent, the Palmaz-Schatz stent. This redesign of the very first stent led the way in a new era of vascular medical device design, with a vast range of new stent designs, materials and adjunct drug therapies subsequently emerging at an ever increasing pace. Now over 25 years on, stents have undeniably become the gold standard in the non invasive treatment of atherosclerosis with 3 million implanted worldwide each year (van Beusekom & Serruys, 2010). To-date, vascular stents have been developed using an extensive range of high grade metals, from tantalum and titanium to the more common medical grade stainless steel, and more recently high yield strength materials such as cobalt chromium and platinum chromium alloys have also been used (Lally et al., 2006; Gopinath et al., 2007; Huibregtse et al., 2011). Self-expanding stents have been developed from shape memory alloys for peripheral anatomies to eliminate the need for expansion using angioplasty balloons (Gopinath et al., 2007). Biodegradable stents have been developed to allow for removal of the stent following successful revascularisation, whilst stents have also been developed to incorporate complementary drug, gene and radiation therapies and even pre-seeded with endothelial cells to lower thrombosis and encourage re-endothelialisation (Serruys et al., 2006; Sharif et al., 2004; Kay et al., 2001; Van der Giessen 1988; Dichek et al., 1989).While many of these new stent designs have offered improvements on their predecessors, no single design has successfully incorporated all of the characteristics of the ideal stent and one significant limitation in the long-term success of stents still remains, namely in-stent restenosis.

In-stent restenosis, which ultimately results in re-occlusion of a stented artery, is effectively an over-zealous wound healing response. It has been identified to comprise mainly of neointimal growth, composed principally of proliferating smooth muscle cells (SMC) and extracellular matrix (Lowe et al., 2002). Stent induced injury to the vessel wall is believed to be a determining factor in the onset and progression of in-stent restenosis (Hoffmann & G. S. Mintz, 2000) and consequently there is increasing evidence that stent design influences restenosis. While the biocompatibility of the metal or surface coating may affect long-term healing in stented vessels, studies have shown that stent geometry designed to optimize expansion and lower recoil is a prerequisite for favourable clinical outcomes (McLean & Eigler 2002). Strut thickness also appears to be an important risk factor, but changing one parameter, such as strut thickness, requires altering other design characteristics, thus altering the overall stent design (McLean & Eigler 2002). Computational models of stent deployment, such as finite element (FE) models, are a very cost effective means of optimising stent designs and can be used to carry out parameterisation studies, whereby the influence of alterations in several stent parameters on the overall stent performance are systematically investigated (Bedoya et al., 2006). Materials changes can be analysed quickly and effectively using numerical modelling techniques such that even the influence that material degradation has on the scaffolding offered by a biodegradable stent can be assessed (Grogan et al., 2011).

FE models of stent expansion enable quantification of the stress-strain field in stents and the vessel wall following stent deployment and therefore provide insights into the various aspects of stent design that are critical in terms of arterial injury (Lally et al., 2005; Holzapfel et al., 2005a). More importantly, however, numerical modelling also provides a means to model the biological response to an implant using mechanobiological models whereby the mechanical environment may be used to dictate the growth and remodelling of vascular cells (Boyle et al., 2011; Zahedmanesh & Lally, 2011). With the emergence of Drug Eluting Stents (DES) and gene delivery stents, however, comes a need to include not only the growth and remodelling of the vessel wall but also the temporal and spatial distribution of such therapeutic agents and their influence on cell growth. Mechanobiological models offer the possibility of including such factors and therefore have the potential to enable future stent designs to be developed such that they combine the best features of conventional bare metal stent designs with the modifications required to facilitate biodegradation or optimum multi-agent drug or gene elution for a variety of vascular applications.

2. The mechanism of in-stent restenosis

Following stent deployment, a healing biological response initiates within the arterial wall which can ultimately lead to renarrowing of the vessel due to excessive migration and proliferation of medial vascular smooth muscle cells (VSMC) towards the vessel lumen. This biological response known as in-stent restenosis consists of four main phases, namely (i) thrombosis (ii) inflammation (iii) proliferation and (iv) remodelling (Edelman et al., 1998). Biomechanical factors which are dictated by the mechanical design of stents have been found to play a key role in all of the aforementioned phases in the development of in-stent restenosis.

During the expansion of the stent, high stresses induced by the stent cause injury to the artery which leads to thrombosis formation in the arterial wall and a cascade of inflammatory events. Close correlation has been observed between the degree of inflammation and neo-intimal thickness which suggests that inflammation caused by the arterial injury plays a central role in the formation of in-stent restenosis (Wieneke et al., 1999; Welt et al., 2002; Mitra et al., 2006). After stent deployment, vessel injury by the stent struts leads to the activation of thrombocytes and the formation of mural thrombus at the injury site. These thrombocytes produce mitogenic factors which contribute to dedifferentiation of medial VSMC, which are in a quiescent and contractile phenotype in the uninjured artery, to a synthetic phenotype. This change of phenotype is followed by a chemotactic migration and proliferation of dedifferentiated medial VSMC towards the lumen and lesion formation, see Figure 1.

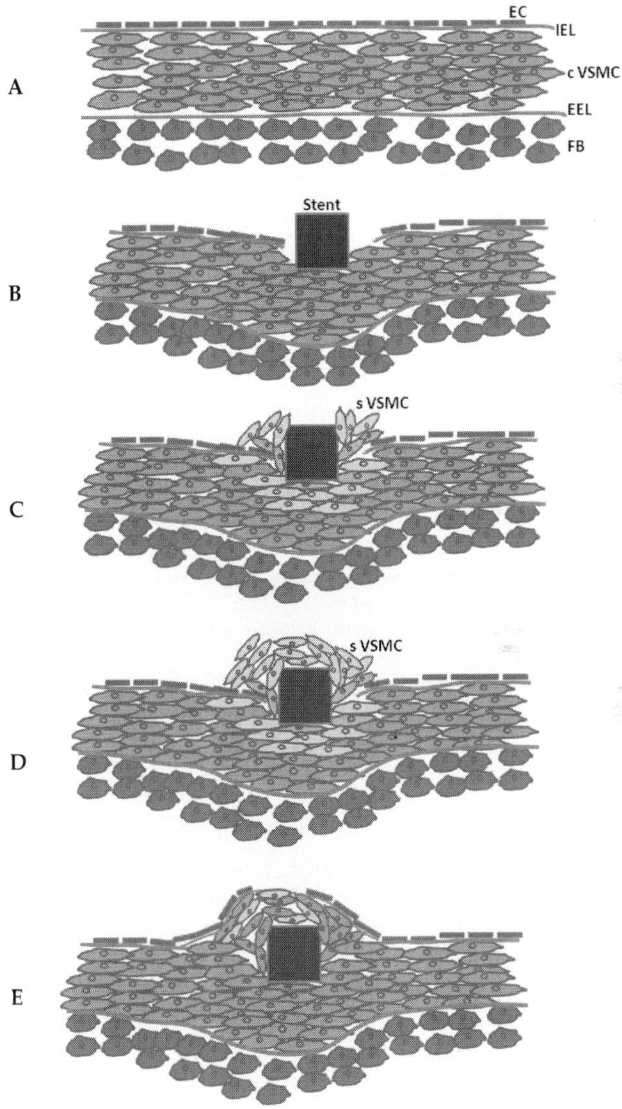

Fig. 1. Development of in-stent restenosis following stent deployment. (A) normal artery (B) de-endothelialisation and injury of the media (C) modulation of medial VSMC phenotype and their migration and proliferation towards the lumen (D) development of in-stent restenosis (E) re-endothelialisation and differentiation of VSMC back to the quiescent phenotype. (EC) endothelial cells, (IEL), internal elastic lamina, (s VSMC) synthetic vascular smooth muscle cell, (c VSMC) contractile vascular smooth muscle cell, (EEL), external elastic lamina.

The cytokines produced by the inflammatory cells not only serve as mitogens for VSMC but also upregulate synthesis of extracellular matrix by the synthetic VSMC (Wieneke et al., 1999; Babapulle and Eisenberg, 2002; Welt et al., 2002; Mitra et al., 2006).

In addition to the stresses induced within the arterial wall and the resulting mechanical injury, flow field perturbations due to stent implantation have also been found to influence the degree to which thrombocytes are recruited and their adhesion to the arterial wall. Specifically, it has been shown that a higher degree of thrombocyte aggregation occurs in locations where the flow field is directed toward the arterial wall rather than away from the wall (Duraiswamy et al., 2005). In addition, stagnant flow patterns adjacent to stent struts, particularly low shear stress, has been found to trigger the recruited inflammatory cells into their activated states (Kroll et al., 1996; Moazzam et al., 1997).

The altered solid mechanical environment following stent deployment also governs the inflammatory and remodelling response. The stent induced lesions are invaded by VSMC with mainly a synthetic phenotype. These cells produce extracellular matrix (ECM) components such as collagen, elastin and proteoglycans which constitute the neointimal tissue and the process usually takes up to 6 months, after which further luminal loss is minimal (Wieneke et al., 1999, Sousa et al., 2005). Intimal hyperplasia is found to be present at increasing thicknesses following injury and lacerations to the internal elastic lamina (IEL), the media, external elastic lamina (EEL) and adventitia (Wieneke et al., 1999; Lowe et al., 2002). An experimental study carried out in pigs identified the degree of injury caused by the implantation of a stent as an independent determinant for estimating the thickness of restenotic growth (Schwartz & Holmes 1994). Consistently, Gunn defined an Injury Score system that determined the degree of injury according to the angle of the IEL at the point of strut contact, the rupture of the IEL or, for extreme cases, rupture of EEL. Gunn applied this scoring system to categorize injury arising from the deployment of a stent in a porcine model (Gunn et al., 2002). The degree of vessel injury is therefore a major determining factor for in-stent restenosis and consequently a key design consideration for stents. In the context of stent optimisation using numerical modelling techniques, the design objective must therefore be to minimise the stress level in the arterial wall following stent deployment (Lally et al., 2005, Holzapfel et al., 2005a).

Several factors are involved in the modulation of VSMC phenotype from a quiescent to synthetic phenotype, including endothelial damage and denudation during stent deployment which is followed by adhesion of thrombocytes which express mitogenic chemokines and result in the chemotactic migration and proliferation of VSMC towards the lumen. Nevertheless, mitogens are not the only factor involved in the phenotypic modulation and activation of medial VSMC. For example, exogenously added fibroblast growth factor (FGF) increases VSMC proliferation in injured arteries, whereas it does not influence VSMC proliferation in uninjured arteries (Lindner & Reidy, 1991; Reidy & Lindner 1991). This observation suggests that other changes related to injury within the vessel may also be involved in the regulation of VSMC activation. In this context, the extracellular matrix (ECM) changes following vessel injury seem to be key regulators of VSMC phenotype and activation. Thyberg et al. (1997) showed that the medial VSMC in injured rat carotid arteries with a synthetic phenotype were enclosed by an incomplete basement membrane compared to normal arteries. These cells were found to migrate into the intima via holes in the internal elastic lamina and to form the neointimal tissue. Ultimately the

VSMC resumed a contractile phenotype as the neointima reached its final size with development of a complete basement membrane. Based on these observations Thyberg et al., (1997) suggested that laminin and other basement membrane components promote differentiation of VSMC towards a quiescent and contractile phenotype whereas their degradation leads into VSMC dedifferentiation and activation. Consistently, several studies have shown the role of collagen type IV, a major component of ECM representing 50% of all basement membrane proteins, in promoting restoration of VSMC to a contractile and quiescent phenotype (Hirose et al., 1999; Aguilera et al., 2003). In addition, exposing VSMC to mechanical loading has been shown to upregulate matrix metalloproteinase (MMP) synthesis by VSMC and mechanical injury upregulates MMP-2 production which is a major proteinase of the basement membrane (James et al.; 1993; Bendeck et al. 1994; Southgate et al., 1996; George et al., 1997) and so does mechanical stretch (Asanoma et al., 2002; Grote et al., 2003). By degrading ECM, MMPs are therefore key regulators of the onset and progression of in-stent restenosis, since they can regulate VSMC phenotype and consequently their behaviour i.e. migration and proliferation.

Finally, it should be noted that the origin of VSMC that accumulate in the neointima in vascular diseases such as in-stent restenosis remains controversial. These cells are a highly heterogeneous cell population with different characteristics and markers, and distinct phenotypes in physiological and pathological conditions. Although, early research on the pathophysiology of in stent-restenosis presents evidence indicating that these cells originate in the host artery (Edelman et al., 1998), several more recent studies have reported a role for bone marrow-derived progenitor cells in vascular maintenance and repair. Moreover, bone marrow-derived smooth muscle progenitor cells have been detected in human atherosclerotic tissue as well as in *in vivo* mouse models of vascular disease. However, it is not clear whether smooth muscle progenitor cells can be regarded as a 'friend' or 'foe' in neointima formation (van Oostrom er al., 2009). The relationship of circulating progenitor cells during stent deployment to the subsequent development of in-stent restenosis has also been evaluated. Bone-marrow- and neural-crest-derived cells, the most dendritic cells, have been found to be consistently present in in-stent restenosis, whilst α-smooth muscle actin positive cells constitute the largest intimal cell pool (Skowasch et al., 2003). Patients with restenosis also have higher numbers of subpopulations of endothelial progenitor cells incorporated into endothelial cells when compared with controls (Pelliccia et al., 2010). Cleary the role of intimal cells and progenitor cells in in-stent restenosis remains to be further elucidated and numerical modelling, and in particular mechanobiological modelling, may provide insights in this area.

3. Numerical modelling as a means to reduce stent induced injury

3.1 Stress/strain analyses of stenting

In addition to being cost effective, computational models often offer the only solution to address some of the important challenges influencing stent design, such as the estimation of stresses induced in the vessel wall and therefore the degree of vascular injury. Several different computational models of stent deployment have been developed in recent years. These models have improved our knowledge on the mechanics of stent-artery interaction (Migliavacca et al., 2002; Wang et al., 2006; Zahedmanesh et al., 2010) and the influence of several different variables of stent geometry such as the influence of stent strut thickness

(Timmins et al., 2007; Zahedmanesh & Lally 2009), plaque composition (Pericevic et al., 2009) and bending in stented peripheral arteries (Early et al., 2009). Balloon expandable stents and self expandable stents have been compared in terms of the level of stresses they induce within the arterial wall and hence the risk of arterial injury using finite element (FE) models (Migliavacca et al., 2004) whilst a number of studies have also been dedicated to investigating hemodynamic related factors in stent design and performance (Wentzel et al., 2000; Wentzel et al., 2001; LaDisa et al., 2006; Duraiswamy et al., 2007; Pant et al., 2010).

One important advantage of computational models of stent deployment over *in-vivo* studies is that they enable the influence of the mechanical parameters of interest to be studied in isolation. Due to the several complex and intertwined biological, chemical and mechanical factors involved *in-vivo*, it is often difficult to associate the outcome of an *in-vivo* trial with one specific mechanical factor. A good example of this is the influence of stent strut thickness on in-stent restenosis. In recent years, several clinical trials have identified stent strut thickness as an independent predictor of restenosis (Kastrati et al., 2001; Briguori et al., 2002; Pache et al., 2003). A clear conclusion from the many clinical studies on stent strut thickness is that stents with thinner struts have a lower restenosis rate, consequently, most of the current generation of stents are produced with thinner struts using high strength materials such as cobalt-chromium alloys (Morton et al., 2004). The ISAR-STEREO clinical trial focussed on the influence of stent strut thickness and compared the restenosis outcome for two stents with the same design but different strut thickness (Kastrati et al., 2001). Although the study highlights the importance of stent strut thickness, it does not clearly elucidate the role and significance of the mechanism by which stent strut thickness could lead to the higher restenosis rate.

From a mechanical perspective the effect of stent strut thickness can be twofold: (i) from a solid mechanical viewpoint strut thickness would influence the stresses induced in the artery during stent deployment and recoil, and (ii) from a hemodynamic viewpoint strut thickness could influence blood flow perturbations. *In-vitro* studies cannot address each of these factors in isolation whilst *in vivo* several biological factors are also involved, such as the higher metal surface exposed to blood flow in thicker strut stents to which platelets can adhere and produce mitogenic growth factors. In contrast, computational models enable each different parameter involved in such a complex process to be studied in isolation. For instance, Duraiswamy et al., (2007) studied the influence of stent strut thickness from a hemodynamics perspective and quantitatively showed that thicker stent struts lead to significantly larger recirculation zones and altered shear stress patterns in the vicinity of struts which can contribute to restenosis. In this context, to further elucidate the influence of stent strut thickness on the vessel wall stresses Zahedmanesh & Lally developed FE simulations of stent deployment procedures and showed that stents with thicker struts induce higher chronic stresses within the vessel wall and also pose a higher risk of injury in the vessel during expansion (Zahedmanesh & Lally 2009). Together, these results elucidate the role of the mechanical environment in the lower restenosis rates observed when using thin strut stents compared to thick strut stents as reported by such clinical trials as the ISAR-STEREO, (Kastrati et al., 2001).

Stent strut thickness is just one of the many factors involved in stent design and the use of finite element method (FEM) is not limited to this factor. FEM can be utilised to study a wide range of design parameters in order to reduce arterial injury. Several studies have investigated the mechanical response of stents using FEM and have suggested different strategies for their simulation (Lee et al., 1992, Rogers et al., 1999, Auricchio et al., 2001, Prendergast et al., 2003, Holzapfel et al., 2005a, Lally et al., 2005, Migliavacca et al., 2002, 2005, 2007, Wang et al., 2006, Gijsen et al., 2008). Given the difficulties involved in construction of the model geometry and the complex contact problem involved in the interaction of a balloon, stent and artery, many simplified methods have been used to model the complex mechanics of stent deployment. Balloons used for stent deployment are initially in a folded configuration. As the balloon unfolds it appears highly compliant, however, as its unfolded shape is reached the balloon becomes highly noncompliant. This complex procedure of balloon unfolding is difficult and very computationally expensive to model. Four main strategies have been used in the literature for numerically modelling balloon expansion of stents which include, (i) direct application of a uniform pressure to the stent luminal surface (Dumoulin & Cochelin 2000; Migliavacca et al., 2005; De Beule et al., 2006; Early et al., 2008), (ii) a rigid cylinder expanded by application of radial displacement (Hall & Kasper, 2006; Takashima et al., 2007; Wu et al., 2007), (iii) stent deployment using a folded balloon model (De Beule et al., 2008; Gervaso et al., 2008; Mortier et al., 2010) and (iiii) pressurisation of simple elastic cylinders with hyperelastic material properties neglecting the balloon folds (Ju et al., 2008; Kiousis et al., 2009).

In a recent study using FE simulation Zahedmanesh et al. (2010) presented a method to create a folded balloon model and utilised the method to numerically model the accurate deployment of a stent in a realistic geometry of an atherosclerotic human coronary artery. Stent deployment is commonly modelled by applying an increasing pressure to the stent, thereby neglecting the balloon and reducing the computational cost and complicated contact between the balloon, stent and artery. This method was compared to the realistic balloon expansion simulation to fully elucidate the limitations of this more simplified procedure. The results illustrated that inclusion of a realistic balloon model is essential for accurate modelling of stent deformation and stent stresses. An alternative balloon simulation procedure was also presented however, which overcame many of the limitations of the applied pressure approach by using elements which restrained the stent as the desired diameter was achieved (Zahedmanesh et al., 2010). This study showed that direct application of pressure to the stent inner surface may be used as an optimal modelling strategy to estimate the stresses in the vessel wall using these restraining elements and hence offer a very efficient alternative approach to numerically modelling stent deployment within complex arterial geometries.

The aforementioned advances in computational modelling when applied to the analysis of the mechanical interaction between stents and the vessel wall provide a robust and efficient tool for stent design optimisation. The models can quantitatively assess the risk of vessel injury by different stents in the early design phase and hence minimise in-stent restenosis in the longer term.

3.2 Mechanobiological models and stenting

The global biological response of vessels to the biomechanical perturbation caused by stent implantation emerges at the tissue level as excessive luminal ingrowth. However, the tissue level response stems from the dynamic changes which occur in the micro-environment of cells deep at the cell level. Cellular behaviours such as differentiation, proliferation, migration, protein and chemokine synthesis and cell death are influenced by the changes in the micro-environmental factors such as extracellular matrix, chemicals, and forces and combine to result in complex responses at the tissue level. This intrinsic multi-scale behaviour of biological systems necessitates a multi scale modelling approach. Therefore, multiscale approaches utilising discrete methods such as cellular automata (CA) (Masselot & Chopard 1998, Ilachinski 2001) and agent based models (ABM) (Wooldridge 2002; Walker et al., 2004) have recently received particular attention for modelling in-stent restenosis.

One prominent example is the multiscale modelling platform developed within the COAST (complex automata simulation technique) project (www.complex-automata.org) which is funded by the European Commision (Evans et al., 2008). The project takes a multiscale and discrete approach towards modelling in-stent restenosis where the growth response of VSMC within the arterial wall is modelled based on the value of wall shear stress (WSS) due to blood flow, the stress level experienced by VSMC within the arterial wall and the concentration of the anti-proliferative drugs diffused from drug eluting stents (Caiazzo et al., 2009). Their model has also been applied to investigate the influence of stent strut size and shape where their simulation results suggest that the growth of the restenotic lesion is strongly dependent on the stent strut cross-sectional profile consistent with the outcome of clinical and animal models (Tahir et al., 2011).

In addition to the approach adopted by the COAST project which is mainly based on discrete methods, a hybrid approach can also be adopted by combining continuum methods such as FEM and discrete methods. FEM is particularly advantageous given that it has proved to be a robust method for quantification of arterial stresses and has been successfully utilised for patient specific modelling of stent-artery interaction (Zahedmanesh et al., 2010, Gijsen et al., 2008). As an example, Boyle et al., (2010) used FE simulations of stent deployment to quantify damage within a stented artery and subsequently used a CA approach to simulate the biological response of the artery to this stent induced damage quantified by the FE model (Boyle et al., 2010, Boyle et al., 2011).

Although the differences between CA and ABM are marginal, the main difference is that a lattice needs to be defined for CA while ABM can be lattice free, meaning that cells can be at any location in the computational domain. This location is usually determined by solving either kinematic or dynamic equations of motion for each individual cell. Hence ABM can yield more realistic results given that no restriction is imposed on the location of the cells in comparison to CA where the cells can only move through certain predefined lattice points and results can therefore be highly dependent on the lattice structure and lattice point density. As a result, a hybrid model utilising ABM, as opposed to CA, and FEM can potentially provide greater simulation capabilities and produce more realistic results. Therefore, a novel hybrid model to simulate in-stent restenosis, using coupled ABM and FEM, will now be presented by the authors. This novel approach has recently been applied to model vascularisation in tissue engineered blood vessels (Zahedmanesh et al., 2011) and is adapted and applied here to model in-stent restenosis.

4. A multi-scale mechanobiological model of in-stent restenosis using coupled agent based models and the finite element method

4.1 Model background

As previously discussed, changes occurring within the arterial wall, particularly ECM changes and degradation of basement membrane around VSMC, play a key role in the dedifferentiation and activation of medial VSMC. Here, a novel mechanistic model is presented which quantitatively captures the processes involved in the degradation and activation of VSMC following stent implantation. The model enables quantitative investigation of the role of stent induced stresses, ECM degradation by MMPs and the subsequent response of VSMC. It can therefore provide insight into the mechanisms involved in the development of in-stent restenosis and it can also be used as a robust and efficient tool to improve the mechanical behaviour of stents in the design cycle. A significant novelty of the presented model is the combination of the FEM with a lattice free ABM which holds significant advantages over the lattice based CA models.

4.2 Materials and methods

4.2.1 Model overview

A mechanobiological modelling framework was developed which comprises of two main coupled modules, (i) a module based on FEM that quantifies von Mises stress to determine the level of arterial damage due to stent deployment and (ii) a biological modelling module based on a lattice free ABM that simulates the key responses of VSMC growth, i.e. migration, proliferation, and ECM degradation and synthesis, in the arterial wall in response to the stent induced damage quantified using the FE analysis, see Figure 2.

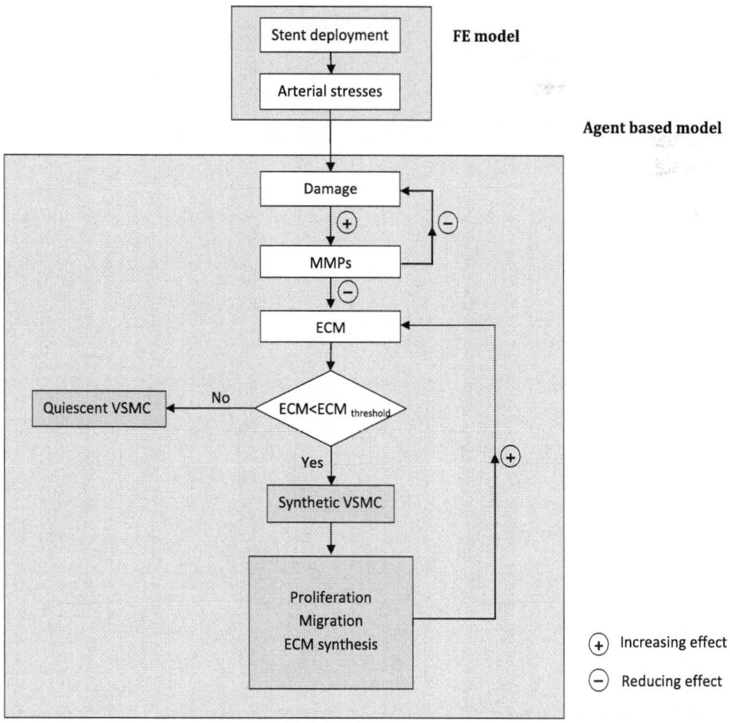

Fig. 2. Overall schematic of the mechanobiological model of in-stent restenosis

The simulation starts in the FE module where the value of the initial stent induced damage is quantified and is transferred to the ABM where the growth of VSMC is simulated. A custom-written routine was developed using python programming language to enable communication between the FE software Abaqus (Simulia, Providence, RI, USA) and the agent-based modelling framework BREVE (www.Spiderland.org). The ABM was programmed using the STEVE language specific to the BREVE agent-based modelling framework.

4.2.2 Finite element model

An axisymmetric hyperelastic FE model of an artery was developed and the influence of stent struts was modelled by application of a radial displacement of 1mm to the luminal surface of the artery where the stent strut contacts the artery, see Figure 3. A pressure of 120 mmHg was applied to the luminal surface to take the systolic arterial blood pressure into account while the two ends of the artery were longitudinally tethered. The model is composed of 3,040 equilateral rectangular axisymmetric elements (Abaqus type CAX4RH). The artery geometry was modelled as 8mm long with a thickness of 0.673mm and a luminal diameter of 4.18mm and was discretised by 190 elements longitudinally and 16 elements radially. This mesh density was chosen based on mesh sensitivity studies.

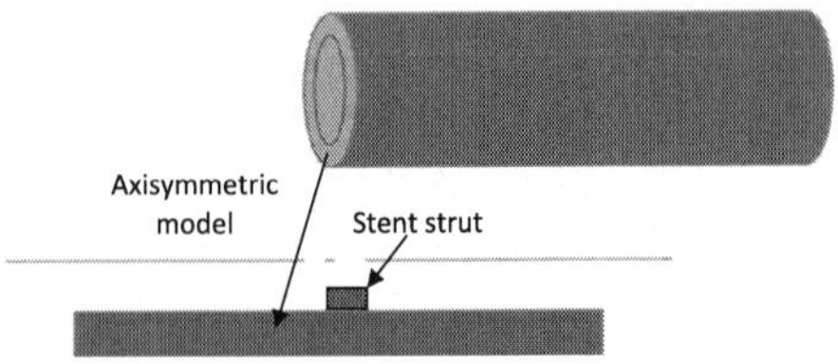

Fig. 3. Axisymmetric representation of the model

The following Ogden hyperelastic equation was used to model the stress-strain response of the artery (Ogden, 1972).

$$\bar{U} = \sum_{i=1}^{3} \frac{2\mu_i}{\alpha_i^2}(\lambda_1^{-\alpha_i} + \lambda_2^{-\alpha_i} + \lambda_3^{-\alpha_i} - 3) \quad (1)$$

Where, $\bar{U}$ is the deviatoric strain energy density, λ_i denotes the deviatoric principle stretches and μ_i and α_i are the hyperelastic constants, see table 1.

Hyperelastic constants	Value
μ_1 (Pa)	-1,231,144.96
μ_2 (Pa)	785,118.59
μ_3 (Pa)	453,616.46
α_1	16.59
α_2	16.65
α_3	16.50

Table 1. Coefficients of the Ogden hyperelastic constitutive models (Zahedmanesh & Lally 2009, Zahedmanesh et al., 2011)

4.2.3 Damage/injury quantification

As a first approach, damage/injury level within the stented artery was quantified with a continuous linear range of 0 to 1. A value of 1 was assigned for the damage in the elements where von Mises stresses exceeded 150kPa. This is a simplified assumption which represents a very first approach to modelling damage accumulation within the artery. This value was chosen given that the intimal layer in human coronary arteries has been reported to have an ultimate tensile strength of 394±223 kPa in the circumferential direction whilst the human medial layer has an ultimate tensile strength of 446±194kPa (Holzapfel et al., 2005b). Therefore, 150kPa represents the lowest value of ultimate tensile strength of these tissues before failure, i.e. one standard deviation below the mean for intimal tissue, and it is therefore deemed a suitable stress level for maximal injury. The authors are currently developing a more sophisticated damage model which will provide a more accurate measure of damage accumulation by defining damage as a continuous function of stent induced stress rather than simply using a threshold stress value. It should be noted that the ABM-FE model presented here can incorporate any range of damage models, with damage accumulation calibrated against clinical or experimental data, such as that proposed by Boyle et al, 2011.

4.2.4 Agent based model

An agent based model of an artery was constructed with VSMC randomly distributed throughout the artery domain. Following the FE analysis the values of the arterial damage at each element of the FE model were exported to the ABM module where the response of VSMC to damage was modelled similar to the approach previously outlined in Zahedmanesh et al., (2011).

The damage induced in the vessel wall due to high stresses upregulates MMP synthesis by VSMC which consequently causes degradation of the ECM. Initially VSMC are in a quiescent and contractile phenotype, degradation of ECM modulates their differentiation toward a synthetic phenotype at the site of damage which ultimately triggers their migration and proliferation, i.e. cells are only allowed to migrate and proliferate when their ECM is degraded to lower than half of the value of ECM in the healthy arteries which for collagen is a value of approximately 3.1×10^{-4} µg/cell (Hahn et al., 2007). In the meantime ECM cleavage and degradation due to MMP upregulation reduces the value of the initially accumulated damage, and hence functions as a negative feedback mechanism leading to recession of the neointimal growth rate. In addition, the proliferating VSMC synthesise ECM and gradually switch back to the contractile phenotype once their value of ECM reaches normal values, see Figure 1. A summary of the relevant parameters used in the ABM and their values is provided in Table 2.

Parameter	Value	Reference
MMP synthesis by VSMC	$\mathrm{MMP}\left(\frac{\mathrm{pg/cell}}{6\mathrm{hour}}\right) = \frac{0.0006}{1+3462\times e^{(-16.3\times \mathrm{dmg})}}$ where dmg is damage value with a range of 0 to 1.	(Kim et al., 2009; Okuno et al., 2002)
ECM degradation rate	50 pg collagen/pg MMP/hour	(Welgus et al., 1980, 1981)

Parameter	Value	Reference
Damage removal by MMPs	0.1/ pg MMP/hour	Set to ensure damage will be fully remove in 15 days
MMP Removal	0.0001pg MMP/element/hour	(Mass balance constraint)
ECM synthesis by VSMC	0.00899 pg collagen/hour/cell	(Kim et al. 1988; Schlumberger et al., 1991; Absood et al., 2004)
Doubling time of synthetic VSMC	35 hours	(Zahedmanesh et al., 2011)
Maximum VSMC migration Speed:	0.001 mm/hr	(Zahedmanesh et al., 2011)

Table 2. Parameters used in the ABM module and their values.

4.3 Results

The mechanobiological model captured the characteristic S-shaped neointimal growth response of arteries to stent deployment previously reported in *in-vivo* studies (Schwartz et al., 1996), see Figure 4. The growth curve comprised a dramatic increase in VSMC number shortly after stent deployment and a plateau region following stabilisation of the healing response. The value of arterial von Mises stresses due to stent deployment was quantified showing high stress concentrations where the stent strut contacted the artery, see Figure 5.

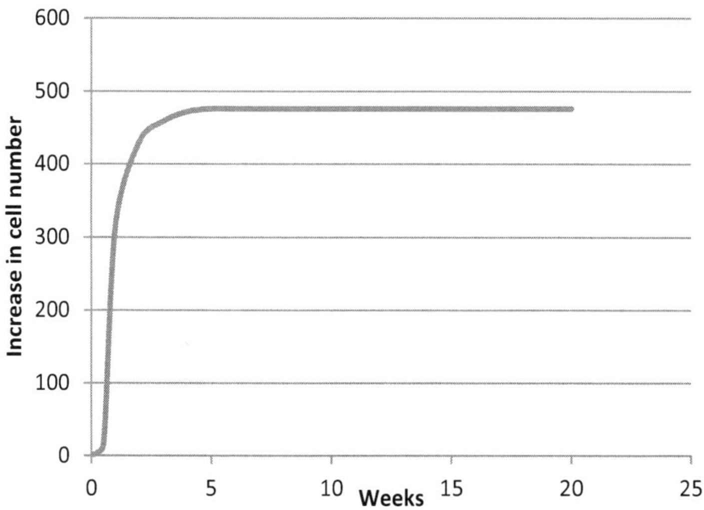

Fig. 4. Increase in the VSMC count in the model due to in-stent restenosis.

A significant area in the vicinity of stent strut showed stresses higher than the threshold stress value for damage and hence a damage value of 1 was automatically assigned to the associated elements. This damage was fully removed following two weeks due to upregulation of MMPs, see Figure 6.

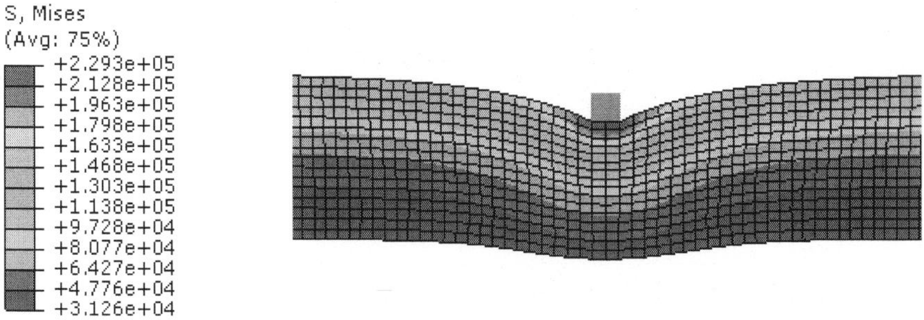

Fig. 5. Distribution of von Mises stresses (Pa) in the arterial wall following stent deployment.

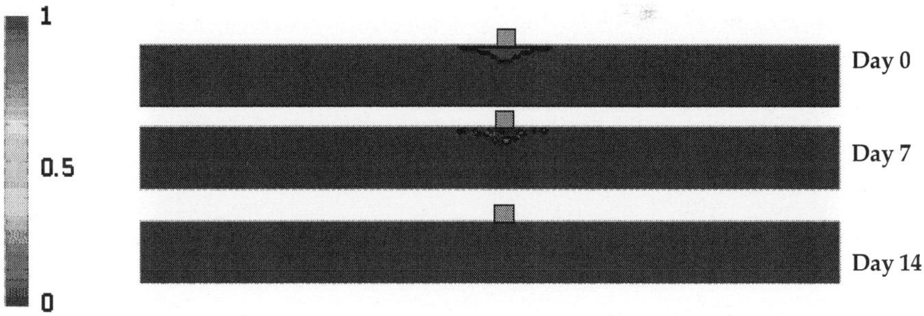

Fig. 6. Damage accumulation in the artery following stent deployment and its reduction due to the healing response.

Following stent deployment, neointimal growth started due to degradation of ECM by MMPs which were upregulated due to the damage accumulation. Neointimal growth reached its maximum following 35 days when the stenosis size reached steady state, see Figures 4 & 7.

The alteration in the ECM distribution and value with time post stent deployment is shown in Figure 7 where ECM is initially degraded due to the damage accumulation and upregulation of MMPs. With the removal of damage and recession of the inflammation, new ECM is synthesised by VSMC, reaching the normal values of ECM in the healthy arteries following 100 days.

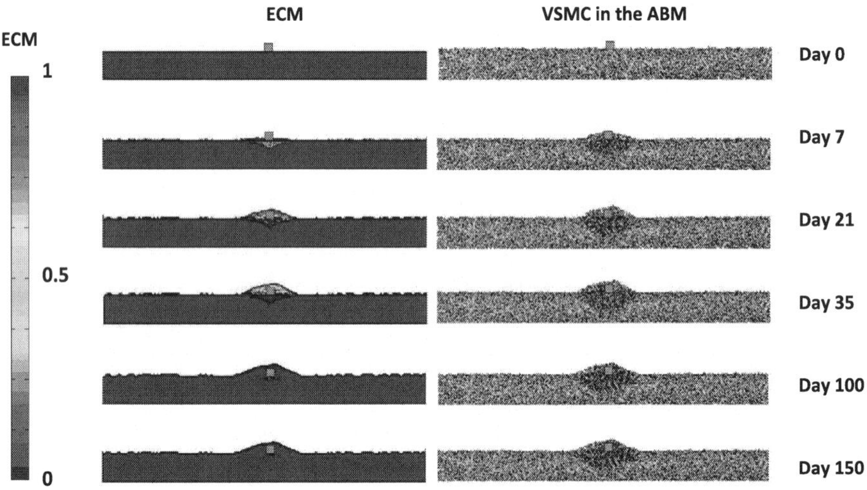

Fig. 7. The development of neointimal tissue with time, (left) alterations of ECM due to degradation and also synthesis by activated VSMC, (right) VSMC growth and distribution.

4.4 Conclusion

Although in a relatively early stage of development, the mechanobiological model presented here successfully captures the key characteristics of the arterial response to stent deployment, specifically the neointimal growth. *In-vivo* studies on the development of intimal hyperplasia in patients due to vascular injury report an exponential increase in the number of neointimal VSMC with a peak in the proliferation rate occurring about two weeks post injury, followed by a reduction in the cell proliferation rate (Schwartz et al., 1996). This characteristic growth response is captured by the mechanobiological model where the cells initially increase at exponential rate followed by a cessation in the cell proliferation and lesion size, see Figure 4 & 7. Nevertheless, this response also depends on the intensity of the mechanical damage and hence it is necessary to further study how different stent designs and deployment parameters influence the development of in-stent restenosis. In this context, when the extent of vascular injury increases, causing laceration to the external elastic lamina and adventitia, the neointimal thickness significantly increases and could necessitate repeat surgical intervention (Wieneke et al., 1999). In addition, endothelial denudation and disruption is observed following stent deployment which has implications for in-stent restenosis given that endothelial cells synthesise nitric oxide which is directly implicated in inducing and maintaining the contractile and quiescent phenotype in VSMC (Lemson et al., 2000). It is therefore also necessary to study the influence of reendothelialisation following stent deployment and this will be addressed with further development of the model and inclusion of endothelial cells.

The presented model is based on the hypothesis that damage accumulation occurs within the ECM, given that ECM components bear the most significant part of the mechanical load. Clearly therefore, it is feasible to hypothesise that mechanical damage accumulation is most significant within ECM and specifically collagen matrix which is the most abundant ECM constituent, making up more than 50% of the basement membrane (Monaco et al., 200). This hypothesis is also supported by comparison to *in-vivo* studies on injured arteries, where it has been shown that VSMC with synthetic phenotype in the injured arteries are encapsulated by an incomplete basement membrane (Thyberg et al., 1997). Whether this observed disruption of the basement membrane is caused by direct mechanical injury or it is due to the increased matrix degradation, it is clear from such *in-vivo* findings that ECM, and specifically the basement membrane, plays a key role in regulation of VSMC phenotype as the main mechanism underlying the development of intimal hyperplasia.

The presented model provides a quantitative evaluation of the ECM alterations occurring within the arterial wall following stent deployment and the resulting neointimal growth. In addition the multiscale mechanobiological model provides a platform for understanding the processes underlying the development of in-stent restenosis. The platform enables new hypotheses on the mechanisms of in-stent restenosis to be tested quantitatively and hence helps to generate key knowledge and insights into the pathophysiology of in-stent restenosis. Knowledge creation is a particular advantage of this modelling framework given that ABMs enable a fully mechanistic approach towards modelling the mechanisms involved in the development of in-stent restenosis. This strength of ABM also facilitates direct translation and incorporation of *in-vitro* and clinical data into the *in-silico* models of in-stent restenosis in a manner which is comprehensible for scientists from diverse backgrounds, such as biologists, clinicians and engineers. As such, ABMs facilitate communication and integration of investigators with diverse backgrounds for a more thorough analysis and understanding of biomedial challenges, which is a crucial requirement for today's multidisciplinary research in the biomedical field. In addition, combining the lattice free ABMs with FE simulations of stent deployment gives a new dimension to the ongoing research on modelling in-stent restenosis by integrating the proven capabilities of FEM in capturing the mechanics of stent-artery interaction with the added value of ABM for mechanistic modelling of the biological response of cells within arteries.

This model clearly has the potential to be used as a robust and efficient tool in the design phase of stents and can be developed further to include additional cell populations such as endothelial cells, the influence of various growth factors, and even drug or gene elution from the stent or stent degradation.

5. Future directions

Whilst stent optimisation studies have advanced considerably in the last 20 years by using numerical modelling techniques, the future of such studies lies in their ability to assess the biological response of the artery to the deployed stent along with the mechanical environment changes induced by the stent. The real power of these models will only be fully realised when inter-patient variability can be incorporated into the models, thereby generating similar data to clinical trials where the probability of stent success in a large population is determined rather than simply one clinical outcome. This can be achieved using patient-specific geometry and material properties in numerical models of stents and such data can currently be obtained from non-invasive medical imaging techniques (Creane et al., 2010). Variations in patient growth responses, and even genetic information can be used to inform such stochastic models (Nowlan & Prendergast, 2005) with advances in computational techniques possibly enabling lesion and patient-specific stents to be designed and manufactured for such patients on the basis of the model results. Ultimately, clinicians may be in a position to prescribe the optimum patient specific stent design, which incorporates drug elution, gene delivery, radiation therapy or a biodegradable stent, to treat a patient specific lesion taking into account the geometry, material properties and growth response of the patient concerned using preclinical predictive models which indicate the best long-term outcome.

6. Acknowledgments

Funding was provided by Irish Research Council for Science Engineering and Technology (IRCSET) under Embark Initiative postgraduate scholarship and Research Frontiers Grant SFI (08/RFP/ENM1378)

7. References

Absood, A., Furutani, A., Kawamura, T. & Graham, L.M. (2004). A comparison of oxidized LDL-induced collagen secretion by graft and aortic SMCs: role of PDGF. *American Journal of Physiology- Heart and Cyrculation Physiology*, Vol. 287, pp. H1200–H1206.

Aguilera, C.V., George, S.J., Johnson, J.L. & Newby A.C. (2003). Relationship between type IV collagen degradation, metalloproteinase activity and smooth muscle cell migration and proliferation in cultured human saphenous vein. *Cardiovascular Research,* Vol. 58, pp. 679-688.

Asanuma, K., Magid, R., Johnson, C., Nerem, R.M. & Galis, Z. (2002). Uniaxial strain upregulates matrix-degrading enzymes produced by human vascular smooth muscle cells. *American Journal of Physiology- Heart and Circulation Physiology,* Vol. 284, pp. 1778-1784.

Auricchio, F., Di Loreto, M. & Sacco, E. (2001) Finite-element analysis of a stenotic revascularization through a stent insertion. *Computer Methods in Biomechanics and Biomedical Engineering,* Vol. 4, pp. 249–264.

Babapulle, M.N. & Eisenberg, M.J. (2002) Coated stents for the prevention of restenosis: Part I. *Circulation,* Vol. 106, pp. 2859-2866.

Bedoya, J., Meyer, C.A., Timmins, L.H., Moreno, M.R. & Moore, J. E. (2006) Effects of stent design parameters on normal artery wall mechanics. *Journal of Biomechanical Engineering*. Vol. 128, pp. 757–765.

Bendeck MP, Zempo, N., Clowes, A.W., Galardy, R.E. & Reidy M.A. (1994). Smooth muscle cell migration and matrix metalloproteinase expression after arterial injury in the rat. *Circulation Research,* Vol. 75, pp. 539–545.

Boyle, C.J., Lennon, A.B., Early, M., Kelly, D.J., Lally, C. & Prendergast, P.J. (2010). Computational simulation methodologies for mechanobiological modelling: a cell-centred approach to neointima development in stents. *Philosophical Transactions of the Royal Society A-Mathematical Physical and Engineering Sciences,* Vol. 368, pp. 2919-2935.

Boyle, C.J., Lennon, A.B. & Prendergast, P.J. (2011) In silico prediction of the mechanobiological response of arterial tissue: application to angioplasty and stenting. *Journal of Biomechanical Engineering,* Vol. 133(8), 081001. doi:10.1115/1.4004492.

Briguori, C., Sarais, C. & Pagnotta, P. (2002). In-stent restenosis in small coronary arteries: impact of strut thickness. *Journal of American College of Cardiology,* Vol. 40, pp. 403–409.

Caiazzo, A., Evans, D., Falcone, J.L., Hegewald, J., Lorenz, E., Stahl, B., Wang, D., Bernsdorf, J., Chopard, B., Gunn, J., Hose, R., Krafczyk, M., Lawford, P.,, Smallwood, R., Walker, D. & Hoekstra, A.G. (2009). Towards a complex automata multiscale model of in-stent restenosis. *Computational Science - ICCS,* Vol. 5544, pp. 705–714.

Creane A., Maher, E., Sultan, S., Hynes, N., Kelly, D., Lally, C. (2010). Prediction of fibre architecture and adaptation in diseased carotid bifurcations. *Biomechanics and Modeling in Mechanobiology,* doi: 10.1007/s10237-010-0277-8.

De Beule, M., Mortier, P., Carlier, S.G., Verhegghe, B., Van Impe, R. & Verdonck, P. (2008). Realistic finite element-based stent design: the impact of balloon folding. *Journal of Biomechanics,* Vol. 41, pp. 383–389.

De Beule, M., Van Impe, R., Verhegghe, B., Segers, P. & Verdonck, P. (2006). Finite element analysis and stent design: reduction of dogboning. *Technology and Health Care,* Vol. 14, pp. 233–241.

Dichek, D.A., Neville, R.F., Zwiebel, J.A., Freeman, S.M., Leon, M.B. & Anderson, W.F. (1989) Seeding of intravascular stents with genetically engineered endothelial cells. *Circulation,* Vol. 80, pp. 1347-1353.

Dumoulin, C. & Cochelin, B. (2000). Mechanical behaviour modelling of balloon-expandable stents. *Journal of Biomechanics,* Vol. 33, pp. 1461–1470.

Duraiswamy, N., Jayachandran, B., Byrne, J. et al. (2005). Spatial distribution of platelet deposition in stented arterial models under physiologic flow. *Annals of Biomedical Engineering,* Vol. 33, pp. 1767–1777

Duraiswamy, N., Schoephoerster, R.T., Moreno, M.R. & Moore J.E. Jr. (2007). Stented artery flow patterns and their effects on the artery wall. *Annual Review of Fluid Mechanics,* Vol.39, pp. 357–382.

Early, M., Lally, C., Prendergast, P.J. & Kelly, D.J. (2008). Stresses in peripheral arteries following stent placement: a finite element analysis. *Computer Methods in Biomechanics and Biomedical Engineering,* Vol.12, pp. 25–33.

Edelman, E.R. & Rogers, C. (1998). Pathobiologic responses to stenting. *American Journal Cardiology,* Vol. 81, pp. 4E–6E.

Evans, D., Lawford, P., Gunn, J., Walker, D., Hose, R., Smallwoodm R., Chopard, B., Krafczyk, M., Bernsdorf, J., Hoekstra, A. (2008). The Application of Multiscale Modelling to the Process of Development and Prevention of Stenosis in a Stented Coronary Artery. *Philosophical Transactions of the Royal Society A,* Vol. 366, pp. 3343–3360.

George, S.J., Zaltsman, A.B. & Newby, A.C. (1997). Surgical preparative injury and neointima formation increase MMP-9 expression and MMP-2 activation in human saphenous vein. *Cardiovascular Research, Vol.* 33, pp. 447– 59.

Gervaso, F., Capelli, C., Petrini, L., Lattanzio, S., Virgilio, L.D. & Migliavacca, F. (2008). On the effects of different strategies in modelling balloon-expandable stenting by means of finite element method. *Journal of Biomechanics,* Vol.41, pp. 1206–1212.

Gijsen, F.J.H., Migliavacca, F., Schievano, S., Socci, L., Petrini, L., Thury, A., Wentzel, J.J., van der Steen, A.F.W., Serruys, P.W.S. & Dubini, G. (2008). Simulation of stent deployment in a realistic human coronary artery. *BioMedical Engineering OnLine,* Vol. 6, pp. 7-23.

Gopinath, M., Feldman, M.D., Patel, D. & Agrawal C.M. (2007) Coronary stents: A materials perspective. *Biomaterials,* Vol. 28(9), pp. 1689-1710.

Grogan, J.A., O'Brien, B.J., Leen, S.B. & McHugh, P.E. (2011) A corrosion model for bioabsorbable metallic stents. *Acta Biomaterialia,* Vol. 7, pp. 3523-3533.

Grote, K., Flach, I., Luchtefeld, M., Akin, E., Holland, S.M., Drexler, H. et al. (2003). Mechanical stretch enhances mRNA expression and proenzyme release of matrix metalloproteinase-2 (MMP-2) via NAD(P)H oxidase-derived reactive oxygen species. *Circulation Research,* Vol. 92, pp. 80e- 86e.

Gunn, J., Arnold, N., Chan, K.H., Shepherd, L., Cumberland, D.C. & Crossman, D.C. (2002). Coronary artery stretch versus deep injury in the development of in-stent neointima. *Heart,* Vol. 88, pp. 401-405.

Hahn, M.S., Mchale, M.K., Wang, E., Schmedlen, R.H. & West, J.I. (2007). Physiologic pulsatile flow bioreactor conditioning of poly(ethyleneglycol)-based tissue engineered vascular grafts. *Annals of Biomedical Engineering,* Vol. 35(2), pp. 190-200.

Hall, G.J., Kasper, E.P. (2006). Comparison of element technologies for modelling stent expansion. *Journal of Biomechanical Engineering,* Vol.128, pp. 751-756.

Hirose, M., Kosugi, H., Nakazato, K. & Hayashi, T. (1999). Restoration to a quiescent and contractile phenotype from a proliferative phenotype of myofibroblasts-like human aortic smooth muscle cells by culture on type IV collagen gels. *Journal of Biochemanics,* Vol. 125, pp. 991-1000.

Hoffmann R. & Mintz G.S. (2000) Coronary in-stent restenosis—predictors, treatment and prevention. *European Heart Journal,* Vol. 21, pp. 1739-1749.

Holzapfel, G.A., Stadler, M. & Gasser T.C. (2005a). Changes in the mechanical environment of stenotic arteries during interaction with Stents: computational assessment of parametric stent designs. *Journal of Biomechanical Engineering -Transactions of ASME,* Vol.127, pp. 166-180.

Holzapfel, GA., Sommer, G., Gasser, C.T. & Regitnig, P. (2005b). Determination of layer-specific mechanical properties of human coronary arteries with nonatherosclerotic intimal thickening and related constitutive modelling. *American Journal of Physiology – Heart and Circulatory Physiology,* Vol.289, pp. 2048-2058.

Huibregtse, B., Dawkins, K.D., Allocco, D.J., Jacoski, M.V. & Mickley, T. (2011) Platinum Chromium Stent Series - The TAXUS™ Element™ (ION™), PROMUS Element™ and OMEGA™ Stents. *Interventional Cardiology,* Vol. 6(2), pp. 134-141.

Ilachinski, A. (2001). Cellular automata: a discrete universe. Singapore: World Scientific.

James, T.W., Wagner, R., White, L.A., Zwolak, R.M. & Brinkerhoff, C.E. (1993). Induction of collagenase gene expression by mechanical injury in avascular smooth muscle cell derived cell line. *Journal of Cellular Physiology,* Vol. 157, pp. 426- 437.

Ju, F., Xia, Z. & Sasaki, K. (2008). On the finite element modelling of balloon-expandable stents. *Journal of the Mechanical Behavior of Biomedical Materials,* Vol. 1, pp. 86-95.

Kastrati, A., Mehilli, J., Dirschinger, J. et al. (2001). Intracoronary stenting and angiographic results: strut thickness effect on restenosis outcome (ISAR-STEREO) trial. *Circulation,* Vol. 103, pp. 2816- 2821.

Kay, I.P., Wardeh, A.J. & Kozuma, K. et al. (2001) Radioactive stents delay but do not prevent in-stent neointimal hyperplasia. *Circulation,* Vol. 103, pp. 14-17.

Kim, Y.J., Sah, R.L., Doong, J.Y. & Grodzinsky, A.J. (1988). Fluorometric assay of DNA in cartilage explants using Hoechst 33258. *Analytical Biochemistry.* Vol. 174, pp. 168–176.

Kim, Y.S., Galis, Z.S., Rachev, A., Han, H.C. & Vito, R.P. (2009). Matrix metalloproteinase-2 and -9 are associated with high stresses predicted using a nonlinear heterogeneous model of arteries. *J. Biomech. Eng.*, Vol. 131, 011009.

Kiousis, D.E., Wulff, A.R. & Holzapfel, G.A. (2009). Experimental studies and numerical analysis of the inflation and interaction of vascular balloon catheter-stent systems. *Annals of Biomedical Engineering*, Vol.37, pp. 315–330.

Kroll, M.H., Hellums, J.D., McIntire, L.V. et al. (1996). Platelets and shear stress. *Blood,* Vol. 88, pp. 1525–1541.

LaDisa, J.F. Jr., Olson, L.E., Douglas, H.A., Warltier, D.C., Kersten, J.R. & Pagel, P.S. (2006) Alterations in regional vascular geometry produced by theoretical stent implantation influence distributions of wall shear stress: analysis of a curved coronary artery using 3D computational fluid dynamics modeling. *Biomedical Engineering Online.* Vol. 5, pp. 40-51. (doi:10.1186/1475-925X-5-40)

Lally, C., Dolan, F. & Prendergast, P.J. (2005). Cardiovascular Stent Design and Vessel Stresses: A Finite Element Analysis. *Journal of Biomechanics*, Vol. 38, pp. 1574–1581.

Lally, C., Kelly D.J. & Prendergast, P.J. (2006) *Stents, Wiley Encyclopedia of Biomedical Engineering,* Metin Akay (Ed), Wiley.

Lee, R.T., Loree, H.M., Cheng, G.C., Lieberman, E.H., Jaramillo N. & Schoen, F.J. (1993). Computational structural analysis based on intravascular ultrasound imaging before in vitro angioplasty: prediction of plaque fracture locations. *Journal of the American College of Cardiology*, Vol. 21, pp. 777–782.

Lemson, M.S., Tordoir J.H.M., Daemen, M.J.A.P., Kitslaar, P.J.E.H.M. (2000). Intimal hyperplasia in vascular grafts. *European Journal of Vascular and Endovascular Surgery,* Vol. 19, pp. 336–350.

Lindner, V. & Reidy, M.A. (1991). Proliferation of smooth muscle cells after vascular injury is inhibited by an antibody against basic fibroblast growth factor. *Proceedings of the National Academy of Sciences of the united states of america,* Vol. 88(9), pp.3739–3743.

Lowe, H.C., Oesterle, S. N. & Khachigian L. M. (2002). Coronary in-stent restenosis: Current status and future strategies *J. Am. Coll. Cardiol.* Vol. 39, pp. 183-193.

Masselot, A. & Chopard, B. (1998). A lattice Boltzmann model for particle transport and deposition. *Europhys. Lett.* Vol. 42, pp. 259–262.

McLean, D.R. & Eigler, N.L. (2002) Stent design: implications for restenosis. *Rev Cardiovasc Med.* Vol. 5, pp. S16–S22.

Migliavacca, F., Gervaso, F., Prosi, M., Zunino, P., Minisini, S., Formaggia, L. & Dubini, G. (2007). Expansion and drug elution model of a coronary stent, *Computer Methods in Biomechanics and Biomedical Engineering*. Vol.10, pp. 63–73.

Migliavacca, F., Petrini, L., Colombo, M., Auricchio, F. & Pietrabissa, R. (2002). Mechanical behavior of coronary stents investigated through the finite element method. *Journal of Biomechanics*, Vol.35, pp. 803–811.

Migliavacca, F., Petrini, L., Massarotti, P., Schievano, S., Auricchio, F. & Gabriele Dubini (2004). Stainless and shape memory alloy coronary stents: a computational study on the interaction with the vascular wall. *Biomechanics and Modeling in Mechanobiology,* Vol. 2, pp. 205-217.

Migliavacca, F., Petrini, L., Montanari, V., Quagliana, I, Auricchio, F. & Dubini, G. (2005). A predictive study of the mechanical behaviour of coronary stents by computer modelling. *Medical Engineering and Physics*, Vol.27, pp. 13–18.

Mitra, A.K. & Agrawal, D.K. (2006). In stent restenosis: bane of the stent era, *Journal of Clinical Pathology*, Vol. 59, pp. 232–239.

Moazzam F, DeLano FA, Zweifach BW, et al. (1997). The leukocyte response to fluid stress. *Proceedings of the National Academy of Sciences of the united states of america* , Vol. 94, pp. 5338–5343.

Monaco, S., Sparano, V., Gioia, M., Spardella D., Di Pierro, D., Marini, S., Coletta, M. (2006) Enzymatic processing of collagen IV by MMP-2 (gelatinase A) affects neutrophil migration and it is modulated by extracatalytic domains *Protein Science*, Vol. 15, pp. 2805–2815.

Mortier, P., Holzapfel, G.A., De Beule, M., Van Loo, D., Taeymans, Y., Segers, P., Verdonck, P. & Verhegghe, B. (2010) A Novel Simulation Strategy for Stent Insertion and Deployment in Curved Coronary Bifurcations: Comparison of Three Drug-Eluting Stents. *Annals of Biomedical Engineering*, Vol. 38, pp. 88-99.

Morton, A.C., Crossman, D. & Gunn, J. (2004). The influence of Physical Stent Parameters Upon Restenosis. *Pathological Biology*, Vol. 52, pp. 196–205.

Nowlan N.C. & Prendergast P.J. (2005). Evolution of mechanoregulation of bone growth will lead to non-optimal bone phenotypes, *Journal of Theoretical Biology* 235, 408-418.

Ogden, R.W. (1972). Large deformation isotropic elasticity: on the correlation of theory and experiment for incompressible rubberlike solids. *Proceedings of the Royal Society of London A- Mathematical and Physical Sciences*, Vol.326, pp. 565–584.

Okuno, T., Andoh, A., Bamba, S., Araki, Y., Fujiyama, Y., Fujiyama, M. & Bamba, T. (2002). Interleukin-1beta and tumor necrosis factor-alpha induce chemokine and matrix metalloproteinase gene expression in human colonic subepithelial myofibroblasts. *Scandinavian Journal of Gastroenterology*, Vol. 37, pp. 317–324.

Pache, J., Kastrati, A., Mehilli, J. et al. (2003). Intracoronary Stenting and Angiographic Results: Strut Thickness Effect on Restenosis Outcome (ISAR-STEREO-2), Trial. *Journal of the American College of Cardiology*, Vol. 41, pp. 1283–1288.

Palmaz, J.C., Sibbitt, R.R., Reuter S.R., Tio F.O. & Rice W.J. (1985) Expandable intraluminal graft: a preliminary study: work in progress. *Radiology*, Vol. 156, pp. 73-77.

Pant, S., Bressloff, N.W., Forrester, A.I. & Curzen, N. (2010) The influence of strut-connectors in stented vessels: a comparison of pulsatile flow through five coronary stents. *Annal of Biomedical Engineering*, Vol. 38, pp. 1893-1907.

Pericevic, I., Lally, C., Toner, D. & Kelly, D.J. (2009). The influence of plaque composition on underlying arterial wall stress during stent expansion: The case for lesion-specific stents. *Med Eng Phys.*, Vol. 31, pp. 428-33.

Prendergast, P.J., Lally, C., Daly, S., Reid, A.J., Lee, T.C., Quinn, D. & Dolan, F. (2003). Analysis of prolapse in cardiovascular stents: a constitutive equation for vascular tissue and finite-element modelling. *Journal of Biomechanical Engineering*, Vol. 125, pp. 692–699.

Reidy, M.A. & Lindner, V. (1991). Basic FGF and growth of arterial cells. *Annals os the New York Academy of Sciences*, Vol. 638, pp. 290-299.

Rogers, C., Tseng, D.Y., Squire, J.C. & Edelman, E.R. (1999). Balloon–artery interactions during stent placement: a finite element analysis approach to pressure, compliance, and stent design as contributors to vascular injury. *Circulation Research*, Vol. 84, pp. 378–383.

Schatz, R.A., Palmaz, J.C., Tio, F.O., Garcia, F., Garcia, O. & Reuter, S.R. (1987) Balloon-expandable intracoronary stents in the adult dog. *Circulation,* Vol. 76, pp. 450-457.

Schlumberger, W., Thie, M., Rauterberg, J. & Robenek, H. (1991). Collagen synthesis in cultured aortic smooth muscle cells. Modulation by collagen lattice culture, transforming growth factor- beta 1, and epidermal growth factor. *Arterioscler. Thromb.* Vol. 11, pp. 1660–1666.

Schwartz, R.S. & Holmes, D.R. (1994). Pigs, dogs, baboons, and man—lessons for stenting from animal studies. *Journal of Interventional Cardiology,* Vol. 7, pp. 355–368.

Schwartz, R.S., Chua, A., Edwards, W.D., Srivatsa, S.S., Simaric, R.D., Isner, J.M. & Holmes, D.R. Jr. (1996). A proliferation analysis of arterial neointimal hyperplasia: lessons for antiproliferative restenosis therapies. *International Journal of Cardiology* Vol. 53, pp. 71-80

Serruys, P.W., Kutryk, M. J.B. & Ong, A.T.L. (2006) Coronary-Artery Stents. *New England Journal of Medicine,* Vol. 354, pp. 483-495.

Sharif, F., Daly, K., Crowley, J. & O'Brien, T. (2004) Current status of catheter- and stent-based gene therapy. *Cardiovascular Res*earch, Vol. 64 (2), pp. 208-216. doi: 10.1016/j.cardiores.2004.07.003

Sousa, J.E., Costa, M.A., Abizaid, A. et al. (2005). Four-year angiographic and intravascular ultrasound follow-up of patients treated with sirolimus-eluting stents. *Circulation,* Vol. 111, pp. 2326–2329.

Southgate, K.M., Fisher, M., Banning, A.P., Thurston, V.J., Baker, A.H., Fabunmi, R.P. et al. (1996). Upregulation of basement-membrane-degrading metalloproteinase secretion following balloon angioplasty of pig carotid arteries. *Circulation Res*earch, Vol. 79, pp. 1177–11 87.

Tahir, H., Hoekstra, A.G., Lorenz, E., Lawford, P.V., Hose, D.R., Gunn, J. & Evans D.J.W. (2011). Multi-scale simulations of the dynamics of in-stent restenosis: impact of stent deployment and design. *Interface Focus,* doi:10.1098/rsfs.2010.0024

Takashima, K., Kitou, T., Mori, K. & Ikeuchi, K. (2007). Simulation and experimental observation of contact conditions between stents and artery models. *Medical Engineering and Physics*, Vol. 29, pp. 326–335.

Thyberg, J., Blomgren, K., Roy, J., Tran, P.K. & Hedin. A. (1997). Phenotype modulation of smooth muscle cells after arterial injury is associated with changes in the distribution of laminin and fibronectin. *J Histochem Cytochem,* Vol. 45, pp. 837-846.

Timmins, L.H., Moreno, M.R., Meyer, C.A., Criscione, J.C., Rachev, A. & Moore J.E. Jr. (2007). Stented artery biomechanics and device design optimization. *Medical and Biological Engineering and Computing,* Vol. 45(5), pp. 505–513.

Van Beusekom, H.M.M. & Serruys, P.W. (2010) Drug-Eluting Stent Endothelium: Presence or Dysfunction. *J Am Coll Cardiol Intv,* Vol. 3, pp. 76-77.

Van der Giessen, W.J., Serruys, P.W., Visser, W.J., Verdouw, P.D., Van Schalkwijl, W.P. & Jongkind, J.F. (1988) Endothelialization of intravascular stents. *Journal of Interventional Cardiology,* Vol. 1, pp. 109-120.

Walker, D.C., Southgate, J., Hill, G., Holcombe, M., Hose, D.R., Wood, S.M., MacNeil, S. & Smallwood, R.H. (2004). The epitheliome: agent-based modelling of the social behaviour of cells. *Biosystems,* Vol. 76, pp. 89–100.

Wang, W.Q., Liang, D.K., Yang, D.Z. & Qi, M. (2006). Analysis of the transient expansion behavior and design optimization of coronary stents by finite element method. *Journal of Biomechanics*, Vol.39, pp. 21-32.

Welgus, H.G., Jeffrey J.J. & Eisen, A.Z. (1981). The collagen substrate specificity of human skin fibroblast collagenase. *Journal of Biological Chemistry*, Vol. 256, pp. 9511-9515.

Welgus, H.G., Jeffrey, J.J., Stricklin, G.P., Roswit, W.T. & Eisen, A.Z. (1980). Characteristics of the action of human skin fibroblast collagenase on fibrillar collagen. *Journal of Biological Chemistry*, Vol. 255, pp. 6806–6813.

Welt, F.G. & Rogers, C. (2002). Inflammation and restenosis in the stent era. *Arteriosclerosis, Thrombosis and Vascular Biology*, Vol. 22(11), pp. 1769–1776.

Wentzel, J.J., Krams, R., Schuurbiers, J.C.H., Oomen, J.A., Kloet, J., van der Giessen, W.J., Serruys, P.W. & Slager, C.J. (2001) Relationship between neointimal thickness and shear stress after wallstent implantation in human coronary arteries. *Circulation*. Vol. 103, pp. 1740–1745.

Wentzel, J.J., Whelan, D.M., van der Giessen, W.J., van Beusekom, H.M.M, Andhyiswara, I., Serruys, P.W., Slager, C.J. & Krams, R. (2000) Coronary stent implantation changes 3-D vessel geometry and 3-D shear stress distribution. *Journal of Biomechanics*. Vol. 33, pp. 1287–1295.

Wieneke, H., Haude, M., Knocks, M., Gutersohn, A., von Birgelen, C., Baumgart, D. & Erbel R. (1999). Evaluation of Coronary Stents in the Animal Model: A Review. *Materialwissenschaft und Werkstofftechnik*, Vol.30, pp. 809–813.

Wooldridge, M. (2002). *Introduction to multiagent systems.*, NY: Wiley, New York.

Wu, W., Wang, W.Q., Yang, D.Z. & Qi M. (2007). Stent expansion in curved vessel and their interactions: a finite element analysis. *Journal of Biomechanics*, Vol.40, pp. 2580–2585.

Zahedmanesh, H. & Lally C. (2011). A multiscale mechanobiological model using agent based models, Application to vascular tissue engineering. *Biomechanics and Modeling in Mechanobiology*, doi:10.1007/s10237-011-0316-0.

Zahedmanesh, H. & Lally, C. (2009). Determination of the influence of stent strut thickness using the finite element method: implications for vascular injury and in-stent restenosis. *Medical and Biological Engineering and Computing*, Vol. 47, pp. 385-393.

Zahedmanesh, H., Kelly, D. & Lally, C. (2010). Simulation of a balloon expandable stent in a realistic coronary artery, Determination of the optimum modelling strategy. *Journal of Biomechanics*, Vol. 43, pp. 2126–2132.

Part 2

Biomechanical Engineering Methods and Applications

11

Functional Significance of Force Fluctuation During Voluntary Muscle Contraction

Kazushige Oshita[1,2] and Sumio Yano[2]
[1]*Department of Sports Science, Faculty of Sports Science, Kyushu Kyoritsu University*
[2]*Graduate School of Human Development and Environment, Kobe University*
Japan

1. Introduction

Human movement is the result of the joint torque or muscle force generated by the contraction of multiple muscles. The force generated during voluntary muscle contraction is not constant, but fluctuates as observed through the variability in movement. The normalised force fluctuation (measured according to the standard deviation (SD) of force) during isometric contractions is referred to as 'steadiness', which influences functional human movement (Carville et al., 2007; Kornatz et al., 2005; Marmon et al., 2011; Salonikidis et al., 2009). For example, Salonikidis et al. (2009) and Kornatz et al. (2005) report that greater fluctuation during voluntary muscle contraction can influence functional human movement in the upper limbs. With regard to the lower limbs, Carville et al. (2007) report that the elderly who tend to fall exhibit less steady knee extension than do both the young and the elderly who do not tend to fall. However, the relationship between force fluctuations in lower limb muscles and human movements for daily activities remains unclear. The ability to control posture during quiet standing is one of the fundamental activities of daily living. Furthermore, the muscle activities of lower limb muscles are important for postural stability during quiet standing. Therefore, this chapter focuses on the relationship between force steadiness in lower limb muscles and postural stability during quiet standing.

1.1 Asymmetry of muscle function in leg muscles

Some studies demonstrate that the asymmetry of muscle function between the 2 legs may influence human movement. For example, Skelton et al. (2002) report that although 'fallers' (20 women living at home, aged >65 years with a history of falls in the past year) and 'non-fallers' (15 age-matched women with no history of falls) have asymmetric lower limb power, the fallers exhibit significantly greater asymmetry. Furthermore, the relationship between the asymmetry of leg strength and walking speed in 1,205 healthy women aged 30–89 years old has been reported (Oshita et al., 2009). Walking speed is fastest when the asymmetries of knee extension and flexion strength are below 5%, as shown in Fig. 1. However, if the asymmetry of one of the parameters (i.e. knee extension or flexion) is more than 10%, walking speed is still reduced. Furthermore, the walking speed is slowest when the asymmetries of knee extension and flexion strength are more than 10% (Fig. 1). Moreover, the asymmetry of leg strength does not affect the walking speed of subjects with higher leg strength (Fig. 2). However, in subjects with low leg strength, walking speed decreases with increasing asymmetry of leg strength.

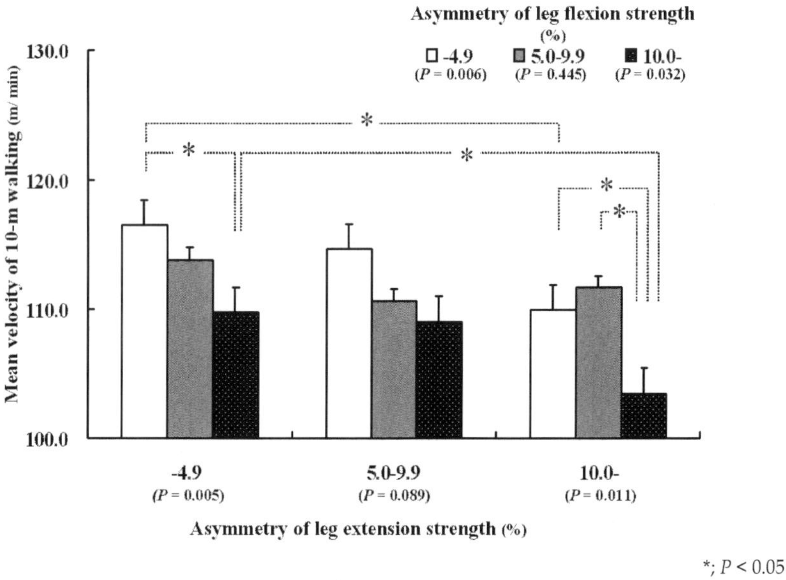

Fig. 1. Relationship between walking speed and asymmetry of leg strength

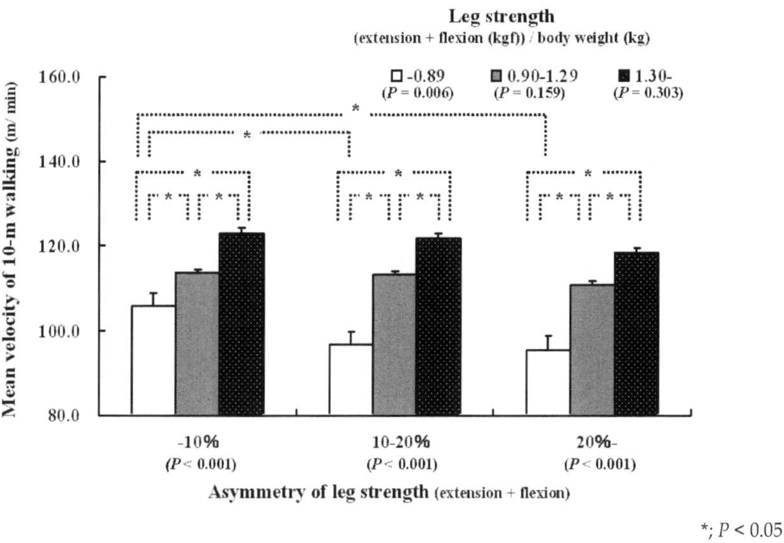

Fig. 2. Relationship between walking speed and leg strength and asymmetry of leg strength

Although these previous studies suggest that the asymmetry of leg strength might affect the human movement regarding postural stability, the intensity of most daily activities is not maximal, but is thought to be less than approximately 20% of maximum voluntary contraction (MVC) (Sawai et al., 2004). These studies lead us to hypothesise that asymmetry in muscle function at less than 20% MVC is an important factor for postural stability. Thus, in section 3, we introduce the asymmetry of force fluctuations during isometric contraction in lower limb muscles during low-intensity muscle contraction.

1.2 Plantar flexor muscles during quiet standing

Based on the dynamics of human quiet standing, numerous studies (i.e. analyses using electromyograms or the model of a single-joint inverted pendulum rotating around the ankle joint) show that the plantar flexor muscles play a significant role in stabilising the body during quiet standing. For example, the activities of the plantar flexors during bipedal quiet stance are coherent with both spontaneous body swaying (Gatev et al., 1999; Masani et al., 2003) and mechanically induced body swaying (Fitzpatrick et al., 1996). Although many factors (e.g. proprioception, control of upper body motion, etc.) are related to postural stability during quiet standing, the plantar flexors (i.e. the soleus muscle) are the most activated muscles in the entire body during quiet standing (Ohnishi et al., 2005; Sawai et al., 2004). These studies lead us to hypothesise that quiet standing is associated with force fluctuation in the plantar flexors. If force fluctuation in the plantar flexors is one of the most important factors for postural stability during quiet standing, the amplitude of force fluctuation will indicate a relationship between ability and posture stability. In section 4, we discuss the relationship between force steadiness of the plantar flexors and the postural sway during quiet standing.

1.3 Practice reduces force fluctuation and improves human movement

In order to increase muscle strength in healthy adults, the American College of Sports Medicine (1998) recommends strength training at least 2-3 times per week. Further, 1 day of exercise per week may not develop into habitual exercise; for example, the definition of habitual exercise according to a national health and nutrition survey is least 2 sessions of exercise per week (Ministry of Health, Labour, and Welfare of Japan, 2011). Although this training frequency is generally recommended for strength training, it might be not necessarily realistic for people aiming to maintain their health or who are unable to devote a considerable amount of time to strength training alone (Ohmori et al., 2010). However, previous studies involving relatively low-frequency strength or functional training (1 session per week or per 2 weeks) demonstrate increases in muscle strength in both normal young adults (Hayashi and Miyamoto, 2009; Ohmori et al., 2010) as well as in normal and functionally limited older adults (Oshita et al., 2008; Sato et al., 2007). The improvement in strength brought about by such low-frequency training is attributed to several neural factors such as motor learning, adjustment of motor function, acquisition of skills, excitability of alpha-motor neurons, increased motor neuron firing rate, and motor unit synchronisation (Ohmori et al., 2010).

In order to reduce force fluctuations in healthy adults, strength training and/or steadiness practice can be used during voluntary contraction of the distal muscles of the upper and lower limbs. Keen et al. (1994) report that in young adults, 4 weeks of strength training of the first dorsal interosseous muscle using a heavy load (80% of maximum) reduces the force fluctuations measured during isometric contraction at 50% MVC. Similarly, steady contractions or force-tracking tasks also reduce force fluctuations. For example, 2 weeks of practicing a steadiness task with a light load (10% of maximum) on the index finger reduces force fluctuations and the discharge rate variability of single motor units in the hand muscles of older adults (Kornatz et al., 2005); similar effects are observed in young adults. Patten and Kamen (2000) report that the ability to match force trajectory in the dorsiflexor muscles improves after 2 weeks of isometric force modulation training. However, the effect of low-frequency steadiness practice (1 day of practice per week) on force fluctuations during isometric contraction is currently unknown. Furthermore, if the force fluctuations in the plantar flexor muscles are associated with postural stability, force steadiness practice should improve postural stability during quiet standing. Thus, in section 5, we discuss the effects of low-frequency steadiness practice in the plantar flexor muscles on force fluctuations during isometric contraction and postural stability during quiet standing.

2. Method

2.1 Experimental setup

Here, we describe the design used for the plantar flexion exercise. Each participant performed a static unilateral plantar flexion exercise (Fig. 3). Participants were instructed to remove all footwear and sit on an insulated straight-backed chair. An additional strap was used to secure the thigh of the leg to the chair. Force was measured with a load cell (LPR-A-S10, Kyowa, Tokyo, Japan) positioned between a metal base plate and the foot. The foot was secured with a strap at the foot lever plate. The strain gauge transducer was aligned between the 2 plates near the distal part of the foot. The exact position of the entire device was carefully adjusted such that the knee was fully extended with the ankle joint angle at 90°. The amount of force produced and the target were displayed on a computer screen (14.1 inches) positioned 1 m away at the level of the participant's eyes to provide visual feedback.

The following paragraph outlines the design used for the knee extension exercise (Fig. 3).

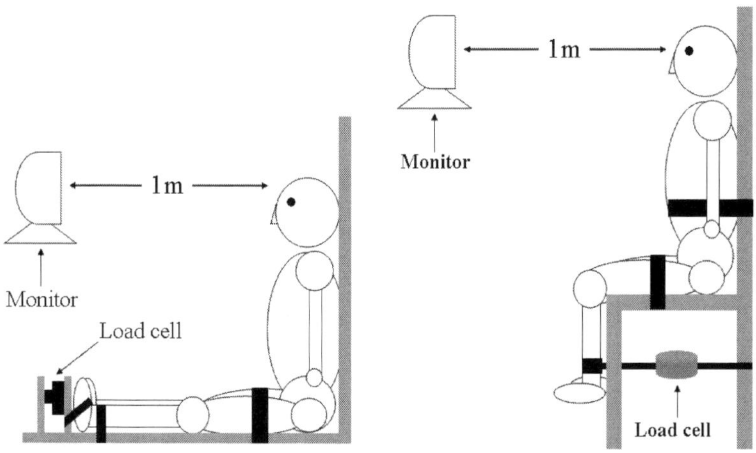

Fig. 3. Schematic drawing of the setup used for the isometric plantar flexion (left) and knee extension (right)

Each participant performed an isometric unilateral knee extension exercise with each leg while in a seated position, with the hip and knee joints both flexed at 90° (full extension = 0°). Throughout the experiment, the participant's upper body was firmly fixed to a chair with a seat belt. The force of the isometric contraction of the knee extensor muscles was measured by a load cell (LTZ-100KA, Kyowa, Tokyo, Japan) attached to the ankle just above the malleolus by a strap. The amount of force produced and the target were displayed on a computer screen (14.1 inches) positioned 1 m away at the level of the participant's eyes to provide visual feedback.

2.2 Muscle strength test (MVC measurement)

Each participant performed MVC for a period of 5 s with encouragement from the investigators. Participants performed 3 trials with subsequent trials performed if the difference in the peak force of 2 MVCs was >5%. Participants were allowed to reject any effort that they did not consider 'maximal'. The trial with the highest peak force was chosen for analysis.

2.3 Force-matching (steady isometric contraction) task

On the basis of the MVC measurements, the participants performed a steady isometric contraction task for 15-20 s at levels corresponding to 10%, 20%, or 30% of the MVC; there was an approximately 30-min rest period between MVC measurement and these tasks. The force signals were obtained by a sensor interface with a 12-bit analogue-to-digital converter at a sampling frequency of 1 kHz (PCD-300A, Kyowa, Tokyo, Japan) and stored on the hard disk of a computer for future analysis. Data were collected for 1 trial with each target, and the order of the target forces was randomised for each participant. There was a rest period of >1 min between trials, and between-trial rest periods of up to 5 min were also allowed at subject's request.

2.4 Postural sway during quiet standing

Each participant was instructed to remove all footwear and maintain quiet standing for 30-40 s on a platform (Fig. 4). The subjects had their arms alongside their body and their feet were kept parallel with the centres of the heels 15 cm apart. To assess the trajectory of the centre of mass displacement (CoMdis) during quiet standing the horizontal position of a lumbar point at L3 was measured by a laser displacement sensor (ANR 1251, SUNX, Japan). The present study focused on anteroposterior CoMdis, because the force produced by the plantar flexor muscles mainly contributes to the body sway in this particular axis (Masani et al., 2003). The signals were acquired at a sampling frequency of 100 Hz with a 16-bit analogue-to-digital converter (AI-1608AY, CONTEC, Japan) and stored on the hard disk of a computer for future analysis.

2.5 Data analysis

The data were processed with SPCANA waveform analysis software (version 4.71, Japan) and Microsoft Excel. For the stored force signals, the data for an 8-s period in the middle portion of the collected data (15-20 s) were selected for analysing individual trials because there was no systematic change in fluctuations within trials. After low-pass filtering (<100 Hz), the SD of the force was calculated to evaluate the amplitude of force fluctuation.

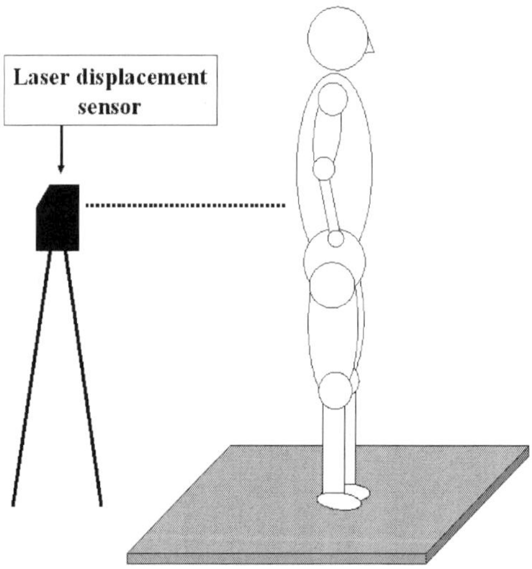

Fig. 4. Schematic drawing of the setup used for the measurement of postural sway

For the CoMdis signals, the data for a 20-s period in the middle portion of the collected data (30-40 s) were selected for analysing individual trials. The velocity of CoMdis (CoMvel) was calculated by numerically differentiating CoMdis as a function of time. This is because the velocity of body sway (i.e. the centre of pressure displacement or CoMdis) in the anteroposterior axis is the most sensitive parameter capable of distinguishing not only children and young adults from seniors, but also middle-aged subjects from seniors (Abrahamova and Hlavacka, 2008; Prieto et al. 1996; Masani et al., 2007). Furthermore, the SD of CoMvel was calculated to assess postural sway during quiet standing.

3. Asymmetry of force fluctuation in leg muscles

3.1 Proximal part (Knee extension)

In this section, we discuss the asymmetry of force fluctuations during isometric knee extension (Oshita and Yano, 2010a). Data were obtained from 12 healthy men (age, 21 ± 1 years). Each participant performed the steady isometric knee extension task for 15 s at levels corresponding to 10% or 20% MVC. Force fluctuations were compared between the stronger and weaker MVC limbs. In all subjects, the right limb was stronger. The MVCs of the stronger and weaker limbs were 688.0 ± 49.6 and 625.8 ± 43.1 N, respectively. Figure 5 shows the force fluctuations during the steady isometric knee extension task. Force fluctuation was significantly greater in the 20% MVC task than in the 10% MVC task in both limbs. However, no significant differences in force fluctuations during the 10% and 20% MVC tasks were observed between the stronger and weaker limbs. Thus, although force fluctuation increased with contraction intensity, no asymmetry of force fluctuation was observed during low-intensity steady isometric knee extension.

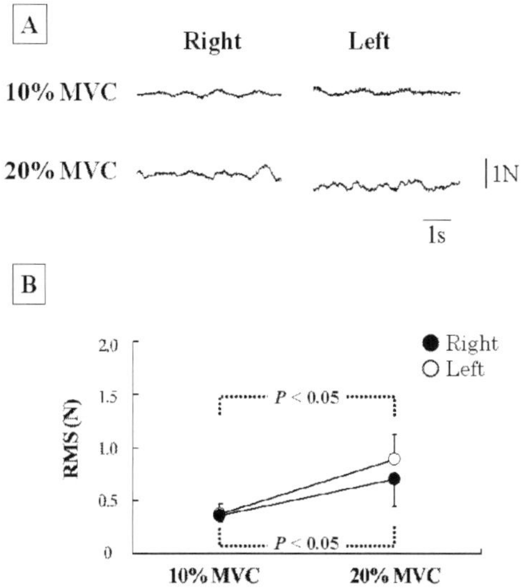

Fig. 5. Representative force fluctuations during isometric knee extension (A) and means and standard errors of the means (B) (Oshita and Yano, 2010a)

Adam et al. (1998) report significantly greater fluctuation in the non-preferred hand than in the preferred hand during a 30% MVC isometric abduction task in the index finger; furthermore, the discharge rate variability during task is greater in the non-preferred hand than in the preferred hand. One of the important factors in the asymmetry differences in the upper limb is their daily preferential use. However, our results indicate that no asymmetry in force fluctuation was observed during steady isometric knee extension at 10 or 20% MVC.

Furthermore, figure 5 and 6 show mechanomyogram signals in vastus lateralis during the steady isometric knee extension task. These results indicate that no asymmetry differences in the mechanical characteristics in the active muscle were observed. In contrast to the upper limb, the role of limb preference in lower limbs is not clear. For example, if a person kicks a ball with their preferred limb, the other limb is often required to support the entire body weight. Therefore, it is unclear which limb is stronger: the limb preferred for daily use or the other limb regularly supporting the body weight over many years. However, our results are consistent with those of Semmler and Nordstrom (1995) who report that no asymmetry of force fluctuation or discharge variability is observed during isometric index finger abduction. The difference in the results of Adam et al. (1998) and Semmler and Nordstrom (1995) is thought to be due to differences in contraction intensity. Although the asymmetry of force fluctuation is observed during 30% MVC (Adam et al., 1998), it is not observed during <10% (Semmler and Nordstrom, 1995), 10%, or 20% MVC (Fig. 5). The force fluctuations observed during isometric contraction are correlated with the discharge rate variability, which is thought to be a major determinant of force fluctuations (Mottram et al., 2005; Tracy et al., 2005). Thus, no asymmetry of force fluctuations might be observed during low-intensity contraction because the variability in the discharge rate is too small. Furthermore, the present results indicate asymmetry of mechanomyogram signals in the active muscle. These results suggest that no asymmetry of force fluctuations during low-intensity isometric knee extension is observed, because there are no differences regarding mechanical characteristics in the active muscle between stronger and weaker legs.

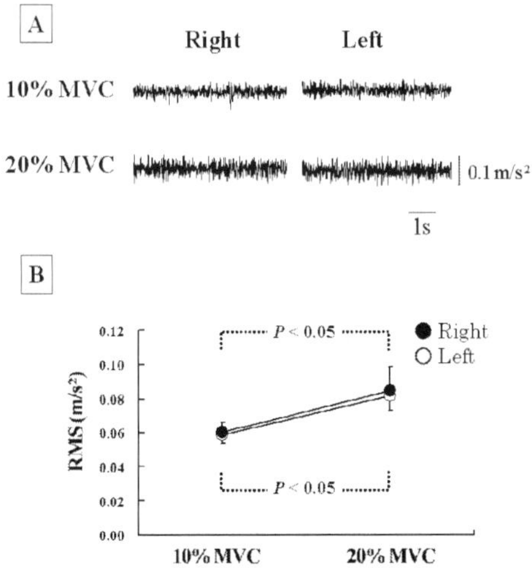

Fig. 6. Representative amplitude of mechanomyogram signal during isometric knee extension (A) and means and standard errors of the means (B) (Oshita and Yano, 2010a)

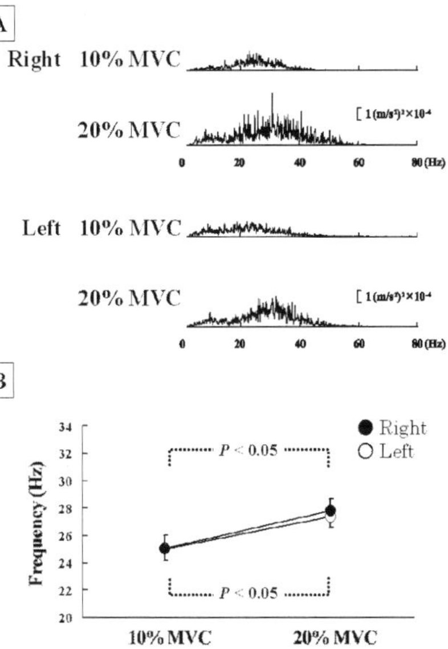

Fig. 7. Representative mean power frequency of mechanomyogram signals during isometric knee extension (A) and means and standard errors of the means (B) (Oshita and Yano, 2010a)

3.2 Effect of contraction intensity

In section 3.1, we found that force fluctuations during isometric knee extension at 10% and 20% MVC were not significantly different between the 2 legs. However, Adam et al. (1998) reported a significantly greater fluctuation for the non-preferred than the preferred hand during a 30% MVC isometric abduction task with the index finger. The different results obtained by Adam, et al. (1998) and Semmler and Nordstrom (1995) are thought to reflect the difference in intensity of contraction. If the asymmetry of force fluctuations is influenced by intensity of contraction, asymmetry of force fluctuation in the lower limbs which was not observed below 20% MVC might be observed above 30% MVC. Furthermore, although the intensity of most daily activities is below 20% MVC, some activities of high intensity are required in daily life (e.g., climbing stairs or walking up or down a slope) or sports activities. Apparently, although Oshita and Yano (2010a) reported the asymmetry of force fluctuation in leg muscle at low intensity, the asymmetry of force fluctuation in the leg muscles at moderate intensity remains unclear. In this section, we discuss the asymmetry of force fluctuation during isometric knee extension at low and moderate intensities (Oshita and Yano, 2011a).

Data were obtained from 11 healthy men (age, 21 ± 1 years). Each participant performed the steady isometric knee extension task for 15 s at levels corresponding to 20% or 30% MVC. Figure 10 shows the force fluctuations during the steady isometric knee extension task. Although force fluctuation was not statistically significantly different between the 2 legs during the 20% MVC task, it was statistically significantly higher in the left leg than in the right leg during the 30% MVC task (Fig. 8). These results indicate asymmetry of force fluctuation during isometric knee extension was observed in the moderate intensity task (30% MVC) but not in the low intensity task (20% MVC). In the section 3.1, we reported the force fluctuations during isometric knee extension at low intensities (10% and 20% MVC) were not significantly different between the 2 legs (Oshita and Yano; 2010a). In the upper limbs, Semmler and Nordstrom (1995) also reported the force fluctuation during isometric abduction of the index finger at below 10% MVC was not statistically significantly different between the 2 hands. These previous data are consistent with the present result; force fluctuation during isometric knee extension at low intensity (20% MVC) was not statistically significantly different between the 2 legs. However, Adam et al. (1998) reported a statistically significantly greater fluctuation for the non-preferred than for the preferred hand during a task with 30% MVC isometric abduction of the index finger. They suggested the different results of Adam et al. (1998) and Semmler and Nordstrom (1995) were influenced by the difference in the intensity of contraction. In the current study, force fluctuation during knee extension which was not different between the 2 legs at low intensity (20% MVC) was statistically significantly different between the legs at moderate intensity (30% MVC). Therefore, the present results were consistent with the suggestion of Adam et al. (1998) that the asymmetry of force fluctuation in lower limbs was also influenced by the contraction intensity.

Several researchers have suggested that a major determinant of the force fluctuation is the variability in motor-unit discharge rate (Mottram et al., 2005; Tracy et al., 2005), viz., the positive association of force fluctuation with variability of the discharge rate during isometric contraction (Mottram, et al., 2005; Tracy, et al., 2005). Although the present study did not measure the activities of motor units directly, the firing rate of the motor unit in active muscle (i.e. vastus lateralis) was evaluated using an mechanomyogram. Further, there was a statistically significant association between the 2 legs' mean power frequency of mechanomyogram signal during the 20% MVC task but not during the 30% MVC task (Fig. 9), so individuals who had higher (or lower) mean power frequency of mechanomyogram signal in the right leg's active muscle also tended to have higher (or lower) mean power frequency in the left leg during isometric knee extension at low intensity (20% MVC). In contrast, mean power frequency of mechanomyogram signal during the moderate intensity (30% MVC) task was uneven between the 2 legs. Thus, the asymmetry of the firing rates of the motor units in active muscle during isometric knee extension is associated with intensity of the contraction.

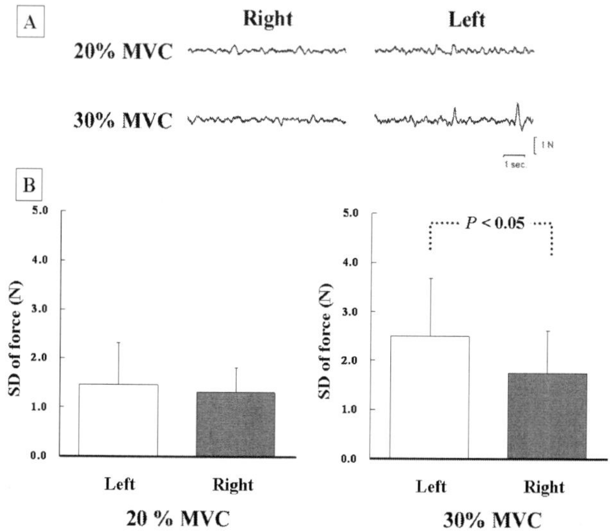

Fig. 8. Representative force fluctuations during isometric knee extension (A) and means and standard errors of the means (B) (Oshita and Yano, 2011a)

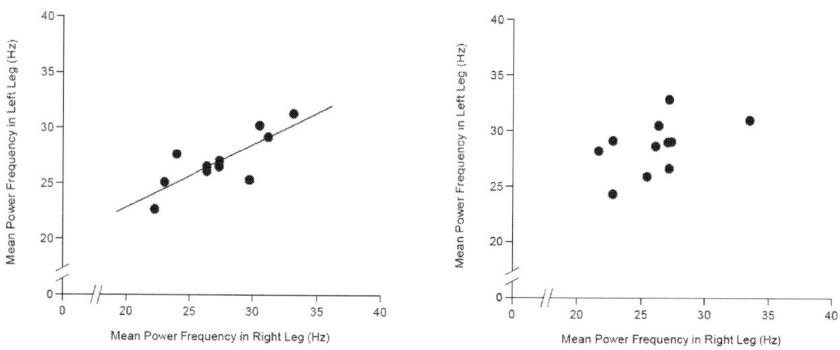

Fig. 9. Relationships regarding mean power frequency of mechanomyogram signal during isometric knee extension at 20% (left) and 30% (rihgt) MVC between the right and left legs (Oshita and Yano, 2011a)

Force fluctuation may influence functional performance of controlling finger or limb movements in daily life. Although the intensity of most daily activities is below 20% MVC, some activities of high intensity are required in daily life or sports activities. Asymmetry of force fluctuation might be important in these motions. Most importantly, although the intensity of most daily activities is below 20% MVC for individuals with normal or high muscle strength, it would be of higher intensity for those with lower muscle strength. Asymmetry of force fluctuation during voluntary contractions of high intensity might affect normal daily activities of individuals with low muscle strength.

3.3 Distal part (Plantar flexion)

Although the force fluctuations were not significantly different between the 2 legs during low-intensity isometric knee extension, the asymmetry of force fluctuations in the plantar flexor muscles is currently unknown. The apparent biomechanical differences between limb segments are reflected in the distinct control of proximal versus distal joints. There are different control loops for distal and proximal muscles in the cerebellum and reflex pathways (Kurata and Tanji, 1986; Nisky et al., 2010). According to previous studies (Lemon and Griffiths, 2005; Davidson and Buford, 2006; Nisky et al., 2010), humans are more accurate in control and perception of the position of endpoint of the limb. Opposite gradients in maximum controllable force and resolution of force control were reported; that is, proximal joints are more successful than distal joints in the control of force (Hamilton et al., 2004; Nisky et al., 2010). Thus, a significant difference in the force fluctuations between the 2 legs might be observed in the plantar flexor muscles. In this section, we discuss the asymmetry of force fluctuations during isometric plantar flexion (Oshita and Yano, 2010b).

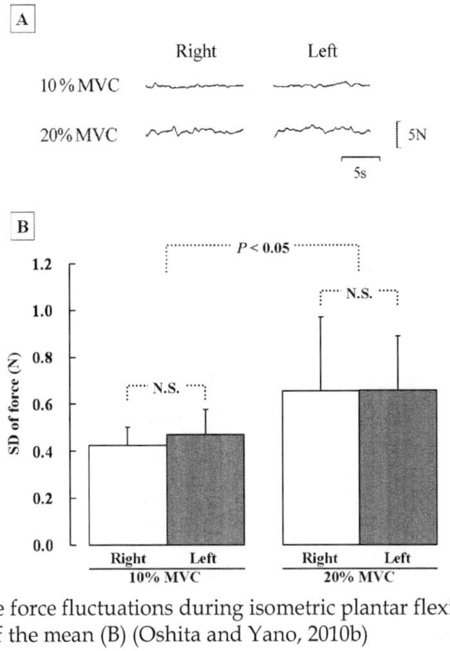

Fig. 10. Representative force fluctuations during isometric plantar flexion (A) and means and standard errors of the mean (B) (Oshita and Yano, 2010b)

Data were obtained from 12 healthy men (age, 21 ± 1 years). Each participant performed the steady isometric plantar flexion task for 20 s at levels corresponding to 10% and 20% MVC. Force fluctuations in the plantar flexors were compared between the stronger (right) and weaker (left) MVC limbs. In all subjects, the right limb was the stronger limb. Figure 10 shows force fluctuations during the steady isometric plantar flexion task. Force fluctuation was significantly greater in the 20% MVC task than in the 10% MVC task in both limbs. However, no significant differences in force fluctuations in both the 10% and 20% MVC tasks were observed between the right and left limbs. Furthermore, the force fluctuation was significantly associated between the 2 legs (Fig. 11). In addition, the participants who had greater (or smaller) force fluctuations in the right limb also had greater (or smaller) fluctuations in the left limb. Although force fluctuation increased with contraction intensity, no asymmetry of force fluctuation was observed during low-intensity steady isometric plantar flexion.

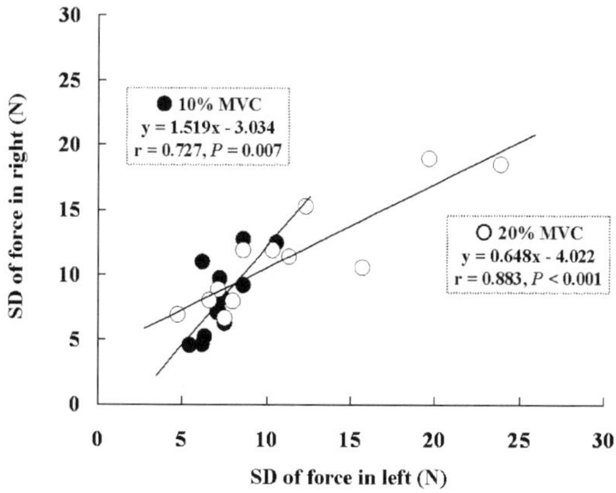

Fig. 11. Relationships regarding force fluctuation during force-matching tasks between the right and left legs (Oshita and Yano, 2010b)

Although there are different control loops for distal and proximal muscles in the cerebellum and reflex pathways, force fluctuations in the plantar flexor muscles were not significantly different between the 2 legs. The present study focuses on investigating the asymmetry of force fluctuations during low-intensity isometric contraction in lower limb muscles. Therefore, the underlying mechanisms of the asymmetry of force fluctuation remain unclear. Future studies are required to determine muscle activity in the antagonist muscle and/or neuromuscular properties (e.g. electromyography, motor unit activity, etc.) in order to clarify the mechanisms of the effects of practice like those reported here.

4. Steadiness in plantar flexion and postural sway

If force fluctuation in the plantar flexors is an important factor for postural stability during quiet standing, the amplitude of force fluctuation will indicate a relationship between ability and postural stability. Thus, in this section, we discuss the relationship between the force steadiness of the plantar flexors and postural sway during quiet standing (Oshita and Yano, in submitting). Data were obtained from 12 healthy men (age, 21 ± 1 years). Each participant performed the isometric unilateral plantar flexion exercise with their preferred leg. The relationship between force fluctuation during isometric plantar flexion and postural sway during quiet standing was evaluated using linear regression analysis. Figure 12 shows the relationship between postural sway during quiet standing and force fluctuation in plantar flexion. Although postural sway was significantly associated with force fluctuation at 10% MVC, it was not significantly associated with that at 20% MVC. These results suggest that the strategy of motor output in the plantar flexor muscles during low-intensity contraction is different between 10% and 20% MVC; moreover, the fluctuation in motor output in the plantar flexor muscles at 10% MVC was associated with postural sway during quiet standing in young adults.

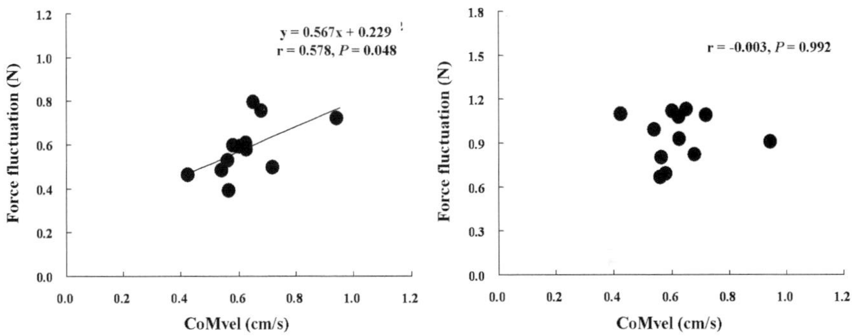

Fig. 12. Relationship between postural sway and force fluctuation during plantar flexion at 10% (left) and 20% (right) MVC

Numerous studies show that the plantar flexor muscles play a significant role in stabilising the body during quiet standing (Masani et al., 2003; Morasso and Schieppati, 1999). Furthermore, we observed a relationship between postural stability during quiet standing and force fluctuations during low-intensity isometric plantar flexion exercise. Therefore, individuals who have greater difficulty controlling plantar flexion force during isometric contraction tend to have greater difficulty controlling their standing posture. We revealed that plantar flexor force fluctuation is associated with postural sway during quiet standing in young adults. These results indicate that the force steadiness in plantar flexor muscles is important for postural stability during quiet standing; this is somewhat consistent with the results of previous studies. Oshita and Yano (2010c) report that force fluctuation during plantar flexion at 20% MVC is associated with postural stability during single-leg quiet standing. Although they report that postural stability is associated with force fluctuation at 20% MVC, the present results show a significant positive correlation between postural sway and force fluctuation at 10% MVC. The discrepancy between these results is thought to be due to the difference in the state of quiet standing. Oshita and Yano (2010c) report that force fluctuation is associated with postural stability during single-leg quiet standing. The activity level of the plantar flexor muscles is approximately 15–20% of MVC during single-leg standing (Sawai et al., 2004); however, it is approximately 10% of MVC during bipedal standing (Ohnishi et al., 2005; Sawai, et al., 2004). Further, we suggest that the significant correlation between postural stability during quiet standing and the plantar flexor force fluctuation is found only at the corresponding contraction intensities for plantar flexor muscles. Therefore, the present results suggest that the neural strategies for plantar flexor muscles during quiet standing are similar to the strategies for controlling plantar flexor force in young adults.

Although the neural strategies at work in the plantar flexor muscles during quiet standing and those controlling plantar flexion forces are similar, the underlying mechanisms of the effects of steadiness practice on postural stability remain unclear. One possibility is that influence of the co-activation of the antagonist muscle (i.e. tibialis anterior) during both a force-matching task and quiet standing. Benjuya et al. (2004) report that subjects with a large postural sway (i.e. elderly adults) exhibit greater co-activation of the tibialis anterior during quiet standing. During the force steadiness tasks in finger muscles, fluctuations can be produced by alternating activation of the agonist and antagonist muscles (Vallbo and Wessberg, 1993). However, some studies (Burnett et al., 2000; Tracy and Enoka, 2002) report conflicting results in that the co-activation of antagonist muscles does not seem to have a major effect on force fluctuations. Thus, it remains unclear whether co-activation influences force fluctuation and postural stability.

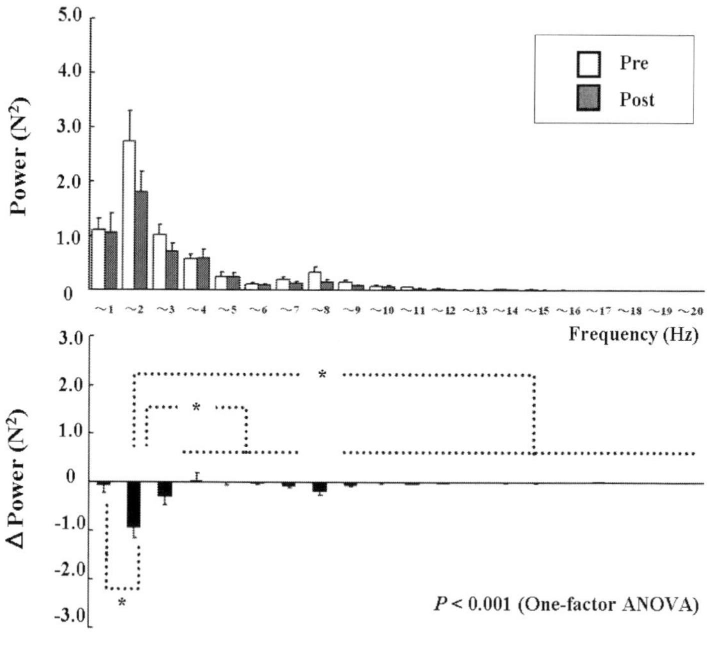

Fig. 13. Power spectral analysis of force fluctuation before and after steadiness practice (Oshita and Yano, 2011b)

Another possibility is that Ia afferent function has the capacity to modulate force fluctuations and postural stability. Ia afferent inputs contribute to force fluctuations in the low-frequency range. Yoshitake et al. (2004) report force fluctuations in the plantar flexor muscles at <2 Hz during low-level contractions (<10% MVC) after prolonged Achilles tendon vibration, a factor known to influence Ia afferent function. Oshita and Yano (2011b) found a reduction in force fluctuation in the frequency range of <2 Hz after force steadiness practice (Fig. 13). Furthermore, postural stability during quiet standing is also influenced by the efficacy of Ia afferent function as reflected by the amplitude of the H-reflex (Tokuno et al., 2007; Tokuno et al., 2008). Thus, force fluctuations might be associated with postural sway as a result of the contribution of Ia afferent function. Future studies are required to determine muscle activity in the antagonist muscle and/or neuromuscular properties (e.g. electromyography, motor unit activity, etc.) in order to clarify the mechanisms of practice effects like those reported here.

In summary, the present results indicate that the significant correlation between postural stability during quiet standing and force fluctuation during plantar flexion is found only at the corresponding contraction intensities for the plantar flexor muscles in young adults. Furthermore, the present results suggest that the neural strategies for plantar flexor muscles during quiet standing are similar to those controlling the plantar flexor force in young adults.

5. Steadiness practice reduces force fluctuation and postural sway

In section 4, we found a significant correlation between postural stability during quiet standing and force fluctuation in plantar flexion. If the force fluctuation in the plantar flexor muscles is reduced by steadiness practice, postural sway during quiet standing would also be reduced. This is because the results presented in section 4 suggest that the neural strategies employed by the plantar flexor muscles during quiet standing are similar to those controlling plantar flexion forces in young adults. Thus, in this section, we discuss the effects of steadiness practice in the plantar flexor muscles on force fluctuation during isometric contraction and postural sway during quiet standing (Oshita and Yano, 2011c).

Data were obtained from 21 healthy men (age, 21 ± 1 years). Participants were randomly assigned to a practice group (n = 14) and a non-exercising control group (n = 7). Practice groups were divided according to the frequency of practice: for 4 weeks, 7 participants practiced once a week while the other 7 practiced twice a week. Participants performed a strength test, force-matching tasks, and a postural stability test before and 4 weeks after the practice program. Strength was assessed by measuring MVC force. Force-matching tasks were performed to maintain isometric contraction. Steady contraction practice was performed as an isometric plantar flexion exercise under conditions identical to those in the experimental session. All practice was performed in the laboratory under supervision with emphasis on performing steady contractions. Practice consisted of 5 sets of practice per session. Verbal encouragement was provided during the sessions. The practice session consisted of the steady contraction task that lasted for 60 s (30 s at 10% and 20% MVC each) followed by a 30-s rest period.

Although MVC values were not significantly different before and after the practice period in the practice group, force fluctuation was significantly lower. Although the practice itself reduced force fluctuation, the frequency of practice did not have an effect (Table 1). Furthermore, there was no statistically significant interaction between practice intervention and frequency (Table 1). These results indicate that force fluctuation is reduced by low-intensity force steadiness practice but does not change the MVC. Moreover, no effect of practice frequency (one or two time per week) was observed between groups.

Strength and steadiness practice reduce force fluctuation during the voluntary contraction of the distal muscles of the upper and lower limbs. Keen et al. (1994) found that 4 weeks of strength practice with the first dorsal interosseous muscle with a heavy load (80% of maximum) in 10 young adults (aged 18–27 years) reduced force fluctuation during isometric contraction at 50% MVC. Patten and Kamen (2000) report that the ability of 6 young adults (aged 18–22 years) to match a force trajectory requiring force modulation up to 60% MVC in the dorsiflexor muscles improved after 2 weeks of isometric force modulation training.

				Practice group		ANOVA		
				Once a week	Twice a week	Frequency	Pre - Post	Interaction
Muscle strength	Right	(N)	*Pre*	470.6 ± 187.9	538.0 ± 252.9	$P = 0.730$	$P = 0.370$	$P = 0.174$
			Post	509.2 ± 164.3	529.6 ± 246.5			
	Left	(N)	*Pre*	474.7 ± 165.2	548.6 ± 238.0	$P = 0.600$	$P = 0.722$	$P = 0.614$
			Post	496.1 ± 165.3	544.9 ± 222.2			
Force Fluctuation	10% MVC Right	(N)	*Pre*	0.559 ± 0.088	0.695 ± 0.279	$P = 0.468$	$P = 0.050$	$P = 0.318$
			Post	0.518 ± 0.157	0.468 ± 0.086			
	10% MVC Left	(N)	*Pre*	0.540 ± 0.055	0.782 ± 0.262	$P = 0.291$	$P < 0.001$	$P = 0.053$
			Post	0.427 ± 0.046	0.426 ± 0.127			
	20% MVC Right	(N)	*Pre*	0.880 ± 0.056	1.142 ± 0.457	$P = 0.297$	$P < 0.001$	$P = 0.253$
			Post	0.720 ± 0.087	0.901 ± 0.399			
	20% MVC Left	(N)	*Pre*	1.096 ± 0.013	1.237 ± 0.327	$P = 0.604$	$P < 0.001$	$P = 0.456$
			Post	0.758 ± 0.120	0.715 ± 0.227			
Postural sway	CoM velocity	(cm/s)	*Pre*	0.593 ± 0.095	0.607 ± 0.060	$P = 0.690$	$P = 0.004$	$P = 0.655$
			Post	0.539 ± 0.045	0.530 ± 0.043			

Table 1. Changes in muscle strength and force fluctuation due to steadiness practice in the practice group (Oshita and Yano, 2011c)

These previous findings corroborate those of the present study. Both the existing literature and present results indicate that strength and steadiness training interventions consistently reduce fluctuations during the low-to-moderate-intensity contractions of the distal muscles of the upper and lower limbs. Furthermore, even though the frequency of practice was relatively low (once a week), it was sufficient to reduce the force fluctuation in the present study.

We also showed that steadiness practice in the plantar flexor muscles reduces the postural sway during quiet standing. In a study involving the upper limbs, Ranganathan et al. (2001) found that skilled finger movement practice improves both the steadiness of the hand muscle and Purdue pegboard test scores. Kornatz et al. (2005) also found that steadiness practice in hand muscles improves the steadiness of the hand muscles and Purdue pegboard test scores. The results of these previous studies led us to hypothesise that steadiness practice in the plantar flexor muscles decreases the force fluctuations of the plantar flexor muscles and improves postural stability. The results of the present study demonstrate that steadiness practice in the plantar flexor muscles reduces postural sway during quiet standing. Therefore, this suggests that the neural strategies employed by the plantar flexor muscles during quiet standing and those controlling plantar flexion forces in young adults are similar.

Figure 14 shows the relationship between pre-practice postural sway and changes in steadiness. Linear regression analysis revealed a significant relationship between pre-practice postural sway and the change in postural sway due to steadiness practice. This result indicates that subjects exhibiting relatively large pre-practice postural sway also exhibit greater reductions in postural sway following force steadiness practice in the plantar flexor muscles. Thus, the effects of practice on postural stability are dependent on pre-practice postural stability. This finding is also consistent with the findings of other reports demonstrating that improvements in steadiness are more frequent in subjects with low initial steadiness levels (Manini et al., 2005; Tracy et al., 2004); this strengthens the notion that the effectiveness of training is dependent on the initial level of steadiness.

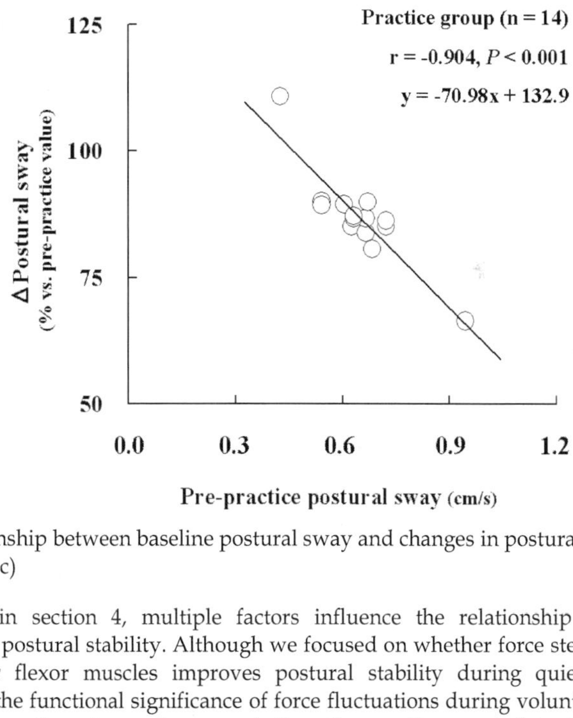

Fig. 14. Relationship between baseline postural sway and changes in postural sway (Oshita and Yano, 2011c)

As indicated in section 4, multiple factors influence the relationship between force steadiness and postural stability. Although we focused on whether force steadiness practice in the plantar flexor muscles improves postural stability during quiet standing, we demonstrated the functional significance of force fluctuations during voluntary contraction. From the perspective of exercise prescription, the results reported in this section also suggest that even low-frequency, (once a week) low-intensity (within 20% MVC) steadiness practice is an effective method for improving human movement.

6. Conclusion

This chapter discussed the relationship between force steadiness in lower limb muscles and postural stability during quiet standing. Although previous studies suggest that the asymmetry of leg muscle functions might affect the human movements (Skelton et al., 2002; Oshita et al., 2009), no significant differences in force steadiness during isometric knee extension or plantar flexion were observed between the 2 legs as shown in section 3. In section 4, a significant correlation between postural stability during quiet standing and force fluctuation during plantar flexion was found only at the corresponding contraction intensities of the plantar flexor muscles in young adults. Furthermore, in section 5, we found that steadiness practice in plantar flexor muscles improves postural stability during quiet standing and that the effects of practice are dependent on pre-practice postural stability. These results will provide useful information to design a training program for postural stability. Usually, the goal of many training programs is improvement of postural stability by an increase in muscle strength (Anderson and Behm, 2005; Holviala et al., 2006). Certainly, strength of the main working muscles to support self body weight is thought to be the most important factor for postural stability. However, MVC in the plantar flexor did not relate with posture sway in our report (Oshita and Yano, 2010c). Further, Kouzaki et al. (2007) reported that postural sway during bipedal quiet standing increases following bed rest despite maintenance of the muscle volume of the main working muscle for human postural standing by strength training. These results indicate that not only muscle strength but also force steadiness is an important factor for postural stability. From the perspective of exercise prescription, the results described in section 5 also suggest that even low-frequency (once a week), low-intensity (within 20% MVC) steadiness practice is an effective method for improving human movement. Therefore, this chapter demonstrates the functional significance of force fluctuations in lower limb muscles.

7. Future direction

So far we have focused on clarifying the relations between postural stability and force steadiness in healthy young men. Regarding the force steadiness, the following investigations are also required:

- To clarify the relationship between force steadiness and various human movements (i.e., walking, to go up (down) stairs, dynamic postural stability, and so on)
- To measure the force steadiness in multiple generations and, possibly, in individuals with neurological disorders.

In particular, unsteady movement or large variability in force output in elderly adults (Galganski, et al., 1993) might lead to difficulties in the performance of daily activities (Kornatz, et al., 2005). By examining the relations between force steadiness and human movement in multiple generations, the findings would more clarify the functional significance of force steadiness and might lead to an understanding of the physiological mechanisms of deteriorations in movement in elderly adult or individuals with neurological disorders.

8. Acknowledgment

These works were supported by following grants

KAKENHI (Grant-in-Aid-for JSPS Fellows (21-2787))
KAKENHI (Grant-in-Aid for Scientific Research "B" (20300235))

9. References

Abrahamova, D. & Hlavacka, F. (2008). Age-related changes of human balance during quiet stance. *Physiological Research*. Vol.57, No.6, 957-964

Adam, A.; De Luca, C.J. & Erim, Z. (1998). Hand dominance and motor unit firing behavior. *Journal of Neurophysiology*. Vol.80, No.3, 1373-1382

American college of sports medicine (1998). American College of Sports Medicine Position Stand. The recommended quantity and quality of exercise for developing and maintaining cardiorespiratory and muscular fitness, and flexibility in healthy adults. *Medicine & Science in Sports & Exercise*. Vol.30, No.6, 975-991

Anderson, K. & Behm, D.G. (2005). The impact of instability resistance training on balance and stability. *Sports medicine*. Vol.35, No.1, 43-53

Benjuya, N.; Melzer, I. & Kaplanski, J. (2004). Aging-induced shifts from a reliance on sensory input to muscle cocontraction during balanced standing. *The Journals of Gerontology. Series A, Biological Sciences and Medical Sciences*. Vol.59, No.2, 166-171

Burnett, R.A.; Laidlaw, D.H. & Enoka, R.M. (2000). Coactivation of the antagonist muscle does not covary with steadiness in old adults. *Journal of Applied Physiology*. Vol.89 No.1, 61-71

Carville, SF.; Perry, M.C.; Rutherford, O.M.: Smith, I.C. & Newham, D. J. (2007). Steadiness of quadriceps contractions in young and older adults with and without a history of falling. *European Journal of Applied Physiology*. Vol.100, No.5, 527-533

Davidson, A. & Buford, J. (2006). Bilateral actions of the reticulospinal tract on arm and shoulder muscles in the monkey: stimulus triggered averaging. *Experimental Brain Research*. Vol.173, No.1, 25–39

Fitzpatrick, R.; Burke, D.; Gandevia, S.C. (1996). Loop gain of reflexes controlling human standing measured with the use of postural and vestibular disturbances. *Journal of Neurophysiology*. Vol.76, No.6, 3994-4008

Galganski, M.E.; Fuglevand, A.J. & Enoka, R.M. (1993). Reduced control of motor output in a human hand muscle of elderly subjects during submaximal contractions. Journal of neurophysiology. Vol.69, No.6, 2108–2115.Gatev, P.; Thomas, S.; Kepple, T. and Hallett, M. (1999). Feedforward ankle strategy of balance during quiet stance in adults. *Journal of Physiology*. Vol.514, No.3, 915-928

Hamilton, A.F.; Jones, K.E. & Wolpert, D.M. (2004). The scaling of motor noise with muscle strength and motor unit number in humans. *Experimental Brain Research*. Vol.157, No.4, 417–430

Hayashi, N. & Miyamoto, T. (2009). Effect of resistance training at a frequency of once a week on muscular strength in college students. *Japan Journal of Physical Education, Health and Sport Sciences*. Vol.54, No.1, 137-143 [in Japanese with English abstract]

Holviala, J.H.; Sallinen, J.M.; Kraemer, W.J.; Alen, M.J. & Häkkinen, K.K. (2006). Effects of strength training on muscle strength characteristics, functional capabilities, and balance in middle-aged and older women. *The Journal of Strength & Conditioning Research*. Vol.20, No.2, 336-344

Keen, D.A.; Yue, G.H. & Enoka, R.M. (1994). Training-related enhancement in the control of motor unit output in elderly humans. *Journal of Applied Physiology*. Vol.77, No.6, 2648-2658

Kornatz, K.W.; Christou, E.A. & Enoka, R.M. (2005). Practice reducesmotor unit discharge variability in a hand muscle and improves manual dexterity in old adults. *Journal of Applied Physiology*. Vol.98, No.6, 2072-2080

Kouzaki, M.; Masani, K.; Akima, H.; Shirasawa, H.; Fukuoka, H.; Kanehisa, H. & Fukunaga, T. (2007). Effects of 20-day bed rest with and without strength training on postural sway during quiet stance. *Acta physiologica*. Vol.189, No.3, 279-292

Kurata, K. & Tanji, J. (1986). Premotor cortex neurons in macaques: activity before distal and proximal forelimb movements. *The Journal of Neuroscience*. Vol.6, No.2, 403–411, 1986.

Lemon, R.N. & Griffiths, J. (2005). Comparing the function of the corticospinal system in different species: organizational differences for motor specialization? *Muscle and Nerve*. Vol.32, No.3, 261–279

Manini, T.M.; Clark, B.C.; Tracy, B.L.; Burke, J. & Ploutz-Snyder, L. (2005). Resistance and functional training reduces knee extensor position fluctuations in functionally limited older adults. *European Journal of Applied Physiology*. Vol.95, No.5-6, 436-446

Marmon, A.R.; Gould, J.R. & Enoka, R.M. (2011). Practicing a functional task improves steadiness with hand muscles in older adults. *Medicine & Science in Sports & Exercise*. Vol.43, No8, 1531-1537

Masani, K.; Popovic, M.R.; Nakazawa, K.; Kouzaki, M. & Nozaki, D. (2003). Importance of body sway velocity information in controlling ankle extensor activities during quiet stance. *Journal of Neurophysiology*, Vol.90, NO.6, 3774-3782

Masani, K.; Vette, A.H.; Kouzaki, M.; Kanehisa, H.; Fukunaga, T. & Popovic, M.R. (2007) Larger center of pressure minus center of gravity in the elderly induces larger body acceleration during quiet standing. *Neuroscience letters*. Vol.422, No.3, 202-206

Ministry of health, labour and welfare of Japan (2011). *The reports of national health and nutrition survey 2008*. Ministry of health, labour and welfare of Japan, Tokyo, 6 [in Japanese]

Morasso, P.G. & Schieppati, M. (1999). Can muscle stiffness alone stabilize upright standing? *Journal of Neurophysiology*. Vol.82, No.3, 1622-1626

Mottram, C.J.; Christou, E.A.; Meyer, F.G. & Enoka, R.M. (2005). Frequency modulation of motor unit discharge has task-dependent effects on fluctuations in motor output. *Journal of Neurophysiology*. Vol.94, No.4, 2878-2887

Nisky, I.; Baraduc, P. & Karniel, A. (2010). Proximodistal gradient in the perception of delayed stiffness. *Journal of Neurophysiology*. Vol.103, No.6, 3017-3026

Ohmori, H.; Kume, T.; Sasaki, K.; Ohyama, B.K.; Takahashi, H. & Kubota, T. (2010). Low-frequency isometric training, 1-day of training every 2 weeks, increases muscle strength in untrained subjects. *Advances in Exercise and Sports Physiology*. Vol.16, No.1, 1-5

Onishi, H.; Ehara, Y. & Soma, T. (2005). EMG analysis of the leg muscles during sit-to-stand. *Journal of Physical Therapy*. Vol.22, No.3, 546-552 [in Japanese]

Oshita, K.; Kashimoto, S.; Ito, H.; Yano, S.; Takahashi, K.; Kawakami, M.; Ebisu, T.; Oshida, Y. & Yanagimoto, Y. (2008). Effects of the low frequency self weight bearing training on the elderly residing in or visiting geriatric health care facilities or special nursing homes. *Journal of Training Science for Exercise and Sport*. Vol.20, No.2, 137-143 [in Japanese with English abstract]

Oshita, K.; Yano, S.; Kashimoto, S.; Takahashi, K. & Kawakami, M. (2009). The relationship between the walking speed and the asymmetry of leg strength in 1205 female aged 30-89 years. *Journal of Physiological Sciences,* Vol.59, Suppl.1, 355

Oshita, K. & Yano, S. (2010a). Asymmetry of force fluctuation in knee extension. *Intarnational Journal of Sports Medicine.* Vol.31, No.5, 342-346

Oshita, K. & Yano, S. (2010b). Asymmetry of force fluctuation during low-intensity isometric plantar flexion. *Transactions of Japanese Society for Medical and Biological Engineering.* Vol.48, No.4, 377-382

Oshita, K. & Yano, S. (2010c). Relationship between force fluctuation in the plantar flexor and sustainable time for single-leg standing. *Journal of Physiological Anthropology.* Vol.29, No.3, 89-93

Oshita, K. & Yano, S. (2011a). Asymmetry of force fluctuation during low and moderate intensity isometric knee extensions. *Perceptual & Motor Skills.* Vol.112, No.3, 860-870

Oshita, K. & Yano, S. (2011b). Transitory effects of one week interval on force fluctuation during isometric knee extension. *The Journal of Clinical Sports Medicine.* Vol.28, No.1, 79-84 [in Japanese]

Oshita, K. & Yano, S. (2011c). Low-frequency force steadiness practice in plantar flexor muscle reduces postural sway during quiet standing. *Journal of Physiological Anthropology.* Vol.30, No.6, 233-239

Oshita, K. & Yano, S. (in submitting). Association of force steadiness of plantar flexor muscles and postural sway during quiet standing by young adults.

Patten, C. & Kamen, G. (2000). Adaptations in motor unit discharge activity with force control training in young and older human adults. *European Journal of Applied Physiology.* Vol.83, No.2-3, 128-143

Prieto, T.E.; Myklebust, J.B.; Hoffmann, R.G.; Lovett, E.G. & Myklebust, B.M. (1996) Measures of postural steadiness: differences between healthy young and elderly adults. *IEEE Transactions on Biomedical Engineering.* Vol.43, No.9, 956-966

Ranganathan, V.K.; Siemionow, V.; Sahgal, V.; Liu, J.Z. & Yue, G.H. (2001). Skilled finger movement exercise improves hand function. *The Journals of Gerontology. Series A, Biological Sciences and Medical Sciences.* Vol.56, No.8, M518-M522

Salonikidis, K.; Amiridis, I.G.; Oxyzoglou, N.; de Villareal, E.S.; Zafeiridis, A. & Kellis, E. (2009). Force variability during isometric wrist flexion in highly skilled and sedentary individuals. *European Journal of Applied Physiology,* Vol.107, No.6, 715-722

Sato, D.; Kaneda, K.; Wakabayashi, H. & Nomura, T. (2007). Some effect of water exercise frequency on functional mobility in nursing care elderly. *Japanese Journal of Physical Fitness and Sports Medicine.* Vol.56, No.1, 141-148 [in Japanese with English abstract]

Sawai, S.; Sanematsu, H.; Kanehisa, H.; Tsunoda, N. & Fukunaga, T. (2004). Evaluation of muscle activity level in daily actions. *Japanese Journal of Physical Fitness and Sports Medicine,* Vol.53 No.1, 93-106 [in Japanese with English abstract]

Semmler, J.G. & Nordstrom, M.A. (1995). Influence of handedness on motor unit discharge properties and force tremor. *Experimental Brain Research.* Vol.104, No.1, 115-125

Skelton, D.A.; Kennedy, J. & Rutherford, O.M. (2002). Explosive power and asymmetry in leg muscle function in frequent fallers and non-fallers aged over 65. *Age and Ageing,* Vol.31, No.2, 119-125

Tokuno, C.D.; Carpenter, M.G.; Thorstensson, A.; Garland, S.J. & Cresswell, A.G. (2007). Control of the triceps surae during the postural sway of quiet standing. *Acta Physiologica*. Vol.191, No.3, 229-236

Tokuno, C.D.; Garland, S.J.; Carpenter, M.G.; Thorstensson, A. & Cresswell, A.G. (2008). Sway-dependent modulation of the triceps surae H-reflex during standing. *Journal of Applied Physiology*. Vol.104, No.5, 1359-1365

Tracy, B.L. & Enoka, R.M. (2002). Older adults are less steady during submaximal isometric contractions with the knee extensor muscles. *Journal of Applied Physiology*. Vol.92, No.3, 1004-1012

Tracy, B.L.; Byrnes, W.C. & Enoka, R.M. (2004). Strength training reduces force fluctuations during anisometric contractions of the quadriceps femoris muscles in old adults. *Joural of Applied Physiology*. Vol.96, No.4, 1530-1540

Tracy, B.L.; Maluf, K.S.; Stephenson, J.L.; Hunter, S.K. & Enoka, R.M. (2005). Variability of motor unit discharge and force fluctuations across a range of muscle forces in older adults. *Muscle & Nerve*. Vol.32, No.4, 533-540

Vallbo, A.B. & Wessberg, J. (1993). Organization of motor output in slow finger movements in man. *Journal of Physiology*. Vol.469, 673-691

Yoshitake, Y.; Shinohara, M.; Kouzaki, M. & Fukunaga, T. (2004). Fluctuations in plantar flexion force are reduced after prolonged tendon vibration. *Journal of Applied Physiology*. Vol.97, No.6, 2090-2097

12

The Influence of Different Elbow Angles on the Twitch Response of the Biceps Brachii Muscle Between Intermittent Electrical Stimulations

Srdjan Djordjevič[1,3], Sašo Tomažič[2],
Gregor Zupančič[1], Rado Pišot[3] and Raja Dahmane[4]
[1]*Department of Biology, Biotechnical Faculty, University of Ljubljana, Ljubljana,*
[2]*Department of Telecommunications, Faculty of Electrical Engineering, University of Ljubljana, Ljubljana,*
[3]*Institute for Kinesiology Research, Science and Research Center of Koper, University of Primorska, Koper,*
[4]*Medical Faculty, Institute of Anatomy, University of Ljubljana, Ljubljana, Slovenia*

1. Introduction

Prolonged or repeated contractions of skeletal muscles lead to impaired muscle action or to a decrease in force-generating ability. This phenomenon is due to fatigue. Fatigue may be caused by factors/processes within the muscle cells (peripheral fatigue) or by diminished activation from the central nervous system (central fatigue). When observing a muscle twitch, decreases in contraction amplitude, decreases in contraction speed, and prolonged relaxation phases are the main indicators of fatigue.

There are several mechanisms involved in muscle fatigue. The variation of responsible mechanisms has been termed the task dependency of muscle fatigue (Enoka, 2002; Mottram, 2005a; 2005b; Baudry, 2010).

The use of different protocols of electrical stimulation can characterize the variety of the task dependency of muscle fatigue. Two examples of the task dependency of fatigue are the phenomena known as low-frequency fatigue (LFF), first described by Edwards et al. (1977), and high-frequency fatigue (HFF), described by Bigland-Ritchie et al. (1979), Jones (1979) and Jones, et al. (1986).

Another possible variable in muscle response could be initial muscle tension/length. Muscle tension can influence the muscle activation pattern and the amplitude of muscle contraction. Two other phenomena also show relation between length of muscle and muscle contraction properties during electrical stimulation "the catchlike property" (Lee et al., 1999; Binder-Macleod and Ketlar, 2005) and "twitch potentiation" (Raissier, 2000; Place, 2005).

The level of fatigue depends on muscle length, in which the contractile response is measured. Using the human tibialis anterior muscle, Sacco et al. (1994) observed that, when the muscle was fatigued at short muscle lengths, the decline in force was more pronounced than when the muscle was fatigued at optimal length. Although this result was confirmed by Gauthier (1993), other researchers (Fitch et al. 1985; McKenzie et al. 1987; Lee et al., 2007) have observed reduced fatigue in short muscle lengths.

In our preliminary study (unpublished data), we observed the influence of different elbow angles on muscle twitch parameters, measured with the tensiomyography (TMG) method on the biceps brachii (BB) muscle during short-acting electrical stimulation (ES). We observed a shorter contraction time in pre-stretched muscles (long muscles, elbow angle 5°) compared to relaxed muscles (short muscles, elbow angle 60°). The question that arose was whether this observation was an isolated phenomenon or whether similar changes would also occur in different circumstances.

Therefore, the present study explored the twitch-to-twitch effect of an intermittent stimulation protocol at variable muscle lengths (different elbow angles) on the muscle twitch response of the human BB muscle.

Our working hypothesis was that the changes in muscle response to intermittent electrical stimulation would be dissimilar at different elbow angles.

2. Materials and methods

2.1 Subjects

Nine healthy, sedentary subjects (6 men, 4 left-handed) ranging from 25 to 45 years old (mean of 32.7 ± 8), with no history of muscle or joint problems, participated in this study. All subjects were informed of the purpose and procedures of the study and gave written, informed consent for their participation.

The local ethics committee approved the tensiomyographical measurements.

2.2 Measurements

The contractile properties of the BB muscles on the left and right side were measured with the TMG method, which is classified as a mechanomyographical (MMG) method based on the 1995 convention (CIBA Foundation Symposium, 1995). TMG is based on a displacement sensor detecting muscle belly enlargement in the radial direction. TMG was invented in 1997 (Valencic et al. 1997) and has since become more established (Dahmane et al. 2001; 2005; 2006; Zagar and Krizaj, 2005; Tous-Fajardo, 2010; García-Manso, 2011).

For the measurements, an inductive sensor, incorporating a spring with a coefficient of 0.17 N/mm, was used. It provided an initial pressure of approximately 1.5×10^{-2} N/mm^2 on the tip area of 1.13 mm^2. The responses of the BB muscles on the right and left sides were compared.

The measured subject sat in a measuring chair. The measured arm was fastened to the frame with two bands to achieve isometric conditions during the measurement. In all of our experiments, isometric conditions were applied within physiological limits. Our referential definition for isometric contraction was "the total length of the muscle tendon complex remains constant." The sensor location for each muscle was determined anatomically, according to Delagi et al. (1975). Maximal muscle amplitude/response was used as an additional criterion for the optimal sensor position. For the BB, the sensor location was at the midpoint of the line between the lateral head of the clavicle and the head of the radius.

Muscle contraction was elicited by single-twitch electrical stimuli. Two self-adhesive electrodes were placed symmetrically around the TMG sensor. The anode was placed distally and the cathode proximally, 20-50 mm from the measuring point. Bipolar ES consisted of a single DC pulse of 1 ms in duration. A typical TMG record with parameters and definitions is shown in Figure 1. The measured parameters are shown in Figure 2. These parameters were the maximal amplitude of the signal (Dm), the delay time from the stimulation to 10% of the maximal contraction (t_d), the time of contraction from 10% to 90% of the maximal contraction (t_c), the time of sustained contraction from 50% contraction to 50% of the relaxation (t_s) and the relaxation time from 10% relaxation to 50% relaxation (t_r).

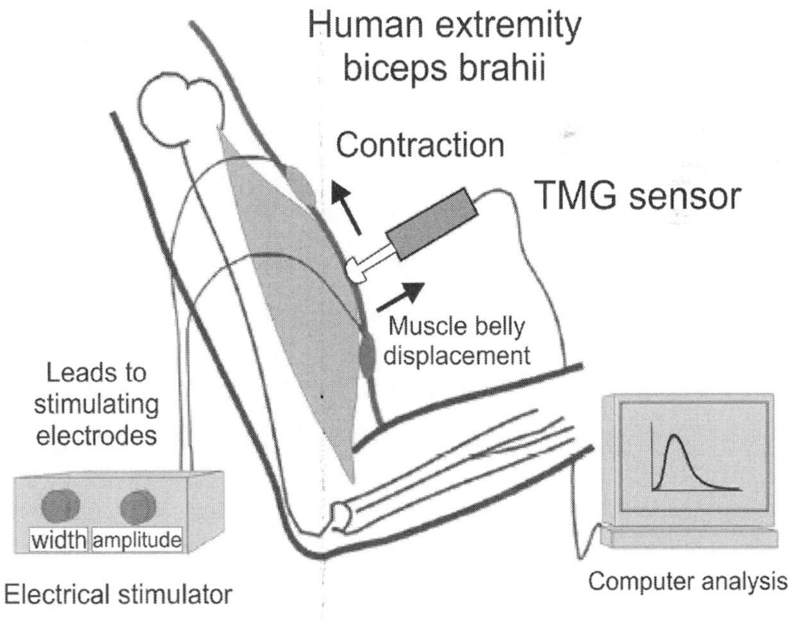

Fig. 1. Experimental setup used to evoke and measure the biceps brachii (BB) isometric twitch contraction responses. The TMG sensor measures muscle radial displacement during twitch contractions induced by short electrical stimuli. The stimulating electrodes are placed directly onto the skin.

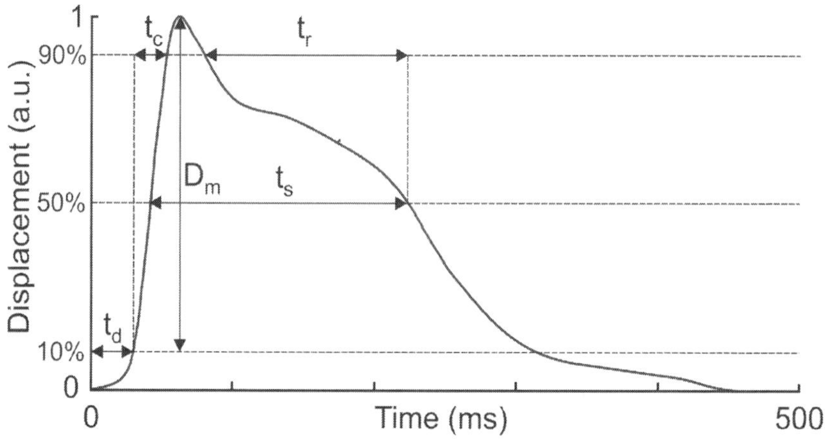

Fig. 2. (a) The parameters that were measured with the TMG signal: Dm - maximum amplitude (displacement), t_d - initial delay time, t_c - contraction time, t_s - sustained contraction time and t_r - half relaxation time.

2.3 Measurement protocols

Throughout the stimulation protocol, muscle activity was monitored with the TMG sensor. The stimulus intensity was set at 66% of a supramaximal twitch that was determined for a single 1-ms electrical impulse, before proceeding with the ES protocol for each muscle.

The electrical intermittent stimulation protocol (ISP) (Figure 3) consisted of 30 100-ms stimulation bouts (100 Hz, 0.1-ms impulse width) with 400-ms pauses between bouts, followed by a 1000-ms pause and an in-between twitch bout (IBT; also 100 Hz, 0.1-ms impulse width; Figures 3 and 4b), followed by a 900-ms pause. The protocol was repeated six times so that the whole stimulation lasted 90 s, which amounted to a total of 180 100-ms stimulation bouts. The entire protocol was flanked by two basic twitch stimuli (TS, single 1-ms impulse), one 3 s before and the other 3 s after end of the protocol.

The data were later read into Matlab (MathWorks, Natick, Massachusetts, USA) and analyzed with that software.

Measurements were performed on the biceps brachii muscles of both arms. On the left arm, the elbow angle was fixed at 5° (intermittent protocol of electrical stimulation at 5° [ISP5]), while the right arm was fixed at 60° (intermittent protocol of electrical stimulation at 60° [ISP60]). The reason for using the BB muscles of both arms was that the recovery from and/or the influence of a certain type of electrical stimulation can be quite prolonged. In severe cases, it may take as long as a few days to achieve full recovery (Jones et al. 1996).

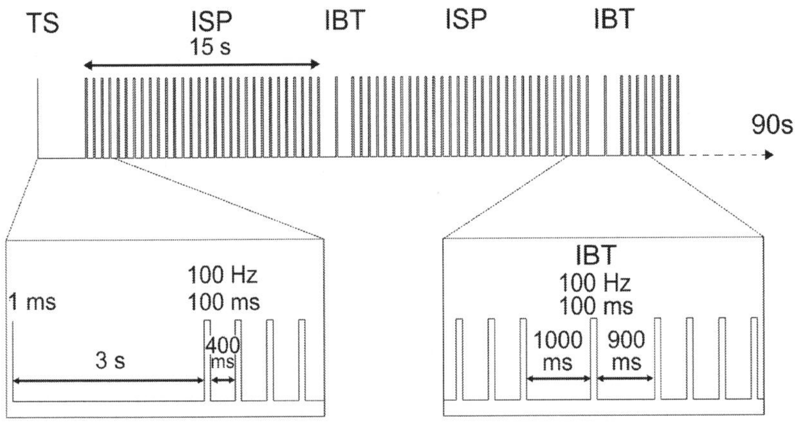

Fig. 3. Fatigue-inducing stimulation protocol: ISP = intermittent electrical stimulation protocol; IBT = in between twitch; TS = basic twitch stimulus.
The ISP was repeated six times so that the whole stimulation lasted 90 s, which amounted to a total of 180 100-ms stimulation bouts. IBT was repeated five times. The entire protocol was flanked by two basic twitch stimuli (a single 1-ms impulse), one 3 s before and the other 3 s after the end of the protocol.

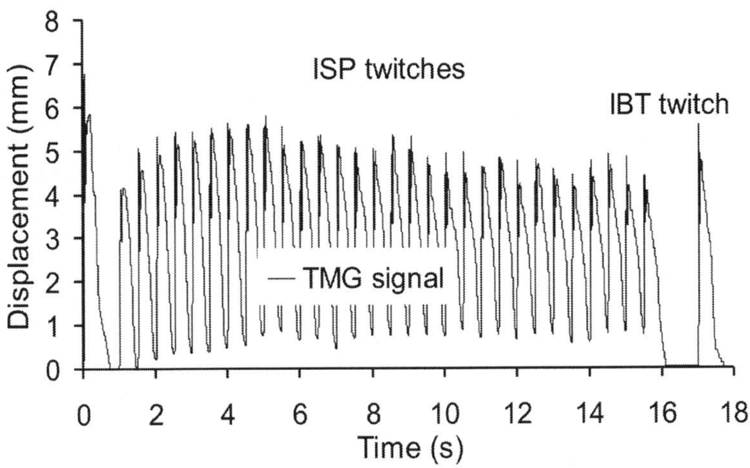

Fig. 4. (a) Muscle twitches between the first 18 s of ISP60, assessed on human BB.

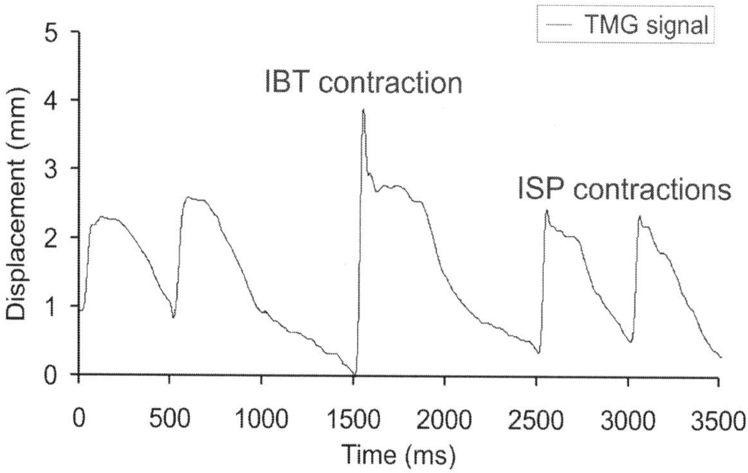

Fig. 4. (b) A detail with two types of twitches: IBT and ISP twitches.

2.4 Statistical Analysis

Paired-samples t-tests were used to compare differences in the changes in contraction parameters t_d, t_c, t_s, t_r, and Dm as well as the differences between the two protocols (ISP5 and ISP60). Paired t-tests have greater power than unpaired tests when the paired units are similar with respect to "noise factors" that are independent of membership. Paired t-test was used to reduce the effects of confounding factors in our study. Significance for all tests was set at $P < 0.05$.

3. Results

A typical muscle response to ISP measured with the TMG sensor is shown in Figure 4a (first 18 s of 90-s intermittent stimulation with an extended or flexed elbow). An evident decrease in the contraction amplitude was observed during both ISPs at 15 to 20 s (Figure 5). There was a statistically significant change in responses during both protocols.

With the ISP5 protocol, we observed a significantly faster decrease in effective contraction amplitudes and, at the same time, a greater difference in amplitude decreases at the end of stimulation, compared to the ISP60 protocol (Figure 5). After 60 s of the ISP60 protocol, the ISP twitch amplitude was statistically unchanged.

The results of basic twitch response measurements before and after the ISP in long and short muscles are shown in Table 1.

The differences between time parameters (t_c, t_d, t_s, and t_r in long [5°] and short [60°] muscles) before the ISP were statistically significant, as shown in Figure 6c and Table 1. The difference between Dm in long (5°) and short (60°) muscles before the ISP was also statistically significant. For example, t_c was statistically shorter (t_c ISP60=26.3±1.1 and t_c ISP5=24.4±2.7, $p<0.05$) and Dm was smaller in long muscles (Dm ISP60=15.1±4.1, Dm ISP5=8.4±2.1, $p<0.001$)

In the basic twitch responses before and after the ISP60 protocol (Figure 6a and Table 1), there were no significant differences in t_c, t_d, t_s, t_r or Dm.

In the ISP5 (Figure 6b) protocol, there were significant changes in t_d, t_s, and t_r and no significant differences in t_c or Dm.

The IBTs had different dynamics of changes compared to those observed in twitches similar to contractions (ISP twitches), during both the ISP5 and ISP60 protocols.

From all the observed parameters in the IBTs during the ISP5 protocol, we found statistically significant differences in Dm only ($p<0.05$). The same pattern of response/changes was found with the ISP60 protocol in Dm only ($p<0.05$).

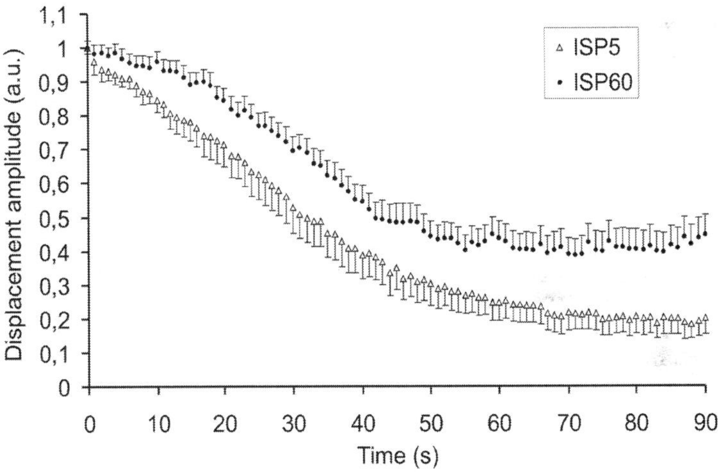

Fig. 5. The time course of the decline of maximal displacement amplitudes, normalized to the initial amplitude, during the 90 s of the stimulation protocol. ISP5 - open triangles ± SE; ISP60 - black circles ± SE. There was a statistically significant difference ($p<0.001$) between the two elbow angles (indicated on the figure).

	t_c(ms) ± SD	t_s(ms) ± SD	t_r(ms) ± SD	t_d(ms) ± SD	Dm(mm) ± SD
ISP60 before	26.34 ± 1.18	153.02 ± 33.47	104.33 ± 36.00	23.75 ± 1.81	15.14 ± 4.22
ISP5 before	24.44 ± 2.67 *	205.71 ± 48.74 ***	169.64 ± 47.88 *	22.31 ± 2.25 *	8.50 ± 2.06 ***
ISP60 before	26.34 ± 1.18	153.02 ± 33.47	104.33 ± 36.00	23.75 ± 1.81	15.14 ± 4.22
ISP60 after	27.01 ± 2.51	136.54 ± 27.73	104.21 ± 27.55	25.47 ± 2.12	13.63 ± 3.06
ISP5 before	24.44 ± 2.67	205.71 ± 48.74	169.64 ± 47.88	22.31 ± 2.25	8.50 ± 2.06
ISP5 after	26.80 ± 5.96	173.48 ± 27.04 §	112.31 ± 26.07 §§	23.84 ± 1.44 §	7.69 ± 1.70

Contraction parameters from ISP60 are significantly different from ISP5 contraction paremeters, * P < 0.05 and *** P<0.001
Contraction parameters from ISP5 before are significantly different from ISP5 after contraction parameters, § P< 0.05 and §§ P<0.01

Table 1. Results of basic twitch response measurements before and after the ISP in long and short muscles.

The dynamics (direction and size of changes) of IBT response during the ISP were not significantly different when comparing the ISP60 and ISP5 protocols.

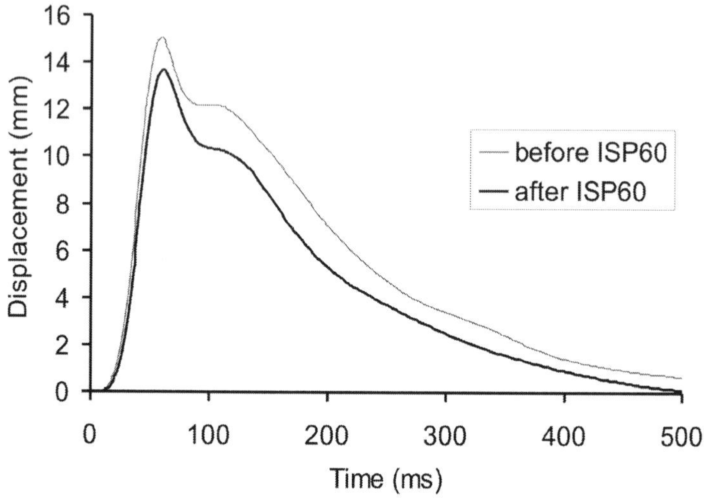

Fig. 6. (a) Twitch responses of the BB before and after ISP60. No statistically significant changes for any of the measured parameters were observed.

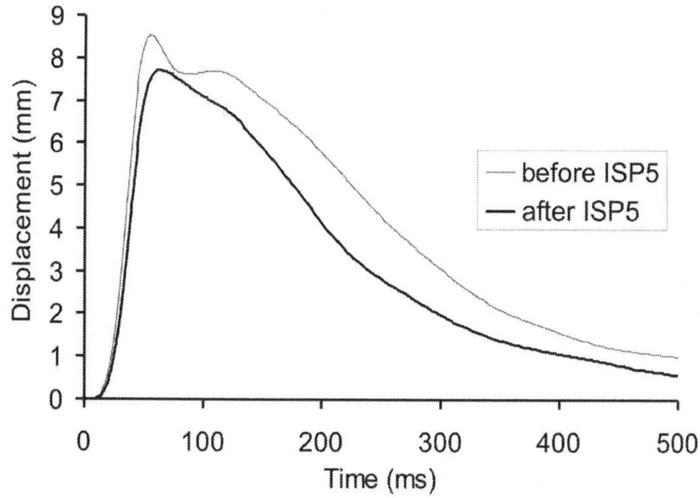

Fig. 6. (b) Twitch responses of the BB before and after ISP5. Statistically significant differences were observed for t_r and Dm ($p<0.05$).

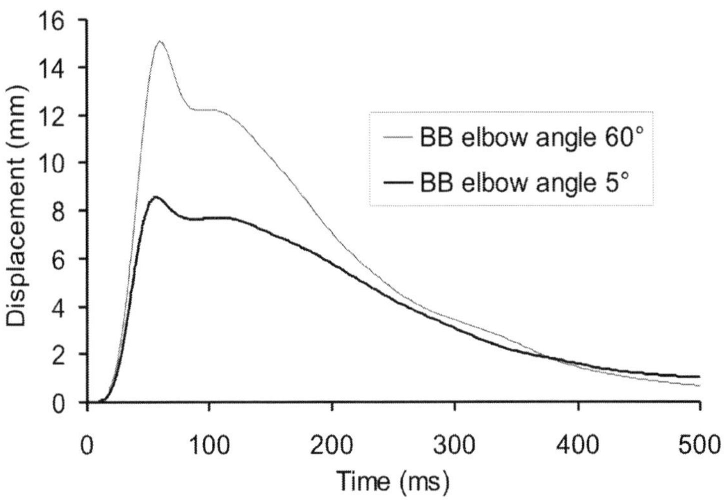

Fig. 6. (c) Twitch responses of the BB in the long muscle (elbow angle 5°) and short muscle (elbow angle 60°). The differences between t_c and Dm in the long (5°) and short (60°) muscles were statistically significant (t_c [60°] = 26.3±1.1, t_c [5°] = 24.4±2.7, $p<0.05$)

4. Discussion

TMG has been used in previous studies in which linear correlations were found between t_c and the percentage of type I muscle fibers (Dahmane et al. 2001) and between relative axial force and muscle belly radial displacement (Djordjevic et al. 2005).

The initial muscle length (length at the beginning of a contraction) is an extremely important modulator of muscle action. It has been established previously that several skeletal muscle physiological parameters depend on initial muscle length. Examples include the production of force/tension (Rassier et al. 1999), changes in motor unit activity (Ballantyne et al. 1993; Van Zuylen et al. 1988; Kennedy 2001), Ca^{2+} sensitivity (Stephenson, 1984) and the development of fatigue (Sacco et al., 1994; Fitch et al., 1987; Gauthier et al., 2000; McKenzie et al. 1987; Rassier, 2000, Lee et al., 2007).

All the cited authors studying the development of fatigue (except Fitch et al. 1987; McKenzie et al. 1987) showed that shortened muscles fatigue more quickly than extended muscles. At first glance, our data were not consistent with most of these studies; however, these studies are difficult to compare, as different measuring approaches were used as well as different muscle groups and stimulation protocols. These differences may explain the inconsistency of the obtained results.

In all previously mentioned studies, tetanic-type electrical stimulation was applied to induce fatigue. For example, in the study by Sacco et al. (1994), a fatigue protocol consisting of 6 15-s tetanic stimulations at 30 Hz (on the tibialis anterior) was applied. Rassier (2000) used a muscle fatigue protocol of nine tetanic contractions (50 Hz, 5 s in duration), with 5-s intervals between contractions, on the quadricep muscle. Gauthier et al. (1993) used tetanic stimulation (train duration = 500 ms, duty cycle = 0.25) decreasing from 100 to 50 Hz with a 250-s duration on the rat diaphragm. In Fitch and McComas's (1993) study, the fatiguing procedure consisted of either indirect tetanic stimulation at 20 Hz or maximal voluntary contractions; each procedure lasted 90 s. Here, the observed muscle was the human ankle dorsal flexor muscle.

An important factor that may be responsible for the effects of stimulation is the recruitment order because this factor would affect the dynamics of fatigue. In our study, we used an intermittent type of transcutaneous electrical stimulation. Bursts of 100 Hz for 100 ms were given twice per second with two types of rest intervals (400 ms in between each pulse train and 1000 ms every 30 stimuli; Figure 3b), which was different from any of the previously published protocols. Our idea was to simulate the moderate cyclic activity of the muscles during fast walking, jogging or cycling. In this type of muscle activity, it is important that there is no overlapping of the contraction and the relaxation phases during fatigue development. Using the intermittent type ES, we wanted to avoid the effects of HFF, which can produce very dramatic losses of force/amplitude of contraction, and it is questionable whether HFF is a "normal" (physiological) fatigue mechanism (Jones 1996).

We believe that twitch intermittent-type ES has similar recruitment patterns to those found during voluntary action. A few studies have supported our contention that the recruitment order due to transcutaneous ES-induced contractions is non-selective (normal recruitment order versus reverse recruitment order) (Adams et al. 1993; Bickel et al. 2003; Binder-Macleod et al. 1995; Dahmane et al. 2005; Feiereisen et al. 1997; Knaflitz et al.1990; Slade et al. 2003).

Nevertheless, with the ISP5 protocol, we observed an almost immediate drop in the twitch amplitude (Figure 3c), while with the ISP60 protocol, a decrease occurred after 10-20 s. This last observation could be attributed to a usual HFF response (Jones 1996). In the time frame of 10-20 s, the difference between the two protocols was most evident. After 60 s with the ISP60 protocol, the twitch amplitude was unchanged, while the twitch amplitude with the ISP5 protocol continued to decrease (Figures 5 and 7).

A statistically significant difference was observed between the two protocols regarding the twitch response of the biceps brachii, while the differences in basic twitches before and after the ISP were not significant, except for t_d, t_s, and t_r when comparing the ISP5 and ISP60 protocols.

This finding can be explained by the different electrical stimuli and by the delay (1 s) at the end of the stimulation protocols before the 1-ms twitch. The reasoning for incorporating the 1-s delay into the protocol following the ISP, as opposed to the normal 400-ms delay between twitches, was to prevent the possibility of twitch fusion. The stimulation protocol is depicted in Figure 4b.

This study showed that the high data acquisition rate during the ISP resulted in a better assessment of the temporal components of the fatigue process. It also revealed that twitch measurements every 15 s (IBT) did not alone show statistically significant differences between the ISP protocols (it is true that the conditions were slightly different: 1000 ms versus 400 ms rest between 100 ms stimulus durations). The applied procedure and the recording method enabled a higher sampling rate (180 ISP twitches versus 7 IBTs), which resulted in a much more precise (statistically significant) detection of changes occurring during the fatigue process. A summary of important results/differences is shown in Figure 7.

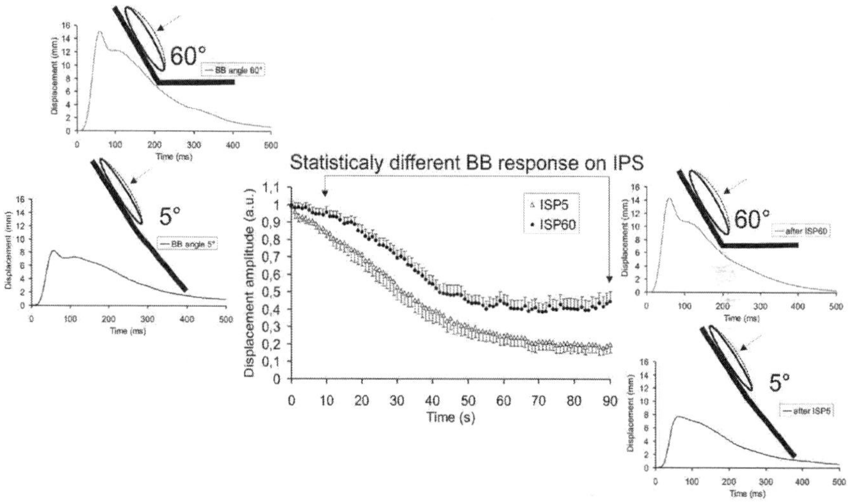

Fig. 7. The IBTs before (a and b) and after the ISP protocol (c and d) were measured at two different lengths of the BB muscle (elbow angle 5 and 60°). Shorter contraction time and faster fatigue (decline of contraction amplitude) were observed in the long muscle (elbow angle 5°). A statistically significant difference in fatigue development during the ISP was observed after 10 s for the two elbow angles (e). During ISP60, after 50 s, the BB displacement achieved a steady state; however, this finding was not observed during ISP5. The influence of muscle length was reflected in muscle contractions and twitch conditions and during fatigue conditions produced by the ISP.

The crucial question that we wanted to answer in this study was whether the shorter contraction times at smaller angles (longer muscle) were related to changed muscle activation patterns (motor unit recruitment order) or whether there were other mechanisms involved. Hence, we expected the fatigue process to be more pronounced if faster twitch fibers were recruteited during contraction. Although this finding would not have been definite proof, it would have indicated that such a hypothesis could not be rejected. The results confirmed our working hypothesis. They showed a higher fatigue rate and a different time course in long muscles using the same ISP protocol. If we accept that the shorter t_c in long muscles means a greater percentage recruitment of fast twitch fibers, then a faster and more pronounced onset of fatigue during the ISP5 protocol seems to be a logical consequence.

5. Conclusion and future directions

Prolonged or repeated contractions of skeletal muscles lead to impaired muscle action or to a decrease in force-generating ability. The present study explores the twitch-to-twitch effect of an intermittent stimulation protocol at variable muscle lengths (different elbow angles) on the muscle twitch response of the human biceps brachii muscle. Results showed a higher fatigue rate and a different time course in long muscles compared to short muscle using the same ISP protocol. For a better understanding of the detected changes and underlying processes, further research, in combination with other methods (EMG ...) and conditions, e.g., normalize(load) cyclic voluntary muscle activation is required.

6. References

[1] Adams, G.R., Harris, R.T., Woodard, D., Dudley, G.A., 1993. Mapping of electrical stimulation using. MRI. J Appl Physiol 74, 532-537.

[2] Ballantyne, B.T., Kukulka, C.G., Soderberg, G.L., 1993. Motor unit recruitment in human medial gastrocnemius muscle during combined knee flexion and plantar flexion isometric contractions. Exp Brain Res 93, 492-498.

[3] Baudry, S., Maerz, A.H., Gould, J-R-, Enoka, R.M., 2011. Task- and time-dependent modulation of Ia presynaptic inhibition during fatiguing contractions performed by humans. J Neurophysiol, 106(1), 265-73.

[4] Bickel, C.S., Slade, J.M., Warren, G.L., Dudley, G.A., 2003. Fatigability and variable-frequency train stimulation of human skeletal muscles. Phys Ther 83, 366-373.

[5] Bigland-Ritchie, B., Jones, D.A., Woods, J.J., 1979. Excitation frequency and muscle fatigue: electrical responses during human voluntary and stimulated contractions. Exp Neurol 64, 414-427.

[6] Binder-Macleod, S.A., Halden, E.E., Jungles, K.A., 1995. Effects of stimulation intensity on the physiological responses of human motor units. Med Sci Sports Exerc 27(4), 556-565.

[7] Binder-Macleod, S.A., Kesar, T., 2005. Catchlike property of skeletal muscle: recent findings and clinical implications. Muscle Nerve 31(6):681-93.

[8] Burger, H., Valencic, V., Marincek, C., Kogovsek, N., 1996. Properties of musculus gluteus maximus in above-knee amputees. Clin Biomech (Bristol, Avon) 11, 35-38.

[9] Dahmane, R., Valenčič, V., Knez, N., Eržen, I., 2001. Evaluation of the ability to make non-invasive estimation of muscle contractile properties on the basis of the muscle belly response. Med Biol Eng Comp 38, 51-56.

[10] Dahmane, R., Djordjevic, S., Simunic, B., Valencic, V., 2005. Spatial fiber type distribution in normal human muscle. Histochemical and tensiomyographical evaluation. J Biomech 38, 2451-2459.

[11] Dahmane R, Djordjevic S, Smerdu V (2006) Adaptive potential of human biceps femoris muscle demonstrated by histochemical, immunohistochemical and mechanomyographical methods. Med Biol Eng Comput 44, 999-1006.

[12] *Delagi, E.F., Perotto, A., Iazzetti, J., Morrison, D., 1975. Anatomic guide for the electromyographer: the limbs. In: Thomas, C.C. (Eds). Springfield, Illinois, pp. 35-43.*

[13] Delitto, A., Brown, M., Strube, M.J., Rose, S.J., Lehman, R.C. 1989. Electrical stimulation of quadriceps femoris in an elite weight lifter: a single subject experiment. Int J Sports Med 10, 187-191.

[14] Djordjevič, S., Simunič. B., 2005. Comparison between parameters of axial force and muscle radial displacement during isometric twitch contraction In Proceedings of the European College of Sport Science, Beograd.

[15] Edwards, R.H., Hill, D.K., Jones, D.A., Merton, P.A., 1977. Fatigue of long duration in human skeletal muscle after exercise. J Physiol 272, 769-778.

[16] Feiereisen, P., Duchateau, J., Hainaut, K., 1997. Motor unit recruitment order during voluntary and electrically induced contractions in the tibialis anterior. Exp Brain Res 114, 117-123.

[17] Fitch, S., McComas, A., 1985. Influence of human muscle length on fatigue. J Physiol 362, 205-213.

[18] García-Manso, J.M., Rodríguez-Ruiz, D., Rodríguez-Matoso, D., De Saa, Y., Sarmiento, S., Quiroga, M., 2011. Assessment of muscle fatigue after an ultra-endurance triathlon using tensiomyography (TMG). J Sports Sci 29(6), 619-25

[19] Gauthier, A.P., Faltus, R.E., Macklem, P.T., Bellemare, F. 1993. Effects of fatigue on the length-tetanic force relationship of the rat diaphragm. J Appl Physiol 74, 326-332.

[20] Jones, D.A., 1979. Change in excitation threshold as a cause of muscular fatigue [proceedings]. J Physiol 295, 90P-91P.

[21] Jones, D.A., 1996. High-and low-frequency fatigue revisited. Acta Physiol Scand 156, 265-270.

[22] Jones, D.A., Bigland-Ritchie, B., Edwards, R.H., 1979. Excitation frequency and muscle fatigue: mechanical responses during voluntary and stimulated contractions. Exp Neurol 64, 401-413.

[23] Kennedy, P.M., Cresswell, A.G., 2001. The effect of muscle length on motor-unit recruitment during isometric plantar flexion in humans. Exp Brain Res 137, 58-64.

[24] Kersevan, K., Valencic, V., Djordjevic, S., Simunic, B. 2002. The muscle adaptation process as a result of pathological changes or specific training procedures. Cell Mol Biol Lett 7, 367-369.

[25] Knaflitz, M., Merletti, R., De Luca, C.J., 1990. Inference of motor unit recruitment order in voluntary and electrically elicited contractions. J Appl Physiol 68, 1657-1667.

[26] Lee, S.C., Gerdom, M.L., Binder-Macleod, S.A., 1999. Effects of length on the catchlike property of human quadriceps femoris muscle. Phys Ther 79(8), 738-48.

[27] Lee, S.C., Braim, A., Becker, C.N., Prosser, L.A., Tokay, A.M., Binder Macleod, S.A., 2007. Diminished fatigue at reduced muscle length in human skeletal muscle. Muscle Nerve 36, 789–797.

[28] McKenzie, D.K., Gandevia, S.C., 1987. Influence of muscle length on human inspiratory and limb muscle endurance. Respir Physiol 67, 171-182.

[29] Mottram, C.J., Christou, E-A., Meyer, F.G., Enoka, R.M., 2005. Frequency modulation of motor unit discharge has task-dependent effects on fluctuations in motor output. J Neurophysiol 94(4), 2878-87.

[30] Mottram, C.J., Jakobi, J.M., Semmler, J.G., Enoka, R.M., 2005. Motor-unit activity differs with load type during a fatiguing contraction. J Neurophysiol, 93(3), 1381-92.

[31] Place, N., Maffiuletti, N.A., Ballay, Y., Lepers, R., 2005. Twitch potentiation is greater after a fatiguing submaximal isometric contraction performed at short vs. long quadriceps muscle length. J Appl Physiol, 98, 429–436.

[32] Rassier, D.E., 2000. The effects of length on fatigue and twitch potentiation in human skeletal muscle. Clin Physiol 20, 474-482.

[33] Rassier, D.E., MacIntosh, B.R., Herzog, W., 1999. Length dependence of active force production in skeletal muscle. J Appl Physiol 86, 1445-1457.

[34] Sacco, P., McIntyre, D.B., Jones, D.A., 1994. Effects of length and stimulation frequency on fatigue of the human tibialis anterior muscle. J Appl Physiol 77, 1148-1154.

[35] Slade, J.M., Bickel, C.S., Warren, G.L., Dudley, G.A., 2003. Variable frequency trains enhance torque independent of stimulation amplitude. Acta Physiol Scand 177, 87-92.

[36] Stephenson, D.G., Wendt, I.R. 1984. Length dependence of changes in sarcoplasmic calcium concentration and myofibrillar calcium sensitivity in striated muscle fibres. J Muscle Res Cell Motil 5, 243-272.

[37] Tous-Fajardo, J., Moras, G., Rodríguez-Jiménez, S., Usach, R., Doutres, D.M., Maffiuletti, N.A., 2010. Inter-rater reliability of muscle contractile property measurements using non-invasive tensiomyography. J Electromyogr Kinesiol 20(4), 761-6.

[38] Valencic, V., Knez, N., 1997. Measuring of skeletal muscles' dynamic properties. Artif Organs 21, 240-242.

[39] Van Zuylen, E.J., Gielen, C.C., Denier van der Gon, J.J., 1988. Coordination and inhomogeneous activation of human arm muscles during isometric torques. J Neurophysiol 60, 1523-1548.

[40] Zagar, T., Krizaj, D. 2005. Validation of an accelerometer for determination of muscle belly radial displacement. Med Biol Eng Comput. 43,78-84.

Experimental Examination on the Effects and Adaptation Condition of the Fibula Excision Method Using the Stress Freezing Method on the Osteoarthritis of the Knee

Nobutaka Maezaki, Tsutomu Ezumi and Masashi Hachiya
Shibaura Institute of Technology, Yokohama Minami Kyousai Hospital
Japan

1. Introduction

The knee joint is a joint where arthropathy occurs frequently. Osteoarthritis of the Knee (: Knee OA) is the most important typical joint disease. In the medical orthopedics field, 900 thousand people regularly go to the hospital annually, of which the frequency of senior citizens is high. Conditions of deformations, such those of the cartilage between the knee joints, wearing out are common. Among Japanese people, pain is common on the inside of the knee. Depending upon the advancement of Knee OA, there are times when walking becomes difficult. The diagnosis of Knee OA generally measures leg alignment. Especially FTA, which measures the angle of the femur and the tibia that form the knee joint, provides a guide for the decisive deformation type and operation invasive quantity through measuring fixed quantities. In FTA measurement, a normal knee shows 172°~176°, inside contravariant shape knee arthropathy (O leg) is above 180°, and outside contravariant shape knee arthropathy (X leg) is below 170°. From previous reports of Knee OA types, among Japanese people, inside contravariant shape knee arthropathy (O leg) is common, and among Europeans and Americans, outside contravariant shape knee arthropathy (X leg) is common. When a mechanical factor related to the cause is common, therapeutic reform of the mechanical state becomes the main purpose. Implementation of operations, such as High tibial osteotomy (: HTO), total knee arthroplasty and (: TKA), in addition to minimally invasive surgery (: MIS), is sometimes necessary depending upon the condition.

Fig.1 shows the Osteoarthritis knee method and fibula excision method. The operation considers for four conditions: (1) The skin it is a little ardently, (2) the damage to the soft section organization is only a little, (3) the bleeding quantity is small, and (4) the bone excision is only a little. Operation requires that all above conditions be satisfied. Along with these four conditions, for the patient there are five: (1) operation time is short, (2) after operating, the pain is light, (3) the operation marks must be small and clean, (4) recovery is quick, and (5) economic burden is light. Presently, there is a fibula excision method for one operation technique of MIS. The object of this operation technique system is inside contravariant shape knee arthropathy (O leg). Especially, from the present condition where a large majority of patients are senior citizens, an optimum operation technique system will have the lowest physical strength burden on the patient. In this technique system, the fibula is revised so that the alignment of the legs reaches the normal position. However, the remedy guidelines of deformation characteristic arthropathy are being investigated presently in the Japanese medical orthopedics field. Especially, the occasion where engineering new technology is introduced in the future, reports regarding physicians on site, where engineering knowledge and experience influence the result, are many in number. For example, the excision quantity, detection angle, etc, of specifications and the bone positions of the affected parts examination and operation invasive quantity decisions, etc, are made at the time of planning before the operation.

In this research, the fibula excision method, which is an MIS was examined. This experiment dealt with the knee joint of a normal state and Osteoarthritis of the Knee before the operation and after the operation. The experiment supposed one foot standing and concerned the resultant stress state. Grasp of the mechanical state is important in operation, so this is useful as a mechanical guide at the time of planning before operation. In addition, mechanical examination of this operation system which can lighten physical strength burden with aging patients as a quite urgent characteristic is high.

Therefore, the remaining state of FTA and the meniscus, which are diagnostic guides of Osteoarthritis of the knee, influence the results of clearing for operation. A hybrid experiment used the 3-dimensional stress freezing method and a pressure gauge to examine the effectiveness and application condition of the fibula excision method.

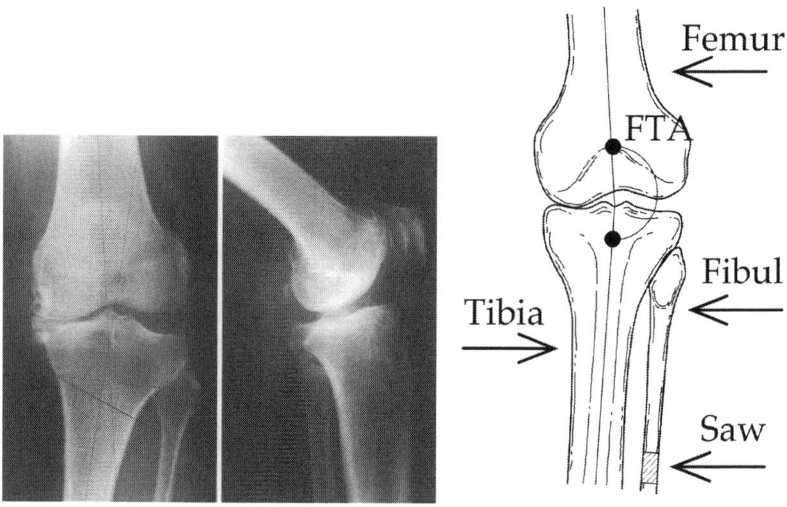

(a) Osteoarthritis of knee method (b) Fibula excision

Fig. 1. Osteoarthritis of knee method and fibula excision method

2. FTA, Mikulicz lineand and osteoarthritis of the knee

2.1 FTA, Mikulicz line

In the knee joint, the inside type (O leg) or outer part type (X leg) in the guide, are used for making a decision. An example is shown in Fig.2 of two Tsugas of FTA and the Mikulicz line. FTA is the angle which consists of the extended shaft direction of the femur and the tibia seen from the front. As for FTA of a normal knee, the range is 173° to approximately 176°. The inside type (O leg) for FTA is above 180°, and the outer part type (X leg) for FTA is below 170°. It is something which the Mikulicz line, the line which ties the thigh antique center and the foot joint center, displays for the leg load line in the standing position. Specifically, this is the line condition of the legs under the arrangement state of the pelvis, femur, tibia and ankle. A normal knee passes by the fog and outside from the center of the knee. As for an O leg, from the center of the knee it passes on the inside. In this research, FTA was utilized, and the leg alignment was decided. Among reports of Knee OA types, in Japanese people, the inside contravariant shape Osteoarthritis of the knee (O leg) is common, and among Europeans and Americans the outside contravariant shape Knee OA (X leg) is common.

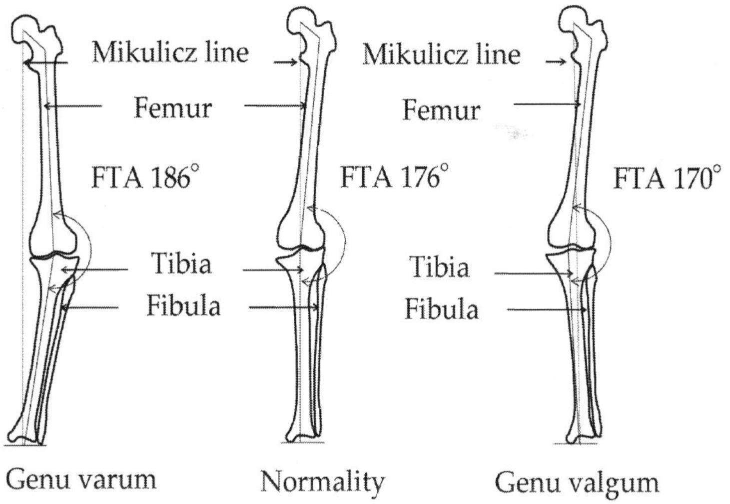

Fig. 2. FTA and Mikulicz line

Osteoarthritis of the knee is classified from appearance and inspection results; inside contravariant shape Knee OA (O leg) and the outside contravariant shape knee arthropathy (X leg). As dangerous factors of emergence there exists: history of external wounds, arthritis, age and obesity as four characteristic items for which Knee OA risk is increased. The emergence ratio becomes high from around 40 years old, and the frequency which emerges in senior citizens is high. As for the male to female ratio of patients, male : female = 1: 4. As a cause, mechanical factors are pointed out (e.g., stress concentrated inside the knee such as an imbalance of muscular strength or becoming fat).

3. Photoelastic theory, experimental model and actual model by epoxy resin

3.1 Photoelastic theory

The similarity rule is generally utilized for model production and analysis method. Production and an experiment must consider and satisfy the following conditions. (1) The experimental model and actual model from examination and supposition must be within the limit of elasticity, (2) Similarity of experimental model and actual model, (3) agreement of load point, load distribution and similarity, (4) similarity to Poisson's ratio ν. Then, when all conditions are satisfied, even with high polymer materials such as the epoxy resin, which was used for the experiment, the stress distribution of actual model of steel, alloy and concrete, etc, agrees. In addition, experimental values which can match the stress values of the actual model by conversion are possible.

However, like this experiment in the case of 3 dimensional photoelasticity, there are times when it does not agree to these under heating. It is necessary to know the characteristics and coping methods of the materials.

(1) the experimental model and examination within the elastic limit of the apparatus are supposed, and (2) the experimental model and similarity of the apparatus, are faults for the stress freezing process with respect to the relationship which utilizes the elastic body of the rubber condition, whereby the elastic coefficient is vitrified because it becomes 1/100, and deformation is easy to become large. In addition, the size of the model differs before the stress freezing and after the freezing, with error due to change in size being easy to occur. There is a deformation revision method as the expedient which removes these faults. This method, expecting the deformation quantity of the specimen beforehand, produces a model of the form which it revises, and stress freezing it is the method for the occasion of making a specified size. With this method, the error which originates in the deformation of geometric form can be made rather small.

As for the photoelastic experiment, other experimental stress analyses inside it are not possible for a single form to discover the pattern of analysis and entire stress distribution of stress simply. On the other hand, an experimental value which utilizes these features has recently become necessary, with experimental stress analysis it is the most effective method.

In addition, the numerical analysis with FEM has become easy, but the experimental data from which photoelasticity in the verification for supporting numerical analysis is of importance.

When analyzing the stress distribution of three dimensional structures, a stress freezing process which utilizes the characteristics of the epoxy resin is generally used, where the epoxy resin reaching a temperature above approximately 120 °C causes a second order transition, and the condition becomes rubber elastic. The load is loaded above this temperature. It makes the temperature fall to approximately room temperature. A distortion state occurs in the rubber elastic range under freezing. As for this distortion removing the load, it continues under freezing. In order to measure this distortion, the model after the stress freezing is sliced into approximately 5mm wide slices. The photoelastic device shown in Fig.3 was used. As for the distortion, which became an isochromatic fringe pattern depending upon the polarized light. Fig.3 shows the construction of the photoelastic device where S is the illuminant, L and L2 are the field lenses, P is the polarizer, A is the analyzer, and Q1 and Q2 are the quarter undulation plates.

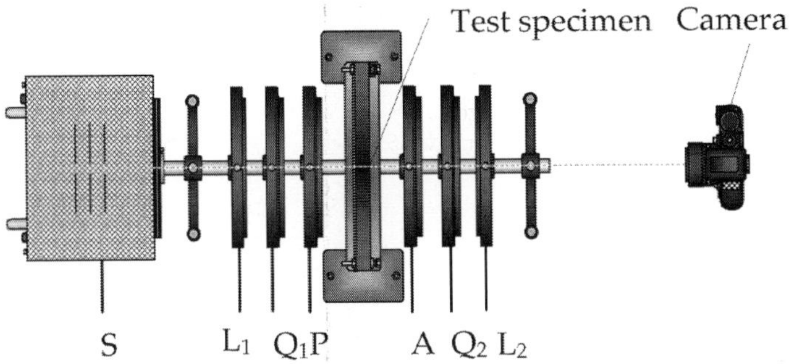

Fig. 3. Circular polariscope

Fringe order and the relationship of principal stress which occurs becomes (1).

$$N = \alpha t(\sigma_1 - \sigma_2) \tag{1}$$

Here, for the N fringe order, t is the thickness of sliced specimen, α is the photoelastic sensitivity, and σ_1 and σ_2 are the principal stresses inside the slices.

In addition, with respect to free boundaries, the σ_1 each of σ_2 becomes 0. Therefore, through (2) the stress state can be known.

$$\sigma = N/\alpha t[\text{MPa}] \tag{2}$$

3.2 Material error of relation between experimental model and actual model

The epoxy resin of the photoelastic material used as the test material is an isotropic homogeneous body, but the organism bone (sponge bone and fine bone, from marrow constitution) is an anisotropic heterogeneous body. Due to this, error occurs in the comparison analysis of the material and the heterogeneous material of which Young's modulus, *E*, is homogeneous. Depending on this, examination becomes necessary by use of epoxy resin concerning the quantitative error of the bone.

Concerning this, Nishida allotted the epoxy resin of Young's modulus, *E*, which differs by layer, and a bend experiment which imitated the bone was performed. The design of the experiment is shown in Fig.4. As a result of the experiment, the error of Young's modulus, *E*, was calculated to be 10% when the experiment was performed on a solid monolayer structure. As the quantitative error is small, quantitative reproducibility can be expected. In addition, for the dynamic quality of the bone, due to a characteristic difference and personal equation, for the femur of an adult male 30~50 years of age, an average tension of 137.30MPa, an elastic limit of 100.82Mpa, and a recovery factor of the distortion due to stress relief with extension of 0.0125 have been reported as representing 95% or more.

As for the bone, to think of the body as being composed of photoelastic material and use a photoelastic experiment is favorable. This method, which is a powerful experimental analysis method in stress distribution visualization of the whole bone, was adopted on the basis of these reports. In addition, mechanical characteristics of the silicon rubber which was used in this experiment showed a hardness of JIS A43, a tensile strength of 2.2MPa, and a growth rate of 170%.

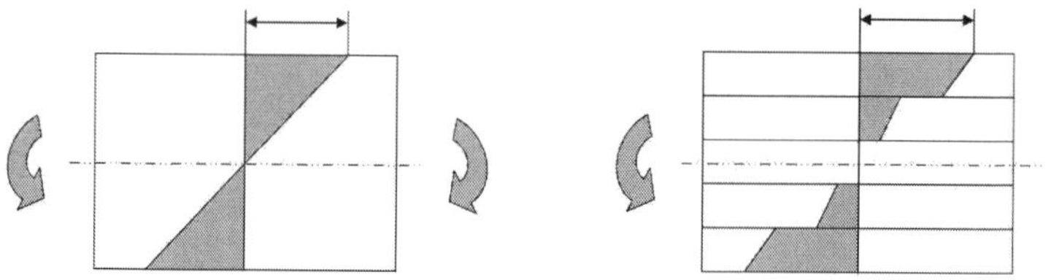

(a) homogeneous (b) unhomogeneous

Fig. 4. Difference between experiment and model

3.3 Experimental summary

3.3.1 Test material and test pieces

In this research, experimental analysis which used three-dimensional stress freezing was performed. A specimen model of the framework which forms the left side of the knee joint ,including the femur, tibia and fibula, was produced using actual equipment and material, making use of the medical organism skeletal model,. The test material selected was an epoxy resin (mixed weight ratio; ARALDITE B CT200: HARDENER HT901=100: 30). The normal temperature (25°C) and high temperature (128°C) against mechanical quality are shown in Table 1.

Organism bone is generally formed by marrow, etc, which does not bear stress from the fine adrenal cortex section and the porous spongin section, and furthermore, shows rigidity. Therefore, it is not possible to handle the homogeneous body, and in addition, the modulus anisotropy of elasticity and strength regarding the same adrenal cortex section must be considered. However, the aforementioned has reproducibility concerns, and error in this research is due to the layer system, so a 3 dimensional photoelastic experimental model was produced as a solid structure.

	Normal temperature [25°C]	High temperature [125°C]
Modulus of longitudinal elasticity *E* (MPa)	2940	13.62
Modulus of transverse elasticity *G* (MPa)	1131	4.59
Poisson's ratio ν	0.30	0.48
Photoelastic stress sensitivity α (mm/ N)	0.1	4.0

Table 1. Properties of the epoxy resin

3.3.2 Experimental method

In this research, the skeletal structure of the knee joint was reproduced, making use of a specimen model of the framework which forms the left side of the knee joint, including the femur, tibia and fibula. The framework for reappearance consisted of the knee joint of the femoral model and the fibula combined with the tibia model. In order for more accurate vertical load to be imposed, the muscular part was produced using silicon as the jig. In the case of stress freezing, 107.8N was loaded as a freezing load. In reappearance of joint cartilage, clay for ceramic art with a hardness of HS29 (Sculpey III American poly- form the corp.) was used. The specimen model is shown in Fig. 5, and the load device is shown in Fig. 6.

After the stress freezing ended, for the standing position state, especially when the FTA was maintained, slices of a 5mm thickness were made. Slices were made from the front of the knee, with the inside as a standard. The slice direction is shown in Fig. 7 (a), and a slice is shown in Fig. 7 (b) and (c).

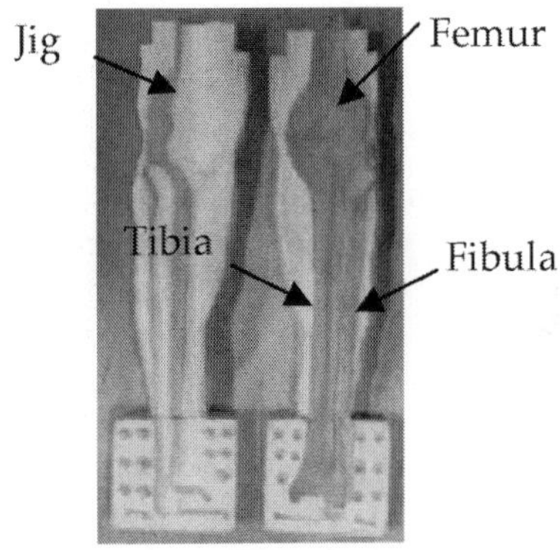

Fig. 5. Model specimen

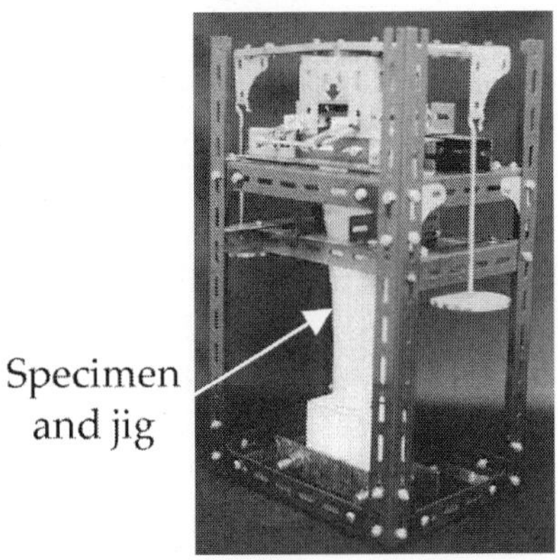

Fig. 6. Load device

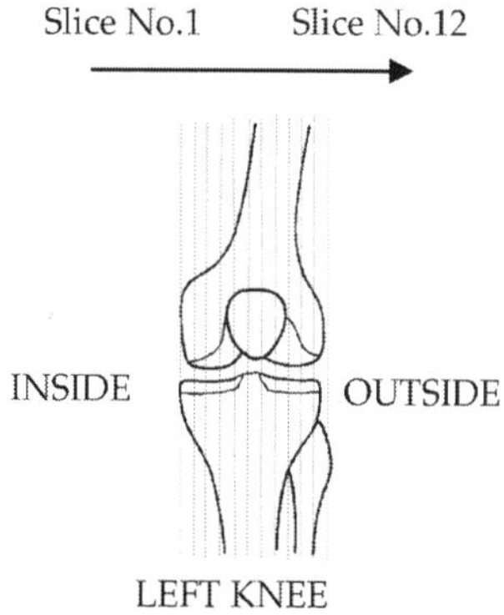

(a) Slice position

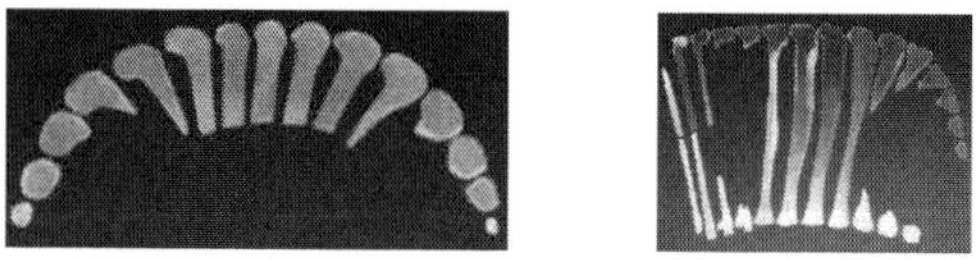

(a) Slice of femur (b) Slice of tibia

Fig. 7. Model slice

4. Relation experimental results converted to actual model

As for stress distribution, if the apparatus and the figure are similar, the distribution is the same regardless of material. However, as it is a model experiment, when Young's modulus, E, differs, conversion of the obtained experimental value and the stress value of the apparatus are necessary. Therefore, a photoelastic material of which the Young's modulus, E, of the apparatus was known was inspected.

Concerning this, a system for the conversion of the stress value obtained from the experiment to the stress value of the actual bone is plural, and was implemented into the program conversion. Here, subscript experiment values: *ex* is the value of the actual bone: *a*.

4.1 Experimental value for the calculation method regarding the stress value of the actual bone

As an outline, the case of a plane surface stress state is written. The ratio, L, of length of the actual model and the experimental model is expressed by (3).

$$L = \frac{Actual\ size}{Experimental\ size} \tag{3}$$

The relation of (4) gives the length ratio, L, of the error ratio and load, W, of the respective stress value, σ, for the model. Depending on this, the stress value for the error ratio, K, of the actual model and the experimental model becomes (5).

$$K = \frac{\sigma_a}{\sigma_{ex}} = \frac{W_a}{W_{ex} L^2} \tag{4}$$

$$\sigma_a = K \cdot \sigma_{ex} \tag{5}$$

Generally, for a three dimensional photoelastic experiment, if Poisson's ratio, v, is almost identical to the experimental result and analogy is for conversion to the apparatus such that:

$$\nu_{ex} \cong \nu_a$$

In the three dimensional problem, it designates the ratio of the length of the model as L_{ratio}, as shown in (6).

$$L_{ratio} = \frac{Experimental\ size}{Actual\ size} = \frac{L_{ex}}{L_a} \tag{6}$$

where the area ratio, A_{ratio}, and specific volume, V_{ratio}, are given by (7),

$$A_{ratio} = L_{ratio}^2,\ V_{ratio} = L_{ratio}^3 \tag{7}$$

and the load ratio, W_{ratio}, given by (8) becomes similar,

$$W_{ratio} = \frac{Experimental\ load}{Actual\ load} = \frac{W_{ex}}{W_a} \tag{8}$$

so that the stress ratio, σ_{ratio}, (9) can be given by:

$$\sigma_{ratio} = \frac{\sigma_{ex}}{\sigma_a} = \frac{W_{ex}}{W_a}\left(\frac{L_{ex}}{L_a}\right)^2 \tag{9}$$

For conversion to the stress ratio $\sigma_{ratio}=1$, knowing a more accurate stress value is desirable, so it is necessary to consider the experimental load well. In addition, after drawing up a stress distribution chart, because the experimental load is computed from Fringe Order, the experimental stress value, σ_{ex}, of the actual bone stress value, σ_a, can be calculated by (10).

$$\sigma_a = \sigma_{ex} \frac{W_{ex}}{W_a}\left(\frac{L_{ex}}{L_a}\right)^2 \tag{10}$$

4.2 Experiment value and the calculation method which uses Young's modulus *E* of the experimental model and Young's modulus *E* of the actual bone

The stress value of the actual bone is able to be calculated by the experimental value and the proportional system which uses Young's modulus, E. If the actual bone and the experimental model are similar figures, the same stress distribution is given regardless of material. However, when Young's modulus differs, conversion is necessary for the obtained experimental value to give the stress value of the actual bone.

Therefore, for the photoelastic material which is used it is necessary to know the Young's modulus, E, of the actual bone which we would like to inspect. Table 3 shows the mechanical characteristics of the femur and tibia. The mechanical characteristics of the epoxy resin are shown in Table 3. For the stress freezing process, Young's modulus, E, of the epoxy resin at the time (freezing) of high temperature was used. Therefore, Young's modulus, E=13.62[MPa].

	Young's modulus E [GPa]	Yield stress [MPa]	Ultimate stress [MPa]
Femur	17s 2	111s 12	129s 6
Tibia	20s 2	124s 8	147s 9

Table 2. Mechanical properties of mechanical characteristics of femur and tibia

	Young's modulus E [MPa]	modules of rigidity G [MPa]	Poisson's ratio ν	photoelastic sensitivity α [mm/ N]
Normal temp.	2940	1131	0.30	0.10
High temp.	13.62	4.59	0.48	4.00

Table 3. Mechanical properties of the epoxy resin

Proportional system (11) can be converted into formula (12), which substitutes the known Young's modulus, E, and experiment stress value, σ_{ex}, respectively, and gives the stress value of the actual bone, σ_a.

$$\sigma_{\max ex} : E_{ex} = \sigma_{\max a} : E_a \tag{11}$$

$$\sigma_{\max a} = \frac{\sigma_{\max ex} \cdot E_{ex}}{E_a} \tag{12}$$

5. Importance of the meniscus

The importance of the meniscus was considered in this experiment. Types I-III were set and compared. The FTA was set at 176°, that of the normal knee, and the meniscus was reproduced using the two materials of silicon rubber and polyurethane resin. In the same way, the meniscus completely wore through, and the femur and the tibia and fibula reached a state where they contacted directly. The laboratory conditions are shown in Table 4, and the experimental parameters are shown in Table 5.

Examples of a photoelastic stripe photograph and a stress distribution chart (principal stress difference at a point of contact) of the femur are shown in Fig. 8. That of the tibia is shown in Fig. 9.

In Fig. 8 and Fig. 9, Types I and II show almost similar stress distribution states. From the fact that the state of the alignment of the normal knee of FTA 176° was reproduced, a normal contact state of the femur, tibia and fibula was established. It was achieved when the meniscus was approximately 60% moisture, much like a sponge which contains water. In addition, there are dynamic functional characteristics of stability for the joint which are quite important for load support, absorption and joint impact load regarding lubrication. For example, in absorbing approximately 20% of the loads which operate the knee joint at the time of knee joint extension, it is thought that it transmits approximately 50%. In addition, it has an influence on the dispersion of the load where the meniscus direction on the outside is thicker than on the inside of the knee joint.

On the one hand, in Fig. 9, Type III can be seen to differ from Type I and II for stress distribution state. In the femur there was a centralization of stress in the contact section, and in the tibia influence in the frame work section was also observed. From this, the meniscus which is between the knee joint not only dispersed the stress of the contact section of the knee joint , but concerning the frame work section, it was found that it plays an important role in bone transmission, e.g., the centralization of stress is eased. A dynamic concentration of stress became a centralized load because it in fact occurred due to a centralized load, and regarding the knee joint, it was found to be in a state where deformation is promoted. In addition, the deformation characteristic of knee OA was the formation of bone spikes, however, it is understood that they were formed due to excessive stress. Type III of the stress distribution state and the stress value reached a higher degree to ease the excess stress, and it is presumed that the location of the bone spike was formed for the purpose of expanding the contact surface area.

Type	FTA	Material of meniscus
I	176°	Silicone rubber
II		Polyurethane
III		No

Table 4. Parameter of Types

Resin	Hardness (JIS A)	Tensile strength (MPa)	Elongation (%)
Silicone rubber	43	2.2	170
Polyurethane	60	15	430

Table 5. Properties of silicone rubber and polyurethane resin

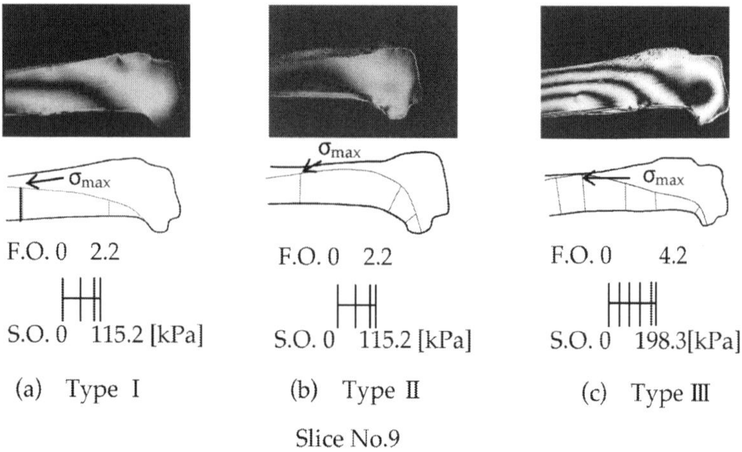

Fig. 8. Isochromatic fringe pattern (Femur)

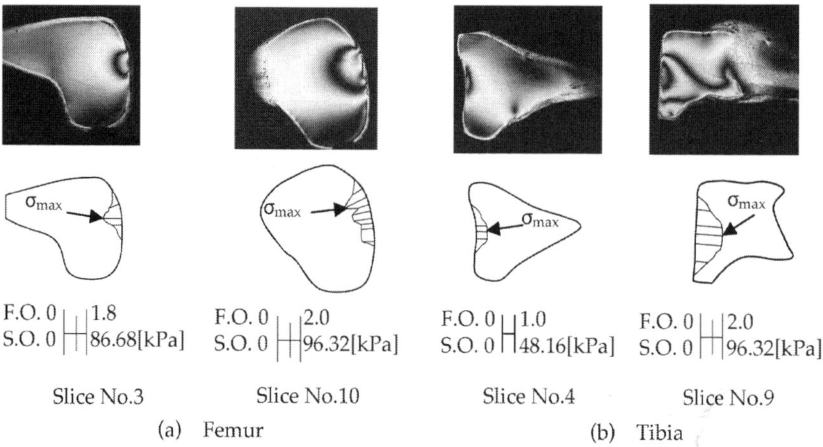

Fig. 9. Isochromatic fringe pattern (Tibia)

6. Examination of the effectiveness of the fibula excision method - Experimental parameter -

In this research, the fibula excision method was examined. The experiment dealt with the knee joint of a normal state, Osteoarthritis of the Knee before and after operation and supposed one foot standing and was concerned with stress state. The state of FTA and remaining meniscus, which are a diagnostic guide of the Osteoarthritis of the knee. In this research examines the influence which these give to an Osteoarthritis of the Knee and operation.

In this experiment, concerning the stress rate, a comparison and examination of a meniscus and the inside of a contravariant shape knee arthropathy (O leg) was done after using the fibula excision method. At that time, the remaining state of the FTA and the meniscus were considered when the laboratory conditions were decided, as shown in Table 3.

Furthermore, the fibula excision method reproduced a state where a 10mm frame work section of the fibula was excised in Types D and E.

Type	FTA	Meniscus	Operation
A	176°	All	No excision
B	186°	All	No excision
C	186°	Half	No excision
D	186°	All	excision
E	186°	Half	excision

Table 6. Parameter of Types A)E

7. Examination of the effectiveness of the fibula excision method -A ~ E type results-

7.1 Mechanical state of a normal knee joint of Type A: Normal knee (FTA176°/extensive meniscus remains)

The isochromatic fringe pattern and stress distribution chart of an example of Type A are shown in Fig. 10 (a) the femur, and (b) the tibia. As for the scale, the upper is the fringe order (: F.O.) and the lower is the stress value (: S.O [kPa]). On the vertical axis are the most compressed stress points, the σmax, and the slice No. are given on the horizontal axis in Fig. 11.

In the femur of a Type A normal knee, regarding Fig. 10, an almost equal stress distribution was shown on the inside and outside. Regarding Fig. 10 (b) of the tibia, on the tibia side, the stress was higher on the inside than on the outside. As for the FTA of 176°, it is thought that this kind of distribution was shown because some of it was transferred to the outer part type (X leg). Regarding Fig. 11, for a normal knee joint, the load was easily imposed on the outside, and the difference of stress which occurred inside and outside was small. Therefore, it was stabilized dynamically. Especially, when the emergence of Knee OA is considered, concentration of stress is difficult to obtain, and wear of the meniscus is thought to not advance.

As for the result, in a healthy knee, for stress to be distributed outside, it must agree with the assumed idea in the orthopedics field that a nearly equal stress distribution is desirable (sharing a load 40 percent inside and 60 percent outside). As the stress value is low overall and the range is wide, the load which falls on the knee joint is efficiently dispersed, making a normal knee joint is stable.

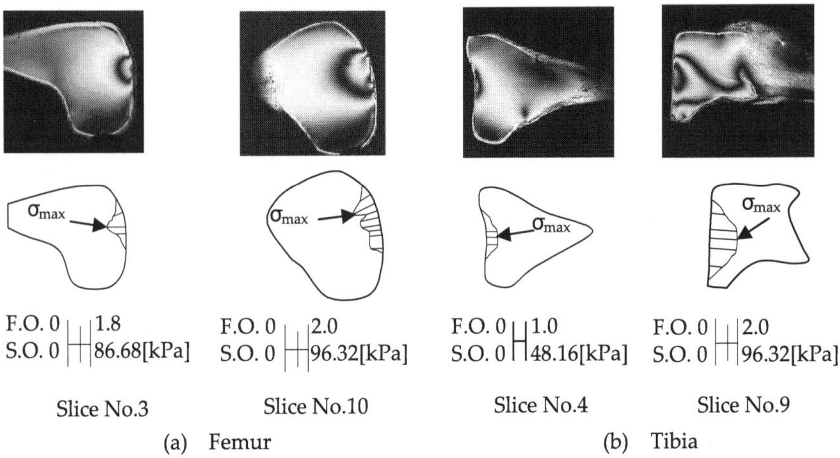

Fig. 10. Isochromatic fringe pattern of Type A

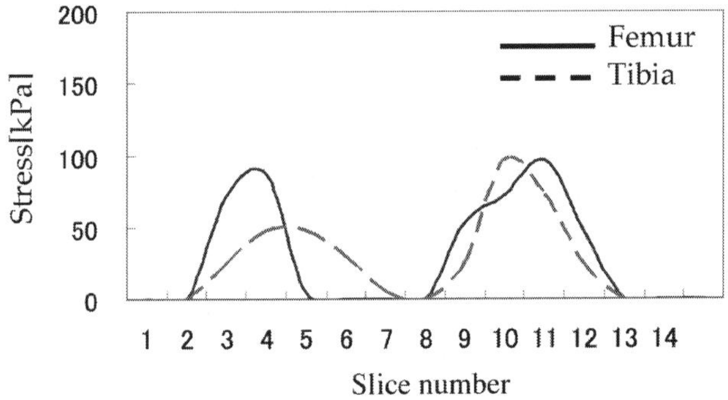

Fig. 11. Stress distribution of Type A

7.2 Contravariant shape knee arthropathy among minor Type B: Osteoarthritis of the knee (FTA186 °/ extensive meniscus remains)

The isochromatic fringe pattern and stress distribution chart of an example of Type B are shown in Fig. 12 (a) the femur, and (b) the tibia. As for the scale, the upper is the fringe order (: F.O.) and the lower is the stress value (: S.O [kPa]). On the vertical axis are the most compressed stress points, the σmax, and the slice No. are given on the horizontal axis in Fig. 13.

In Fig. 12 (b), the tibia, the stress distribution inside the peak of the tibia is narrower than that of Type A. The meniscus extensively remained, but the FTA was 186°. It is thought that 60% of the stress was distributed outside the knee. When walking where impacts occur over time, like the of ascent or descent of a stairway, it is expected that high stress occurs inside the knee. If during this the FTA is not normal, the meniscus cannot disperse the load equally, it is presumed that the change in FTA is strongly related to the wear and deformation of the meniscus.

From the graph in Fig. 13, in the femur, as for stress inside and outside, they were almost the same as in the tibia stress outside. We assumed that in an O leg high stress occurs inside, but, from the result, the cartilage remains even with the O leg, and with the point which only a dead load is loaded, it does not mean that stress is distributed to the inside and outside.

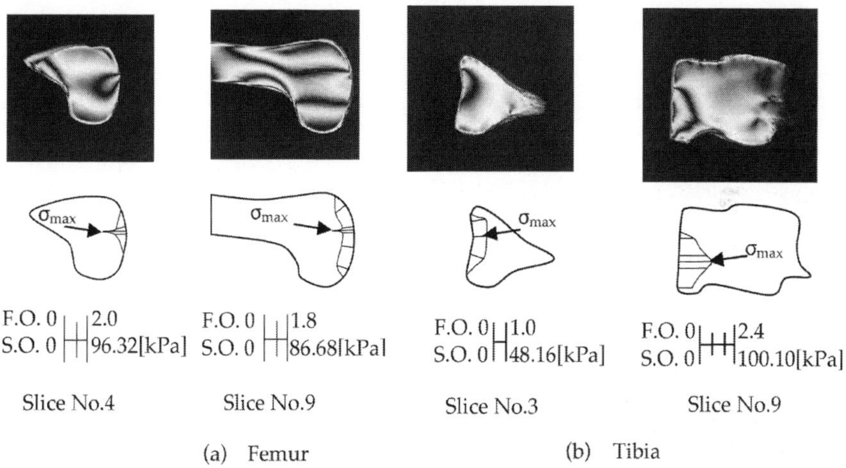

Fig. 12. Isochromatic fringe pattern of Type B

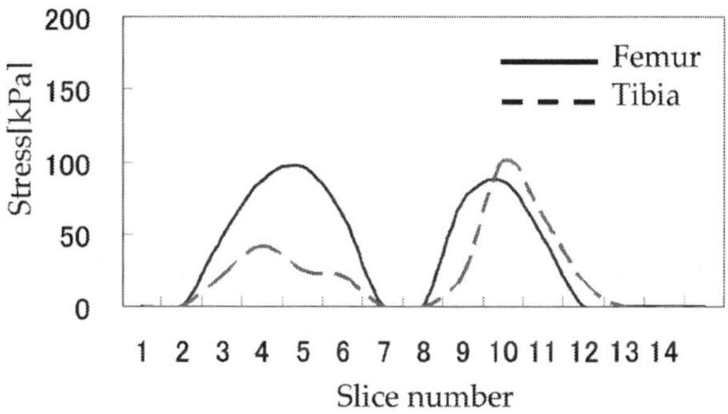

Fig. 13. Isochromatic fringe pattern of Type B

7.3 Type C: Seriousness osteoarthritis of the knee (FTA186°/ on ly outside meniscus remains)

The isochromatic fringe pattern and stress distribution chart of an example of Type C are shown in Fig. 14, the femur, and Fig. 15, the tibia. As for the scale, the upper is the fringe order (: F.O.) and the lower is the stress value (: S.O [kPa]). On the vertical axis are the most compressed stress points, the σmax , and the slice No. are given on the horizontal axis in Fig. 15.

Concentration of stress of higher-order was verified for Type C from Figs. 14 and 15, which show inside the knee where the meniscus disappeared. As for this, the load dispersion role of the meniscus was not fulfilled, and it is thought that the stress was concentrated.

In the tibia in Fig. 16, concentration of stress of higher-order was verified originally in the condylar between bulging sections which existed on the center of the tibia, which did not cause direct contact. This is related to the occurrence of bone spikes which are a feature of Knee OA. These contact states have been expressed as two peaks, one of which is on the left side in the graph. When the meniscus wears, the bones collide, are damaged, and when bending and stretching, the motion causes pain. In the inside contravariant shape knee OA, the result is exemplified by the pain, which agrees with the opinion within the orthopedics field that spikes occur in the condylar between bulging section of the tibia.

Depending, in order for the bone not to contact, it is necessary to perform a remedy which revises FTA and excises the bone spike. The stress which occurs in the knee joint from the abovementioned conditions of Knee OA differs. The stress which occurs in the knee joint from the abovementioned conditions of OA also differs. Especially, as the cartilage wear causes concentration of stress, contact in the condylar between bulging sections occurs, and it is important to prevent wear of the meniscus. FTA is related to the wear of the meniscus, and it is thought that the revision of FTA is connected to preventive methods.

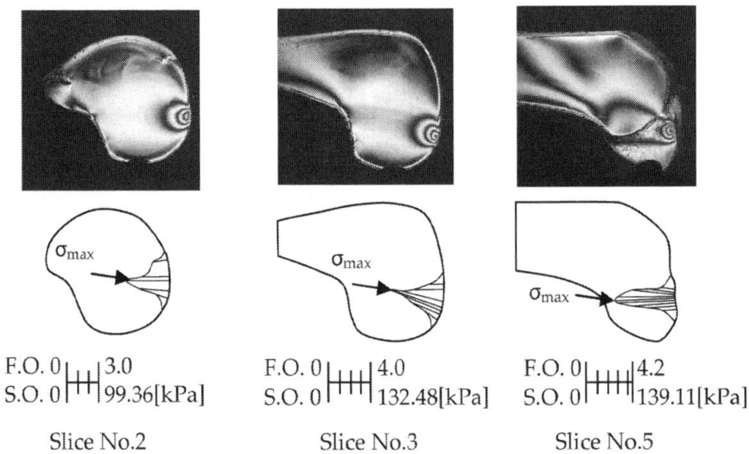

Fig. 14. Isochromatic fringe pattern of Type C (Femur)

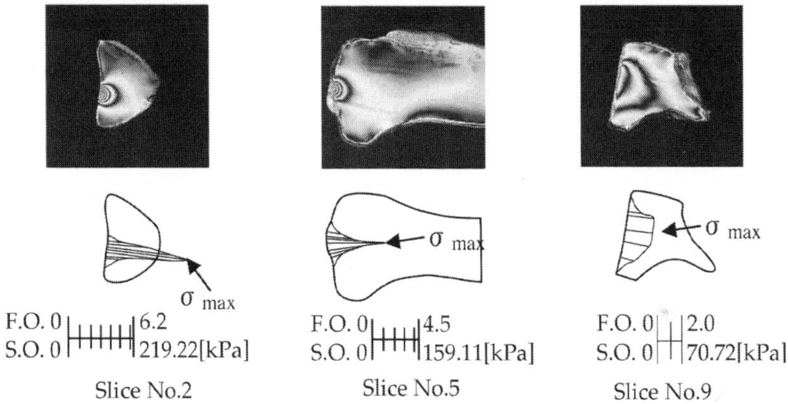

Fig. 15. Isochromatic fringe pattern of Type C (Tibia)

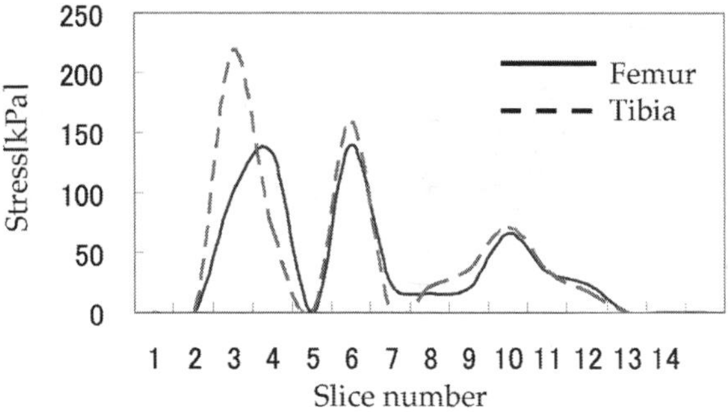

Fig. 16. Stress distribution of Type C

7.4 Type D: After the operation of the fibula excision method for minor OA (FTA176 °/ meniscus extensive remains)

The isochromatic fringe pattern and stress distribution chart of an example of Type C are shown in Fig. 17, the femur, and Fig. 18, the tibia. As for the scale, the upper is the fringe order (: F.O.) and the lower is the stress value (: S.O [kPa]). On the vertical axis are the most compressed stress points, the σmax, and the slice No. are given on the horizontal axis in Fig. 19.

From Figs. 17 and 18, for Type D the stress was distributed equally inside and outside the knee. From Fig. 19, the stress value and stress distribution state were similar to the normal knee (Type A), and were mechanically stability. Correction of FTA was indicated by removal of a fibula. Therefore, the mild OA knee became mechanically stable by the fibula excision method, achieving a mechanical position equal to the normal knee. Depending on the case, the fibula excision method effectiveness is suggested in cases of minor OA knees.

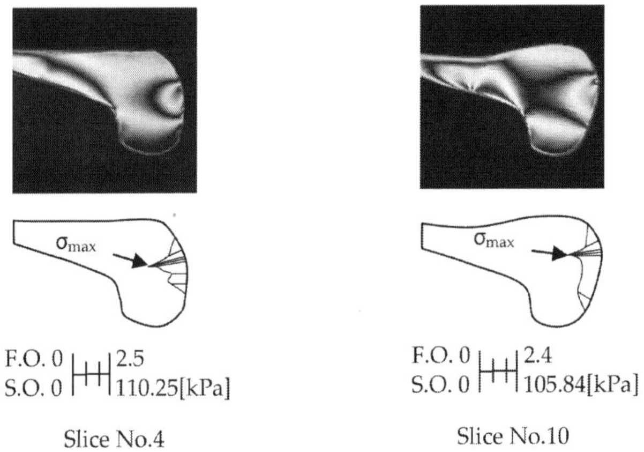

Fig. 17. Isochromatic fringe pattern of Type D (Femur)

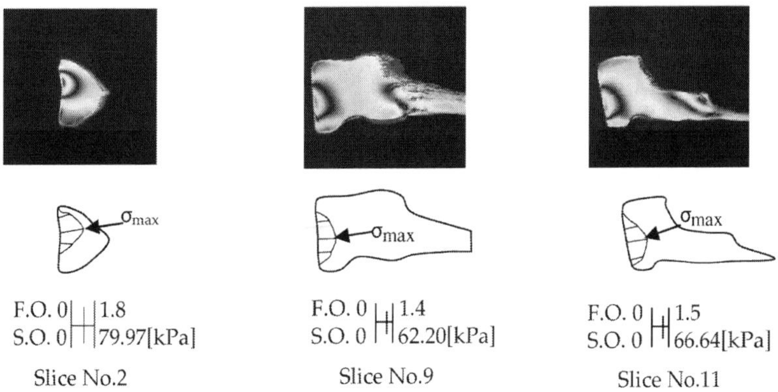

Fig. 18. Isochromatic fringe pattern of Type D (Tibia)

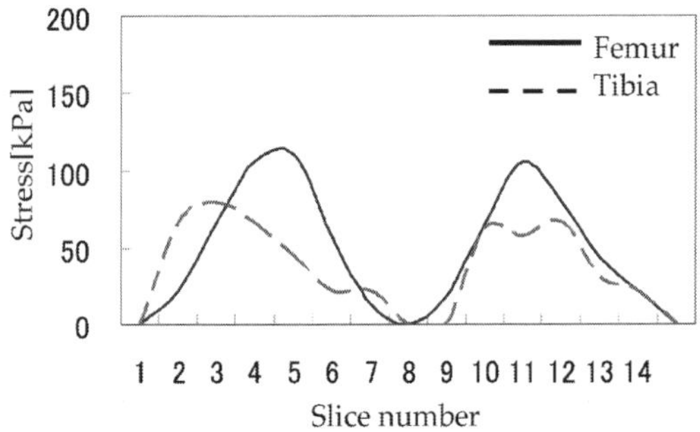

Fig. 19. Stress distribution of Type D

7.5 Type E: After the operation of the fibula excision method for severe osteoarthritis of the knee (FTA176°/ only outside meniscus remains)

The isochromatic fringe pattern and stress distribution chart of an example of Type D are shown in Fig. 20 (a), the femur, and (b), the tibia. As for the scale, the upper is the fringe order (: F.O.) and the lower is the stress value (: S.O [kPa]). On the vertical axis are the most compressed stress points, the σmax, and the slice No. are given on the horizontal axis in Fig. 21.

From Fig. 20 (a), the femur, and (b), the tibia, high order stress concentration was confirmed inside the knee for Type E. In addition, there was concentration of stress on the femur and the tibia. As for this stress distribution state was similar to Type C before the fibula excising, and there was no improvement. However, from Fig. 21, the stress regarding the contact of the condylar between bulging sections of the tibia was not verified to show improvement. From these, there is no improvement in minor Knee OA (Type D) in the contravariant shape knee arthropathy among serious illnesses. Only for the pain of the intercondylar eminence part was the effectiveness observed. However, remarkable improvement for Mild Knee OA cannot be anticipated for Severe Knee OA.

From the above, the fibula excision method is effective as a minor contravariant shape knee arthropathy remedy. In serious Knee OA, the revision of FTA was not obtained at a level of sufficient effect. In serious contravariant shape knee arthropathy, remedy by high tibial osteotomy (: HTO) and similar procedures are presumed to remedy FTA properly. In addition, in performing revision of FTA by the fibula excision method, it was found that the curative effect differs depending upon the state of the remaining meniscus.

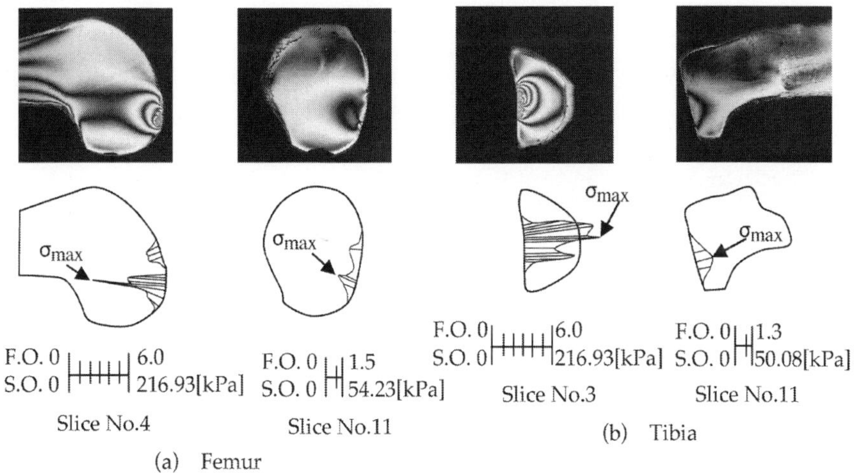

Fig. 20. Isochromatic fringe pattern of Type E

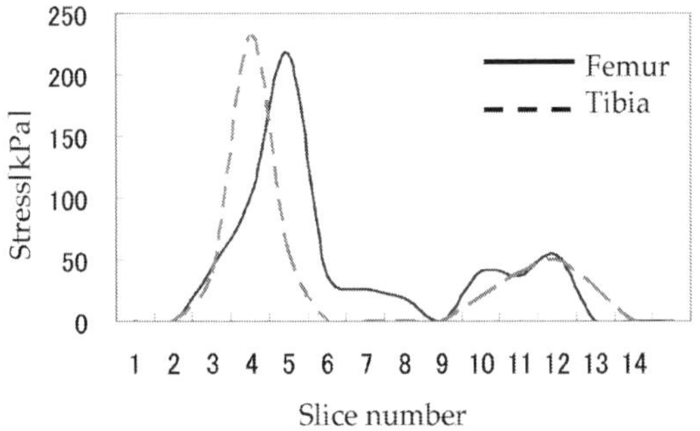

Fig. 21. Stress distribution of Type E

8. Examination about the adaptation condition of the fibula excision method

In this research, other than the photoelastic stress freezing method, pressure of the knee joint was measured by a small-sized pressure sensor. The advantage of using a pressure gauge is that it can obtain results continually. (Segmented type small-sized pressure sensor with a thickness of 2mm and a diameter of 6mm :Kyouwa dengyou * PSM) In this experiment, FTA was changed gradually, and the influence on the knee joint was observed. As for the test-piece, a similar epoxy resin model to that used for stress freezing method was used. Similarly, the amount of remaining meniscus was considered. Similar load equipment and loads 9.8N, which is 1/11 at the time of the stress freezing method from the special quality of the pressure sensor, was used. The pressure sensor was installed in the occurrence position of the principal stress max from the result of the stress freezing method. In Fig. 22 the pressure sensor position and pressure gauge are shown.

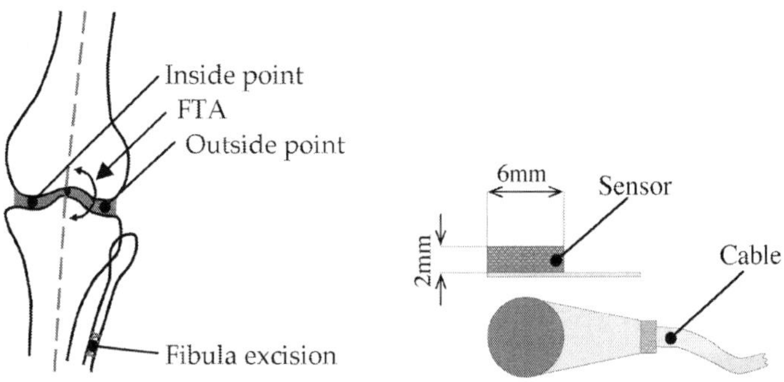

Fig. 22. Pressure sensor position and pressure gauge

8.1 Examination of normal knee joint

Fig. 23 shows the results of the experiment on a normal knee joint. Fig. 26 shows the results after the fibula excision method. In the graph, the vertical axis represents the pressure value, and on the horizontal axis FTA is shown. The solid line indicates inside the knee joint, and the broken line shows the pressure outside.

From Fig. 23, in the healthy knee joint, when FTA was small, (X leg tendency), a small high pressure occurred outside. As FTA (O leg tendency) became larger, it decreased the pressure outside and pressure inside increased. As for pressure inside and outside becoming equal, it was verified that it is at approximately FTA 178°. Optimum FTA, at which the knee joint is stabilized, is therefore approximately 178°. Also, this result was similar to the result in the above photoelastic stress freezing method.

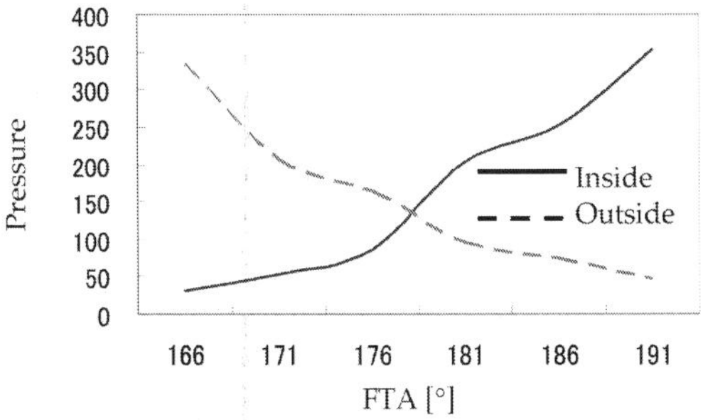

Fig. 23. Pressure distribution of no excision

8.2 Examination after the fibula excision method

From Fig. 24, after the fibula excision method, it can be seen that when FTA was small, (X leg tendency) pressure was increased outside, and when FTA was large, (O leg tendency) pressure increased inside. Pressure inside and outside became equal near the FTA 173°~183°, a wide range compared to before the fibula excision method. As for this, FTA was revised by the fibula excision method, and it is thought that the range of FTA at which the knee joint was stabilized became wide.

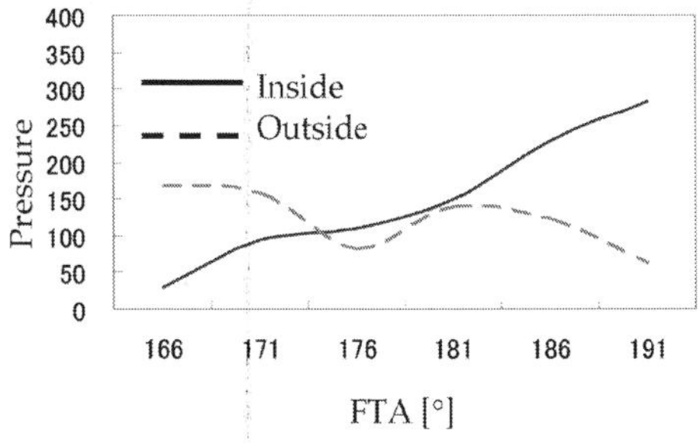

Fig. 24. Pressure distribution of fibula excision

8.3 Examination of FTA and the adaptation condition

The pressures inside and outside the knee were added, and the overall pressure was calculated. The percentage pressure on the inside and the outside were calculated. A result for a normal knee joint is indicated in Fig 25, and that after the fibula excision method is indicated in Fig 26. The vertical axis ratio is the pressure (%), and on the horizontal axis FTA is shown. The percentage on the pressure inside the knee joint is given by a solid line, and the percentage of the pressure on the outside is shown as a broken line.

From Fig. 25, it can be seen that in the normal knee joint, the ratio of pressure inside and outside almost became equal at approximately FTA 178°, but, when FTA changed, that ratio changed suddenly. Especially, the FTA change in ratio was large within the range of 171°~181°. It is thought that 1° or 2° of change in FTA produces a great effect on the knee joint.

However, after the fibula excising, results in Fig. 26, the FTA ratio of pressure was almost 174°~183°, and remarkable reduction in pressure both inside and outside the knee could be seen. The knee joint was mechanically stabilized. In addition, it was found that the pressure which is loaded outside was lightened mechanically. Depending on this, it can be effective concerning the outside contravariant shape knee arthropathy (X leg).

Therefore, as for the fibula excision method, it is thought to be especially effective for adaptation concerning minor OA patients of FTA 174° ~ FTA 183°.

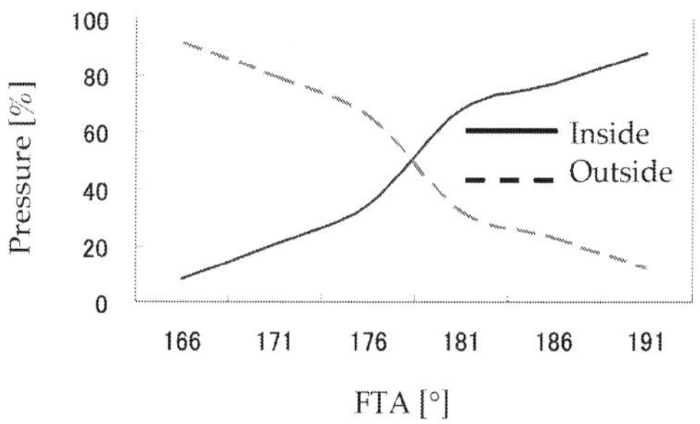

Fig. 25. Percentage of pressure in no excision

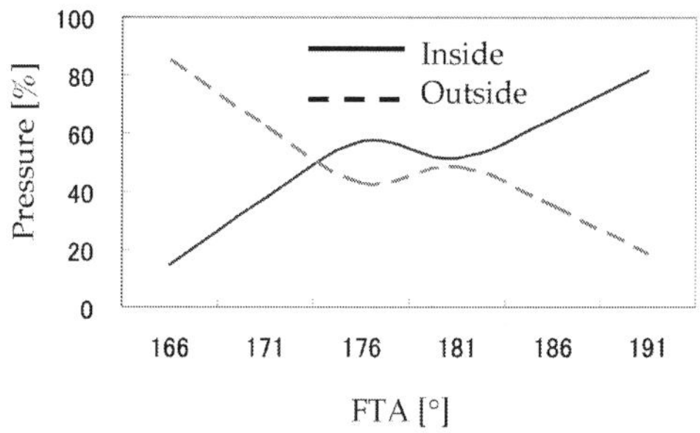

Fig. 26. Percentage of fibula excision

9. Conclusion

In this research, the fibula excision method was examined. The experiment dealt with the knee joint of a normal state, Osteoarthritis of the Knee before and after operation and supposed one foot standing and was concerned with stress state. The state of FTA and remaining meniscus, which are a diagnostic guide of the Osteoarthritis of the knee, clearly influenced the result of the operation.

Experimental conditions of 5 types of experimental hybrids, A-E, used the 3-dimensional stress freezing method and pressure gauge to examine the effectiveness and application conditions of the fibula excision method.

As a result, the knowledge below was obtained:

1. The fibula excision method showed validity for Mild inside type Osteoarthritis of the knee and is suitable for cases of FTA 186 ° and much remaining meniscus.
2. Doing the revision of FTA, the curative effect of the fibula excision method differs depending upon disease condition. The effect is related in the remaining state of the meniscus.
3. As for the fibula excision method, it is suggested to be suited for the remedy of outside contravariant shape knee arthropathy (X leg).

10. Future direction

The photoelastic experiment the analysis of principal stress and singular point is possible too. This analysis is the major feature which only photoelastic experiment is possible. This research utilizes this feature and would like to use in remedy and development of the bone and the artificial joint.

11. References

Asano S., Ezumi T. and Hachiya M. (2004). *A Study on The Characteristics of The Dynamics of Osteoarthritis Treatment Using Photoelastic Method,* Journal of Japanese Non Distractive Inspection, Vol53, No.9, (09. 2004), pp566-571,ISSN0367-5866

Burstein, A, H. & Wright,M,T. M. &Kurosawa,H. &Yamanoi, T.&Yamakoshi,K.(1997). *Fandamentals of Orthopedics Biomechanics*+Nankoudou, ISBN978-4524216215, Tokyo, Japan

Fischer K. J. & Jacobs, C, R. & Levenston, M, E. & Carter, D, R. (1998). Annals of biomedical engineering. *Observations of Convergence and Uniqueness of Node-Based Bone Remodeling Simulations,*Vol. 25,No.2 (08.1997). pp.261-268, ISSN0090-6964

Fujiki, H. & Ishikawa, H. & Yshuda, K. (1999). The Japan Society Of Mechanical Engineers, *Change and the influence of knee joint contact force by the total knee replacement,* Thesis collection A, Vol65, No.629, (01.1999), pp.187-193, ISSN03875008

Hachiya,M. & Huji,H. &Yamada, K. (1999). Joint Surgery. *The method of Salter's Innominate Osteotomy and Pemberton's Pericapsular Osteotomy for the Residual Subluxation of the Hip,* Vol.18, No.2, (02.1999), pp.229-235, ISSN0286-5394

Hayashi, K.(2000). Biomechanics, Coronasha, ISBN978-4381100818, Tokyo, Japan

Ikada,Y. (1994) . *Bio Material Engineering*+ISBN978-4782880012, Tokyo, Japan

Ikeda,K. & Shimazu,H. (2000). *Bio Physical Properties / Medical Mechanical Engineering,*Gakken Medical Shujunsha (Shujunsha), ISBN978-4879622259, Tokyo, Japan

Isekame,F. & Suenaga,M. &Mizushima,I. (1975). Clinical Orthopedic Surgery. *The Circumference of the Occurrence of Osteoarthritis of the Knee,* Vol.10, No.4, (04.1975), pp.303-313, ISSN05570433

Kawai,H. & Morisaki, N. (1985). *Orthopedics Traumatology.* (The 4th edition), Bunkodo, ISBN9784830627019, Tokyo, Japan

Koshino, T. (1992). Orthopedic. *Etiology, Diagnosis and Treatments for Osteoarthritis of the Knee,* NO.43, (10.1992), pp.1629-1638,ISSN0030-5901

Kurokawa,T. & Hujikawa K. & Yamamoto,H. (1999). *Orthopedic Operation No.5*, Operation of a Knee joint, Igakushoin, ISBN 4-521-46121-2, Tokyo, Japan

Li, G & Kawamura, K & Barrance, P & Chao, EY & Kaufman, K. (1998). Annals of biomedical engineering. *Prediction of Muscle Recruitment and Its Effect on Joint Reaction Forces during Knee Exercises. Vol. 26,No.4, (08.1998),pp.725-733, ISSN0090-6964*

Maezaki, N. & Ezumi T. & Hachiya M. (2005). The Japan Society of Mechanical Engineers, *Experimental Examination on the Therapeutic Postoperative Course of Ospharthrosis by Stress Freezing Method,* Thesis collection A, Vol71, No.703, (03. 2005), pp. 500-506, ISSN03875008

Maezaki, N. & Ezumi T. & Hachiya M. (2010). The Japan Society of Mechanical Engineers, *Clarification on Mechanical Characteristic in State of Stress of Osteoarthritis of the Hip joint using Stress Freezing Method,* The Japan Society of Mechanical Engineers, Journal of Solid Mechanics and Materials Engineering Vol.4, No.7 Special Issue of APCMM2009 II, (2010), pp.946-952 ISSN1880-9871

Maezaki, N. & Ezumi T. & Hachiya M. (2008). The Japan Society of Mechanical Engineers, *Experimental Examination on the Effects and Adaptation Condition of the Fibula Excision Method using the Stress Freezing Method on the Osteoarthritic knee,* Thesis collection A, Vol74, No.804, (05. 2008), pp. 101-108, ISSN03875008

Mansour, J, M. & Wentorf, F, A, & Degoede, K, M. (1998). Annals of biomedical engineering. *In Vivo Kinematics of the Rabbit Knee in Unstable Models of Osteoarthrosis.* Vol. 26,No.3, (08.1998),pp.353-360 , ISSN0090-6964

Murakami, T.(2008). *Introduction to Bioengineering,* ISBN978-4339070873, Tokyo, Japan

Ooi,T.&Hatsuyama,Y.&Mahuji,Y.(1987). *Rehabilitation Medicine,* Asakura-shoten, ISBN978-4254320909, Tokyo, Japan

Peter, S,W,. (1977). *Human Joints and Their Artificial Replacements,* Thomas, ISBN978-0398036157, Illinois, USA

Tadano, S. & Ukai, T. & Ochiai, H & Sasaki, T. (1999). The Japan Society of Mechanical Engineers, *Three-Dimensional Stress Analysis in Femur Before and After Total Hip Replacement* , Thesis collection A, Vol60, No.569, (01.1994), pp.278-284, ISSN03875008

Takahashi, S. & Sawa, Y. & Nogata, H. & Shimura, S. & Ezumi, T. & Morimoto, Y. & Shimamoto, K. & Suetsugu, M. & Yamaguchi, I. & Toyooka, R. & Suzuki, S. & Kurita, M. & Umesaki, E.(1997). *Photo Mechanics,* Sankaidou, ISBN978-4381100818, Tokyo, Japan

Takeishi,Y. (2000). *Introduction,* Journal of the Japanese Society for Non Destructive Inspection, Vol49, No.7, (06. 2000), p. 409, ISSN0367-5866, Tokyo, Japan

Terayama,K. & Tsuji,H.(1999). *Standard Orthopedics* (The 7th edition), Igakushoin, ISBN978-4260125819, Tokyo, Japan

The Japan Society of Mechanical Engineers.(1997). *Bio Mechanical Engineering,* The Japan Society of Mechanical Engineers, ISBN 978-4888980814, Tokyo, Japan

Tsuji, J. & Nishida, M. & Kawata, K. (1957). *Photoelasticity Experiment Method,* Nikkan Kogyo Shimbun, ISBN-non nomber, Tokyo, Japan

Xerogeanes, J, W, & Fox R. J. & Takeda, Y. & Kim, H.-S. & Ishibashi, Y. & Carlin, G, J. & Woo S, L,-Y. (1998). Annals of biomedical engineering. *A Functional Comparison of Animal Anterior Cruciate Ligament Models to the Human Anterior Cruciate Ligament,*Vol. 26,No.3 (06.1998). pp.345-352, ISSN0090-6964

Yan, X. & Kakunai, S. & Sakamoto, T. & Murakami, A. & Ikeda, D. & Fujiwara, H. (2003). The Japan Society of Mechanical Engineers, *Mechanical Evaluation of Trochanteric Fracture Fixation Methods : Comparison of Mechanical Properties Between Gamma Nail and Compression Hip Screw,* Thesis collection A, Vol69, No.681, (01. 2003), pp. 952-957, ISSN03875008

14

Motor Unit Potential Train Validation and Its Application in EMG Signal Decomposition

Hossein Parsaei and Daniel W. Stashuk
Department of Systems Design Engineering, University of Waterloo Canada

1. Introduction

Electromyographic (EMG) signal decomposition is the process of resolving an EMG signal into its constituent motor unit potential trains (MUPTs). The purpose of EMG signal decomposition is to provide an estimate of the firing pattern and motor unit potential (MUP) template of each active motor unit (MU) that contributed significant MUPs to the EMG signal. The extracted MU firing patterns, MUP templates, and their estimated feature values can assist with the diagnosis of neuromuscular disorders (Stalberg & Falck, 1997; Tröger & Dengler, 2000; Fuglsang-Frederiksen, 2006; Pino et al., 2008; Farkas et al., 2010), the understanding of motor control (De Luca et al. 1982a, 1982b; Contessa et al.,2009), and the characterization of MU architecture (Lateva & McGill, 2001), but only if they are valid trains. Depending on the complexity of the signal being decomposed, the variability of MUP shapes and MU firing patterns, and the criteria and parameters used by the decomposition algorithm to merge or split the obtained MUPTs, several invalid MUPTs may be created.

An extracted MUPT is considered valid when it accurately represents the activity of a single MU and is contaminated by low numbers of false-classification errors (FCEs). Alternatively, an invalid MUPT either represents the activity of more than one MU (i.e., it is a merged MUPT) or contains a high percentage of FCEs (i.e., it is a contaminated MUPT).

Unfortunately, the MUP template shapes and MU firing patterns of invalid MUPTs cannot be easily distinguished from those of valid trains. Often, the MUP template shape of an invalid train looks similar to that of a valid train; nevertheless, the train does not represent the MUPs of a single MU. As such, the variability of MUP shapes and possibly the MU firing pattern are greater for invalid trains compared to valid trains. If such inaccurate information is not detected and excluded from further analysis, it could improperly suggest an abnormal muscle when interpreted clinically or it may contribute to scientific misstatements. Consequently, the first and most critical step in the quantitative analysis of MUPTs is assessing their validity.

Detecting invalid trains during decomposition can assist with improving the performance of these decomposition methods in terms of estimating the correct number of MUPTs constituting an EMG signal as well as reducing the number of missed-classification errors (MCEs) and FCEs in the extracted trains. At the end of each pass of assigning MUPs to detected MUPTs, invalid MUPTs are detected and then either have their FCEs corrected or are split into valid trains. Such corrections can help find the correct number of constituent

MUPTs, lead to better estimates of the MUP template and MU firing pattern statistics of each train, and also allow more MUPs to be correctly assigned to the obtained trains (i.e., reduce MCEs) during the next steps of decomposition. Consequently, MUPT validation can improve decomposition accuracy.

The majority of the existing MUPT validation methods are either time consuming or related to operator experience and skill (see Section 3). More importantly, they cannot be executed during automatic decomposition of EMG signals to assist with improving decomposition results. To overcome these issues, an automated system is presented to estimate the validity of MUPTs extracted from an EMG signal using a decomposition algorithm. The presented system to estimate the validity of a MUPT uses both its MU firing pattern information and its MUP shape information. MU firing pattern information is employed by a supervised classifier that determines MU firing pattern validity by assessing MU firing pattern consistency and MU firing pattern variability of the train under question. MUP shape information is used by a cluster validation-based algorithm that assesses the MUP shape consistency in the given train to determine its MUP shape validity. A train is considered valid based on a combination of its MU firing pattern and MUP shape validity. The MUP validation system can be used both during EMG signal decomposition and once the process is completed.

The effectiveness of using the developed MUPT validation systems and the MUPT editing methods during EMG signal decomposition was investigated by integrating these algorithms into a certainty-based EMG signal decomposition algorithm. During decomposition, invalid MUPTs are detected and then either have their FCEs corrected or are split into valid trains before decomposition continues. The minimum assignment threshold for each extracted MUPT is adjusted based on the estimated validity. With these modifications, the decomposition accuracy on average was improved 9% on average.

This chapter includes a brief review of the composition and decomposition of EMG signals, a discussion of MUPT validation concepts, a description of a system developed for automatic validation of MUPTs during EMG decomposition, and a discussion of a decomposition system that uses the proposed MUPT validation algorithm to merge or split MUPTs and to adjust the assignment threshold for each MUPT adaptively. Evaluation results using several simulated and real EMG signals and a discussion of the results will be presented at the last section.

2. EMG signal composition and decomposition

To appreciate the concepts of EMG signal decomposition, it is crucial to be familiar with the composition of an EMG signal. This section presents the fundamentals of EMG signal composition followed by a discussion of EMG signal decomposition.

2.1 EMG signal composition

An EMG signal is the sequence of voltages detected from a contracting muscle over time. The potentials are detected in the voltage field generated by the active muscle fibres of a contracting muscle. The muscle fibres of a muscle are organized into groups for the control of muscle force with each muscle fibre of a group being connected to an α-motor neuron. Each muscle fibre of a group is activated concurrently by the α-motor neuron to which they are connected. Formally, a single α-motor neuron, its axon and the set of connected muscle fibres are called a MU (Basmajian & De Luca, 1985). The summation of the muscle fibre potentials created by the spatially and temporally dispersed depolarization and repolarization of all of the excited fibres of a single MU is known as MUP.

During a muscle contraction, MUs fire repetitively to maintain the force of the muscle contraction. Consequently, each active MU generates a train of MUPs during a muscle contraction known as MUPT. A MUPT is mathematically described as (De Luca, 1979; Basmajian & De Luca, 1985; Stashuk, 2001; Parsaei et al., 2010):

$$\mathrm{MUPT}_j(t) = \sum_{i=1}^{M} \mathrm{MUP}_{ji}\left(t-\delta_{ji}\right) \tag{1}$$

where M is the number of times that the jth motor unit fires, δ_{ji} is the ith firing time of motor unit j, and $\mathrm{MUP}_{ji}(t)$ is the ith MUP generated by motor unit j during its ith firing.

Assuming K MUs were active during a muscle contraction, the detected EMG signal can be mathematically represented as (De Luca,1979; Basmajian & De Luca, 1985; Stashuk, 2001; Parsaei et al., 2010):

$$\mathrm{EMG}(t) = \sum_{j=1}^{K} \mathrm{MUPT}_j(t) + n(t) \tag{2}$$

where $\mathrm{MUPT}_j(t)$ is the MUPT generated by the jth motor unit, and $n(t)$ is background noise.

Fig.1 shows both an anatomical and physiological model for an EMG signal. In this figure, $h_i(t)$ is a filter with impulse response MUP_i, and the impulses represent action potentials emerging from an α- motor neuron to innervate the connected muscle fibers. As shown, an EMG signal is in fact the superposition of the MUPTs created by MUs active during a muscle contraction and background noise.

The characteristics of a detected EMG signal depend on several factors such as the level of contraction, the shape and size of the electrode used, and the position and orientation of the electrode relative to the muscle fibres of the active MUs (De Luca, 1979; Basmajian & De Luca, 1985). In addition, the characteristics of an EMG signal detected from a contacting muscle are related to the anatomical and physiological features of the muscle and therefore to its age and state of health or fatigue(Stalberg & Falck, 1997; Tröger & Dengler, 2000; Fuglsang-Frederiksen, 2006; Pino et al., 2008; Farkas et al., 2010). Some parameters of EMG signals for normal and abnormal muscles are compared in Table 1. Consequently, analyzing EMG signals provides information that can be used clinically or for physiological investigation. The technique of detecting, evaluating, and analyzing EMG signals is known as electromyography. One useful technique in electromyography is EMG signal decomposition.

2.2 EMG signal decomposition

EMG signal decomposition is the process of resolving a detected EMG signal into is constituent MUPTs. This process that is conceptually shown in Fig.2 is implemented by employing digital signal processing and pattern recognition techniques in four/five steps:

signal preprocessing, signal segmentation and MUP detection, feature extraction, and then clustering and possibly supervised classification of detected MUPs (Stashuk, 2001; Parsaei et al., 2010).The first step is to remove background noise and low-frequency information from the detected EMG signal, to shorten the duration of MUPs and decrease MUP temporal overlap, and to sharpen the MUPs and increase discrimination between them. The second step is to section the signal into segments containing possible MUPs that were generated by active MUs that contributed significantly to the detected EMG signal. The detected MUPs are represented by a feature vector in the third steps and finally are sorted into MUPTs using clustering and/or supervised classification technniques. If a full or complete decomposition is required, superimposed MUPs (SMUPs) are resolved into their constituent MUPs in another step. For clinical use of EMG signal decomposition results, where only mean MU firing rate and MU firing rate variability are to be studied, resolving SMUPs is not essential (Stashuk,1999,2001) because the desired MU firing parameters can be estimated from incomplete discharge patterns (Stashuk & Qu, 1996b; Stashuk, 1999). However, for detailed studies of MU control and muscle architecture, SMUPs must be resolved. A recent comprehensive review of the algorithms developed for the decomposition of indwelling EMG signals is provided by Parsaei et.al. (2010).

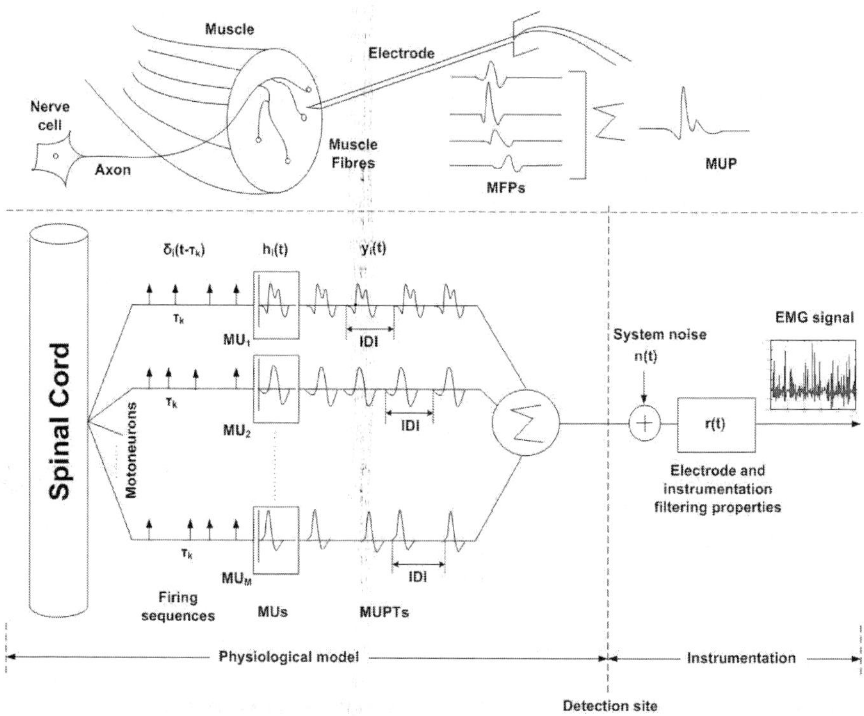

Fig. 1. Anatomical and physiological model for an EMG signal (from Rasheed et al., 2010).

EMG parameter	Normal	Myogenic	Neurogenic
Interference pattern	Full 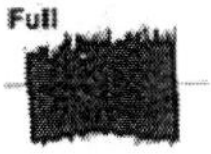	Full 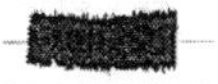 Low Amplitude	Reduced 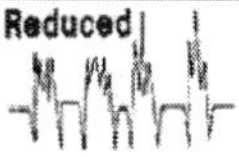 High Amplitude
Motor unit potential	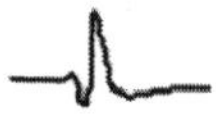	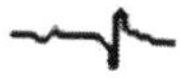 Small Unit	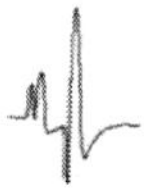 Large Unit

Table 1. Some parameters of EMG signals for normal and abnormal muscles.

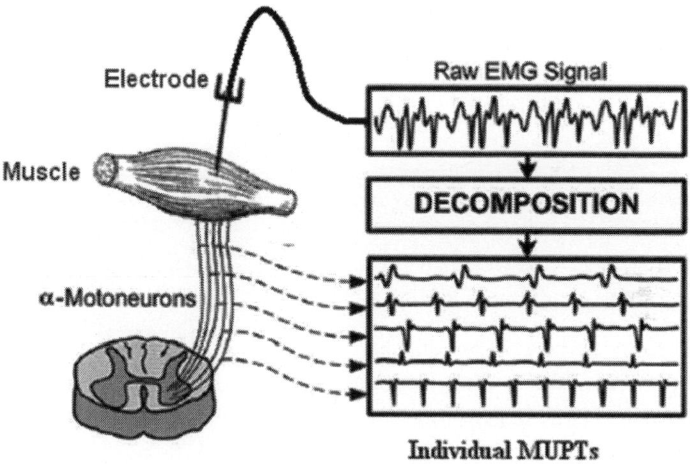

Fig. 2. A schematic representation of EMG signal decomposition (adapted from De Luca et al. 2006; 1982a).

Once the decomposition process is completed, the prototypical MUP shape (MUP template) and MU firing pattern statistics for each extracted MUPT are estimated for future analysis (especially for quantitative electromyography). This provides information, regarding the temporal behaviour and morphological layout of the MUs that significantly contributed to the detected EMG signal, which can assist with the diagnosis of various neuromuscular diseases and the study of MU control, and lead to a better understanding of healthy, pathological, ageing or fatiguing neuromuscular systems (De Luca et al., 1982a, 1982b; Stalberg & Falck, 1997; Tröger & Dengler, 2000; Stashuk, 2001; Fuglsang-Frederiksen, 2006; Calder et al., 2008; Farkas et al., 2010). However, this is achieved only when this information is valid. In fact, before using decomposition results and the MUP shape and MU firing pattern information for either clinical or research purposes the validity of the extracted MUPTs needs to be confirmed.

3. MUPT validation

In general, validating a MUPT is a process of determining whether a given MUPT accurately represents the activity of a single MU or not. The validity of a MUPT can be defined using two different criteria: MU firing pattern validity, and MUP shape validity.

MU firing pattern validity of a MUPT is determined by assessing its inter-discharge interval (IDI) histogram (density function) and the instantaneous firing rate of the corresponding MU versus time. The MU discharges corresponding to a valid MUPT occur at regular intervals and in general, have a Gaussian-shaped IDI histogram while for invalid MUPTs the IDIs have large variations and will not have a Gaussian-shaped IDI histogram. Even though some researchers have demonstrated that the IDI distribution of a MU may not actually be Gaussian (De Luca & Forrest,1973; Matthews, 1996), for MUPTs of MUs that are consistently recruited, the Gaussian density is an appropriate approximation (Clamann, 1969; McGill et al., 1985; McGill & Dorfman, 1985; Stashuk, 1999; Moritz et al., 2005; Rasheed et al., 2010;Parsaei et al.,2011). If an extracted MUPT represents the firing of a single MU and has suitably low percentage of FCEs (FCE rate), it has MU firing pattern validity. As an example, the first two MUPTs shown in Fig. 3 have MU firing pattern validity, but the third MUPT does not have firing pattern validity.

To determine MUP shape validity, a given train is assessed using the shapes of its MUPs. Assuming the MUPs generated by a single MU are homogeneous in shape, the MUPT under study can be assumed to have MUP-shape validity when its MUPs have consistent shapes. As an example, MUPTs shown in the first and third rows of Fig. 3 have MUP-shape validity; however, the MUPT given in the second row does not have MUP–shape validity.

Finally, a train can be considered valid based on a combination of its MU firing pattern and MUP shape validity. For example, the first MUPT shown in Fig. 3, which has both MU firing pattern and MUP shape validity, is considered valid, but the MUPTs shown in rows 2 and 3 will be labelled invalid because they do not have MUP–shape or MU firing pattern validity.

To date, MUPT validation is mainly conducted qualitatively by an expert operator. The MUP shape validity of a MUPT is assessed by an expert using raster/shimmer plots of its assigned MUPs (Doherty & Stashuk,2003; Stashuk, 2001; Stashuk et al., 2004; Boe et al., 2005, Calder et al., 2008; Parsaei et al., 2010). MU firing pattern validity of a MUPT is determined by viewing and qualitative evaluation of its IDI histogram and the plots of the firing rate as a function of time. The accuracy of such qualitative MUPT evaluations, as with other methods that need operator supervision, depends on operator experience and skill. In addition, such evaluations are too time consuming to be practically completed in a busy clinical environment. More importantly, manual MUPT validation methods cannot assist with improving the performance of automatic EMG signal decomposition algorithms. To overcome these issues, methods need to be developed to automatically estimate the validity of a given MUPT.

McGill and Marateb (2010) developed a rigorous statistical method for assessing the validity of MUPTs extracted by decomposing an EMG signal. The evaluation results are encouraging, but due to the computational complexity of the procedures used in this method, the algorithm is only efficient for assessing the decomposition accuracy of 5-second-long, low-complexity signals composed of at most 6 MUPTs. In addition, full decomposition in required in this method. Therefore, this method cannot be used during decomposing or in a busy clinical environment.

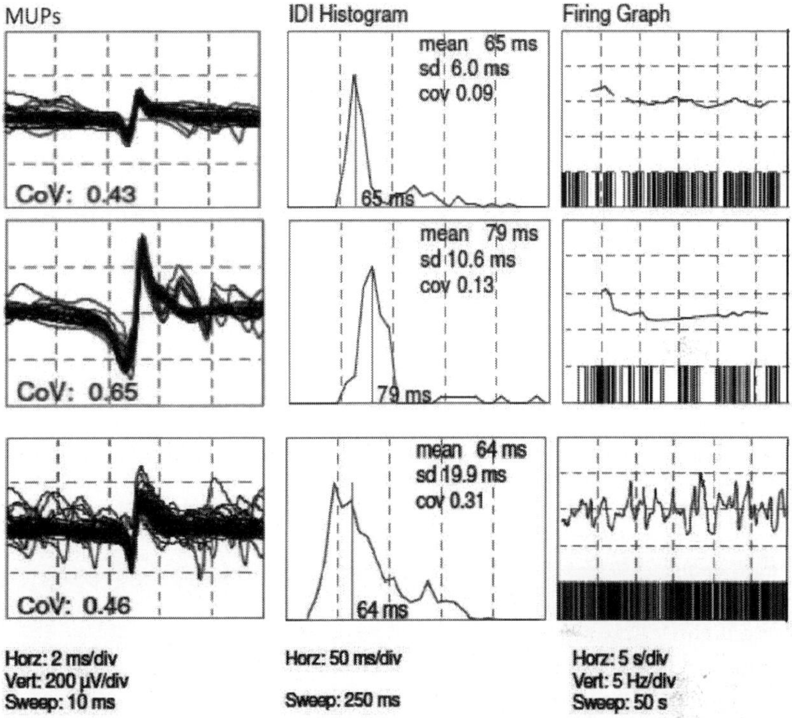

Fig. 3. Example of valid and invalid MUPTs. Column one shows the the shimmer plot of the MUPs assigned to each MUPT. Column two shows the IDI histogram and corresponding statistics for each extracted MUPT. Column three illustractes the discharge patterns and instantaneous firing rates for each MU.

Parsaei and his co-workers (Parsaei et al., 2011; Parsaei&Stashuk, 2011a) developed several methods for automatic validation of MUPTs extracted by a decomposition algorithm: a MU firing pattern based validation method, and a MUP shape based validation method. Across the sets of real and simulated data used for evaluating each of these two MUPT validation methods, the methods performed well in categorizing a train correctly. In addition these methods are fast enough to be used during the decomposition process. However, the accuracy of the firing pattern validity system in correctly classifying invalid trains decreases as the MCE rate (percentage of MCEs) in the MUPTs increases such that this accuracy was reduced to < 60% when the MCE rate was >80%. Likewise, the accuracy of the MUP-shape validation methods decreases as the separability between the trains used to create an invalid train decreases such that the methods failed to detect the majority (>80%) of invalid trains composed of MUPTs with highly similar MUP templates. In this work, using both the MU firing pattern and MUP shape information of a MUPT to estimate its validity was explored with the hope of overcoming these two issues; the achievements of these efforts are presented in this chapter. The objective of developing such methods was to: 1) facilitate the use of intramuscular EMG signal decomposition results for clinical applications of quantitative electromyography by providing the overall validity of MUPTs and excluding or highlighting invalid MUPTs; 2) assist with improving the accuracy and completeness of decomposition results. Using the characteristics of the IDI distribution, MU firing patterns, and within train MUP shape variability of invalid MUPTs two methods based on a combination of feature extraction, cluster validation techniques and supervised classification algorithms were developed; details are presented in the following Section.

4. An automated system for estimating MUPT validity

As discussed in the previous section and illustrated in Fig.3, the characteristics of IDI histograms, MU firing rates over time, and within-train MUP shape inconsistencies of invalid trains differ from those of valid trains. These facts motivate the development of an automated system to determine whether a given MUPT accurately represents the activity of a single MU (i.e., is valid) or not. With the developed MUPT validation method, a given train is considered valid if it has both MU firing pattern validity and MUP-shape validity; otherwise, the train is labelled invalid. MU firing pattern validity is estimated by a firing pattern validity classifier (FPVC) that uses a supervised classifier along with several features extracted from the IDI histo-gram and instantaneous firing rate of the MUPT. MUP-shape validity is determined by assessing the homogeneity of the wave shape of the MUPs of the given train using a MUP-shape validity system that is mainly based on a cluster validation technique. The overall procedure of the system is illustrated in Fig.4. Both the MU firing pattern system and MUP-shape validation system used are discussed below.

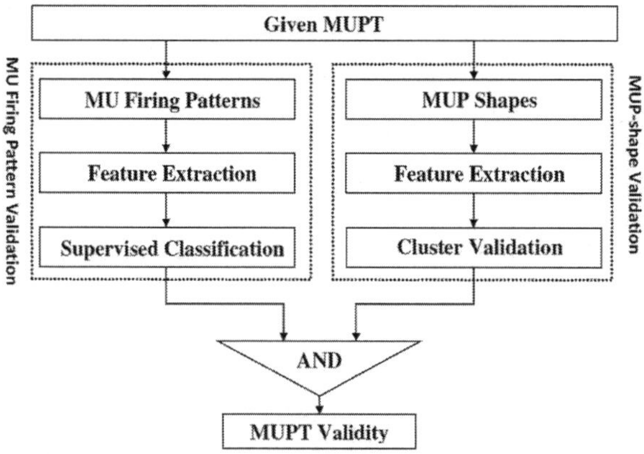

Fig. 4. The procedure of the developed MUPT validation system that estimates the validity of a MUPT by combining its MU firing pattern validity and MUP shape validity estimated using a supervised classifier and a cluster validation technique.

4.1 Firing pattern validity classifier

The overall procedure of the developed FPVC is shown in Fig. 5. The goal of using the FPVC is to determine whether a MUPT accurately represents the firings of a single MU or not. This categorization is performed by a supervised classifier that uses nine features extracted from the IDI histograms and MU firing rates of the given MUPT.

The features used in this work are listed in Table 2; detailed definitions and calculation methods for these features are presented in (Parsaei et al., 2011; Parsaei, 2011). In short, the majority of these features are extracted from the IDI distribution of the given MUPT and target the left side of this distribution, where short IDIs (i.e., the errors of interest) are reflected. The identification rate targets the right side of the IDI distribution to measure the MCE rate in the MUPT. The firing rate mean consecutive difference measures the variation in the instantaneous firing rate over time. The instantaneous firing rate at each MUP occurrence in a MUPT is defined as the inverse of a local IDI that is obtained by applying a normalized Hamming filter of length 11 to the IDIs of the train.

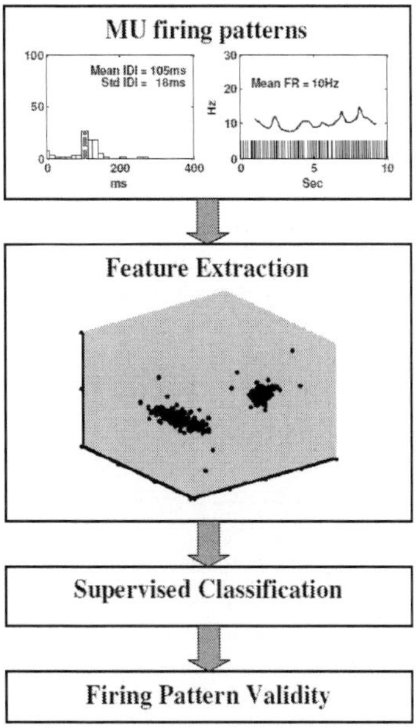

Fig. 5. The steps for the firing pattern validity classifier

Feature	Description
CV	Coefficient of variation
CV_L	Lower coefficient of variation
CV_L/CV_U	The ratio of lower and upper CV
PI	Percentage of inconsistent IDIs
$LIDI_R$	Lower IDI ratio
1stSCorr	First coefficient of serial correlation
Skewness	A measure of symmetry of the IDI histogram
ID- rate	Identification rate
FR-MCD	Firing rate mean consecutive difference
IDI-MCD	IDI mean consecutive difference

Table 2. Firing pattern features used for the firing pattern validity classifier.

For supervised classification, a support vector machine (SVM) classifier (Vapnik, 1999), which uses a Gaussian radial basis function (Eq.3) as a kernel, was employed.

$$K(x,x') = \exp(-\frac{\|x-x'\|^2}{2\sigma^2}) \quad (3)$$

where x is an input data point to a SVM, x' is the centre of the kernel and σ^2 is the width of the kernel specified a priori by the user. In training a SVM, in addition to σ^2 there is another parameter that has to be selected by the user, the cost parameter, C. This parameter, which is also known as the regularization parameter, controls the trade off between allowing training errors and the complexity of the machine. For the objectives of this work, σ^2 and C were determined experimentally using cross-validation.

4.2 MUP –shape validity system

Assuming the MUPs generated by a single MU are homogeneous in shape (but with possibly different degrees of variability across different MUs), the MUP-shape validity of a MUPT can be estimated by assessing the shape consistency of its MUPs. Overall, the process of EMG signal decomposition can be considered a clustering problem because neither the number of MUPTs (i.e., clusters) nor the labels of the MUPs are known in advance. During EMG signal decomposition, detected MUPs are clustered into groups called MUPTs. Therefore, the MUP-shape validation of a MUPT extracted by a decomposition algorithm can be considered a cluster validity problem and the decision to be made is whether the extracted MUPT represents one cluster in terms of the shapes of the assigned MUPs or not. For this purpose, in this work the Beal method (Gordon, 1999), and the Duda and Hart (DH) method (Duda et al., 2000), which are presented for estimating the numbers of clusters in a data set, were employed to develop two automated MUP-shape validation systems. Although numerous methods have been developed to estimate the number of groups in a dataset (Milligan & Cooper, 1985; Gordon, 1999), the majority of these methods cannot be used for assessing MUP-shape validity of a MUPT because of one of these two reasons: a) they cannot be used for testing one cluster versus multiple clusters in a dataset; b) they are computationally too expensive to be used for online validation of MUPTs and especially during EMG signal decomposition (Parsaei, 2011; Parsaei & Stashuk, 2011a).

For a data set consisting of N observations (patterns) each of which repented by d uncorrelated feature values, both the Beal and DH methods test the existence of clusters in the data set by comparing its within cluster dispersion (W_1) to the resulting within cluster dispersion when it is partitioned into two clusters using a clustering algorithm (W_2). The parameter W_K (k=1,2) is usually given by

$$W_K = \sum_{i=1}^{K} \sum_{X \in C_i} (X - m_i)(X - m_i)^T \quad (4)$$

where X is a vector of features representing each object of the given data set, m_i is the sample mean of the N_i objects assigned to cluster C_i.

For the Beal method (Gordon, 1999), the null hypothesis of a single cluster is rejected in favor of multiple clusters if:

$$Bi = \frac{\left(\frac{W_2 - W_1}{W_2}\right)}{\left(\frac{N-1}{N-2}\right)2^{2/d} - 1} > F_{critical} \tag{5}$$

where the value for $F_{critical}$ is obtained from an $F_{d,(N-2)d}$ distribution at an α level of significance.

For the DH method (Duda et al., 2000), the null hypothesis of one cluster is rejected if

$$J = \frac{\left(-\frac{W_2}{W_1} + 1 - \frac{2}{\pi d}\right)}{\sqrt{\frac{2\left(1 - \frac{8}{\pi^2 d}\right)}{Nd}}} > z \tag{6}$$

where z is given by $\alpha = 50\left(1 - erf(\frac{z}{\sqrt{2}})\right)$.

The effectiveness of Beal and DH methods in estimating the MUP–shape validity of a MUPT was investigated using some simulated MUPTs (see Section 6 for the description of the simulated data). For a given MUPT, each of its MUPs is represented using the 80 low-pass differencing (LPD) filtered data samples centred about its peak value (i.e., d=80) and then the MUP– shape validity of the given train was determined using one of these two methods. To split the given train into two clusters, the K-means algorithm was used.

The LPD filtered samples were used instead of unfiltered samples because they discriminate between the MUPs generated by different MUs better than the raw. The 1st-order LPD filter (McGill et al., 1985) used is, in fact, a two-point central difference algorithm (Semmlow, 2004) that acts as a differentiator for the lower frequencies and as a low-pass filter for higher frequencies. Given that x[n], n=1,2, ..,80 are the discrete time samples of a MUP, the LPD filtered output for these time samples, y[n], are calculated as

$$y[n] = \frac{x[n+L] - x[n-L]}{2LT_s} \tag{7}$$

where L is the skip factor and T_S is the sampling interval.

It is worth pointing out that a 2nd-order LPD filter was also evaluated for filtering the MUPs, but the accuracy obtained for classifying valid MUPTs was drastically decreased compared to the accuracy obtained when the MUPs are filtered using a 1st-order LPD filter. Therefore, a 1st-order LPD filter is preferred to a 2nd-order one.

Preliminary tests showed that when representing MUPs using LPD filtered time samples, neither the Beal method (Gordon, 1999) nor the DH method (Duda et al., 2000) (each with α =0.05) was accurate in correctly classifying valid trains. Their accuracy for classifying a valid train correctly was only 5% while that for an invalid train was 99%. The reason for the low accuracy for valid MUPTs were discovered to be: 1) the 80 LPD filtered time samples used as features are highly correlated; 2) the algorithms are sensitive to the inherent MUP shape variability in the valid MUPTs caused by jitter or jiggle (Stålberg & Sonoo, 1994); valid MUPTs with high jitter or jiggle are erroneously classified as invalid trains. To overcome these two issues, an adaptive method based on a combination of feature extraction techniques and the Beal orDH method was developed. An overview of the system is given in Fig. 6. A brief description of each step is given below, detailed discussion can be found elsewhere (Parsaei, 2011; Parsaei & Stashuk, 2011a).

4.2.1 Prepossessing

Preprocessing was completed to increase the signal-to-noise ratio (SNR) of the MUPs, sharpen MUPs, and ultimately enhance the discrimination between the MUPs created by two or more different MUs but mistakenly assigned to one MUPT. For this purposes, MUPs of a MUPT each of which represented using 80 time samples are filtered using a LPD filter (Eq. 7). Fig. 7 shows the effectiveness for a MUPT that consists of the MUPs of two MUs. As shown, LPD filtering increased the distinguishability of the MUPs and ultimately clarified that the given train is an invalid train.

4.2.2 Feature extraction

The feature extraction step is to extract/select effective, uncorrelated, and discriminative features out of the 80 LPD filtered sample points used to represent the MUPs of a MUPT. These features can be extracted using principal component analysis (PCA), however due to computational complexity of the PCA, a PCA-based MUPT validation algorithm will be slow and ultimately will not be efficient to be used during EMG decomposition (Parsaei, 2011; Parsaei &Stashuk, 2011a). In this work a gap-based feature selection technique which is based on the way that a human would assess the validity of a MUPT using its MUP shimmer plot was employed for feature extraction. A human operator visually assesses the consistency of the shapes of the MUPs assigned to a MUPT by inspecting the existence of any gap or obvious differences between specific MUP time sample values. With the proposed gap-based feature selection, the regions in which the MUPs of a MUPT are significantly different are identified first and then the m samples for which the MUPs are significantly differ from each other are identified and used as the effective features representing the MUPs of the MUPT. Such regions that are called here "active parts" for the MUPT under study are determined by calculating gap values (GVs) for the train. Let $y_i[n]$ n=1,2,...,80 represent the 80 LPD filtered time samples of the ith MUP in the given MUPT. At each n, the largest adjacent change in the N sorted $y_i[n]$ values is GV[n]. An active part is a consecutive set of GV[n] values greater than the baseline noise. More details for estimating gap values for a MUPT are given in (Parsaei, 2011; Parsaei &Stashuk, 2011a).

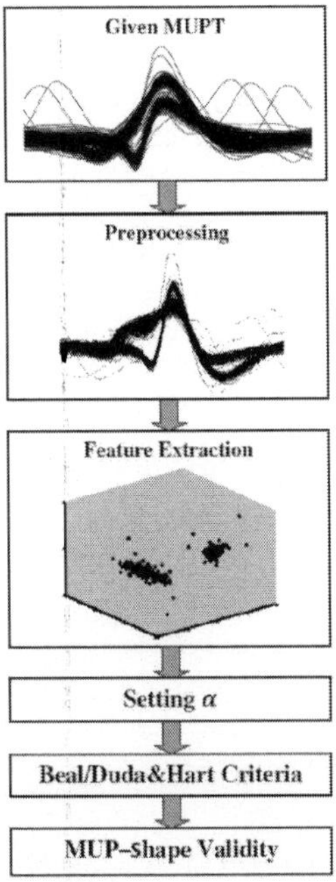

Fig. 6. An overview of the MUP–shape validation system.

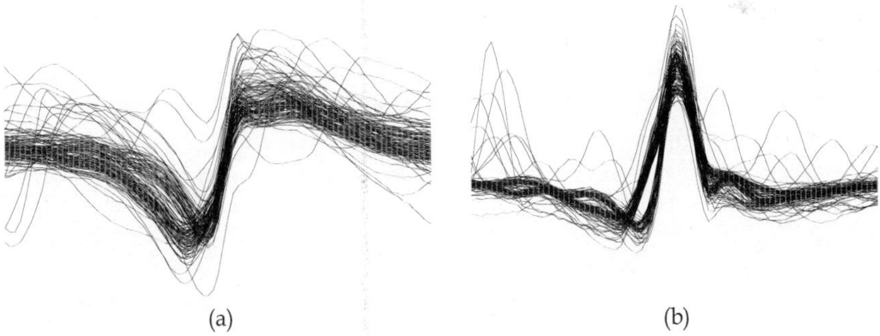

Fig. 7. The effect of preprocessing the MUPs of a MUPT. (a) raw MUPs , (b) LPD filterd MUPs. Such a figure previously presented by McGill et al. (1985).

Given gap values and active parts are respectively estimated and identified for the MUPT under study, the sample corresponding to the maximum gap value in each active part is chosen as an effective feature. Consequently, the number of selected features will be equal to the number of active parts. Additional features, if required are selected based on their gap-values and also their intervals from the previous selected features. Each feature should have the maximum gap value among the remaining samples and also be at least eight samples (i.e. 0.26 ms) before or after any selected features.

4.2.3 Setting the parameter α

The objective of setting the value for parameter α, that is the significance level for rejecting the null hypothesis of valid train, is to make the algorithm less likely to reject the MUP-shape validity of a given MUPT when its MUPs are very similar to each other, and more likely to reject this null hypothesis when the MUPs of a MUPT are less similar to each other. To achieve this, the value of parameter α is set adaptively by first splitting a considered MUPT into two sub-trains using the K-means algorithm. The pseudo-correlation (PsC) between the MUP templates of the two sub-trains is then calculated as a measure of their similarity. Denoting S_1 and S_2 as the MUP templates of the two sub-trains, the PsC value between these templates is defined as (Florestal et al., 2006):

$$\mathrm{PsC} = \max\left\{0, \frac{\sum_{i=1}^{80}\left(S_1[i].S_2[i+t] - \left|S_1[i] - S_2[i+t]\right| \max\left\{S_1[i], S_2[i+t]\right\}\right)}{\sum_{i=1}^{80} \max\left\{S_1[i], S_2[i+t]\right\}^2}\right\} \tag{8}$$

where $S_1[i]$ and $S_2[i]$ are the samples of the two templates S_1 and S_2, respectively. When calculating PsC, t ranges from -5 to +5 (corresponding to 0.32 ms) and the maximum value is selected.

Having a PsC value, the parameter α is defined as follows (Parsaei&Stashuk, 2011a):

$$\alpha = \begin{cases} 0.03 & PsC \geq 0.75 \\ 0.05 & 0.4 \leq PsC < 0.75 \\ 0.1 & 0.3 \leq PsC < 0.4 \\ 0.2 & PsC < 0.3 \end{cases} \tag{9}$$

4.2.4 Estimating MUP–shape validity

The MUP–shape validity which in this work is "1" when the shapes of the MUPs of a train are consistent and "0" vice versa is estimated using either Beal criterion or DH criterion as follows:

a. Using the Beal criteria: If Bi $< F_{d,(N-2)d}$ at an α level of significance, MUP–shape validity=1; otherwise MUP–shape validity=0.
b. Using DH method: If J<z, MUP–shape validity=1; otherwise MUP–shape validity=0.

In the remaining of this Chapter, the MUP–shape validation system that is based on the Beal criterion (Gordon,1999) is called the SVB method and the one developed using the Duda and Hart criterion (Duda et al., 2000) is called SVDH method.

5. Application of MUPT validation in EMG decomposition

The hypothesis is that if invalid trains are detected and corrected during EMG decomposition, especially during the classification step, the decomposition accuracy will be improved. The effectiveness of using the developed MUPT validation system during EMG signal decomposition was studied by integrating this system into a certainty-based EMG signal decomposition algorithm used in the DQEMG (Stashuk, 1999). In the original certainty-based EMG signal decomposition, the detected MUPs are grouped into several MUPTs using a shape and temporal-based clustering (STBC) algorithm (Stashuk&Qu, 1996a) and a supervised certainty-based classifier (CBC). The STBC algorithm is a customized K-means clustering method that uses both MUP shape and MU firing pattern information to cluster MUPs. In the STBC, MUPTs are split or merged based on several heuristic criteria. Assuming the MUPTs provided by the STBC algorithm are valid, they are augmented by the CBC algorithm (Stashuk&Paoli, 1998) in which a MUP is assigned to the MUPT that has the greatest certainty value, if this value is greater than a certainty assignment threshold (C_{AT}). Otherwise, the MUP is left unassigned. In the CBC algorithm, two MUPTs are merged if the resulting MUPT satisfies several predefined heuristic criteria but the MUPTs are not split nor assessed for splitting. The new decomposition system presented in this chapter employs the developed MUPT validation system —instead of those heuristic, user defined criteria—to merge or split MUPTs. The new system also adjusts the C_{AT} value for each individual MUPT adaptively based its validity. The new decomposition program, which is called the validity-based EMG decomposition system, consists of four major steps: signal preprocessing, MUP detection, and clustering and supervised classification of the detected MUPs.

5.1 Signal preprocessing

The signal preprocessing step is involved with filtering the signal to improve the SNR of the signal, decrease MUP temporal overlap, to accentuate the differences between MUPs created by different MUs, and to increase the separation between MUPs and the background noise. For this purpose, a 1st-order LPD filter (McGill et al., 1985) is employed. Fig.8 shows the effectiveness of LPD filtering an EMG signal. As shown, filtering flattens the signal baseline and makes the MUPs more narrow and recognizable.

5.2 MUP detection

MU detection identifies the position of the MUPs in a given EMG signal. The positions of suitable MUPs in the filtered signal are detected using a threshold crossing technique by which the prefilterd EMG signal is scanned and the peaks that satisfy several criteria (Stashuk, 1999) are detected and considered as the occurrence times of MUPs. In general, the amplitudes of detected MUPs are higher than the baseline noise. Fig. 8 illustrates the segmentation procedure for an EMG signal.

For clustering and supervised classification, each detected MUP is represented using the 80 filtered data samples (i.e., 2.56 ms at 31250 Hz sampling rate), centered about its peak value (i.e., about the position of maximum slope of the unfiltered MUP data).

5.3 Clustering of the detected MUPs

Detected MUPs are clustered to obtain the initial information required for supervised classification such as estimates of the number of MUPTs, their prototypical MUP shapes (or templates), and their MU firing pattern statistics. To extract such information, the MUPs detected in a specified portion (a 5 second interval with the highest number of detected MUPs) of the EMG signal are input to the STBC algorithm (Stashuk & Qu, 1996a) that groups the detected MUPs into several MUPTs using both firing time and shape information across multiple iterations. The initial estimate of the number of clusters (number of active MUs) is equal to the maximum number of MUPs and the initial cluster centers are the actual MUPs in the 30 ms interval within the selected 5 second interval. Having estimates for the number of clusters and their centers, each detected MUP is assigned to the closest cluster, if its distance to the core of the closest cluster is smaller than 0.25 times that of the second smallest distance from the candidate MUP and the cluster centers. In the STBC, a MUPT will be split into two trains if it includes a MU firing pattern inconsistency. Similar MUPTs are merged if their MUP templates are close and the firing pattern of the merged MUPT satisfies several criteria. The MUP assignment, cluster splitting, editing, and merging steps are repeated until the resulting MUPTs are stable. Details of the STBC algorithm can be found in (Stashuk & Qu, 1996a).

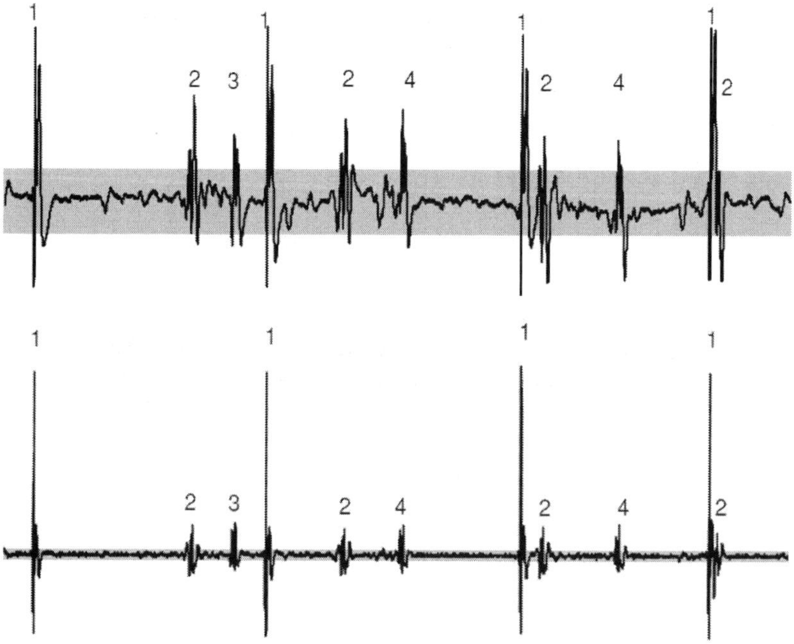

Fig. 8. The effectiveness of LPD filtering and the segmentation procedure for an EMG signal. A portion of the signal containing ten MUPs (top row). The LPD filtering results for this portion. Gray region shows the estimated level of baseline noise.

5.4 Supervised classification of detected MUPs

Having the initial information about possible MUPTs provided by the clustering step, the detected MUPs are assigned to MUPTs using a supervised classifier. The objective here is to assign each MUP to the MUPT for which the MUP's time of occurrence and shape are more consistent with respect to the MU firing times and MUP shapes of the selected MUPT, respectively, than to the other MUPTs. Each of the MUPTs should have low MCE and FCE rates and represent the activity of a single MU that contributed detected MUPs to the given EMG signal. In this work, a new adaptive certainty-based classifier was developed for this purpose.

The CCB (Stashuk & Paoli, 1998) is a supervised classifier that combines both MUP shape and MU firing pattern information to calculate the confidence of assigning a candidate MUP (let's say MUP_j) to a MUPT. The certainties for assigning MUP_j are evaluated for the two trains that have the most and the next most similar MUP templates found by calculating the Euclidian distance between MUP_j and the MUP template of each MUPT. The certainties are calculated by combining MUP shape and MU firing pattern certainties. MUP shape certainty includes normalized absolute shape certainty (C_{ND}) and relative shape certainty (C_{RD}). The first represents the distance from MUPj to the template of a train, normalized by the energy of the template. The second represents the distance from MUP_j to the most similar MUP template relative to the distance of MUP_j to the next most similar MUP template. Firing pattern certainty, C_{FC}, measures the consistency of the occurrence time of MUP_j relative to the established MU firing pattern of a MUPT. Having the shape certainties and the firing pattern certainty, the overall certainties for assigning the MUP_j to one of the two selected MUPTs are estimated by multiplying the shape and firing pattern certainties as

$$C_i^j = C_{ND\ i}^j \times C_{RD\ i}^j \times C_{FC\ i}^j ;\ i = 1,2 \tag{10}$$

where C_i^j is the overall certainty of assigning MUP_j to $MUPT_i$ which is one of the two closest MUPT to MUP_j. Having C_i^j, MUP_j is assigned to the MUPT that has the greatest certainty value, if this value is greater than a C_{AT}. Otherwise, the MUP is left unassigned.

In order to accommodate non-stationarity in MUP shapes, the algorithm updates the MUP templates with each MUP assignment. The MUP templates are calculated using a moving average for which the weights are the certainties with which MUPs are assigned to the MUPTs. If MUP_j is assigned to $MUPT_i$ with certainty C_i^j higher than the updating threshold (0.6 in this work) the template of $MUPT_i$ (S_i) is updated as (Stashuk & Paoli, 1998):

$$S_i^{New} = \frac{S_i + C_i^j \times a_j}{1 + C_i^j} \tag{11}$$

where a_j is the feature vector of MUP_j .

Once each classification pass through the set of detected MUPs is completed and before decomposition (the next pass) continues, the validity of each extracted MUPT is assessed using the system discussed in Section 4. Invalid trains are detected, corrected and have their C_{AT} values adjusted. Merged MUPTs are split into valid trains using the K-means clustering algorithm; contaminated MUPTs have their FCEs corrected using an automated MUPT editing algorithm (Parsaei&Stashuk, 2011b).

To decrease the number of MCEs and FCEs in the MUPTs, the C_{AT} value for each MUPT is adjusted based on its validity (i.e., an adaptive adjustment of the assignment threshold). For invalid MUPTs (either merged or contaminated), the C_{AT} is increased by a step of 0.005 while the C_{AT} of valid trains is decreased by 0.005. The C_{AT} value of a MUPT is not decreased or increased below 0.005 or above 0.990, respectively.

In addition to splitting or editing invalid MUPTs, the chance of merging single MUPTs is evaluated. Pairs of MUPTs that have similar MUP templates (PsC ≥ 0.4) are merged if the resulting train is valid.

The MU firing pattern statistics of each MUPT are estimated using an error-filtered estimation algorithm that provides accurate estimates of these IDI statistics of a MUPT even when contaminated by a high MCE rate (Stashuk&Qu, 1996b). The MUP assignment and MUPT splitting, editing, and merging steps are repeated until either, the maximum number of iterations is exceeded or the MUPTs are stable. If trains are merged or split at least one more supervised classification pass will be completed.

6. Evaluation

The performance of both the MUPT validation system and the new decomposition algorithm was evaluated using both simulated and real data. For this purpose, the simulated and real reference data described in (Parsaei&Stashuk, 2011a) were used.

The simulated data was generated using a physiologically-based EMG signal simulation algorithm [54]. Two hundred and sixty one, 30-second-long, EMG signals with different levels of intensity, ranging from 24 to 193 pulses per second (pps), with MUP jitter values ranging from 50 to 150μs, with IDI variability (i.e., IDI-CV) ranging from 0.10 to 0.45, and with various myopathic or neurogenic degrees of involvement ranging from 0 to 50% were created.

The real data was comprised of three sets of EMG signals: single-channel EMG signals provided by Nikolic (2001); single-channel EMG signals provided by McGill (n.d.); and multi-channel (6 to 8) EMG signals provided by Florestal et al. (2009). In using the multi-channel EMG signals, the signals detected by each electrode were considered as single-channel EMG signals. These three data sets allowed us to study the performance of the developed methods across signals detected using different electrodes and instruments.

6.1 Evaluating MUPT validation system

For evaluting MUPT validation system, the simulated EMG signals were decomposed using the DQEMG algorithms (Hamilton-Wright & Stashuk, 2005). The resulting MUPTs were assessed visually and classified as valid or invalid. Additional valid trains were generated by selecting valid MUPTs with greater than 100 MUPs and randomly splitting them into sub-trains of at least 50 MUPs. Additional invalid trains that are representative of invalid trains likely to be produced by a decomposition algorithm were generated by merging valid trains having similar MUP templates (PsC ≥ 0.5). In total 20,386 MUPTs (18,000 valid and 2386 invalid trains) were generated.

The same analysis as with the simulated data was completed using these signals. However, in analyzing the EMG signals provided by Florestal et al. (2009) and McGill (n.d.), the results of manual decomposition completed by an expert investigator were used. As with the simulated data, the valid trains in these three data sets were split into sub-trains of at least 50 MUPs and those valid trains having similar MUP templates were merged to generate invalid trains. Consequently, 14,632 MUPTs (13,024 valid and 1,608 invalid trains) were generated.

Considering the reference MUPTs as the gold standard, the performance of the developed MUPT validation systems was evaluated in terms of correctly classifying valid and invalid trains. Three accuracy indices were defined for this purpose: accuracy for valid trains (A_V), accuracy for invalid train (A_{IV}), and total accuracy (A_T). These three indices are given by:

$$A_V\% = \frac{\text{Number of valid MUPTs correctly classified}}{\text{Total number of valid MUPTs}} \times 100 \tag{12}$$

$$A_{IV}\% = \frac{\text{Number of invalid MUPTs correctly classified}}{\text{Total number of Invalid MUPTs}} \times 100 \tag{13}$$

$$A_T\% = \frac{\text{Number of MUPTs correctly classified}}{\text{Total number of MUPTs}} \times 100 \tag{14}$$

6.2 Evaluating decomposition system

For evaluating the performance of the developed MUPT validity-based EMG decomposition system, parts of the simulated and real EMG signals discussed in above were used. For each EMG signal used for this evaluation, the MU discharge patterns provided either by the EMG signal simulator used or by a human expert operator were used as reference.

For real data, the real EMG signals provided by Nikolic (2001) were not considered in this evaluation because the true decomposition results for this data were not known. A group of the real EMG signals provided in (Florestal et al., 2009; McGill, n.d.) were employed for this evaluation. Of the MUs contributed to each EMG signal used only the discharge patterns of those MUs that were selected by the expert as accurately identified patterns and the amplitude of the slope of their MUP templates were >0.01V/S were considered as reference and used for evaluation.

Four indices as defined below were used for evaluation: assignment rate (A_r), accuracy (A_c), correct classification rate (CC_r), and error in finding the correct number of MUPTs (E_{NMUPTs}).

$$A_r\% = \frac{\text{Number of MUPs assigned}}{\text{Number of MUPs detected}} \times 100 \tag{15}$$

$$A_c\% = \frac{\text{Number of MUPs correctly classified}}{\text{Total number of MUPs classified}} \times 100 \tag{16}$$

$$CC_r\% = \frac{\text{Number of MUPs correctly classified}}{\text{Total number of MUPs detected}} \times 100 \tag{17}$$

$$E_{NMUPTs} = \text{Number of extracted MUPTs - Number of expected MUPTs} \tag{18}$$

where the number of expected MUPTs equals to the number of MUPTs identified by the human expert or identified by the simulator as significant.

7. Results and discussions

7.1 MUPT validation system

The calculated means and standard deviations for the three accuracy indices used to evaluate the developed MUPT validation methods are summarized in Table 3. The numbers were obtained by testing each method using both simulated and real data sets when each set is split into the ten different data subsets. In this table VB stands for the MUP validation system developed by combing the FPVC and SVB outputs using AND logic. Likewise, VDH stands for the MUP validation system developed by combing the FPVC and SVDH outputs using AND logic.

As shown in Table 3, the accuracy in detecting invalid trains (i.e., in terms of A_{IV}) significantly improved when both MU firing pattern and MUP-shape information is employed for estimating the validity of a MUPT. However, the accuracy of both VB and VDH in correctly classifying valid MUPTs decreased compared to that of the FPVC, which only assesses the firing patterns of the MUPTs.

Figures 10 and 11 illustrate the advantage of using both MU firing pattern and MUP shape information for MUPT validation compared to using just MU firing pattern or MUP shape information.

Method	Simulated data			Real data		
	A_V (%)	A_{IV} (%)	A_T (%)	A_V (%)	A_{IV} (%)	A_T (%)
FPVC	**99.8±0.1***	95.9±0.7	**99.4±0.1**	**98.2±0.6***	96.2±1.4	**98.0±0.5***
SVB	92.2±0.3	66.5±0.8	89.2±0.3	95.0±0.6	74.5±1.7	92.8±0.5
SVDH	93.8±0.3	73.9±1.0	91.5±0.3	96.7±0.3	80.4±1.2	94.9±0.5
VB	98.2±0.2	**98.6±0.3***	98.4±0.2	**98.0±0.6***	**99.1±0.3***	**98.3±0.3***
VDH	93.7±0.7	**99.1±0.2***	96.4±0.5	95.2±0.7	**99.7±0.2***	94.4±0.3

Table 3. Mean and standard deviations for the accuracy of the different MUPT validation methods applied to both simulated and real data. In each column of the table, individual or groups of methods bolded and indicated by an '*' had significantly better performance than the others as determined using analysis of variance, at a 5% significance level and the Tukey-Kramer honestly significant difference test for pair-wise comparison of the mean values.

Fig.10 presents A_{IV} values versus the PsC between the templates of the two MUPTs selected for generating an invalid train for the methods studied. The PsC value represents a measure of the average similarity of the MUPs of the two trains selected to create an invalid train; high values of PsC indicate highly similar MUP templates. As shown, A_{IV} values of the two MUP-shape validation methods (SVB and SVDH) decreases drastically as the PsC between the MUP templates of the constituent MUPTs increases; the methods failed to detect > 80% of invalid trains composed of two MUPTs with PsC > 0.8. On the other hand, the A_{IV} values of both the VB and VDH methods were > 90% for most cases. For the worst case (high PsC), the accuracy of these two methods were > 80%, which is 57.6% higher than that of the SVB and SVDH methods. On average, the A_{IV} was improved by a factor of 1.3.

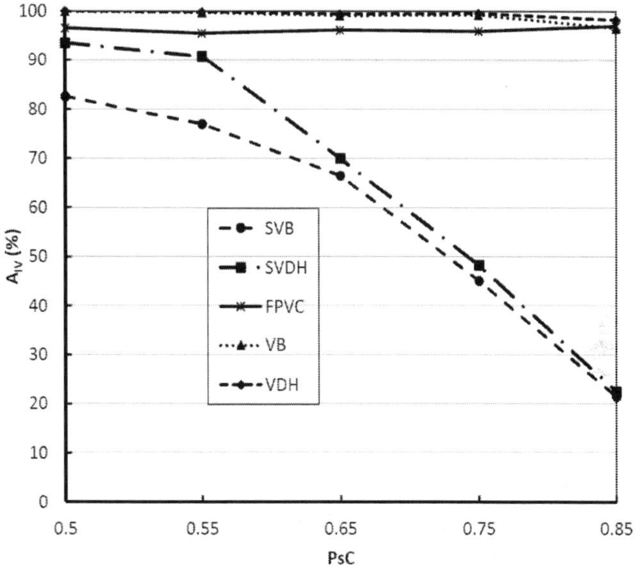

Fig. 9. A_{IV} values for the studied MUPT validation methods versus the pseudo-correlation (PsC) between the templates of two valid MUPTs merged to generate an invalid train.

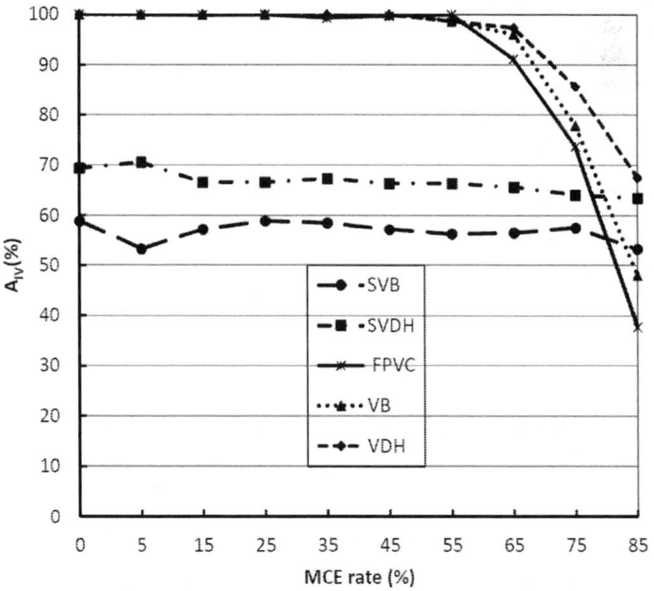

Fig. 10. A_{IV} values for the studied MUPT validation algorithms versus the MCE rate in the invalid trains. The MCE rate represents the sparsity of the MUPT.

Fig.11 demonstrates the advantages of using the VB and VDH algorithms (especially the VDH algorithm), which uses both MU firing pattern and MUP shape information in assessing the validity of a MUPT, over the FPVC that uses just MU firing pattern information. As shown, A_{IV} for the FPVC decreases as the MCE rate in the trains increases such that the algorithm misclassified around 60% of the invalid trains having a MCE rate > 80%. One reason for the drop in A_{IV} is that the accuracy with which the MU firing pattern statistics can be estimated and consequently the accuracy of the MU firing pattern features used decreases as a train becomes sparse (Parsaei et al. 2011). The VBDH method performed significantly better than the FPVC for invalid trains with MCE rate > 80%. The A_{IV} values of the VBDH method for such invalid trains was 31% higher than the A_{IV} of the FPVC, which is a significant improvement in detecting invalid trains especially during the early stages of an EMG signal decomposition.

Based on the results presented in Table 3 and Fig.11, the VDH method can be used in early stage of the decomposition when MCE rate >55%, as it is most accurate method in detecting highly-sparse invalid MUPTs. In the latter stage of the decomposition or for the MUPTs with MCE rate <55%, to avoid duplication of valid MUPT the other methods (VB or FPVC) that had higher A_V values than the VDH can be used to assess the validity of the extracted MUPTs. Overall, it is recommended to use only the FPVC at the final stage of the decomposition or for trains with MCE rate <30%, because VB misclassified valid trains with high MUP shape variability and ultimately cause duplication of such trains (Parsaei; 2011).

7.2 EMG decomposition system

Performance results for the validity-based decomposition system and that of the original decomposition algorithms of DQEMG for both simulated and real data are summarized in Tables 4 and 5, respectively. For each data set, the performance for each signal used along with the mean and standard deviation (STD) for the performance indices over all signals used is reported. Statistical comparison of the average values was conducted using paired t-tests (α= 0.05), while comparison of the STD values was conducted using F-tests (α= 0.05).

			Original DQEMG				Validity-based system			
Signal	Intensity (pps)	No. of MUPTs	A_r (%)	A_c (%)	CC_r (%)	E_{NMUPTs}	A_r (%)	A_c (%)	CC_r (%)	E_{NMUPTs}
1	54.0	6	92.6	98.0	90.7	0	95.4	99.1	94.5	0
2	59.4	7	90.7	95.9	87.0	0	93.8	98.5	92.4	0
3	61.4	6	78.0	96.4	75.2	2	90.5	98	88.7	0
4	68.2	7	90.2	96.4	86.9	0	94.6	97.4	92.1	0
5	70.7	7	73.3	96.9	71.0	3	90.3	96.5	87.1	0
6	79.3	8	91.0	82.3	74.9	0	93.6	95.1	89.0	0
7	82.5	8	83.5	89.8	75.0	2	89.2	96.3	85.9	1
8	85.2	9	92.3	80.3	74.1	-1	93.2	96.9	90.3	0
9	91.7	7	80.5	85.8	69.0	1	85.8	96.2	82.5	1
10	97.5	10	87.6	84.8	74.3	1	91.8	95.8	87.9	0
	Mean		**86.0**	**90.7**	**77.8**	**1.0**	**91.8**	**97.0**	**89.1**	**0.2**
	STD		**6.8**	**6.9**	**7.5**	**1.1**	**2.9**	**1.3**	**3.5**	**0.4**

Table 4. The performnace of the validity-based decomposition system compared to that of the original decomposition algorithms of the DQEMG applied to the simulated data.

Overall, the validity-based decomposition system has significantly improved decomposition results in terms of all four performance indices (p<0.03); except for the real data that A_C for both decomposition system was statistically equal. In addition, the validity-based system has lower STD for all performance measures (p<0.02), which shows that the system has better overall and less variable performance. The improvement in decomposition results (especially for CC_r) increases as the complexity of the signal increases, such that for the last two signals in Table 4, the CC_r values are improved by at least 13.4 %.

Signal	Intensity (pps)	No. of MUPTs	Original DQEMG A_r (%)	Original DQEMG A_c (%)	Original DQEMG CC_r (%)	Original DQEMG E_{NMUPTs}	Validity-based system A_r (%)	Validity-based system A_c (%)	Validity-based system CC_r (%)	Validity-based system E_{NMUPTs}
1	48.9	5	93.0	99.9	92.9	0	96.9	100.0	97.9	0
2	63.9	6	99.3	99.8	99.1	0	99.8	100.0	99.8	0
3	71.7	7	84.7	99.8	84.4	1	98.2	98.7	97.3	1
4	79.4	8	91.7	99.4	91.2	0	95.7	99.2	97.0	0
5	80.2	8	95.1	97.8	93.1	0	96.3	98.5	94.9	0
6	115.8	9	94.6	98.9	93.5	0	97.2	98.2	96.3	1
7	105.0	10	95.7	99.9	95.6	0	97.9	98.7	98.6	0
8	116.2	10	96.4	72.3	69.7	-3	98.8	96.4	97.2	0
9	112.4	11	82.7	97.0	80.2	4	92.0	96.4	86.7	1
10	114.3	11	86.6	98.8	85.6	1	93.8	97.2	93.1	0
	Mean		**92.0**	**96.4**	**88.5**	**0.9**	**96.7**	**98.3**	**95.0**	**0.3**
	STD		**5.5**	**8.5**	**7.8**	**1.4**	**2.4**	**1.3**	**3.1**	**0.5**

Table 5. The performnace of the validity-based decomposition system compared to that of the original decomposition algorithms of the DQEMG applied to the 10 real EMG signals.

Increases in MU firing pattern or MUP shape variability can decrease the performance of a decomposition system. Nonetheless, for the EMG signals with relatively high jitter or IDI-CV values studied (e.g., simulated EMG signal #10 which jitter value 100μs), the improvement gained using the validity-based system was significant.

Both DQEMG and the validity-based system are for decomposing intramuscular EMG signals mainly for clinical application; therefore, low amplitude MUPs, which are composed of low frequency components and created by MUs with no muscle fibers close to the electrode detection surface, are neither detected nor considered for clustering and supervised classification. If such MUPs were detected and then considered for clustering and supervised classification, the accuracies of both systems may not be as high as those presented in Tables 4 and 5. Finally, the accuracies of both DQEMG and the validity-based system for EMG signals contaminated by high levels of noise may be lower than the values reported for the simulated and real EMG signals used in this work.

Finally, both DQEMG and the validity-based system assume the mean and standard deviation of the IDIs of the MUs that contributed to the signal being decomposed did not change during signal detection. Such assumptions are valid for EMG signals detected during short-term isometric contraction; however, these assumptions may not be realistic for signals detected during either force-varying or long contractions. Such limitations restrict the use of both DQEMG and the validity-based system for research applications where the decomposition of signals detected during non-isometric or long-term contractions are required. Nevertheless, DQEMG has been useful for the decomposition of intramuscular EMG signals acquired for clinical applications (Stashuk,1999; Doherty & Stashuk, 2003; Boe et al., 2005; Pino et al.,2008; Calder at al.,2008)

8. Conclusions and future work

Decomposition of an EMG signal may result in several invalid MUPTs that do not accurately represent the activity of a signal MU; such invalid MUPTs must be identified and then either corrected or excluded before extracted MUPTs are quantitatively analyzed. Characteristics of IDI histograms, MU firing rates over time and within-train MUP shape inconsistencies of MUPTs extracted during EMG decomposition can be used to estimate their validity. The existing qualitative MUPT validation methods, which typically need human operator supervision, are time consuming, related to operator experience and skill, and cannot assist with improving the performance of automatic EMG decomposition systems. To overcome these issues, in this chapter an automated MUPT validation system that estimate the validity of a MUPT is estimated using both its MU firing pattern and MUP shape information is presented.

Based on the results obtained, the developed methods with overall A_T >91.5% performed well in classifying MUPTs extracted by a decomposition system. Nevertheless, the methods that use only shape or only firing pattern information did not perform as well as the ones that used both types of information, especially for invalid trains. Of the method studied, the VDH method is the most accurate method in classifying sparse invalid trains, but the FPVC and VB are more accurate than the VDH in classifying valid MUPTs. Therefore, using VDH when MCE rate of the train >55% and VB or FPVC when MCE rate < 55% and even FPVC when MCE rate < 30% in the optimum scheme of using the proposed validation methods.

Finally, it was revealed that using the proposed MUPT validation system during decomposition will improve the results in terms of finding the correct numbers of MUPTs that constitute a given signal as well as decreasing the MCE and FCE rates in the extracted trains. Overall, the decomposition accuracy for 20 EMG signals (10 simulated and 10 real) was improved by 9.0%. For these 20 signals, the validity-based decomposition system with average E_{NMUPTs} 0.3 was better able to estimate the number of constituent MUPTs than the previous system, with average E_{NMUPTs} of 0.9. The improvement gained using the validity-based system for dificult- to- decompose EMG signals was even higher. Such improvements, especially in E_{NMUPTs}, along with the confidence that the extracted MUPTs will be valid encourage using the validity-based decomposition system for decomposing intramuscular EMG signals for clinical application.

Future work will address: a) further analysis of the developed decomposition system, especially using clinical EMG signals acquired from myopathic and neurogenic muscles; b) improving the performance of the developed MUPT validation system in terms of both accuracy and computational time.

9. Acknowledgment

The authors would like to gratefully thank Dr. A. Ghodsi for his helpful discussion, on clustering and cluster validation methods, Dr. M. Nicolic, Dr. K.C. McGill, Dr. J.R. Florestal, Dr. P.A. Mathieu, Dr. Z. Lateva, and Dr. H.R. Marateb for sharing several EMG signals and the decomposition results of these signals. Financial support from the Natural Sciences and Engineering Research Council of Canada (NSERC) is gratefully acknowledged.

10. References

Basmajian, J.V. & Luca, C.J.D., 1985. *Muscles alive: their functions revealed by electromyography* (*5th* ed.), Williams & Wilkins.

Boe, S. G.; Stashuk, D. W.; Brown, W. F.& Doherty, T. J. (2005). Decomposition-based quantitative electromyography: effect of force on motor unit potentials and motor unit number estimates. *Muscle Nerve,* 31(3), pp.365-373.

Calder, K.M.; Stashuk, D.W. & McLean, L. (2008). Physiological characteristics of motor units in the brachioradialis muscle across fatiguing low-level isometric contractions. *J Electromyogr Kinesiol.,* vol. 18,no. 1, pp.2-15.

Clamann, H.P. (1969). Statistical analysis of motor unit firing patterns in a human skeletal muscle. *Biophysical Journal,* vol. 9, no. 10, pp.1233-1251.

Contessa, P.; Adam, A. & De Luca, C. J. (2009). Motor unit control and force fluctuation during fatigue. *J Appl Physiol,* vol. 107,no.1, pp.235-243.

Doherty,T. J. & Stashuk, D.W. (2003). Decomposition-based quantitative electromyography: methods and initial normative data in five muscles. *Muscle Nerve,* vol. 28,no. 2, pp.204-211.

Duda, R.O., Hart, P.E. & Stork, D.G. (2000). *Pattern classification* 2nd ed., Wiley-Interscience.

Farkas, C. et al., (2010). A review of clinical quantitative electromyography. *Crit Rev Biomed Eng.,* vol. 38,no.5, pp.467-485.

Florestal, J.R.; Mathieu P. A.& Malanda A. (2006). Automated decomposition of intramuscular electromyographic signals. *IEEE Trans Biomed Eng.,* vol. 53, no. 5, pp. 832-839.

Florestal, J.R.; Mathieu, P. & and Mcgill, K.C. (2009). Automatic decomposition of multichannel intramuscular EMG signals. *J. Electromyogr Kinesiol.,* 695 vol. 19, no. 1, pp. 1–9.

Fuglsang-Frederiksen, A. (2006). The role of different EMG methods in evaluating myopathy. *Clin Neurophysiol.,* vol. 117, no. 6, pp.1173-1189.

Gordon, A.D., 1999. *Classification,* 2nd ed., Chapman & Hall/CRC.

Hamilton-Wright ,A. & Stashuk, D.W.(2005). Physiologically based simulation of clinical EMG signals. *IEEE Trans Biomed Eng.,* vol. 52, no. 2, pp. 171–183.

Lateva, Z.C. & McGill, K C, 2001. Estimating motor unit architectural properties by analyzing motor unit action potential morphology. *Clin Neurophysiol.,* vol. 112,no.1, pp.127-135.

De Luca, C. J. et al., (1982b). Control scheme governing concurrently active human motor units during voluntary contractions. *J Physiol.,* 329, pp.129-142.

De Luca, C. J.& Forrest, W.J.(1973). Some properties of motor unit action potential trains recorded during constant force isometric contractions in man. *Kybernetik,* vol. 12,no.3, pp.160-168.

De Luca, C. J.(1979). Physiology and mathematics of myoelectric signals. *IEEE Trans Biomed Eng.,* vol. 26, no. 6, pp. 313-325.

De Luca, C. J.; LeFever, R. S.;. McCue, M. P.& Xenakis, A. P. (1982a). Behaviour of human motor units in different muscles during linearly varying contractions. *J Physiol.,* vol. 329,no. 1, pp.113-128.

De Luca, C.J.; Adam, A.& Wotiz, R.(2006).Decomposition of surface EMG signals. *J Neurophysiol,* vol. 96,no. 3, pp.1646-1657.

Matthews, P.B. (1996). Relationship of firing intervals of human motor units to the trajectory of post-spike after-hyperpolarization and synaptic noise. *J Physiol.,* 492(Pt 2), pp.597-628.

McGill, K. & Marateb, H. (2011). Rigorous a-posteriori assessment of accuracy in EMG decomposition. *IEEE Trans Neural Syst Rehabil Eng,*vol.19, no. 1, pp. 54–63.

McGill, K. C. (n.d.) Dataset R005 Available: http://www.emglab.net.

McGill, K. C., Cummins, K.L. & Dorfman, L.J. (1985). Automatic decomposition of the clinical electromyogram. *IEEE Trans Biomed Eng.,* vol. 32,no. 7, pp.470-477.

McGill, K.C. & Dorfman,L.J. (1985). Automatic decomposition electromyography (ADEMG): validation and normative data in brachial biceps. *Electroencephalogr Clin Neurophysiol.*, vol. 61,no. 5, pp.453-461.

Milligan, G. & Cooper, M., 1985. An examination of procedures for determining the number of clusters in a data set. *Psychometrika*, vol. 50,no. 2, pp.159-179.

Moritz, C.T. et al., 2005. Discharge rate variability influences the variation in force fluctuations across the working range of a hand muscle. *J Neurophysiol.*, vol. 93,no. 5, pp.2449 -2459.

Nikolic, M. (2001). *Detailed analysis of clinical electromyography signals EMG decomposition, findings and firing pattern analysis in controls and patients with myopathy and amytrophic lateral sclerosis.* PhD dissertation, University of Copenhage, Copenhagen, U.K .

Parsaei, H. & Stashuk, D. W. (2011a).Adaptive motor unit potential train validation using MUP shape information. *Med Eng Phys.*, vol. 33, no. 5, pp. 581-589.

Parsaei, H. & Stashuk, D.W. (2011b). A method for detecting and editing MUPTs contaminated by false classification errors during EMG signal decomposition. in *Proc. 33rd IEEE Annu Int Conf Eng Med Biol Soc.*, 2011, Boston, USA.

Parsaei, H., 2011. *EMG signal decomposition using motor unit potentail train validity.* PhD dissertation, Waterloo, Ont.: University of Waterloo.

Parsaei, H., Nezhad, F., Stashuk,D.W. & Hamilton-Wright, A. (2011). Validating motor unit firing patterns extracted by EMG signal decomposition. *Med Biol Eng Comput.*, vol. 49, no. 6, pp. 649–658.

Parsaei, H., Stashuk, D. W.; Rasheed, S., Farkas, C.& Hamilton-Wright, A. (2010). Intramuscular EMG signal decomposition. *Crit Rev Biomed Eng.*, vol. 38, no. 5, pp.435-465.

Pino, L.J.; Stashuk, D.W. & Podnar, S. (2008). Bayesian characterization of External Anal sphincter Muscles using Quantitative Electromyography. *Clin Neurophysiol.*, vol. 119,no. 10, pp.2266-2273.

Rasheed; S.; Stashuk, D. W.& Kamel, M. S. (2010). Integrating heterogeneous classifier ensembles for EMG signal decomposition based on classifier agreement. *IEEE Trans Inf Technol Biomed*, vol. 14, no. 3, pp. 866-882.

Semmlow, J.L. (2004). *Biosignal and Biomedical Image Processing: Matlab-based Applications*, CRC Press.

Stalberg, E.V. & Falck, B. (1997). The Role of Electromyography in Neurology. *Electroencephalogr Clin Neurophysiol.*, vol. 103,no. 6, pp.579-598.

Stålberg, E.V. & Sonoo, M.(1994). Assessment of variability in the shape of the motor unit action potential, the "jiggle," at consecutive discharges. *Muscle Nerve*, vol. 17,no.10, pp.1135-1144.

Stashuk D. W. (2001). EMG signal decomposition: how can it be accomplished and used? *J Electromyogr Kinesiol.*, vol. 11,no. 3, pp.151-173.

Stashuk, D. W. & Paoli, G. (1998). Robust supervised classification of motor unit action potentials. *Med Biol Eng Comput.*, vol. 36, no. 1, pp.75-82.

Stashuk, D. W. (1999). Decomposition and quantitative analysis of clinical electromyographic signals. *Med Eng Phys.*, vol. 21.no. 6, pp.389-404.

Stashuk, D.W & Qu, Y.(1996a). Adaptive motor unit action potential clustering using shape and temporal information. *Med Biol Eng Comput.*, vol. 34, no.1, pp.41-49.

Stashuk, D.W. & Qu, Y. (1996b). Robust method for estimating motor unit firing-pattern statistics. *Med Biol Eng Comput.*, vol. 34,no. 1, pp.50-57.

Tröger, M. & Dengler, R. (2000). The role of electromyography (EMG) in the diagnosis of ALS. *Amyotroph Lateral Scler*, vol. 1, no. 2, pp.33-40.

Vapnik,V.(1999). *The Nature of statistical learning theory*, 2nd ed. Springer.

15

Role of Biomechanical Parameters in Hip Osteoarthritis and Avascular Necrosis of Femoral Head

Veronika Kralj - Iglič[1], Drago Dolinar[1], Matic Ivanovski[1], Ivo List[1] and Matej Daniel[2]
[1]*Laboratory of Clinical Biophysics, Faculty of Medicine, University of Ljubljana*
[2]*Laboratory of Biomechanics, Faculty of Mechanical Engineering, Technical University in Prague*
[1]*Slovenia*
[2]*Czech Republic*

1. Introduction

It is considered that living organisms are subject to physical laws. Forces and stresses importantly influence the development of tissues and cells. In order to manipulate physiological and patophysiological states of the organism, it is necessary to understand the underlying mechanisms. Experience has led to mechanical hypothesis stating that some diseases or disorders are a consequence of unfavorable load distribution which is expressed by biomechanical parameters (e.g. forces, stresses, load - bearing areas). Since 1993 we have considered contact stress in the hip joint. We took part in development of a mathematical model for determination of the contact hip stress distribution (Iglič (1993b); Ipavec (1999)) and in population studies which were performed to validate the model. Different diseases and disorders of the hip were considered by this model: hip dysplasia (Mavčič (2002; 2008); Pompe (2003; 2007)), slipped epiphysis of the femoral head (Zupanc (2008)), avascular necrosis of the femoral head (Daniel (2006); Dolinar (2003)), postoperative changes in hip geometry (Herman (2002); Kralj (2005); Vengust (2001)) and osteoarthritis of the hip (Rečnik (2007; 2009a;b)). The method HIPSTRESS was put forward consisting of mathematical model for resultant hip force (Iglič (1990; 1993a)), mathematical model for contact hip stress (Iglič (1993b); Ipavec (1999)) and the corresponding software. The models require as an input geometrical parameters of the hip and pelvis. These parameters can be assessed from images as for example from standard anteroposterior radiograms. As appropriate images are available from clinical practice and from the archives, prospective and retrospective studies of the development of different diseases can be performed. A thorough survey on resultant hip force and the corresponding stress has recently been published (Daniel (2011)).

Albeit the HIPSTRESS method is of limited repeatability and accuracy, the population studies have shown that biomechanical parameters are useful in reaching better understanding of mechanisms taking place in different diseases and in predicting the outcome of the treatment, on the level of populations. In particular, the results indicated that long lasting elevated contact stress is connected to degeneration of the hip articular cartilage and development of hip osteoarthritis (Dolinar (2003); Kralj (2005); Mavčič (2002; 2008); Pompe (2003); Rečnik (2007; 2009a;b)).

The physical content of the model for hip stress used in these studies is simple and clear. The model states that the resultant hip force is distributed over the load - bearing area according to the corresponding normal stress in the cartilage which is subject to Hooke's law. The equations that must be solved to obtain the relevant forces, stresses and load - bearing area are transparent while the solution of the problem is almost analytical. Moreover, a user - friendly software HIPSTRESS was developed which by fast determination of biomechanical parameters of the hip and pelvis enables analyses of large populations of hips.

However, due to space limitations in journals, the full derivation of the model equations was not encouraged in our previously published papers. Presenting only the final short and elegant equation for determination of stress parameters may lead the readers to think that the model itself is also simple. To elucidate the derivation and the model assumptions, we present in the first part of this work a detailed derivation of the model for contact hip stress distribution within the HIPSTRESS method, and indicate the connection between an unfavorable stress distribution and osteoarthritis development. In the second part, we present new results indicating the contact hip stress distribution as an etiological factor in avascular necrosis of the femoral head.

2. Determination of hip stress distribution by mathematical model

The femoral head is represented by a fraction of a sphere (the femoral head sphere) and the acetabulum is represented by a half of a spherical shell (the acetabular sphere). An articular spherical surface is imagined. This spherical surface is an abstract object rather than a physical one and extends beyond the load - bearing area. The load - bearing area is however a part of the articular spherical surface.

The shear stresses in the hip joint are neglected because of the small value of the frictional coefficient corresponding to forces acting in the hip joint (Eberhardt (1991); Lipshitz (1979); McCutchen (1962)) so that only the normal stress is considered. We refer to the normal stress as to the contact hip stress.

When the hip is unloaded, the femoral head sphere and the acetabular sphere are concentric (Fig.1A). Upon loading the femoral head moves towards the acetabulum thereby squeezing the cartilage in between (Fig.1B). The femoral head sphere and the acetabular sphere are no longer concentric and the surfaces are shifted with respect to each other. The point on the articular sphere corresponding to the closest approach of the femoral head sphere and the acetabular sphere is called the stress pole (denoted by P in Fig.1B).

The radius vector from the centre of the femoral head sphere to the selected point at the acetabular sphere after the loading is denoted by $\mathbf{r}$, the respective radius vector before the loading is denoted by $\mathbf{r}'$ and the penetration of the centre of the femoral head is denoted by $\mathbf{d}$. The coordinate system is rotated so that the side view plane is defined by the three vectors.

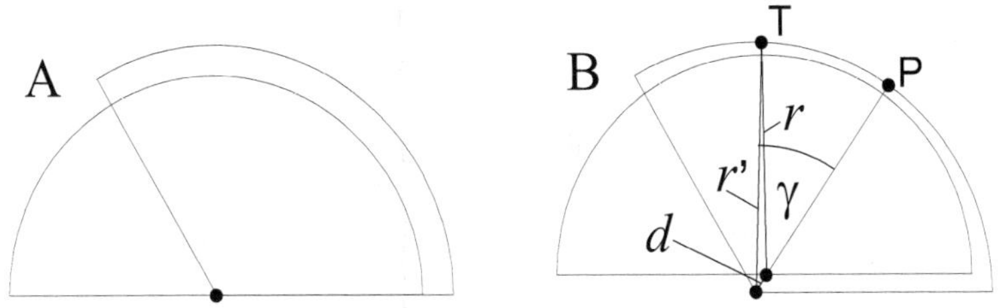

Fig. 1. Schematic presentation of the relative shift of the acetabular sphere and the femoral head sphere. A: before loading, the two spheres are concentric. B: after loading, the femoral head sphere penetrates towards the acetabular sphere.

It follows from trigonometric relations that

$$r^2 = r'^2 + d^2 - 2r'd\cos\gamma \tag{1}$$

where γ (Fig. 1B) is the angle between the radius vector from the origin of the coordinate system at the centre of the articular sphere to the pole and the radius vector to the selected point on the articular surface while r, r' and d are the magnitudes of the vectors $\mathbf{r}$, $\mathbf{r}'$ and $\mathbf{d}$. It is considered that the deformation of the cartilage is very small i.e. that the distance of penetration d is much smaller than distances r and r', so we can neglect the quadratic term in Eq.(1),

$$r = \sqrt{r'^2 - 2r'd\cos\gamma} \tag{2}$$

and use the approximation for small x, $\sqrt{1+x} \simeq 1 + x/2$,

$$r = r'(1 - \cos\gamma\frac{d}{r'}). \tag{3}$$

The deformation and the strain of the cartilage are proportional to the difference $r' - r$,

$$r' - r = d\cos\gamma. \tag{4}$$

As the normal stress at a particular point on the articular sphere (p) is taken proportional to strain in the cartilage, it can be written as (Brinckmann (1981))

$$p = p_0\cos\gamma \tag{5}$$

where the proportionality constant p_0 is the value of stress at the pole.

Considering the resultant hip force $\mathbf{R}$ to be known, it is connected to the hip stress distribution by

$$\int p_0\cos\gamma\,\mathbf{dS} = \mathbf{R}, \tag{6}$$

where $\mathbf{dS}$ is the vector form of the area element pointing in the direction normal to the surface. The integration is performed over the load - bearing area.

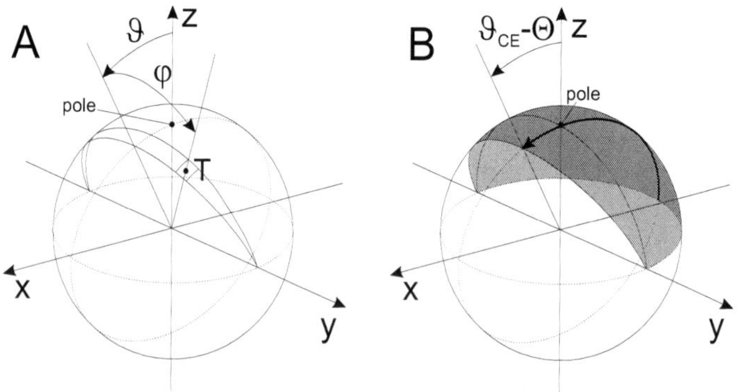

Fig. 2. Schematic presentation of the articular sphere and the coordinate system.

The coordinate system is adjusted to the geometry of the load-bearing area. The coordinates of a selected point (T) are (Fig.2A)

$$x = r\cos\varphi\sin\vartheta, \tag{7}$$

$$y = r\sin\varphi, \tag{8}$$

$$z = r\cos\varphi\cos\vartheta. \tag{9}$$

The infinitesimal element of the surface area is given by

$$\mathbf{dS} = r^2\cos\varphi(\cos\varphi\sin\vartheta, \sin\varphi, \cos\varphi\cos\vartheta)\mathrm{d}\varphi\mathrm{d}\vartheta. \tag{10}$$

The space angle γ is the angle between the radius vector to the stress pole and the radius vector to the selected point on the articular surface, hence we can use the dot product to define the angle,

$$\cos\gamma = \frac{\mathbf{r}\cdot\mathbf{r}_{\mathrm{pole}}}{r^2}, \tag{11}$$

where

$$\mathbf{r} = r(\sin\vartheta\cos\varphi, \sin\varphi, \cos\vartheta\cos\varphi), \tag{12}$$

and

$$\mathbf{r}_{\mathrm{pole}} = r(\sin\Theta\cos\Phi, \sin\Phi, \cos\Theta\cos\Phi). \tag{13}$$

The dot product yields

$$\mathbf{r}\cdot\mathbf{r}_{\mathrm{pole}} = r^2(\sin\vartheta\cos\varphi\sin\Theta\cos\Phi + \sin\varphi\sin\Phi + \cos\vartheta\cos\varphi\cos\Theta\cos\Phi) \tag{14}$$

so that

$$\cos\gamma = \sin\vartheta\cos\varphi\sin\Theta\cos\Phi + \sin\varphi\sin\Phi + \cos\vartheta\cos\varphi\cos\Theta\cos\Phi. \tag{15}$$

In the chosen coordinate system, the position of the pole is given by two angles (Φ and Θ). However, for clarity and simplicity we rotate the hip in the coordinate system so that the pole is at the top of the articular sphere (Fig.2B),

$$\cos\tilde{\Theta} = 1, \tag{16}$$

and

$$\sin\tilde{\Theta} = 0, \tag{17}$$

while $\tilde{\Phi} = 0$ so that

$$\cos\tilde{\Phi} = 1, \tag{18}$$

and

$$\sin\tilde{\Phi} = 0. \tag{19}$$

It follows from Eqs.(15) and (16)– (19) that in the rotated system

$$\cos\gamma = \cos\varphi\cos\vartheta. \tag{20}$$

2.1 Contact hip stress in relation to resultant hip force

Using expressions (5), (6), (10) and (20), the components of the vector equation for the resultant hip force in the rotated system are expressed as

$$R_x = p_0 r^2 \int \cos^3\varphi \mathrm{d}\varphi \int \cos\vartheta\sin\vartheta \mathrm{d}\vartheta, \tag{21}$$

$$R_y = p_0 r^2 \int \cos^2\varphi\sin\varphi \mathrm{d}\varphi \int \cos\vartheta \mathrm{d}\vartheta, \tag{22}$$

$$R_z = p_0 r^2 \int \cos^3\varphi \mathrm{d}\varphi \int \cos^2\vartheta \mathrm{d}\vartheta. \tag{23}$$

In order to calculate the coordinates of the pole Θ and Φ and the value of stress at the pole p_0 we must solve the above system of equations. For this we must define the boundaries of the load - bearing area within the articular surface.

We take for simplicity that the lateral border of the load - bearing area is defined by the lateral rim of the acetabulum. Neglecting the detailed anatomy of the border and taking that the rim presents a part of a circle on the sphere with the centre at the centre of the sphere, the rim is described by an intersection of the articular sphere and a plane passing through the center of the sphere. The plane is inclined by an angle ϑ_L with respect to the vertical axis. The coordinate system is then rotated for an angle $-\Phi$ so that the lateral border is symmetric with respect to the frontal plane through the centre of the articular sphere. Stress represents loading only if it is positive. Therefore the medial border of the load - bearing area is defined at points on the articular sphere where stress vanishes,

$$\cos\gamma = 0. \tag{24}$$

This condition includes points which are for $\pi/2$ away from the stress pole.

Consider a hip with the lateral coverage ϑ_L and the pole of stress (given by angles Θ and Φ) located laterally with respect to the sagittal plane through the centre of the femoral head. The coordinate system is rotated for angles $-\Theta$ and $-\Phi$, so in the rotated system, the lateral border is at $\vartheta = \vartheta_L - \Theta$. As the pole is at the top of the rotated system, the medial border in the rotated system is at $\vartheta = -\pi/2$. Parameter φ is bounded within the interval $[-\pi/2, \pi/2]$.

Taking into account that

$$\int \cos^3 \varphi d\varphi = \sin \varphi - \frac{1}{3} \sin^3 \varphi, \tag{25}$$

$$\int \cos \vartheta \sin \vartheta d\vartheta = \frac{1}{2} \sin^2 \vartheta, \tag{26}$$

$$\int \cos^2 \varphi \sin \varphi d\varphi = -\frac{1}{3} \cos^3 \varphi, \tag{27}$$

$$\int \cos \vartheta d\vartheta = \sin \vartheta, \tag{28}$$

$$\int \cos^2 \vartheta d\vartheta = \frac{1}{2}(\vartheta + \frac{1}{2} \sin 2\vartheta), \tag{29}$$

and considering the boundaries, the components of the force are

$$R_x = -p_0 r^2 \frac{2}{3} \cos^2(\vartheta_L - \Theta) \tag{30}$$

$$R_y = 0 \tag{31}$$

and

$$R_z = p_0 r^2 \frac{2}{3} (\vartheta_L - \Theta + \frac{\pi}{2} + \frac{1}{2} \sin 2(\vartheta_L - \Theta)). \tag{32}$$

The resultant hip force is given by the vector

$$\mathbf{R} = R(-\sin \vartheta_R \cos \varphi_R, \sin \varphi_R, \cos \vartheta_R \cos \varphi_R) \tag{33}$$

which is in the rotated system expressed as

$$\mathbf{R} = R(-\sin(\vartheta_R + \Theta), 0, \cos(\vartheta_R + \Theta)) \tag{34}$$

since

$$\Phi = -\varphi_R. \tag{35}$$

The ratio R_x/R_z yields

$$\tan(\vartheta_R + \Theta) = \frac{\cos^2(\vartheta_L - \Theta)}{(\vartheta_L - \Theta + \frac{\pi}{2} + \frac{1}{2} \sin 2(\vartheta_L - \Theta))}. \tag{36}$$

Eq.(36) is a nonlinear equation for Θ which can be solved numerically, for example by using the Newton method. The value of stress at the pole is then expressed from Eqs.(30) and (34),

$$p_0 = \frac{3R}{2r^2} \frac{\sin(\vartheta_R + \Theta)}{\cos^2(\vartheta_L - \Theta)}. \tag{37}$$

The solution (Eqs.(36) and (37)) first appeared in (Ipavec (1999)). Due to the geometry of the articular sphere, the first choice of coordinates were spherical coordinates. In such coordinate system, the load - bearing area was subject to boundaries in which the two angles were related, so the load - bearing area had to be divided into 6 segments with different types of boundary shapes. Although yielding the same relatively simple result (Eq.(36)), the calculation was tedious and due to many terms in the integrals the probability of making the mistake was increased. The derivation of the result was practically inaccessible by simply following the instructions given in (Ipavec (1999)). Probably this added to the fact that a typing mistake in the equations in (Ipavec (1999)) was deleterious for potential users of the model. The authors are indebted to W. Wilson and B.V. Rietbergen from Eindhoven University of Technology, who found the mistake while they were trying to repeat the derivation. An erratum was published in J. Biomech. (Ipavec (2002)), however, a thorough description of the model is still required as to help the potential users of the model to verify all steps.

In attempting to develop models with slightly more sophisticated load - bearing areas (such as after the Chiari osteotomy in which additional load - bearing area is created by a roof created by the cut iliac bone) the spherical coordinates used in (Ipavec (1999)) were found of practically no use and finding a more convenient coordinate system was prerequisite for description of the system. The coordinates presented above yielded considerably simpler derivation which was then first published in (Herman (2002)).

It can be seen that the simple, transparent and almost analytical form of the system of equations (35) - (37) does not mean that the model and the derivation of equations are simple. The simplicity and elegance of the result is primarily a consequence of the symmetry of the load - bearing area and of the stress distribution function.

It can also be mentioned that another choice of configuration preceded the above models. Inspired by Brinckmann et al., (Brinckmann (1981)), we chose the configuration in which the system was rotated so that the resultant hip force would point in the vertical direction (Iglič (1993b)). This model was however restricted to resultant hip force lying in the frontal plane of the body. It was a major achievement of the improved model described in (Ipavec (1999)) that regardless of the direction of the resultant hip force, within the described model, a coordinate system can always be found in which the above defined load-bearing area is symmetric.

To assess contact hip stress by a single numerical value, peak stress on the load - bearing area $p_{\max}$ is given. If the stress pole is located inside the load - bearing area, $p_{\max}$ is equal to the value of stress at the pole p_0. If the stress pole lies outside the load - bearing area, contact stress is the highest at the point of the load - bearing area which is closest to the stress pole and can be determined by using Eq.(5).

$$p_{\max} = p_0 \cos(\vartheta_{\mathrm{L}} - \Theta). \tag{38}$$

2.2 Index of the hip stress gradient and functional angle of load-bearing area

Not only stress, but also stress differences between adjacent cell layers can be important in development of tissues (Daniel (2003)). These differences are expressed by the stress gradient,

$$\nabla p = (\frac{\partial p}{\partial r}, \frac{1}{r}\frac{\partial p}{\partial \theta}, \frac{1}{r \sin\theta}\frac{\partial p}{\partial \phi}) \tag{39}$$

where r is the magnitude of the radius vector while θ and ϕ are the polar and the azimuthal coordinates of the spherical system (Fig.3).

In this system

$$x = r \cos\phi \sin\theta, \tag{40}$$

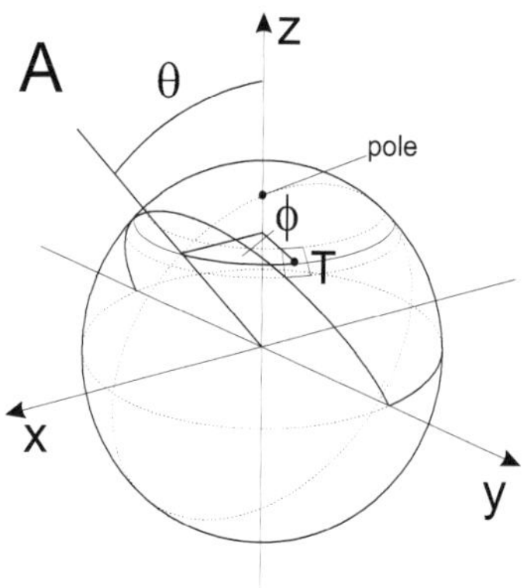

Fig. 3. Schematic presentation of the articular sphere in the spherical coordinate system.

$$y = r \sin\phi \sin\theta \tag{41}$$

and

$$z = r \cos\theta, \tag{42}$$

while the coordinates of the pole are

$$x_{\mathrm{p}} = r \cos\phi_{\mathrm{p}} \sin\theta_{\mathrm{p}}, \tag{43}$$

$$y_{\mathrm{p}} = r \sin\phi_{\mathrm{p}} \sin\theta_{\mathrm{p}} \tag{44}$$

and

$$z_{\mathrm{p}} = r \cos\theta_{\mathrm{p}}. \tag{45}$$

The space angle derived from the dot product is

$$\cos\gamma = \cos\theta \sin\phi \cos\phi_{\mathrm{p}} \sin\theta_{\mathrm{p}} + \sin\phi \sin\theta \sin\phi_{\mathrm{p}} \sin\theta_{\mathrm{p}} + \cos\theta \cos\theta_{\mathrm{p}}. \tag{46}$$

As in the rotated system the stress pole is at the top of the sphere, $\tilde{\theta}_{\mathrm{p}} = \tilde{\phi}_{\mathrm{p}} = 0$, the above expression simplifies into

$$\cos\gamma = \cos\theta. \tag{47}$$

It follows from Eqs.(39) and (47) that the gradient is

$$\nabla p = (0, -\frac{p_0}{r} \sin\theta, 0). \tag{48}$$

Here, r is the radius of the articular sphere. The stress gradient is a vector pointing in the direction of strongest change of stress. It would however be convenient to assess the gradient by a single numerical value. By mapping the three dimensional problem onto two dimensions we introduced the index of the hip stress gradient at the lateral acetabular rim G_p (Daniel (2002); Pompe (2003)),

$$G_p = -\frac{p_0}{r} \sin(\vartheta_{\mathrm{L}} - \Theta). \tag{49}$$

The absolute value of G_p is equal to the magnitude of stress gradient ∇p at the lateral acetabular rim. If the pole of stress distribution lies outside the load - bearing area (i.e., if

$\Theta > \vartheta_L$) then $G_p > 0$. If the pole of stress distribution lies inside the load - bearing area (i.e., if $\Theta < \vartheta_L$) then $G_p < 0$.

We defined another biomechanical parameter which describes the size of the load - bearing area: the functional angle ϑ_F. The functional angle is equal to the load - bearing area divided by $2r^2$,

$$\vartheta_F = \frac{\pi}{2} + \vartheta_{CE} - \Theta. \tag{50}$$

The index of the hip stress gradient at the lateral acetabular rim G_p is in a simple way connected to the size of the load-bearing area which is proportional to the functional angle of the load-bearing area,

$$G_p = \frac{p_0}{r} \cos \vartheta_F. \tag{51}$$

2.3 Clinical relevance of hip stress with respect to osteoarthritis development

Population studies have shown that long lasting high peak stress is unfavorable and leads to osteoarthritis of the hip, however, even if the peak stress is not very high, large positive index of the hip stress gradient at the lateral acetabular rim and small functional angle of the load - bearing area express unfavorable stress distribution.

Index of the hip stress gradient at the lateral acetabular rim G_p characterizes the slope of the contact stress distribution at the lateral border of the load - bearing area while the functional angle of the load-bearing area ϑ_F describes the amount of the articular sphere occupied by the load - bearing area. To illustrate these parameters Fig.4 presents stress distribution and parameter ϑ_F in two hips with different pelvic geometry: normal hip (A) and dysplastic hip (B). In hip A the pole of stress distribution lies within the load - bearing area and contact stress increases from the lateral edge in the medial direction, reaches its maximum and then decreases towards the medial border of the load - bearing area. The corresponding value of G_p is negative and the functional angle of the load - bearing area ϑ_F is large. In hip B the pole lies outside the load - bearing area so that at the lateral edge of the load - bearing area stress steeply decreases in the medial direction. The corresponding value of G_p is positive and the functional angle of the load - bearing area ϑ_F is small. The lower (more negative) the index of gradient and the larger the functional angle of the load - bearing area, the more favorable is stress distribution. In a population study it was shown (Pompe (2003)) that the change of sign of G_p correlates well with clinical evaluation of hip dysplasia, i.e. positive values of G_p correspond to dysplastic hips. The functional angle of the load-bearing area ϑ_F which does not critically depend on the size of the pelvis and femur was proved the most relevant in samples with large scattering in the size of the geometrical parameters, as for example in a group of children (Vengust (2001)) or if there is a possibility that the magnification of radiographs varies considerably. In these cases the effect of the parameters R, p_{max} and G_p (strongly dependent on the magnification of radiographs) can not be envisaged due to large scattering and concomitant poor statistical significance.

Population studies have shown that in dysplastic hips, the peak stress is on the average for a factor 2 higher than in healthy hips (Mavčič (2002)) while the index of stress gradient at the lateral acetabular rim is negative in normal hips and positive in dysplastic hips (Pompe (2003)). The differences were statistically significant ($p < 0.001$). In a study including 65 hips

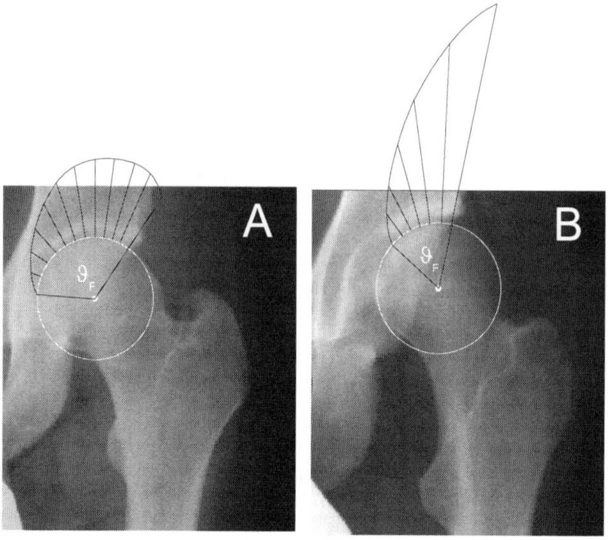

Fig. 4. Stress distribution in a frontal plane through the centre of the femoral head. The length of the line indicates the value of stress. The functional angle of the load - bearing area is shown. A: normal hip, B: dysplastic hip.

that underwent total hip replacement due to idiopathic osteoarthritis of the hip, the age at the replacement negatively correlated with peak stress ($p < 0.001$) (Rečnik (2009a)). These results indicate that contact hip stress plays an important role in progression of osteoarthritis.

3. Hip stress as etiological factor for avascular necrosis of femoral head

3.1 Introduction

Avascular necrosis of the femoral head (AN) is characterized by deterioration of the bone tissue (Figs.5,6). It represents together with secondary osteoarthritis a serious orthopaedic problem affecting mostly young and middle - aged populations (Mont (1995)). In spite of numerous studies, mechanisms leading to ischemic and necrotic processes are not yet understood. In about one third of patients the risk factors cannot be determined (Mahoney (2005)) while disorders and risk factors connected to the onset of AN include alcoholism (Mont (1995)), corticosteroid therapy in patients with connective tissue diseases and transplants (Mont (1995)), sickle cell anemia (Herndon (1972)), HIV (Miller (2002); Mahoney (2005)), antiphospholipid syndrome (Tektonidou (2003)) pregnancy (Cheng (1982); Mahoney (2005)) and some others (Bolland (2004); Macdonald (2001); Rollot (2005)). It was suggested that recidivant microfractures in the region of highly loaded femoral head may lead to microvascular trauma and thereby induce development of AN (Kim (2000)). A question can therefore be posed whether biomechanical parameters such as stresses in the hip are important in the onset of AN. It is the aim of this work to investigate the role of the above biomechanical parameters in the onset of AN.

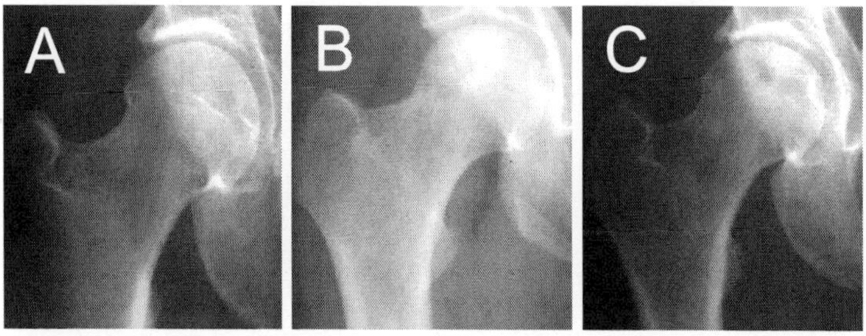

Fig. 5. A: healthy hip, B: initial phase of avascular necrosis of the femoral head when the femoral head is still spherical, C: advanced phase of avascular necrosis of the femoral head in which the femoral head is deformed while the femoral head is unable to bear load.

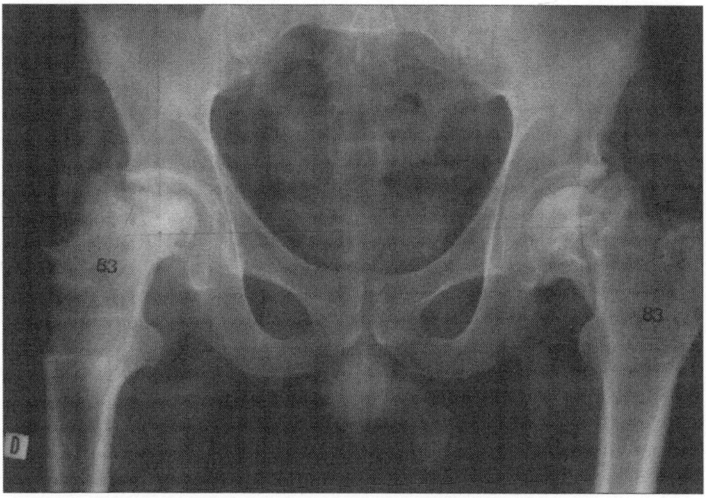

Fig. 6. Bilateral necrosis of the femoral head in an advanced stage.

3.2 Methods

From the archive of the Department of Orthopaedic Surgery, Ljubljana University Medical Centre we selected standard anterior - posterior radiograms of pelvis and proximal femora of 32 adult male persons (32 hips) who were treated due to AN between 1972 and 1991. It was assumed that prior to necrosis both hips had had the same geometry. As the necrotic process had already caused changes in the geometry of some hips, the hips contralateral to the necrotic ones were considered in the study. For comparison, we selected radiograms of 23 male persons (46 normal hips) pertaining to patients who had had a radiogram of the pelvic region taken at the same institution for reasons other than hip joint disease (e.g. lumbalgia). In our study we have considered only male hips. As the values of peak hip stress importantly depend on the gender (Kersnič (1997)) it is important to have gender-matched groups in statistical analysis.

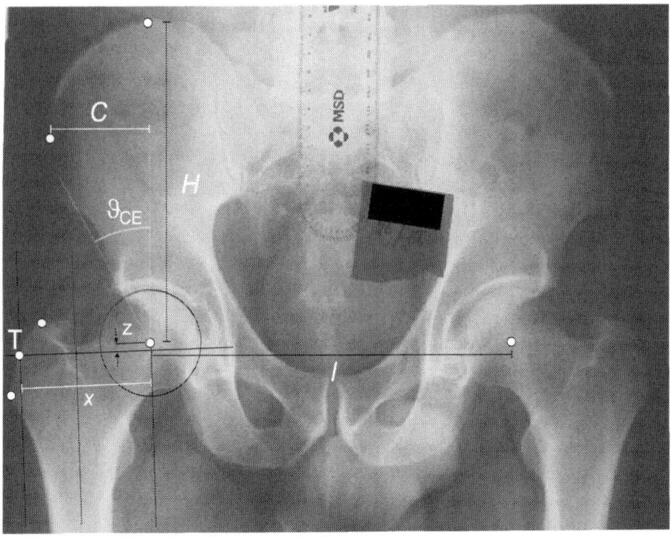

Fig. 7. Geometrical parameters of hip and pelvis which are needed to determine the resultant hip force within the HIPSTRESS method.

The three-dimensional biomechanical model for resultant hip force (Iglič (1993a)) and the above described model for hip stress were used to estimate the magnitude of the resultant hip force in the representative body position (one - legged stance) (Debevec (2010)). The contact stress distribution was given by its peak value p_{max}, location of its pole Θ, index of the contact stress gradient at the lateral acetabular rim G_{p} and functional angle of the load - bearing area ϑ_{F}. The input parameters of the model for the resultant hip force are geometrical parameters of the hip and pelvis: interhip distance l, pelvic height H, pelvic width laterally from the femoral head center C and coordinates of the effective insertion point of abductors on the greater trochanter (point coordinates T_x, T_z) in the frontal plane (Fig.7).

The model of the resultant hip force is based on the equilibria of forces and torques acting between the body segments. To calculate the resultant hip force the three-dimensional reference coordinates of the muscle attachment points were taken from the work of Dostal and Andrews (Dostal (1981)) and scaled with regard to the pelvic parameters (l, C, H, T_x, T_z). To calculate stress, additionally, the radius of the articular surface (taken as the radius of the femoral head) and the angle of the lateral coverage of the femoral head (taken as the centre - edge angle of Wiberg $\vartheta_{\mathrm{L}} \equiv \vartheta_{\mathrm{CE}}$) were assessed from anterior - posterior radiograms for each individual subject. In some radiograms of the patients with AN the upper part of the pelvis was not visible. In these patients the contour was extrapolated on the basis of the visible parts. As in some hips with AN the femoral head was considerably flattened superiorly, centers of rotation on both sides corresponding to the pre - necrotic situation were determined by circles fitting the outlines of the acetabular shells.

To describe stress distribution, we determined biomechanical parameters R, p_{max}, G_p and ϑ_{F} for each hip. The parameters R, p_{max} and G_p were normalized to the body weight (W_{B})

to outline the influence of hip geometry on stress. The respective average values in the test group and the control group were compared by the pooled two - sided Student t - test.

3.3 Results

Parameter (SD)	Test group	Control group	Δ (%)	p
ϑ_F [degrees]	105 (13)	113 (13)	7	0.008
Θ [degrees]	15.4 (7.2)	11.8 (7.6)	27	0.037
G_p/W_B [10^3 m^{-3}]	-17.32 (17.16)	-26.05 (16.85)	40	0.028
p_{max}/W_B [m^{-2}]	2172 (785)	2090 (502)	4	0.604
R/W_B	2.49 (0.21)	2.53 (0.18)	2	0.382

Table 1. Mean biomechanical parameters with standard deviation in brackets in the test group (32 hips contralateral to the necrotic hips) and in the control group (46 normal hips).

Table 1 shows the biomechanical parameters: functional angle of the load bearing area ϑ_F, position of the stress pole, normalized index of the contact stress gradient (G_p/W_B), normalized peak stress (p_{max}/W_B) and normalized resultant hip force (R/W_B) in the test group and in the control group. Hips in the test group are on average less favorable with respect to ϑ_F, G_p/W_B and p_{max}/W_B. The differences in ϑ_F (7%), Θ (27%) and G_p/W_B (40%) are statistically significant ($p = 0.008$, $p = 0.037$ and $p = 0.028$, respectively) while the difference in p_{max}/W_B (4%) is not statistically significant ($p = 0.604$). The magnitude of the resultant hip force R is smaller (more favorable) in the test group, however the difference is very small (2%) and statistically insignificant ($p = 0.382$).

Parameter (SD)	Test group	Control group	Δ (%)	p
C [mm]	60.0 (10.0)	58.5 (8.6)	3	0.463
H [mm]	163.0 (19.6)	162.4 (9.8)	0.4	0.867
l [mm]	203.1 (17.5)	199.6 (8.9)	2	0.305
T_x [mm]	12.5 (7.6)	7.6 (6.4)	49	0.002
T_z [mm]	74.7 (11.3)	69.7 (7.7)	7	0.033
r [mm]	28.5 (3.1)	27.7 (1.7)	3	0.187
ϑ_{CE}[degrees]	30.4 (5.6)	34.7 (6.1)	13	0.002

Table 2. Mean geometrical parameters with standard deviation in brackets in the test group (32 hips contralateral to the necrotic hips) and in the control group (46 normal hips).

In order to better understand the differences in biomechanical parameters, the differences in geometrical parameters used in the models for the above biomechanical parameters were studied (Table 2). The center-edge angle ϑ_{CE} is smaller (less favorable) in the test group than in the control group, the difference (13%) is statistically significant ($p = 0.002$). The lateral position of the insertion point of the effective muscle on the greater trochanter (T_z) is statistically significantly more favorable in the test group than in the control group ($p = 0.033$), while its inferior position (T_x) is considerably (49%) and statistically significantly more favorable in the control group ($p = 0.002$). The differences in other geometrical parameters are small and statistically insignificant.

3.4 Discussion

Our results show that the peak contact hip stress $p_{\max}/W_B$ in the group of hips contralateral to necrotic ones and in the group of normal hips are not statistically significantly different, however, the shape of the stress distribution (given by parameters ϑ_F and G_p/W_B) is statistically significantly less favorable in the group of hips contralateral to necrotic ones.

The differences in the biomechanical parameters can be explained by the differences in the geometrical parameters. The difference in pelvic height H and width C and in the interhip distance l were very small (below 3%) and statistically insignificant while the difference in the vertical coordinate of the insertion of the effective muscle on the greater trochanter (T_x) was statistically significant, but this parameter does not influence much the biomechanical parameters (Daniel (2001)). The differences in the remaining three parameters (lateral coordinate of the insertion of the effective muscle on the greater trochanter, radius of the femoral head and center-edge angle) can however contribute to the explanation of the differences in biomechanical parameters. The centre - edge angle CE is the most important parameter in determination of contact stress distribution. Larger CE corresponds to lower $p_{\max}/W_B$ and smaller G_p/W_B. Table 2 shows that ϑ_{CE} is statistically significantly lower in the test group (p = 0.002) indicating that $p_{\max}/W_B$ and G_p/W_B would be higher in hips contralateral to the necrotic ones. However, $p_{\max}/W_B$ and G_p/W_B strongly depend also on the radius of the femoral head ($p_{\max}/W_B$ is inversely proportional to the square of r and G_p/W_B is inversely proportional to the third power of r). Although the difference in the radii of the two groups is not statistically significant (p = 0.187), the difference (3%) is in favor of hips in the test group. Further, the lateral position of the insertion of the effective muscle is for 7% statistically significantly larger (more favorable) in the test group than in the control group (p = 0.002). The effect of the smaller center-edge angle is therefore counterbalanced by the effect of larger femoral head and more laterally extended greater trochanter. The shape of the stress distribution (described by ϑ_F and G_p/W_B) is on average considerably and statistically significantly different in both groups. In the test group the distribution is steeper, the pole lies more laterally, the gradient index is larger (less negative) and the functional angle of the load-bearing area is smaller than in the control group. This renders hips with increased risk for AN less favorable regarding the stress distribution. However, we did not find a statistically significant difference in $p_{\max}/W_B$.

The magnification of the radiograph was not known, as no unit with known length was visible in the picture. As the magnification may vary considerably contributing to the scattering in the measured distances, poor statistical significance in parameters $p_{\max}/W_B$ and R/W_B can be the consequence of the lack of knowledge of magnification of the radiograms.

It has been hypothesized that transient osteoporosis of the bone marrow oedema syndrome may be the initial phase of osteonecrosis of the femoral head (Hofmann (1994)) and that there may be a common patophysiology. Transient osteoporosis is connected to recidivant microfractures and microvascular trauma at highly loaded regions of the bone leading to the ishemia of the affected part of the bone (Ficat (1981)). Higher contact hip stress may increase the probability and extent of microfractures of the affected bone thereby making the repair more difficult. Furthermore, the replicative capacity of osteoblast cells of the intertrochanteric area of the femur in osteonecrosis patients was found to be significantly reduced compared to patients with osteoarthritis (Gangji (2003)). Thereby, stresses in the hip including the contact hip stress could contribute to the acceleration of the processes leading to AN.

4. Conclusion

Unfavorable stress distribution importantly influences development of the hip and may present a risk factor for osteoarthritis progression as well as for progression of the avascular necrosis of the femoral head.

5. Acknowledgement

Authors are indebted to A. Iglič for discussions and to R. Štukelj and L. Drobne for technical assistance.

6. References

Bolland, M.J., Hood, G., Bastin, S.T., King, A.R., Grey, A., (2004). Bilateral femoral head osteonecrosis after septic shock and multiorgan failure. *J Bone Min Res*, 19, (517-520), ISSN 0884-0431

Brand, R.A., Iglič, A., Kralj-Iglič, V., (2001). Contact stresses in human hip: implications for disease and treatment. *Hip Int*, 11, (117-126), ISSN 1120-7000

Brinckmann, P., Frobin, W., Hierholzer, E.,(1981). Stress on the articular surface of the hip joint in healthy adults and persons with idiopathic osteoarthrosis of the hip joint. *J Biomech*, 14, (149-156), ISSN 0044-3220

Cheng, N., Burssens, A., Mulier, J.C., (1982). Pregnancy and post-pregnancy avascular necrosis of the femoral head. *Arch Orthop Trauma Surg*, 100, (199-210), ISSN 0936-8051

Daniel, M., Antolič, V., Iglič, A., Kralj Iglič., V., (2001). Determination of contact hip stress from nomograms based on mathematical model. *Med Eng Phys*, 23, (347-357), ISSN 1350-4533

Daniel, M., Sochor, M., Iglič, A., Herman, S., Kralj-Iglič, V., (2002). Gradient of contact stress in normal and dyplastic human hips. *Acta Bioeng Biomech, Suppl.* 1, (280-281), ISSN 1509409X

Daniel, M., Sochor, M., Iglič, A., Kralj-Iglič, V., (2003). Hypothesis of regulation of hip joint cartilage activity by mechanical loading. *Medical Hypotheses*, 60, (936-937), ISSN 0306-9877

Daniel, M., Dolinar, D., Herman, S., Sochor, M., Iglič, A., Kralj-Iglič, V., (2006). Contact stress in hips with osteonecrosis of the femoral head. *Clin Orhop Rel Res*, 447, (92-99), ISSN 0009-921X

Daniel, M., Iglič A., Kralj - Iglič, V., (2011). Human hip joint loading - mathematical modeling.Reaction forces and contact pressures. *VDM Verlag Dr. Müller e.K.*, ISBN 978-3-639-26120-2

Debevec, H., Pedersen, D. R., Iglič, A., Daniel, M. (2010). One-legged stance as a representative static body position for calculation of hip contact stress distribution in clinical studies *J Appl Biomech* , ISSN 1065-8483

Dolinar, D., Antolič, V., Herman, S., Iglič, A., Kralj-Iglič, V., Pavlovčič, V., (2003). Influence of contact hip stress on the outcome of surgical treatment of hips affected by avascular necrosis. *Arch Orthop Trauma Surg*, 123, (509-513), ISSN 0936-8051

Dostal, W.F., Andrews, J.G., (1981). A three-dimensional biomechanical model of the hip musculature. *J Biomech*, 14, (803-812), ISSN 0021-9290

Eberhardt, A.W., Lewis, J.L., Keer, L.M., (1991). Contact of layered elastic spheres as a model of joint contact: effect of tangential load and friction. *J Biomech Eng*, 113, (107-108), ISSN 0148-0731

Ficat RP, Arlett, J., (1981). Functional investigation of bone under normal conditions. In: Hungerford, D.S., (ed): Ishemia and necrosis of bone. Baltimore, Williams and Wilkins; 29-52.

Gangji, V., Hauzeur, J.P., Schoutens, A., Hinsenkamp, M., Appelboom, T., Egrise, D., (2003). Abnormalities in the replicative capacity of osteoblastic cells in the proximal femur of patients with osteonecrosis of the femoral head. *J Rheumatol*, 30, (348-351), ISSN 0884-0431

Herman, S., Jaklič, A., Herman, S., Iglič A., Kralj-Iglič, V., (2002). Hip stress reduction after Chiari osteotomy. *Med Biol Eng Comput*, 40, (369-375), ISSN 0009-921X

Herndon, J.H., Aufranc, O.E., (1972). Avascular necrosis of femoral head in the adult. A review of its incidence in a variety of conditions. *Clin Orthop Rel Res*, 86, (43-62), ISSN 0009-921X

Hofmann, S., Engel, A., Neuhold, A., Leder, K., Kramer, J., Plenk, H. Jr., (1994). Bone-marrow oedema syndrome and transient osteoporosis of the hip. An MRI-controlled study of treatment by core decompression. *J Bone Joint Surg*, 76-B, (993-994) ISSN 0301-620X

Iglič, A., Srakar, F., Antolič ,V., Kralj-Iglič, V., Batagelj, V., (1990). Mathematical analysis of Chiari osteotomy. *Acta Orthop Iugosl*, 20, (35-39), ISSN 0350-2309

Iglič, A., Srakar, F., Antolič, V., (1993). Influence of the pelvic shape on the biomechanical status of the hip. *Clin Biomech*, 8, (223-224), ISSN 0268-0033

Iglič, A., Kralj-Iglič, V., Antolič, V., Srakar, F., Stanič, U.,(1993). Effect of the periacetabular osteotomy on the stress on the human hip joint articular surgace. *IEEE T Rehabil Eng*, 1, (207-212), ISSN 1063-6528

Ipavec, M., Brand, R.A., Pedersen, D.R., Mavčič, B., Kralj-Iglič, V., Iglič, A., (1999). Mathematical modelling of stress in the hip during gait. *J Biomech*, 32, (1229-1235), ISSN 0021-9290

Ipavec, M., Brand, R.A., Pedersen, D.R., Mavčič, B., Kralj-Iglič, V., Iglič, A., (2002). Erratum to: Mathematical modelling of stress in the hip during gait, [Journal of Biomechanics, 32(11) (1999) 1229-1235]. *J Biomech*, 35, (555), ISSN 0021-9290

Kersnič, B., Iglič, A., Kralj-Iglič, V., Srakar, F., Antolič, V., (1997). Increased incidence of arthrosis in female population could be related to femoral and pelvic shape. *Arch Orthop Trauma Surg*, 116, (345-347), ISSN 0936-8051

Kim, Y.M., Oh, H.C., Kim, H.J., (2000). The pattern of bone marrow oedema on MRI in osteonecrosis of the femoral head. *J Bone Joint Surg*, 82-B, (837-841), ISSN 0301-620X

Miller, K.D., Masur, H., Jones, E.C. et al., (2002). High prevalence of osteonecrosis of the femoral head in HIV infected adults. *Ann Intern Med*, 137, (17-25), ISSN 0003-4819

Kralj, M., Mavčič, B., Antolič, V., Iglič, A., Kralj-Iglič, V., (2005). The Bernese periacetabular osteotomy: clinical, radiographic and biomechanical 7-15 year follow-up in 26 hips. *Acta Orthop*, 76, (833-840), ISSN 1745-3674

Lipshitz, H., Glimcher, M.J., (1979). In vitro studies of the wear of articular cartilage. II Characteristics of the wear of articular cartilage when worn against stainless steel plates having characteristic surfaces. *Wear*, 52, (297-339), ISSN 0043-1648

Macdonald, A.G., Bissett, J.D., (2001). Avascular necrosis of the femoral head in patients with prostate cancer treated with cyproterone acetate and radiotherapy. *Clin Oncol*, 13, (135-137), ISSN 0936-6555

Mahoney, C.R., Glesby, M.J., DiCarlo, E.F., Peterson, M.G., Bostrom, M.P. (2005). Total hip arthroplasty in patients with human immunodeficiency virus infection: pathologic findings and surgical outcomes. *Acta Orthop*, 76, (198-203), ISSN 1745-3674

Mavčič, B., Pompe, B., Antolič, V., Daniel, M., Iglič, A., Kralj-Iglič, V., (2002). Mathematical estimation of stress distribution in normal and dysplastic human hips. *J Orthop Res*, 20, (1025-1030), ISSN 0736-0266

Mavčič, B., Iglič, A., Kralj-Iglič, V., Brand, R.A., Vengust, R., (2008). Cumulative hip contact stress predicts osteoarthritis in DDH. *Clin Orthop Rel Res*, 466, (884-891), ISSN 0009-921X

McCutchen, C.W., (1962). The frictional properties of animal joints. *Wear*, 5, (1-17), ISSN 0043-1648.

Mont, M.A., Hungerford, D.S. (1995). Non-traumatic avascular necrosis of the femoral head. *J Bone Joint Surg*, 77-A, (459-469), ISSN 0021-9355

Pompe, B., Daniel, M., Sochor, M., Vengust, R., Kralj-Iglič, V., Iglič, A., (2003). Gradient of contact stress in normal and dysplastic human hips. *Med Eng Phys*, 25, (379-385), ISSN 1350-4533

Pompe, B., Antolič, V., Mavčič, B., Iglič, A., Kralj-Iglič, V., (2007). Hip joint contact stress as an additional parameter for determining hip dysplasia in adults: Comparison with Severin's classification. *Med Sci Monitor*, 13,(CR215-219), ISSN 1234-1010

Rečnik, G., Kralj-Iglič ,V., Iglič, A., Antolič,V., Kramberger, S., Vengust, R., (2007). Higher peak contact hip stress predetermines the side of hip involved in idiopathic osteoarthritis. *Clin Biomech*, 22, (1119-1124), ISSN 0268-0033

Rečnik, G., Vengust, R., Kralj-Iglič, V., Vogrin, M., Kranjc Z., Kramberger, S., (2009). Association between Sub-clinical acetabular dysplasia and a younger age at hip arthroplasty in idiopathic osteoarthritis. *J Int Med Res*, 37, (1620-1625) ISSN 0300-0605

Rečnik, G., Kralj-Iglič, V., Iglič, A., Antolič, V., Kramberger, S. , Rigler, I., Pompe, B., Vengust, R., (2009). The role of obesity, biomechanical constitution of the pelvis and contact joint stress in progression of hip osteoarthritis. *Osteoarthr Cartilage*, 3, (879-882), ISSN 1063-4584

Rollot, F., Wechsler, B., du Boutin, le T.H., De Gennes, C., Amoura, Z., Hachulla, E., Piette, J.C., (2005). Hemochromatosis and femoral head aseptic osteonecrosis: a nonfortuitous association. *J Rheumatol*, 32, (376-378), ISSN 0315-162X

Tektonidou, M.G., Malagari, K., Vlachoyiannopoulos, P.G., Kelekis, D.A., Moutsopoulos, H.M., (2003). Asymptomatic avascular necrosis in patients with primary antiphospholipid syndrome in the absence of corticosteroid use: A prospective study by magnetic resonance imaging. *Arthritis Rheum*, 48, (732-736), ISSN 0004-3591

Vengust, R., Daniel, M., Antolič, V., Zupanc, O., Iglič, A., Kralj-Iglič, V., (2001). Biomechanical evaluation of hip joint after Salter innominate osteotomy: a long-term follow-up study. *Arch Orthop Trauma Surg*, 121, (511-516), ISSN 0936-8051

Zupanc, O., Križančič, M., Daniel, M., Mavčič, B., Antolič, V., Iglič, A., Kralj-Iglič, V., (2008). shear stress in epiphyseal growth plate is a risk factor for slipped capital femoral epiphysis. *J Pediatr Orthoped*, 28, (444-451), ISSN 0271-6798

16

Development and Clinical Application of Instruments to Measure Orofacial Structures

Amanda Freitas Valentim,
Renata Maria Moreira Moraes Furlan, Tatiana Vargas de Castro Perilo,
Andréa Rodrigues Motta, Monalise Costa Batista Berbert,
Márcio Falcão Santos Barroso, Cláudio Gomes da Costa,
Iracema Maria Utsch Braga and Estevam Barbosa de Las Casas
Universidade Federal de Minas Gerais
Brazil

1. Introduction

The human body consists of a series of systems, which work in an integrated way for perfect functioning. One of these systems, the muscular system, consists of a set of muscles that are able to contract and relax, resulting in the generation of diverse and varied movements that allow the person to walk, eat and talk, and perform many other actions.

The muscle groups that integrate the human body have different characteristics. There are long muscles, which are powerful but not so precise in their movements, while another set of muscles is described by their small size and high accuracy in generated movements.

The muscles which compose the orofacial system are characterized by their small sizes and the ability to generate highly precise and differentiated movements that includes a series of rapid shape changes. This is made possible due to the large amount of innervations and the complex organization of the muscle fibers. These muscles play an essential role in mastication, swallowing, speech, breathing and suction, functions that require fast and complex movements. They also contribute to the orientation of facial bone growth and maintenance of teeth position.

Like all systems that constitute the body, many diseases can cause changes in the structures that compose the muscular system. Changes, such as muscle weakening, that interfere in tongue and lips movements can hamper activities related to various physiological processes. When any disorder or other conditions causes an improper functioning of orofacial muscles, it is necessary to rehabilitate the impaired muscle group. This muscular rehabilitation work, named myotherapy, includes orientations and rehabilitative exercises and it shall be carefully planned in order to achieve fast and effective results. However, to organize a work plan it is essential to perform a well-structured assessment of muscular condition.

Currently, the evaluation by speech-language pathologists of these muscles is routinely made in a qualitative way. One of the current evaluation techniques consists of asking the patient to perform a contraction against an imposed obstacle, such as a gloved finger. Based on experience, the speech-language pathologist classifies the force as normal or not.

For several years, an effective method has been sought to quantify the force or pressure that orofacial structures are able to exert. This method would allow comparing the values with the parameters obtained in the qualitative evaluation and to measure performance during the main functions and exercises. A quantitative evaluation can improve diagnosis, especially in cases of slight changes in force and is more sensitive in detecting the small differences in strength observed with the progression of the disease or therapy.

The field of Biomechanical Engineering combines engineering with biology and physiology, using principles of mechanics to design, model, develop and analyze equipment and systems. In Brazil there are Biomechanics research groups in different regions of the country, although mostly concentrated in Southeast of the country. In this region is the Biomechanics Engineering Group from the Universidade Federal de Minas Gerais, an interdisciplinary group, was created in 1998, and includes researchers from the fields of engineering and health care. The purpose of the group is to study the mechanical behavior of tissues, organs and biomaterials under the action of external loads and other types of actions using computational and experimental techniques. In 2002, a professor and a few Speech Language Pathology undergraduate students joined the group with a project that aimed to develop instruments for quantifying the forces of orofacial structures in order to help in orofacial myology assessment. The first instrument created was FORLING, to measure tongue force. After that, the group started to grow, with more undergraduate and graduate students, and started a new project: the development of an instrument to measure lips force, FORLAB. Both of them were intended to be used in the stages of diagnosis, prognosis and therapeutic follow-up.

This chapter focuses on describing the development of devices and quantitative techniques created by the Group, to quantify forces and improve the assessment of orofacial muscles. It also includes an analysis of the obtained values of tongue and lip forces and a discussion on the consequences of the obtained data on clinical practice.

2. Tongue

2.1 Anatomy and physiology of the tongue

The tongue is a highly specialized organ of the body and a focal point for many professionals from several fields of knowledge. It actively participates in functions such as sucking, mastication, swallowing and speech, which are fundamental in maintaining the quality of life. It is a mobile structure that can take many shapes and positions, in extremely fast sequences, due to its high innervations and complex organization of muscle fibers (Zemlin 1997).

It is characterized as being essentially a muscular organ, which occupies the functional space of the oral cavity. It is formed by striated muscle tissue and covered by a flat mucosa in the lower part and is irregular on the top due to the large number of papillae (Aprile et al. 1975).

The tongue can be divided into body and root, or, based on its relationship with the palate, into apex and body. The body can be subdivided into the front and back part. The apex of the tongue is the part closest to the anterior teeth; the region just below the hard palate is the front and the region located below the soft palate is the posterior (Zemlin 1997).

The dorsum of the tongue is divided by the longitudinal sulcus, which is continuous from the back to an orifice called the foramen cecum. From the foramen cecum, a shallow V-shaped sulcus, called terminal sulcus, has its anterior and laterally path toward the edges of the tongue. This is the anatomical reference point that separates two anatomically and functionally distinct regions, the anterior two thirds and the posterior third of the tongue. In the anterior two thirds, the dorsum has a rough surface and contains the taste papillae, while the posterior third of the tongue looks smoother and contains numerous mucous glands and lymph vessels that form the lingual tonsil (Zemlin 1997).

The lingual septum divides the tongue into halves and its muscles are considered in pairs. The muscles of the tongue are classified as extrinsic and intrinsic. The extrinsic muscles (Figure 1) originate in adjacent structures and are inserted into the tongue, being responsible for movement in different directions. They are: genioglossus, styloglossus, palatoglossus and hyoglossus. The genioglossus is the largest of the extrinsic muscles and is fan-shaped. The contraction of the posterior fibers moves the tongue forward, protruding the apex, while the contraction of the anterior fibers causes tongue retraction and the contraction of the whole muscle moves the tongue down. The styloglossus, during its contraction, moves the tongue upward and backward, and along with the superior longitudinal muscle, directs the sides of the tongue upward to make the dorsum concave. The function of the muscle palatoglossus is to lower the soft palate or to raise the back of the tongue grooving the dorsum. The hyoglossus retracts and depresses the tongue (Zemlin 1997).

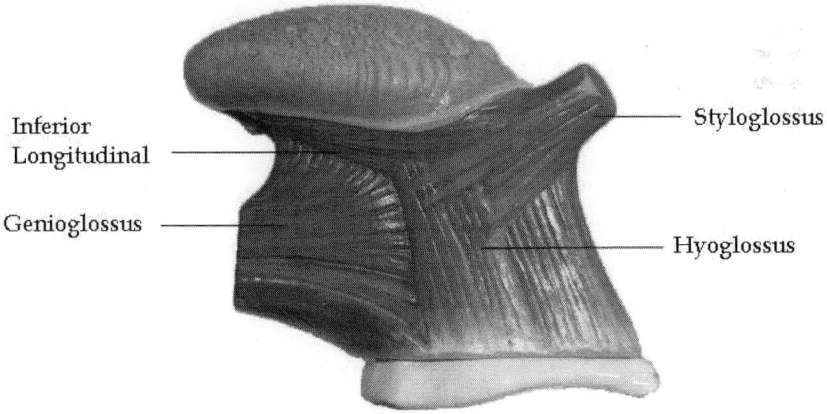

Fig. 1. Extrinsic tongue muscles and the inferior longitudinal

The intrinsic muscles (Figure 2) are contained in the tongue itself and are responsible for changing the shape of the organ. They are: superior longitudinal, inferior longitudinal, transverse and vertical. The superior longitudinal muscle shortens the tongue and turns its apex upward. The oblique fibers help turn the side margins up, leaving the back concave. The inferior longitudinal shortens the tongue, pushes the apex downward and leaves the dorsum convex. The vertical muscle flattens and extends the tongue, while the transverse muscle narrows and lengthens the body (Zemlin 1997).

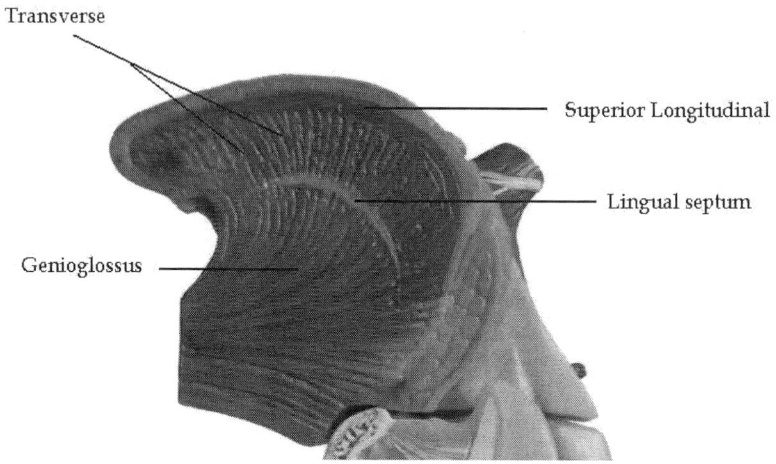

Fig. 2. Intrinsic tongue muscles and genioglossus

Although the genioglossus muscle is considered the most powerful extrinsic lingual muscle (Zemlin 1997), in cases of a protruding tongue against a resistance, genioglossus activation plays an important role, but not a primary one. It actually provides a stable platform against which the intrinsic muscles of the tongue in the anterior part can develop strength (Pittman and Bailey 2009).

Both intrinsic and extrinsic tongue muscles are innervated by the hypoglossal nerve (cranial nerve XII) (Zemlin 1997); Douglas 2002), except the palatoglossus muscle, which is innervated by the glossopharyngeal (the ninth pair of cranial nerves) (Douglas 2002). As for sensitivity, the tongue presents refined taste activity, which results from the action of some nerves, such as the trigeminal nerve, which provides the overall sensitivity of the anterior two-thirds, the glossopharyngeal nerve, responsible for the overall sensitivity of the posterior third and the facial nerve, which is responsible for taste in the anterior two-thirds (Dangelo and Fattini 1998).

2.2 Instruments described in the literature to measure tongue force/pressure

Kydd (1956) quantified tongue force of an edentulous 30-year-old man using a device composed of a denture base made of methyl methacrylate, whose vertical dimensions were maintained between the bases by four vertical rods embedded in the lower denture base. There were three blocks of methyl methacrylate between the rods, positioned to replace the lingual surface of the lower incisor area and second premolar-first molar areas. Electric resistance strain gauges were attached to these blocks. The pressure exerted by the tongue on the block produced a deformation on the gauge, modifying its resistance. An alternating current amplifier and a multichannel pen recorder were used to provide dynamic as well as static recordings. It was found that 23.13 N was the maximum force exerted anteriorly, and 11.56 N and 10.23 N laterally in the right and left lower first molar-second premolar areas, respectively.

Posen (1972) measured maximum tongue force in subjects with and without problems in occlusion. The instrument was made of a gauge to give a reading of up to 50 N when pushing a spring that was attached to the gauge. At the other end of the spring, there was a concave piece where the tongue exerted force. Subjects with normal occlusion exerted forces between 6 N and 25 N.

Dworkin (1980) measured tongue strength using one semiconductor strain gauge welded to a tubular stem for easy insertion into the mouth and a single channel pen-writing portable recording system. The force transducer could be positioned anteriorly between the upper and lower incisor teeth, or laterally, between the canine and first bicuspid teeth, and the subject was requested to bite down on the stem and apply tongue pressure against the transducer with the tongue tip. The maximum force exerted by normal subjects was 20 N anteriorly and 16 N laterally.

Scardella et al. (1993) measured tongue force using a force transducer that translated direct compression forces generated by the tongue into an active arm outside the mouth connected to a strain gauge with a linear response for forces between 50 gf and 100 gf, which was incorporated into a two-arm active bridge circuit. Five normal male subjects (ages 21 to 36) were evaluated. The maximum force ranged between 9.50 N and 16.33 N, with an average maximum force of 12.67 ± 1.25 N.

Mortimore et al. (1999) used a transducer consisting of a machined nylon hand grip and a mouthpiece. The mouthpiece consisted of a 1-cm diameter nylon plate behind which was positioned a 6 kgf button load cell, which responded to tension and compression. Behind the plate, the mouthpiece consisted of a groove approximately 2-mm deep and 2-mm wide. Subjects were asked to rest their upper and lower incisor teeth against the groove in order for the transducer to reach steady state. The force was then exerted on the plate by the subject's tongue. The transducer was connected to a linear visual scale displaying the force in Newton (N) or as a percentage of the subject's maximum force (measured during a previous trial). Eighty-six females and eighty-one males aged between 42 and 62 years were evaluated. An average maximum force of 26 ± 8 N for men and 20 ± 7 N for women was recorded.

Bu Sha et al. (2000) measured tongue force using a custom-designed lingual force transducer housed in a piece of polyvinyl chloride tube. The tube was bisected lengthwise and a latex balloon catheter was mounted between the two halves of the tube and secured in place with dental impression material. The balloon was positioned so that when it was inflated with 4 mL of saline, it protruded 1.0 cm beyond the end of the tube. A 2-mm thick rubber sheath covered the end of the tube, providing the subject a soft, stable surface to bite when producing protrusion efforts. The sheath was marked at 0.5 cm intervals from the balloon end of the tube over a length of 4.0 cm. The balloon catheter was connected to a pressure transducer and the output was amplified, recorded and reconverted into force. The subject held the transducer in the mouth and bit down on the tube. With the tip of the tongue on the balloon, increasing or decreasing the depth of the transducer in the oral cavity increased or decreased the length of the tongue muscle fibers. The maximum measured force was 28.0 ± 2.0 N. Most subjects had a maximum force at a transducer position of 2.5 cm.

A study was conducted with a device developed by the Biomechanical Engineering Group of UFMG named FORLING. It was composed of a piston-cylinder assembly attached to a double silicon protector and to a head that connected it to the cylinder. The oral protector was inserted and fitted in the mouth of the patient, who was required to push the cylinder head with the tongue with the maximum force he could exert for 10 seconds. This procedure was repeated three times, with 1-minute intervals between them. The cylinder head hydraulically transmitted the produced force to a pressure sensor. The pressure sensor measurements were transmitted through a data acquisition device to a personal computer. The method was tested with four healthy subjects, two women and two men aged from 23 to 32 years. The obtained results for the maximum force were 25.7 N, 21.7 N, 21.6 N and 21.1 N, while those for the average force were 20.6 N, 18.2 N, 17.4 N and 18.6 N (Motta et al. 2004).

Another group measured tongue protrusion force using a force transducer (Grass FT10 Force Displacement Transducer) trapped in a vertical surface. The instrument had a piece that was to be placed in the oral cavity. This piece had a cushion for teeth positioning, which the subjects had to bite and press the tongue against a round 20-mm diameter button connected to the force transducer by a cylindrical steel beam of 5 mm diameter and 50 mm length. The button protruded 25 mm from the cushion inside the oral cavity. The maximum protrusion force in voluntary contraction was measured for 5 seconds and the percentage of the force related to maximum force was shown in an oscilloscope to provide visual feedback. The measurements were performed in 12 male subjects with an average age of 23 years, and the maximum obtained force was 24.3 ± 6.7 N (O'Connor et al. 2007).

The palatal plate developed by Kieser et al. (2008) was designed to simultaneously measure pressure at diverse locations in the mouth and was constructed from a chrome-cobalt alloy. To measure pressure during swallowing, an anterior pair of gauges measured lingual and labial contact against the left central incisor tooth, while two pairs of gauges measured pressure contributions of the lateral tongue margin and cheeks on the canine and first molar teeth. Finally, lingual pressure on the midline of the palate was measured by two gauges, one at the position of the premolars and one on the posterior boundary of the hard palate. The 8-channel output was gathered simultaneously and then recorded and displayed on a computer. They recorded intraoral pressures in five adult volunteers during swallowing of 10 mL of water. The pressure ranged from 13.05 kPa to 289.75 kPa.

Utanohara et al. (2008) used a tongue pressure measurement device consisting of a disposable oral probe, an infusion tube as a connector and a recording device. The probe was assembled with a small, partially inflated bulb made from medical grade latex, a plastic pipe as a connector and a syringe cylinder for the patient to hold on. A recording device with a manual autopressurization system was used. By pushing the pressurization button, the probe was inflated with air at an initial pressure of 19.6 kPa. This pressure was taken as the standard and measurements were performed after zero calibration. The subjects were asked to place the bulb in their mouth, holding the plastic pipe at the midpoint of their central incisors with closed lips, to raise the tongue and compress the bulb onto the palate with maximum voluntary effort, and the maximum value was recorded. Tongue pressure was measured in 843 subjects between 20 and 79 years old. The average maximum tongue pressure was 41.7 ± 9.7 kPa in subjects between 20 and 29; 41.9 ± 9.9 kPa (30 to 39 years old); 40.4 ± 9.8 kPa (40 to 49 years old); 40.7 ± 9.8 kPa (50 to 59 years old); 37.6 ± 8.8 kPa (60 to 69 years old) and 31.9 ± 8.9 kPa (70 to 79 years old).

Another study made with FORLING (Barroso et al. 2009) quantified tongue force of 10 subject aged between 14 and 80 years whose tongues were classified as normal or as having a small deficit in force and found average force values between 3.55 N and 13.24 N and maximum force values between 4.97 N and 19.96 N.

A study used the Iowa Oral Performance Instrument (IOPI) to measure tongue pressure of 39 young adults (17 men and 22 women). IOPI is a commercially available tongue pressure measurement system composed of an air-filled bulb connected to a pressure transducer. The bulb was placed in three different positions in the oral cavity, so that they could measure tongue protrusion, lateralization and elevation. In the last two positions, a blade was used to hold the bulb. Three measurements were made for each subject and the higher value was considered the maximum pressure. The average maximum tongue pressures found for all subjects were around 55 kPa for lateralization, 62 kPa for elevation and 65 kPa for protrusion (Clark et al. 2009).

The Myometer 160 used by Lambrechts et al. (2010) contained a probe consisting of two plates that were screwed together on one side. On the other side (probe tip), the two plates could be pushed towards each other. The applied force was measured by an electronic device installed between the plates and shown on a bar graph. To measure tongue force, the patient placed the lips around the opening of the plate and protruded the tongue as hard as possible against the probe tip. Tongue pressure of 107 subjects (63 females and 44 males) between 7 and 45 years old were measured. The average tongue pressure was 1.66 N.

2.3 Instrument proposed to measure tongue force

The prototype of the device developed by the Group of Biomechanics of UFMG for measuring the force of the tongue, Portable FORLING, has the following characteristics: good fixation and stability in the patient's mouth; portability; lightweight; low cost; simple operation; reliable indication of tongue force protrusion; a wide range of force; good repeatability; small size; immune to external influences (temperature or voltage fluctuation); comfortable for the patient; made of biocompatible material; resistant to crashes and easy to sanitize.

Portable FORLING is shown in Figure 3. It consists of two parts, one that goes in the mouth of the patient (where the sensor is located) and another for the data acquisition system.

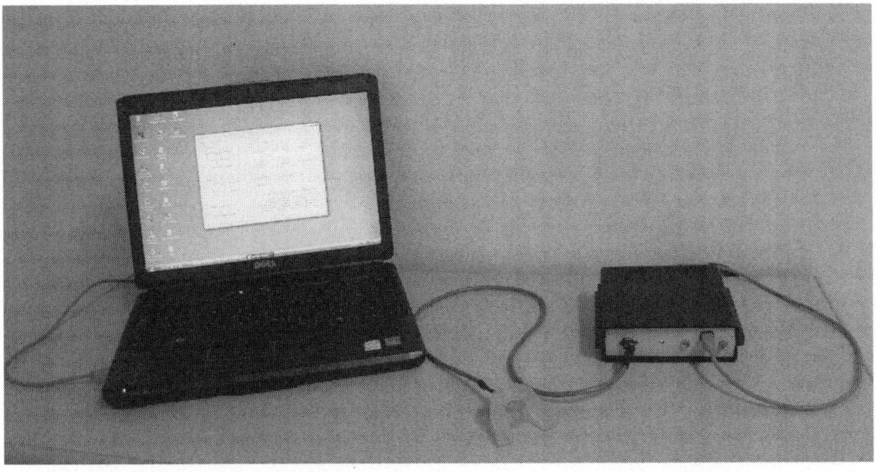

Fig. 3. Portable device for measuring the force of the tongue: Portable FORLING.

The mouthguard consists of a commercially available double mouth protector used by boxers, with an anatomical shape composed of a biocompatible, nontoxic, lightweight and flexible material so as not to cause discomfort, and allows reuse. It is made of moldable material, acquiring the shape of dental arches, which makes it adaptable to patients with malocclusion.

The function of the mouthguard is to keep the device stable in the patient's mouth, so that the position of the force applicator plate is always the same for a given patient. It is also important to guarantee that the relative motion of the patient's body does not interfere with the force measurement. The dimensions of the mouthguard coincide with the teeth, length of dental arches and relationships between the positions of the tooth centers, as described in the literature (Wheeler and Major 1987; Silva and Pecora 1998; Proffit et al. 2007). The mouthguard has a cutout to accommodate the upper and lower lip frenulum and an opening in its front to accommodate the base piece.

There is a set of small pieces at the inner surface of the mouthguard, which consists of a base, a force sensor, an applicator pin, a holder and a force applicator. This set is positioned this way to absorb the force of protrusion of the tongue. All components of the prototype are biocompatible. The mouthguard and its internal parts are shown in Figure 4. The sensor is positioned between the base and pin applicator.

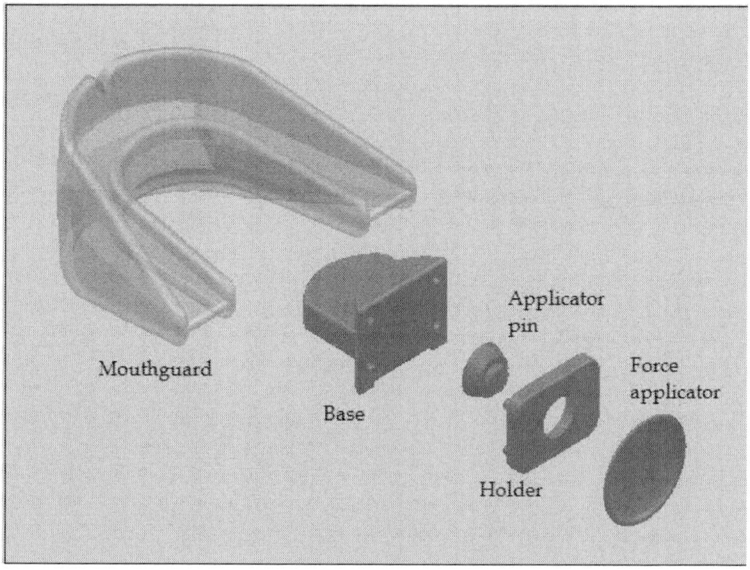

Fig. 4. Illustration of the mouthguard and its internal parts.

The inner parts of the mouthguard were made by stereolithography in epoxy, providing the required mechanical characteristics of stiffness and strength.

The prototype was designed to use small size, thinness, lightness, flexibility and low-cost force sensors, the FlexiForce type A201. A picture of the sensor used is shown in Figure 5.

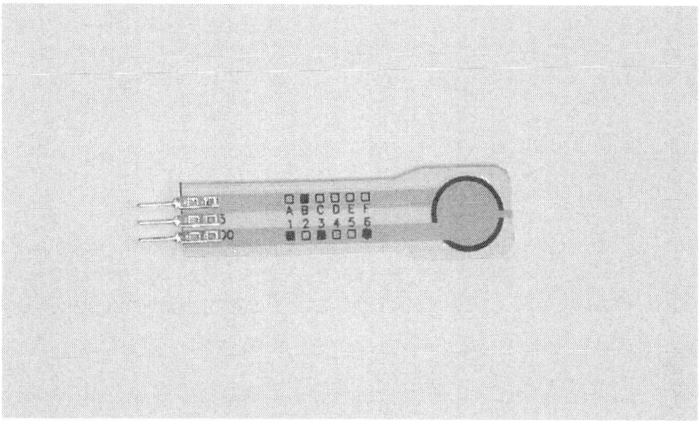

Fig. 5. FlexiForce Sensor (Tekscan) Model A201.

FlexiForce sensors use technology based on resistivity. The application of a force in a sensitive area elicits a change in resistance of a sensing element inversely proportional to the applied force.

The sensors are encapsulated and their movements are restricted to prevent errors in the generated force signal. In addition, there is an adequate guide to the force applicator.

To ensure accurate and repeatable readings of force, care has to be taken to assure that the applied load is evenly distributed in the sensitive area of the sensor and is not supported by the external area.

The signal conditioning is made using operational amplifiers for signal linearization and conversion of electrical resistance into electrical voltage. The signal goes through an amplification system to ensure the adequate quality of the result, since the data acquisition system is at a considerable distance from the measuring point.

The data acquisition system is composed of three main modules:

- Antialiasing filter;
- Analog to digital converter;
- Serial communication.

The sampling rate is 10 Hz, ensuring compatibility with the characteristics of USB communication and is sufficient to obtain the desired information about tongue force.

Communication with the personal computer is controlled by software as well as the timing between the data and the computer, which is used as a monitoring system, storage system control and data acquisition.

The software was developed by one of the researchers at the Universidade Federal São João Del Rei, using a Matlab platform that allows the evaluator to conduct the evaluation process and store all relevant information.

At the end of three measurements, a report is generated that presents the force profile of the patient. This report records the graphics of force over time (profile) of the three measurements taken, as well as the values of maximum and average forces of each measurement, the overall mean and standard deviation of these parameters.

3. Lips

3.1 Anatomy and physiology of the lips

The orbicularis oris muscle (Figure 6) is the facial muscle responsible for the lips shape and function. Its motor innervation is provided by the facial nerve and its sensitivity by the trigeminal nerve (Cosenza 2005). The orbicularis oris is elliptical, and consists of upper and lower fibers, which form the upper and lower lips that interact in the region of the labial commissure (Figun and Garino 2003). Each of those parts consists of pars peripheralis and pars marginalis segments. The pars marginalis fibers have narrow diameters and are localized in the vermilion area of the lip. When this pars contracts, it presses the lip to the maxillary teeth or inverts it, making the lip cover the incisal and occlusal borders of the teeth. The pars peripheralis consists of horizontal, oblique and longitudinal fibers and surrounds the pars previously described. Contraction of this pars results in labial elevation, an action involved in both facial expression and speech (Rogers et al. 2009).

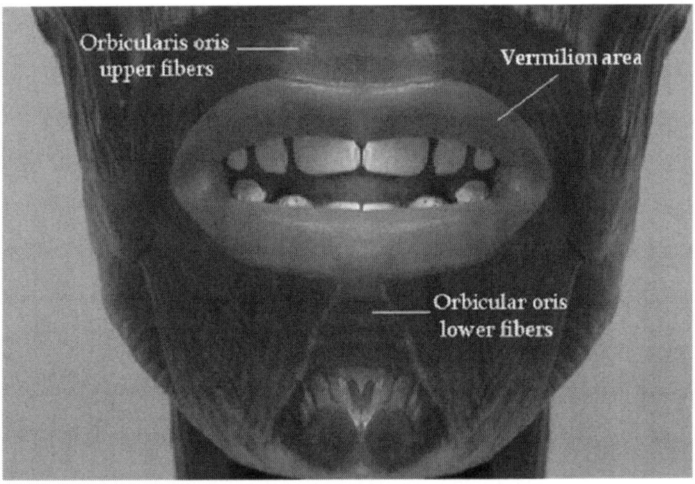

Fig. 6. Orbucularis oris muscle and vermilion area

Lips contraction is essential for many oral functions as it produces closure of the mouth and is necessary in speech, food prehension and swallowing. Lips also participate in the actions of blowing, sucking, kissing and whistling (Figun and Garino 2003). In suction and swallowing, the sealing of the lips is necessary to promote intraoral pressure; in speech, lips work by interrupting the air flow, favoring the pronunciation of different phonemes such as /f/, /v/, /b/, /p/ and /m/ (Douglas 2002), or modifying the shape of the oral cavity, changing voice resonance and helping to produce the vowels.

Since the inferior lip position depends on mandibular movements, this is the more mobile of the two and also the faster. Most of the facial expression muscles are inserted into the lips, which contribute to the great variability of labial movements (Zemlin 1997).

Another important function of the lips is to exert pressure on the teeth in the superior and inferior dental arch. The lips balance the force made by the tongue on teeth. Tongue muscles push the teeth outwards while the lips, when closed, provide resistance to that force, as their contraction presses teeth intraorally. This force balance allows dental elements to erupt and remain in the correct position in the oral cavity (Proffit and Fields 2002). The orbicularis oris together with other muscles act like a muscle strip, orienting growth of the jaws. When the lips are not sealed, there is no action of this muscle strip, possibly leading to some dysfunctions in jaw growth and teeth eruption (Gonzalez and Lopes 2000).

Dysfunctions in lip muscles can initiate important functional problems, one of which is speech distortion characterized chiefly by imprecision of the sounds that require orbicularis oris contraction (Farias et al. 1996). Another one is a dysfunction in feeding functions, like mastication and swallowing, in which the non-closure of the lips leads to difficulties in maintaining food in the oral cavity and generating negative intraoral pressure, which is indispensable for correct food propulsion (Biazevic et al. 2010).

3.2 Instruments described in the literature to measure lips force

The first studies on lips force measurement are from the 1970s. Although the efforts to obtain a numerical value are valid, it is important to observe the agreement with clinical practice diagnosis. Garliner (1971) described the use of a dynamometer, which was adapted into a shirt button attached to a wire. An important question about that study, although it measured values of force, is that traction of the wire was made by the patient, which introduced a subjective element, since the applied force varied from patient to patient and did not allow the establishment of appropriate relationships between individuals.

Posen (1976) reported the development of a device to measure the force of the perioral muscles using a rigid rod and a small circular shaped insert. In this case, the patient was asked to position the lips surrounding this insert and impose traction with the head against the rod as hard as possible. The author evaluated 170 women and 166 men aged between 8 and 18 years with normal occlusion, and categorized the measurements carried out as follows: 160 g to 175 g for individuals with weak lips; 180 g to 195 g for individuals with slightly weak lips; 200 g to 215 g for those with moderate lips force; 220 g to 235 g for those with slightly increased lips force and 240 g to 260 g for individuals classified as having increased lips force. The subjective component was still considerable because head movement was used in addition to the lips.

A study aimed to determine whether advancing age could significantly interfere with the generation of oral forces. Forty women aged between 20 and 100 years were evaluated. For that, leverage force sensors coupled to the incisor teeth were used in both the upper and lower dental arches. The contraction time required for each examination was 5 seconds. Measurements were made during oral functions and maximum voluntary contraction of the lip muscles. The subjects were separated into subgroups according to their age. The mean values of maximal contraction of the upper lip were about 5.8 N for women aged 20 to 60 years, and 4.0 N for women between 80 to 100 years old. For the lower lip, these values ranged from 11.0 N for the first group and 10.0 N for the second. There were significantly higher strength values for the lower lip compared with the upper lip. However, little differences were observed between the subgroups (McHenry et al. 1999).

In the same way, two groups of researchers (Cantero et al. 2003 and Gonzalez et al. 2004) described a method of assessing lips force based on an instrument constructed using a dynamometer. A stainless steel plate was adapted into the dynamometer and the subjects could bite the plate, having a mouthguard as support that was sterilized after use. No further details were given about the methodology. The authors described three measurements for each subject and the analyzed parameter was the highest value of the three trials. In one of these studies, Cantero et al. (2003) evaluated lips force of 90 children before and after speech-language therapy. The measured force values significantly increased after orofacial myofunctional therapy, ranging from 1.68 N to 1.82 N before treatment and from 2.05 N to 2.34 N after treatment. Using the same methodology, another group (Gonzalez et al. 2004) evaluated 180 children between 5 and 12 years old, 90 with lip seal and another 90 with incompetent lip seal. Two measurements were made in children who had incompetent lip seal, one before and one after treatment. The results indicated force values ranging from 1.57 N to 2.15 N before treatment and 2.03 N to 2.72 N after treatment. Moreover, boys presented higher lips forces.

Another usual goal is the verification of malocclusion. Jung et al. (2003) evaluated 32 male students, who had Angle Class I and obtained an average force varying from 3.3 N to 13.1 N, while the maximum force ranged from 4.3 to 20.3 N. Earlier, Unemori and colleagues (1996) examined two individuals before and after orthognathic surgery and obtained force values ranging from 1.0 to 2.2 gf/mm^2.

Hägg and Anniko (2008) recently conducted a retrospective study involving 30 subjects aged between 49 and 88 years who had suffered a stroke. They measured lips force using the Lip Force Meter (LF100). This instrument consists of a transducer that is placed between the lips and teeth and is attached to a steel wire, which is connected to a load cell. After acclimatization, the examiner held the instrument and asked the subjects to contract their lips in order to pull the wire. Lips strength evaluation and swallowing performance analyses were done. The evaluations were conducted pre and post myotheraphic intervention. The average lips force was 7 N before starting treatment and 18.5 N after the intervention and this correlation was statistically significant. An improvement in the ability of swallowing after therapeutic intervention was also observed.

3.3 Instrument proposed to measure lips force

The FORLAB lips measurement system (Figure 7) is composed of an intralips insert, against which the patient presses the lips to generate a counter-resistance force. This force is transmitted to the load cell, by mechanical coupling. The load cell generates an analog signal in tension that is treated, transmitted, processed and saved.

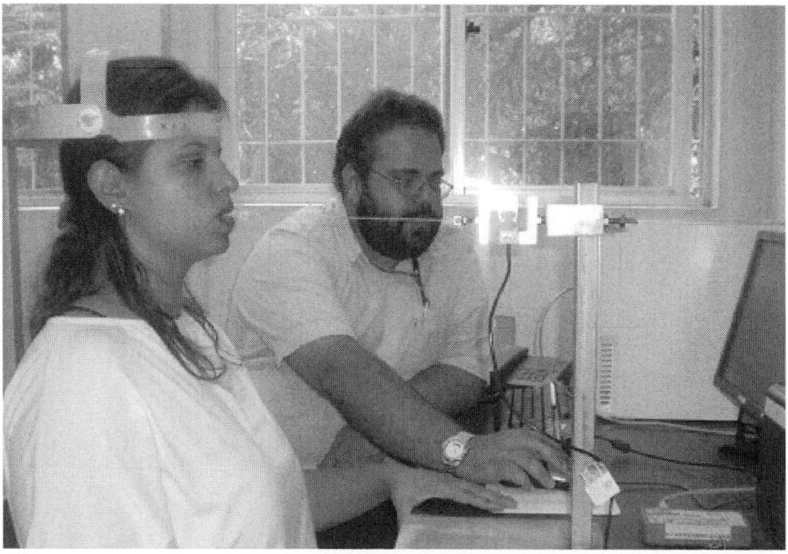

Fig. 7. Portable device for measuring the force of the lips: FORLAB.

The insert (Figure 8) has an elliptical shape with parabolic curvature and a lateral dimension of 60 mm. The manufacturing process was rapid prototyping using nontoxic polymers, which follows the biosafety recommendations for use in human beings.

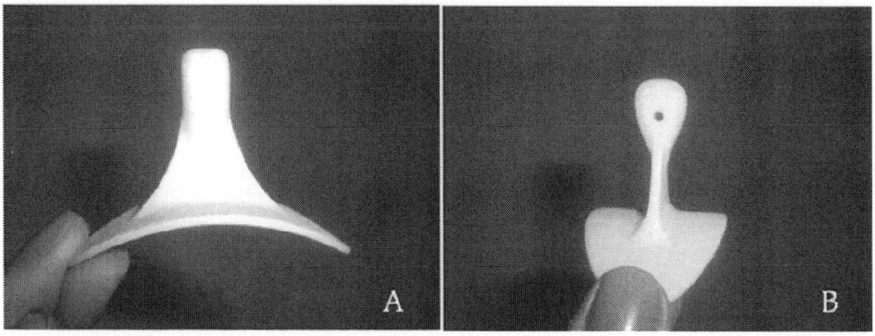

Fig. 8. Frontal (A) and lateral (B) view of the insert.

The insert is positioned as in the qualitative evaluation, leaving a gap between the lips and the dental arch, so that the patient can pull it with the lips (Figure 9), thereby generating a resistance force. This force is transmitted to the load cell by mechanical coupling, in this case, provided by a steel wire. The load cell has a capacity of 50 N, is electronically connected in bridge and generates an analog signal when pulled in traction. A head support is used to prevent the person from generating the force with the head instead of the lips.

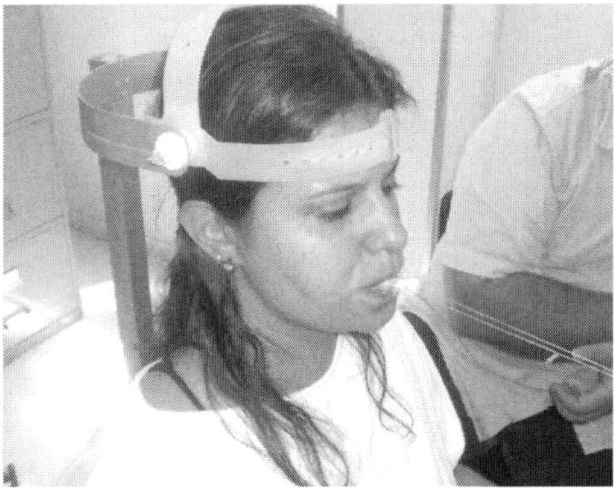

Fig. 9. FORLAB in detail.

The transmission, processing and storage system was especially developed for this study. It is composed of a data acquisition board (Ontrak), an electronic coupling system and an IBM-PC personal computer. The measurement system interacts with the evaluator by a human-machine interface that uses high level programming language and is distributable in a Windows® platform. The stored signals are used to characterize the force profile of the subject. Besides the force x time curve (profile), it is possible to evaluate relevant typical points like maximum force, average force and variations that characterize the lips force of the subject.

4. Studies made with the proposed devices

The initial studies accomplished using FORLING and FORLAB devices aimed to describe the characteristics of the tongue and lips in healthy subjects without any disturbance to the structures or functions of the oral sensorimotor system.

4.1 Methodology

The studies were conducted with approval of the Human Ethics Committee from the Universidade Federal de Minas Gerais. The sample was composed of 20 young women aged between 21 and 33 years with no history of swallowing, respiratory or speech impairments. Moreover, they had no existing medical condition or medication use that could potentially influence orofacial performance or sensation, and no cognitive or intellectual dysfunction.

After providing their informed consent, the subjects first underwent a qualitative evaluation of tongue and lips force. In the qualitative evaluation of tongue force, the subjects had to press the tip of their tongue against the finger of the examiner and against a tongue blade for 10 seconds, with resistance provided by the examiner (Figure 10A). The qualitative evaluation of lips force was done by palpating the musculature at the resting position and in centric isometric contraction, as well as evaluating the strength of resistance against the finger of the examiner placed in the oral vestibule, also for 10 seconds (Figure 10B).

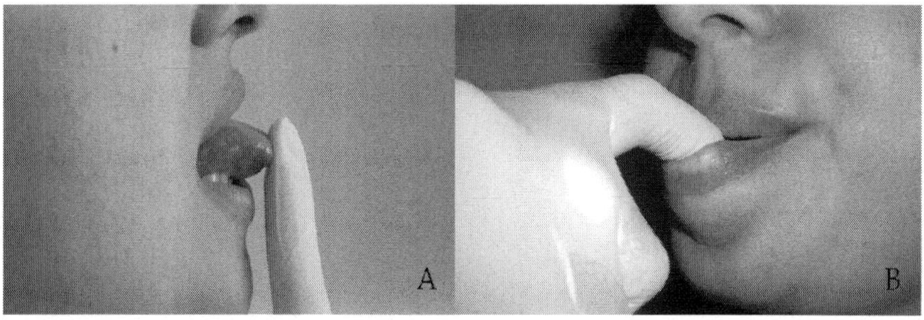

Fig. 10. Qualitative evaluation of tongue (A) and lips (B) force.

After qualitative analysis, the women classified as having normal force according to the judgment of two speech language pathologists were directed to a quantitative assessment of tongue or lips force. These structures were classified as having normal force when they were able to perform protrusion movements against strong resistance exerted by the blade and/or the finger and maintain the force without shaking and deformation.

Ten women were randomly selected to participate in the tongue research using Portable FORLING, and ten women were selected to participate in the lips research using FORLAB.

Measurements were made in a clinical room at the Speech-Language Pathology Ambulatory of the University. Participants were seated comfortably in an upright position and instructed to fit the device into the oral cavity with the help of the examiner. The patients had one minute for acclimatization before undergoing three consecutive trials, in which they performed isometric muscle contractions sustained for 10 seconds, the same period of time for the qualitative assessment. It is important to consider that a very long time of sustained maximal contraction can cause muscle fatigue and thereby compromise the results. One-minute time intervals were given between trials to avoid fatigue.

The interval time for rest and the time for sustained force were controlled by software specially developed for each of the instruments and a beep indicated each of these steps. The sampling rate was 10 Hz.

4.2 Results and discussion

The results obtained by the clinical application of FORLING and FORLAB are presented below. The parameters analyzed were average force and maximum force obtained in the determined period of sustained muscle contraction. Information about data dispersion as standard deviation and coefficient of variation were also recorded. The strength profile of both structures was compared, as well as the stability characteristics.

There were notable differences in the curves of the force over the period of sustained contraction. The tongue's profile can be described as presenting an initial peak of force that gradually decreases. On the other hand, the analysis of data concerning lips force showed a profile characterized by little amount of variability over time and without any noticeable peaks. The decay in the lips' profile curve was slower than that of the tongue. The decay in the tongue/lips strength curve can be explained by physical causes such as muscle fatigue or motivational causes such as mental fatigue and lack of interest. Figure 11 shows typical curves obtained from the quantitative evaluations of the tongue and lips.

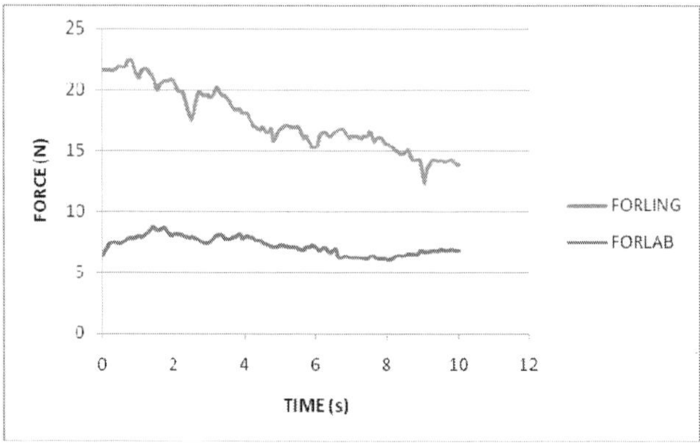

Fig. 11. Profile of the tongue and lips force over time.

The tongue force was higher than that of the lips, in the analysis of both average force and maximum force. Table 1 presents the results of the trials. It was verified that both parameters increased over successive trials, indicating that there is a learning effect.

	TONGUE			LIPS		
	Trial 1	Trial 2	Trial 3	Trial 1	Trial 2	Trial 3
Maximum Force (N)	19.9	21.9	22.5	10.6	11.1	11.1
Maximum force SD	5.5	6.7	5.6	2.5	2.4	2.7
Average Force (N)	15.8	16.9	17.0	9.3	9.0	9.3
Average Force SD	4.9	6.1	4.6	2.6	2.5	2.4

N = Newton; SD= Standard Deviation.

Table 1. Maximum force and average force of tongue and lips.

For the analysis of stability, the coefficient of variation (CV) was used, which is a dimensionless value that provides information about the homogeneity of the results. CV is the result of the division of the standard deviation by the average value, involving data from the same series. The lower the magnitude of CV, the greater is the uniformity of results. A CV lower than 10% was considered low, between 10 and 20 % was considered medium, between 20 and 30% was high and above 30% was thought of as very high.

Tables 2, 3 and 4 present the average force values and the analysis of dispersion of these values for each participant in trials 1, 2 and 3, respectively.

The average tongue force had a high CV compared to lips force, which were classified as low or medium. This can be explained by the characteristics of each of these structures, since the tongue is composed of a set of muscles that contract in a coordinated way, while the lips comprise only one muscle. In an attempt to keep the contraction over ten seconds, the participants exerted peaks of force interspersed with regions of decay in the force measured by Portable FORLING, while FORLAB showed a more stable signal.

Participant	Structure evaluated	Average force (N)	Standard deviation	Coefficient of variation (%)
1	Tongue	12.3	2.2	17.84
2	Tongue	7.8	1.9	24.27
3	Tongue	18.0	1.6	9.00
4	Tongue	11.6	2.3	19.88
5	Tongue	10.6	1.5	14.27
6	Tongue	5.8	1.8	30.24
7	Tongue	11.0	1.8	16.47
8	Tongue	20.5	3.0	14.74
9	Tongue	18.7	1.4	7.26
10	Tongue	13.6	2.6	18.97
11	Lips	13.2	1.0	7.68
12	Lips	7.5	0.4	4.85
13	Lips	7.0	0.4	5.45
14	Lips	12.5	0.9	6.95
15	Lips	5.8	1.0	17.65
16	Lips	10.2	0.6	5.67
17	Lips	9.1	0.5	5.99
18	Lips	8.3	0.8	9.91
19	Lips	7.5	0.6	7.80
20	Lips	12.2	0.3	2.47

N = Newton.

Table 2. Measurements of central tendency and dispersion of force values obtained in Trial 1.

Participant	Structure evaluated	Average force (N)	Standard deviation	Coefficient of variation (%)
1	Tongue	16.4	2.0	12.18
2	Tongue	11.8	2.0	16.79
3	Tongue	19.8	2.6	13.06
4	Tongue	12.6	2.8	22.46
5	Tongue	11.2	1.5	13.58
6	Tongue	7.7	2.6	33.16
7	Tongue	9.9	1.0	9.86
8	Tongue	16.4	4.2	25.32
9	Tongue	18.5	1.7	9.10
10	Tongue	14.9	2.4	16.39
11	Lips	14.4	1.5	10.67
12	Lips	7.2	0.7	9.75
13	Lips	7.7	0.5	6.47
14	Lips	10.6	1.1	10.09
15	Lips	8.7	0.9	10.55
16	Lips	10.9	0.7	6.36
17	Lips	8.2	0.8	9.38
18	Lips	10.2	1.4	13.53
19	Lips	8.2	0.5	5.76
20	Lips	11.0	0.4	4.16

N = Newton.

Table 3. Measurements of central tendency and dispersion of force values obtained in Trial 2.

Participant	Structure evaluated	Average force (N)	Standard deviation	Coefficient of variation (%)
1	Tongue	14.8	2.6	17.68
2	Tongue	14.2	2.5	17.49
3	Tongue	18.5	1.6	8.58
4	Tongue	12.8	3.5	27.00
5	Tongue	11	1.7	15.06
6	Tongue	9.6	2.4	24.90
7	Tongue	12.6	1.7	13.42
8	Tongue	18.4	3.7	19.91
9	Tongue	18.1	2.3	12.49
10	Tongue	13.4	3.1	22.95
11	Lips	14.7	1.3	9.24
12	Lips	9.0	0.4	4.74
13	Lips	7.3	0.5	6.30
14	Lips	11.7	2.2	18.51
15	Lips	7.1	0.4	5.17
16	Lips	9.8	1.8	17.99
17	Lips	9.5	1.4	14.45
18	Lips	7.4	1.0	13.56
19	Lips	7.5	0.6	8.17
20	Lips	8.8	0.5	5.57

N = Newton.

Table 4. Measurements of central tendency and dispersion of force values obtained in Trial 3.

The variability of the signals is due to the complexity of the biological systems. According to Gill (1987) as cited in Judice et al. (1999), a lot of biological characteristics have a CV between 5 and 50%. The wide variation in the amplitude of lingual force values has also been reported by others (Frohlich et al. 1990; Robinovitch et al. 1991). Robinovitch et al. (1991) also attributed tongue slippage and neural-based fluctuations in causing this variation.

By analyzing the values of maximum force (Table 5), it is noteworthy that 90% of the participants showed higher values in Tests 2 and 3. Therefore, the learning factor can be a reasonable explanation for these results.

Many instruments have been developed to quantify tongue force using different technologies, such as dynamometers (Posen 1972; Trawitzki et al. 2010), bulbs (Bu Sha et al. 2000; Hayashi et al. 2002; Clark et al. 2003; Ball et al. 2006; Utanohara et al. 2008), palatal plates (Hori et al. 2006; Hewitt et al. 2008; Kieser et al. 2008), strain gauges (Kydd 1956; Sanders 1968; Dworkin 1980; Robinovitch et al. 1991; Scardella et al. 1993) and others. Each one has its advantages and disadvantages and can measure maximum tongue force in a different direction and sometimes force during function.

Portable FORLING measures tongue protrusion force. It is believed that from the measurement of the ability of the individual to exert a horizontal force towards the outside of the oral cavity (protrusion force), it is eventually possible to infer about the capacity of the tongue to perform other tasks (Motta et al. 2004). This is because the muscles involved in tongue protrusion, the genioglossus and intrinsic tongue muscles, also act during functions of mastication, swallowing and speech among others. Furthermore, the ability to exert protrusion force can indicate the ability to exert forces in other directions, as shown by some authors (Dworkin and Aronson 1986). In their study about tongue force in the anterior and lateral directions, the results indicated that subjects presenting higher force values in one direction also did so in the other directions, and the same happened to those who showed lower forces. However, the main reason for choosing protrusion force was that it is the force direction usually evaluated by speech pathologists in clinical assessment. Thus, it is possible to establish comparisons between the qualitative and quantitative evaluations. Similarly, the quantitative evaluation of lips has the same principle as that of the qualitative assessment.

Participant	Structure evaluated	F max T1 (N)	F max T2 (N)	F max T3 (N)
1	Tongue	16.1	19.8	19.7
2	Tongue	11.4	15.0	18.1
3	Tongue	20.7	23.8	21.9
4	Tongue	15.0	17.5	18.8
5	Tongue	13.7	15.0	14.2
6	Tongue	11.1	12.3	13.2
7	Tongue	14.2	12.3	16.0
8	Tongue	26.1	23.3	25.6
9	Tongue	22.4	23.1	23.6
10	Tongue	17.2	19.3	19.1
11	Lips	14.5	16.1	16.0
12	Lips	8.1	8.7	9.7
13	Lips	8.1	9.1	8.4
14	Lips	14.0	13.0	14.2
15	Lips	8.0	10.2	7.9
16	Lips	11.6	12.2	11.3
17	Lips	9.9	10.1	12.1
18	Lips	9.9	13.2	9.4
19	Lips	8.7	9.2	9.0
20	Lips	12.8	12.3	12.3

F max= Maximum force; N= Newton ; T1= Trial 1; T2= Trial 2; T3= Trial 3.

Table 5. Maximum force in each trial.

Data obtained in this research was compared to other studies that used the same assessment direction in maximum voluntary contraction (Kydd 1956; Posen 1972; Dworkin et al. 1980, Mortimore et al. 1999; Motta et al. 2004; Barroso et al. 2009; Lambrechts et al. 2010). The values obtained in this research were similar to the ones achieved by Kydd (1956) (maximum force: 23.13 N), Posen (1972) (maximum force between 6 N and 25 N), Dworkin et al. (1980) (maximum force was 32.9 N for men and 27.5 N for women), Mortimore et al. (1999) (maximum force: 26± 8N for males and 20± 7N for females), and Motta et al. (2004) (maximum force between 21.1 N and 25.7 N and average force between 17.4 N and 20.6 N), and higher than those obtained by Barroso et al. (2009) (average force between 3.55 N and 13.24 N) and by Lambrechts et al. (2010) (average force 1.66± 0.06 N). However, in the study by Barroso et al. (2009), the sample was composed of subjects with tongue strength classified as normal or slightly reduced in the qualitative assessment, which probably resulted in lower tongue force values, combined with the fact that the age range of the sample included individuals older than 60 years. According to Crow and Ship (1996), a reduction in muscle mass happens after 60 years of age due to atrophy and loss of motor neurons. Lambrechts et al. (2010) included children, who had lower tongue strength than adults due to their stage of developmental maturation in muscle morphology and the central nervous system (Potter et al. 2009; Potter and Short 2009). Moreover, the authors did not provide information about the qualitative evaluation of their participants.

It can be argued that several problems are encountered in the process of measuring the strength of the oral structures, such as lips and tongue. This is because they are structures within the complex biological orafacial system, susceptible to environmental, behavioral and anatomical changes. Therefore, as stressed by Ingervall and Janson (1981), assessing the strength of the lips in a quantitative way is not an easy task. There are different methodological approaches for assessing labial force as presented in the literature. Most of these studies have generated a solution by adapting dynamometers (Garliner 1971; Posen 1976; Ingervall and Janson 1981; Thuer and Ingerval 1990; Cantero et al. 2003; Gonzalez et al. 2004). The disadvantage of this line of instrumentation is the need for a person to conduct stabilization or move the traction device pulling the lips, in order to measure the strength of this structure. This introduces subjective components into the process, since each professional will act slightly differently when supporting the instrument. Moreover, the possibility of evaluating different directions of lip contractions makes comparison between the findings of different studies unreliable. Some researchers have sought to evaluate the lip closing force from the closing of a plate positioned horizontally between the upper and lower lips (Jung et al. 2010). When using this instrument, great attention should be given to controlling the action of compensatory muscles, such as the mentalis. Other assessing instruments reported in the literature use force or pressure lip sensors attached to the teeth (Gentil and Tournier 1998; McHenry et al. 1999; Ruan et al. 2007). These electrodes are fixed by special glues or dental adhesive. The disadvantage of these instruments is the difficulty in accommodating the idealized electrodes at points and in the positioning of the electrodes for comparative reassessments. The ultimate goal of researchers using sensors supported on the teeth is to assess the action of these muscles on the correct teeth positioning as well as studying the balance of power between the lips and tongue. A study in the literature (Hägg and Anniko 2008) evaluated the lip force of contraction in the same way as that proposed by the FORLAB report, but with a population of patients who had suffered a stroke. Considering the results obtained by the authors after the process of force lip rehabilitation, higher average values (18.5 N) were observed when compared to those obtained in the measurements performed with FORLAB. It is important to consider that a muscle group exposed to specific training will gain strength in a manner that can also generate greater force against resistance. It is believed that even subjects without functional complaints and with adequate lip strength during qualitative assessment, like the subjects evaluated with FORLAB, can increase their capacity of generating force after being submitted to muscular training.

It is known that clinical evaluation, which is considered subjective as it does not quantify the force values and depends on the clinical experience of the evaluator, is the reference assessment for professionals in this area. The proposal is to develop instruments that can help this assessment by offering quantitative data. The presented systems follow the same principles as those of clinical evaluation, analyzing the same type of force (counter-resistance). This makes comparisons between the two assessments (qualitative and quantitative) possible and consistent. All the subjects analyzed in this study presented normal tongue strength. Future studies are being planned to compare alterations in clinical assessment (diminished or enhanced force) with numerical values.

Considering the clinical application of FORLAB, some difficulties were found, such as the standardization of the distance between the insert and the frontal teeth, and the correct positioning of the steel wire (mechanic coupling). The distance to the position of the insert was measured subjectively from the region the insert touched the teeth. The traction made by the evaluator caused a displacement of 10 mm, generating a slight projection of the lips. To allow correct mechanical coupling, the wire positioning was also made subjectively. The evaluator adjusted the system parts so that the wire would be as strained as possible. These problems can be solved by substituting the steel wire for a rigid mechanical coupling, like a metal rod, and the marking of a point that allows the visualization of the distance between the teeth and the insert. A new version of this instrument is in development to resolve these problems.

In both instruments, intra-subject analysis presented more significant results, since evaluating biological systems involves the consideration of many particularities and peculiarities. Thus, the quantitative analysis of tongue and lips force can be an efficient instrument in comparing the changes in a patient during therapy.

5. Future direction

More research is needed in the Biomechanics area, especially related to orofacial structures. The Biomechanics Engineering Group is already developing a new version of FORLAB, which will be portable like Portable FORLING, and will eliminate most of the restrictions associated to the first version. The portable FORLAB will also be able to detect differences in force generated by each side of the orbicular oris muscle which is especially important in the evaluation of patients with facial palsy.

Next studies in tongue and lips force will explore other parameters beyond maximum and average force: the average force application rate, which is the speed that the force reaches the higher peak, and the area under the graphic, which is related to the energy dissipated during the task. These parameters are also important to characterize tongue and lips force profile and they need to be investigated in a high number of individuals with different classifications of force, in order to create standard values for each of these groups.

Cheeks form the lateral boundary of the buccal cavity, and display continuity with the lips. They participate, together with the tongue, in the acts of suction, swallowing and mastication. A device to measure cheeks force is also being developed in collaboration with UFRGS (Universidade Federal do Rio Grande do Sul), a university in the Brazilian city of Porto Alegre. It is being based in the same principles of trying to represent the current evaluation technique, proving reliable results and a safe and portable basis. Other devices under development involve gadgets to train and rehabilitate tongue, cheek and lip forces.

These developments show an important potential, as they intend to allow pathologists to be sure of how much load the patient is training with, and to make possible to alter the clinical procedure when required, fixing the ideal force value to be used in training as well as the duration and the number of exercise series. It will also be possible to make biofeedback therapy.

6. Conclusion

To effectively rehabilitate orofacial muscles it is important to consider their characteristics. They have precise and complex movements that are specific to function they are responsible for. The tongue for example is constituted not only of one muscle, but of a set of small muscles which are organized in different directions and work in synchrony promoting a wide range of refined movements. The amount of movements can be justified by the complexity of the functions directly related to the tongue, like speech, mastication and swallowing. On the other hand, the lips muscle has quite different characteristics. It has reduced caliber and its movements are not as elaborated as the ones of the tongue. Knowing these features will enable the rehabilitation process to be directed to each muscle group affected.

Tongue and lips are very important in orofacial functions. To be able to perform the functions properly, they need to be able to generate appropriate force. Thus, it is very important to measure tongue and lips force, especially in patients that have orofacial dysfunctions. This chapter presented the development and application of two instruments developed by the Biomechanics Engineering Group that measure forces of orofacial structures. The Portable FORLING measures tongue force and is composed of a mouthpiece, a base, a resistive sensor, pin and force applicator and a holder, all connected to a data acquisition and processing system. FORLAB measures lips force and is composed of an intralips insert, a stainless steel wire, a load cell and data acquisition and processing system. They were used in studies with normal subjects and proved to be effective and helpful for speech pathologists to improve their assessment. In subjects with normal tongue and lips strength in clinical evaluation, average tongue force was 16.6 N, with average CV of 17.3% and average lips force was 9.2 N with average CV of 7.4%. The tongue presents a force profile over time that is characterized by a force peak followed by the decay of force values, while lips demonstrate stability while maintaining maximum contraction over time. Those results indicate that forces of the lips are lower, but more stable than the ones of the tongue. The described developments were possible due to the multidisciplinary character of the group, including an active exchange between professionals of different background and institutions with the common goal of providing useful and reliable solutions for relevant problems in orofacial myology.

7. References

Aprile, Humberto, Mario Figun, and Ricardo Garino. 1975. *Anatomia: Anatomia Odontológica Oro-cérvico-facial*. Buenos Aires: Ateneu.

Ball, Sarah, Olga Idel, Susan Cotton, and Alison Perry. 2006. "Comparison of two Methods for Measuring Tongue Pressure During Swallowing in People with Head and Neck Cancer." *Dysphagia* 21(1):28-37.

Barroso, Márcio, Cláudio Costa, Jorge Saffar, Estevam Las Casas, Andréa Motta , Tatiana Perilo, Monalise Batista, and, Vivian Brito. 2009. "Desenvolvimento de um Sistema Protótipo para Medição Objetiva das Forças Linguais em Humanos." *Sba Controle & Automação* 20(2):156-63.

Biazevic, Maria, José Antunes, Janina Togni, Fabiana Andrade, Marcos Carvalho, and Victor Wünsch-Filho. 2010. "Survival and Quality of Life of Patients with Oral and Oropharyngeal Cancer at 1-year Follow-up of Tumor Resection." *Journal of Applied Oral Sciences* 18(3):279-84.

Bu Sha, Brett, Sandra England, Richard Parisi, and Richard Strobel. 2000. "Force Production of the Genioglossus as a Function of Muscle Length in Normal Humans." *Journal of Applied Physiology* 88:1678-84.

Cantero, Luis, Brismayda Gonzalez, and Mariela Fernandez. 2003. "La Fuerza Labial Superior y sus Variaciones con la Mioterapia." *Revista Cubana de Estomatologia* 40(3).

Clark, Heather, Katy O'Brien, Aimee Calleja, and Sarah Corrie. 2009. "Effects of Directional Exercise on Lingual Strength." *Journal of Speech, Language and Hearing Research* 52:1034-47.

Clark, Heather, Pamela Henson, Willian Barbe, JulieStierwalt, and Michel Sherrill. 2003. "Relationships among Subjective and Objective Measures of the Tongue Strength and Oral Phase Swallowing Impairments." *American Journal of Speech-Language Pathology* 12:40-50.

Cosenza, Ramon. 2005. *Fundamentos de Neuroanatomia.* 3rd Ed. Rio de Janeiro: Guanabara Koogan.

Crow, Heidi, and Jonathan Ship. 1996. "Tongue Strength and Endurance in Different Aged Individuals." *The Journals of Gerontology. Series A, Biological Sciences and Medical Sciences* 51(5):M247-50.

Dangelo, José, and Carlos Fattini. 1998. *Anatomia Humana Sistêmica e Segmentar.* 2nd Ed. Rio de Janeiro: Atheneu.

Douglas, Carlos. 2002. *Tratado de Fisiologia aplicada à Fonoaudiologia.* São Paulo: Robe.

Dworkin, James, and Arnold Aronson. E. 1986. "Tongue Strength and Alternative Motion Rates in Normal and Dysarthric Subjects." *Journal of Communication Disorders* 19:115-32.

Dworkin, James, Arnold Aronson, and Donald Mulder. 1980. "Tongue Force in Normal and in Dysarthric Patients with Amyotrophic Lateral Sclerosis." *Journal of Speech and Hearing Research* 23(4):828-37.

Dworkin, James. 1980. "Tongue Strength Measurement in Patients with Amyotropic lateral sclerosis: Qualitative vs Quantitative Procedures." *Archives of Physical Medicine and Rehabilitation* 61:422-4.

Farias, Samira , Clara de Ávila, and Marilena Vieira. 2006. "Relação entre Fala, Tônus e Praxia Não-verbal do Sistema Estomatognático em Pré-escolares." *Pró-Fono Revista de Atualização Científica* 18(3):267-76.

Figún, Mario, and Ricardo Garino. 2003. *Anatomia Odontológica: Funcional e Aplicada.* Porto Alegre: Artmed.

Frohlich, Katrin, Urs Thuer, and Bengt Ingervall. 1990. "Pressure from the Tongue on the Teeth in Young Adults." *Angle Orthodontics* 61:17-24.

Garliner, D. 1971. *Myofunctional Therapy in Dental Practice.* 2nd Ed. New York: Bartel Dental Book Inc.

Gentil, Michèle, and Claire Tournier. 1998. "Differences in Fine Control of Forces Generated by the Tongue, Lips and Fingers in Humans." *Archives of Oral Biology* 43:517-23.

Gonzalez, Brismayda, Luis Cantero, Buenaventura Basnueva, and Jaime Betancourt. D. 2004. "Fuerza Labial Superior em Niños." *Revista Habanera Ciências Médicas* 3(8).

Gonzalez, Nidia, and Lucy Lopes. 2000. *Fonoaudiologia e Ortopedia Maxilar na Reabilitação Orofacial: Tratamento Precoce e Preventivo – Terapia Miofuncional*. São Paulo: Santos.

Hagg, Mary, and Matti Anniko. 2008. "Lip Muscle Training in Stroke Patients with Dysphagia." *Acta Oto-laryngologica 128(9):* 1027-33.

Hayashi, Ryo, Kazuhiro Tsuga, Ryuji Hosokawa, Mitsuyoshi Yoshida, Yuuji Sato, and Yasumasa Akagawa. 2002. "A Novel Handy Probe for Tongue Pressure Measurement." *International Journal of Prosthodontics* 15(4):385-8.

Hewitt, Angela, Jackeline Hind, Stephanie Kays, Mark Nicosia, John Doyle, Willis Tompkins, Ronald Gangnon, and JoAnne Robbins. 2008. "Standardized Instrument for Lingual Pressure Measurement." *Dysphagia* 23(1):16-25.

Hori, Kazuhiro, Takahiro Ono, and Takashi Nokubi. 2006. "Coordination of Tongue Pressure and Jaw Movement in Mastication." *Journal of Dental Research* 85(2):187-91.

Ingervall, Bengt., and Tomas Janson. 1981. "The Value of Clinical Lip Strength Measurements." *Am Journal of Orthodontics* 80(5):496-507.

Judice, Marcelo, Joel Muniz, and Roberto Carvalheiro. 1999. "A Avaliação do Coeficiente de Variação na Experimentação com Suínos." *Ciência e Agrotecnologia* 23(1):170-3.

Jung, Min-Ho, Won-Sik Yang, and Dong-Seok Nahm. 2003. "Effects of Upper Lip Closing Force on Craniofacial Structures." *American Journal of Orthodontics and Dentofacial Orthopedics* 123(1):58-63.

Jung, Min-Ho, Won-Sik Yang, and Dong-Seok Nahm.2010. "Maximum Closing Force of Mentolabial Muscles and Type of Malocclusion." *Angle Orthodontics* 80(1):72-9.

Kieser, Jules, Bhavia Singh, Michael Swain, Ionut Ichim, Neil Waddell, Daniel Kennedy, Kylie Foster, and Victoria Livingstone. 2008. "Measuring Intraoral Pressure: Adaptation of a Dental Appliance Allows Measurement During Function." *Dysphagia* 23:237-43.

Kydd, William. 1956. "Quantitative Analyses of Force of the Tongue." *Journal of Dental Research* 35(2):171-4.

Lambrechts, Heleen, Evelyne De Baets, Steffen Fieuws, and Guy Willems. 2010. "Lip and Tongue Pressure in Orthodontic Patients." *European Journal of Orthodontics* 32(4):466-71.

McHenry, Monica, John Minton, Leila Hartley, Karen Calhoun, and Steven Barlow. 1999. "Age-related Changes in Orofacial Force Generation in Women." *The Laryngoscope* 109(55):827-30.

Mortimore, Ian, Pamela Fiddes, Susie Stephens, and Neil Douglas. 1999. "Tongue Protrusion Force and Fatiguability in Male and Female Subjects." *European Respiratory Journal* 14:191-5.

Motta, Andréa, Juliana Perim, Tatiana Perilo, Estevam Las Casas, Cláudio Costa, Francisco E Magalhães, Jorge Safar. 2004. "Método Objetivo para a Medição de Forças Axiais da Língua." *Revista CEFAC* 6:164-9.

O'Connor, Ciara, Madeleine Lowery, Liam Doherty, Michael McHugh, Cormac O'Muircheartaigh, John Cullen, Philip Nolan, Walter McNicholas, and Mark O'Malley. 2007. "Improved Surface EMG Electrode for Measuring Genioglossus Muscle Activity." *Respiratory Physiology and Neurobiology* 159:55–67.

Pittman, Lora J, and E Fiona Bailey. 2009. "Genioglossus and Intrinsic Electromyographic Activities in Impeded and Unimpeded Protrusion Tasks." *Journal of Neurophysiology* 101(1):276-82.

Posen, Aaron. 1972. "The Influence of Maximum Perioral and Tongue Force on the Incisor Teeth." *The Angle Orthodontist* 42(4):285-309.

Posen, Aaron. 1976. "The Application of Quantitative Perioral Assesment to Orthodontic case Analysis and Treatment Planning." *The Angle Orthodontist* 46(2):118-43.

Potter, Nancy, and Robert Short. 2009. "Maximal Tongue Strength in Typically Developing Children and Adolescents." *Dysphagia* 24:391-7.

Potter, Nancy, Raymond Kent, and Jo-Anne Lazarus. 2009. "Oral and Manual Force Control in Preschool-Aged Children: Is there Evidence for Common Control?" *Journal of Motor Behavior* 41(1):66-81.

Proffit, William, and Henry Fields Jr. 2002. "A Etiologia dos Problemas Ortodônticos." In *Ortodontia Contemporânea*, ed. Proffit, William R, and Henry W Fields Jr, 105-34. 3rd Ed. Rio de Janeiro: Guanabara Koogan.

Proffit, William, Henry Fields, and David Sarver. 2007. *Ortodontia Contemporânea.* 4th Ed. Rio de Janeiro: Elsevier.

Robinovitch, Stephen, Cecil Hershler, and Douglas Romilly. 1991. "A Tongue Force Measurement System for the Assessment of Oral-phase Swallowing Disorders." *Archives of Physical Medicine and Rehabilitation* 72:38-42.

Rogers, Caroline, Mark Mooney, Timothy Smith, Seth Weinberg, Bridget Waller, Lisa Parr, Beth Docherty, Christopher Bonar, Lauren Reinholt, Frederic Deleyiannis, Michael Siegel, Mary Marazita, and Anne Burrows. 2009. "Comparative Microanatomy of the Orbicularis Oris Muscle Between Chimpanzees and Humans: Evolutionary Divergence of Lip Function." *Journal of Anatomy* 214(1):36–44.

Ruan, Wen-rua, Ji-mei Su, and Xiao-wei Ye. 2007. "Pressure from the Lips and the Tongue in Children with Class III Malocclusion." *Journal of Zhejiang University* 8(5):296-301.

Sanders, Lois Joan. 1968. "Instrumentation for Measurement of Lingual Strength." *Journal of Speech and Hearing Research* 11(1):189-93.

Scardella, Anthony, Natalia Krawciw, Jefferey Petrozzino, Mark Co, Teodoro Santiago, and Norman Edelman. 1993. "Strength and Endurance Characteristics of the Normal Human Genioglossus." *American Review of Respiratory Disease* 148:179-184.

Silva, Ricardo Gariba, and Jesus Djalma Pécora. 1998. *Anatomia dental: dentes permanentes.* São Paulo: Santos.

Thuer, Urs., and Ingervall, Bengt. 1990. "Effect of Muscle Exercise with an Oral Screen on Lip Function." *European Journal of Orthodontics* 12(2):198-208.

Trawitzki, Luciana Vitaliano Voi, Clarissa Günther Borges, Lilian Dias Giglio, and João Batista da Silva. 2011. "Tongue Strength of Healthy Young Adults." *Journal of Oral Rehabilitation* Doi: 10.1111/j.1365-2842.2010.02182.x.

Unemori, Mikako, Junji Sugawara, Mitsuhiko Kawauchi, and Hideo Mitani. 1996. "A pressure-Distribuition Sensor (PDS) for Evaluation of Lip Functions." *American Journal of Orthodontics and Dentofacial Orthopedics* 109(5):473-480.

Utanohara, Yuri, Ryo Hayashi, Mineka Yoshikawa, Mitsuyoshi Yoshida, Kazuhiro Tsuga, and Yasumasa Akagawa. 2008. "Standard Values of Maximum Tongue Pressure Taken Using Newly Developed Disposable Tongue Pressure Measurement Device." *Dysphagia* 23:286–90.

Wheeler, Russel, and Ash Major. 1987. *Wheeler´s Anatomia, Fisiologia e Oclusão Dental.* São Paulo: SANTOS.

Zemlin, Willard. 1997. *Speech and Hearing Science: Anatomy and Physiology*. 4th Ed. Boston: Allyn & Bacon.

Part 3

Biochemical Engineering Methods and Applications

17

In Vitro Blood Flow Behaviour in Microchannels with Simple and Complex Geometries

Valdemar Garcia[1], Ricardo Dias[1,2] and Rui Lima[1,2]
[1]*Polytechnic Institute of Bragança, ESTiG/IPB, C. Sta. Apolonia, Bragança,*
[2]*CEFT, Faculty of Engineering of the University of Porto (FEUP), R. Dr. Roberto Frias, Porto, Portugal*

1. Introduction

Over the years, various experimental methods have been applied in an effort to understand the blood flow behaviour in microcirculation. The development of optical experimental techniques has contributed to obtain possible explanations on the way the blood flows through microvessels. In recent years, due to advances in computers, optics, and digital image processing techniques, it has become possible to combine a conventional particle image velocimetry (PIV) system with an inverted microscope and consequently improve both spatial and temporal resolution. The present review outlines our most relevant studies on the flow properties of blood at a microscale level by using current micro-PIV and confocal micro-PIV techniques.

Blood flow in both microvessels and microchannels has been measured by several measurements techniques such as: double-slit photometric (Nash & Meiselman, 1983), laser-Doppler anemometer (Uijttewaal et al., 1994), video-based methods (Parthasarathi et al., 1999). Although the past research findings have been encouraging, detailed studies on the way blood flow behaves at a microscopic level have been limited by several factors such as poor spatial resolution, difficulty to obtain accurate measurements at such small scales, optical errors arisen from walls of the microvessels, high concentration of blood cells, and difficulty in visualization of results due to insufficient computing power and absence of reliable image analysis techniques. In recent years, due to advances in computers, optics, high-speed imaging and image processing techniques, it has become possible to combine a conventional particle image velocimetry (PIV) system with an inverted microscope and consequently improve both spatial and temporal resolution (Santiago et al., 1998; Koutsiaris et al., 1999). This system, known as micro-PIV (see Fig.1), has been applied to study the flow behaviour in several research fields in science and engineering. In the biomedical field, Sugii and his co-workers, by using a conventional micro-PIV system, they have used red blood cells (RBCs) as tracer markers to measure their velocities in straight (Sugii et al., 2002) and they found that the velocity profiles were markedly blunt in the central region. However, later they measured both tracer particles and RBCs through a 100 µm glass capillary and they reported that by using in vitro blood with about 20% Hct the velocity profiles were parabolic (Sugii et al., 2005). By using a microchannel close to a rectangular shape, Bitsch and his co-workers (Bitsch et al., 2005) have reported blunt profiles. More recently, by using liposomes tracer particles the blood-plasma velocity was measured in the beating heart of a chicken embryo (Vennemann et al., 2006). Kim and Lee (2006) have analysed the flow behaviour of blood through a circular opaque microchannel by using an X-ray PIV technique. Their measurements have shown typical non-Newtonian flow characteristics of blood such as yield stress and shear-thinning effects. In addition, Chiu et al. (2003) have also applied the conventional micro-PIV system to analyse the effect of flow in monocyte adhesion to endothelial cells cultured in a vertical step flow chamber. Although, micro-PIV systems are gaining widespread among the biomicrofluidics community due to its high spatial and temporal resolution, the employment of conventional microscope leads to the entire illumination of the flow field resulting in high levels of background noise and consequently errors on the flow measurements (Meinhart et al., 2000). These errors can be partially removed by using a spinning disk confocal microscope (SDCM), i. e., by combining a SDCM with a laser, the emitted light intensity is significantly improved and as a result, it is possible to obtain adequate signal to noise ratio to detect the motion of the RBCs in both diluted and concentrated suspensions (Tanaami et al., 2002; Park et al., 2004, 2006; Lima et al., 2006, 2007, 2008). Moreover, in contrast to the conventional microscope where the entire flow region is illuminated, the confocal systems have the ability to obtain in-focus images with optical thickness less than 1 μm (optical sectioning effect). As a result, confocal systems due to its spatial filtering technique and multiple point light illumination system, confocal micro-PIV has become accepted as a reliable method for measuring in vitro blood flow through microchannels.

In this chapter, our recent studies about in vitro blood flow behaviour in microchannels both in straight and with complex geometries are presented. In straight microchannels we present some phenomena such as Fahraeus effect and Fahraeus-Lindqvist effect, the flow of particles and red blood cells (RBCs) in diluted suspensions, the flow of RBCs in concentrated suspensions, the cell-free layer and sedimentations effects. The most recent studies in blood flow through complex geometries such as bifurcations, confluences and stenosis are also reviewed. By using a chromatographic method, the flow of RBCs through a network of microcapillaries is presented.

2. Conventional micro-PIV and confocal micro-PIV/PTV

The main components of a conventional micro-PIV system consists of a microscope, a high resolution objective lens, optical filters, a high power light source for flow illumination and a high speed camera. Briefly, the light enters the inverted microscope and is reflected by a dichromatic mirror to be transmitted through the objective lens which illuminates the entire flow volume. The light emitted from fluorescent trace particles travels back to the dichromatic mirror and filters out all reflected light only allowing to pass the emitted light from the particles. Finally, the signals from the trace particles are recorded by a high speed camera and then by using a PIV cross-correlation method it is possible to obtain velocity fields of the working fluid (see schematic illustration of a conventional micro-PIV in Figure 1). The resolution of a micro-PIV system is influenced by many factors such as out-of-focus particle images from volume illumination, density and size of the tracer particles, size and optical characteristics of the microchannel and image quality (Lima, 2007).

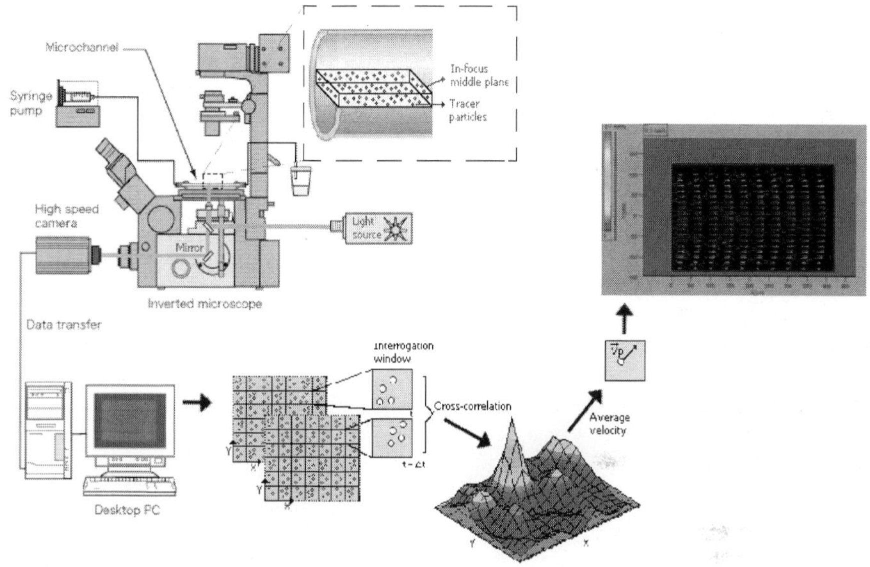

Fig. 1. Experimental setup of a typical conventional micro-PIV system and PIV cross-correlation method.

For the case of a confocal micro-PIV system, the main components of consists of a microscope combined with a confocal scanning unit (CSU), a high resolution objective lens, a high power light source for flow illumination and a high speed camera. In brief, the light emitted by the laser enters the CSU and then is conducted to the microscope to illuminate the microchannel from below the microscope stage. The light emitted from fluorescent particles travels back into the CSU, where a dichromatic mirror reflects it onto a high-speed camera to record the confocal images and by using a PIV cross-correlation method to obtain the velocity fields of the flowing trace particles (see Figure 2).

The main advantages of using a confocal spinning disk (CSD) are: the ability to obtain thin in-focus images, improve image definition and contrast of the trace particles (see Figure 3). As a result confocal micro-PIV systems have potential to obtain three-dimensional information about the fluid flow and also to obtain accurate flow-field measurements. In this way it is possible to study complex blood flow phenomena that often occur in two-phase flows (Lima, 2007).

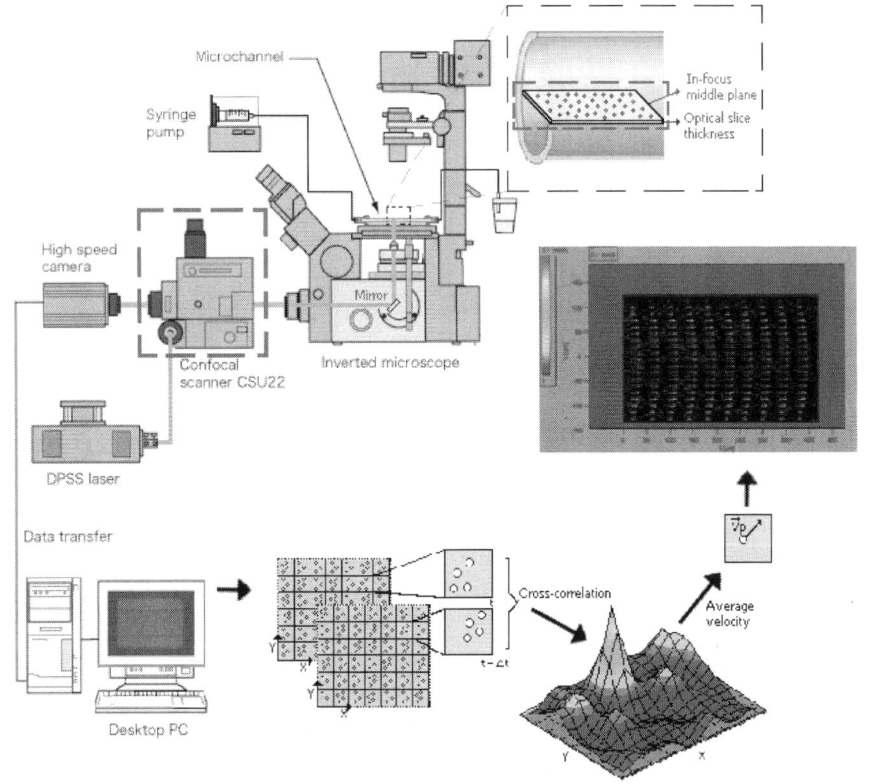

Fig. 2. Experimental setup of a confocal micro-PIV system and PIV cross-correlation method.

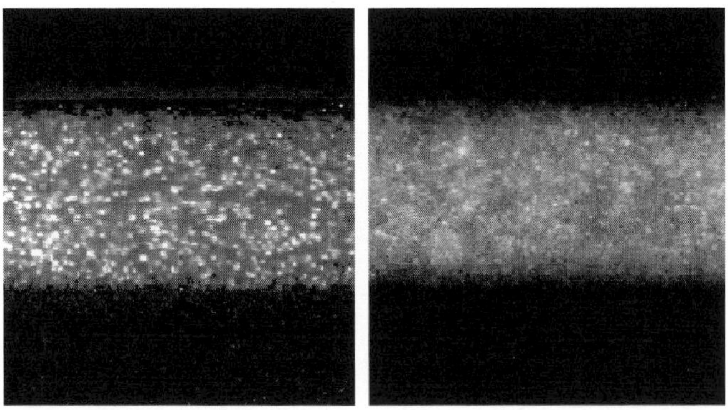

a) b)

Fig. 3. Comparison of trace particles images from both confocal (a) and conventional micro-PIV (b) for pure water.

The density of particles in the recorded images determines the most adequate PIV methodology to obtain the velocity fields. When the concentration of particles is high enough that every interrogation window contains at least three particles, this method is called high-image-density PIV mode (Adrian, 1991). However, for the case of physiological fluids with high concentrations of cells, the amount of tracer particles captured within the fluid is often very low. Hence, if the number of particles within the interrogation area is small, it is recommended to measure the displacements by tracking individual particles in a Lagrangian way. This low-image-density PIV method is often referred as particle tracking velocimetry (PTV) (Adrian, 1991). The main advantage of PTV method is the ability to obtain detailed quantitative information on the motion of particles and cells flowing within the working fluid. This method is becoming essential in several biomedical fields such as cell biology and microcirculation. The present review will show several examples using a micro-PTV method to investigate in vitro blood flow behaviour in microchannels with both simple and complex geometries. A schematic illustration of a confocal micro-PTV is shown in Figure 4.

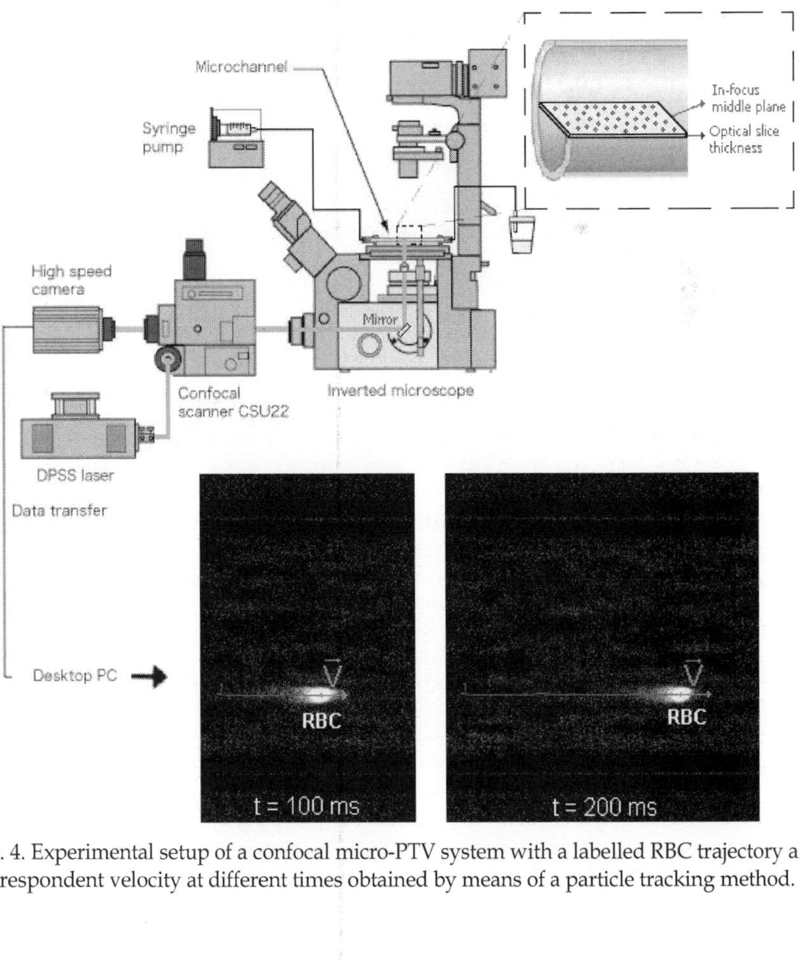

Fig. 4. Experimental setup of a confocal micro-PTV system with a labelled RBC trajectory and correspondent velocity at different times obtained by means of a particle tracking method.

3. Blood composition

In microcirculation, which comprises the smallest arteries and veins, the flow behaviour of individual blood cells and their interactions provide the microrheological basis of flow properties of blood at a macroscopic level. As a result, in microcirculation it is fundamental to study the flow behaviour of blood at cellular level. Thus, blood is not a homogeneous fluid, but one composed of a suspension of cells, proteins and ions in plasma. In normal blood, three types of cells comprise about 46% of its volume. These cells are the red blood cells (RBCs) (also known as erythrocytes) representing 45% of volume, white blood cells (WBCs) (also known as leukocytes) and platelets (also known as thrombocytes) (see Figure 5).

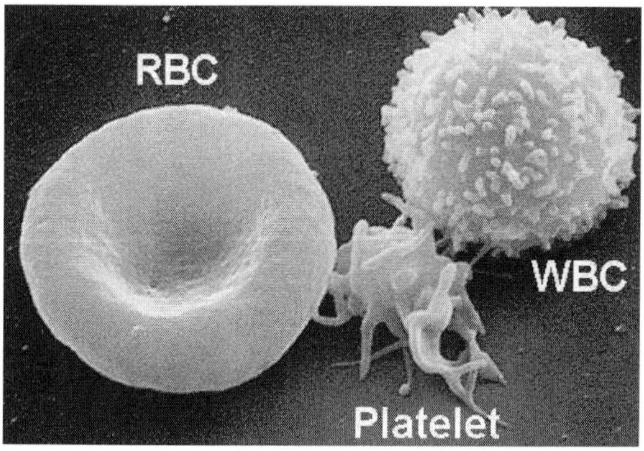

Fig. 5. Scanning electron micrograph of a white blood cells (WBC), a platelet and a red blood cell (RBC) (adpated from NCI-Frederick, 2005).

In vitro blood flow behaviour in microchannels is strongly influenced by the RBCs, since they occupy almost half of whole blood volume. RBCs are formed in the bone marrow and during maturation they lose their nuclei before entering the circulatory system. When suspended in an isotonic medium RBCs has a biconcave discoid shape, with a major diameter of about 8 μm. The density of a RBC is about 1.08×10^3 kg.m^{-3} and its major cellular components are the cytoplasm and a thin membrane composed of lipid bilayer and protein molecules. There is experimental evidence that healthy RBCs are extremely deformable into a variety of shapes in flowing blood in response to hydrodynamic stresses acting on them. Figure 6 shows a RBC deformation in a capillary (Lima et al., 2012).

The WBCs are nucleated cells that represent the major defence mechanism against infections. Generally, their shape is roughly spherical but their surface is not normally smooth (see Figure 5). The diameter of WBCs ranges from about 7 up to 22 μm, depending on its type. Healthy blood contains normally less than 1% of WBCs of the total volume of blood cells (Lima et al., 2012). Little is known about the effect of the WBCs on the blood flow behaviour in microcirculation. The blood flow under pathological conditions may increase amount of WBCs within the flow and consequently they may disturb the flow behaviour in microvessels (see Figure 7).

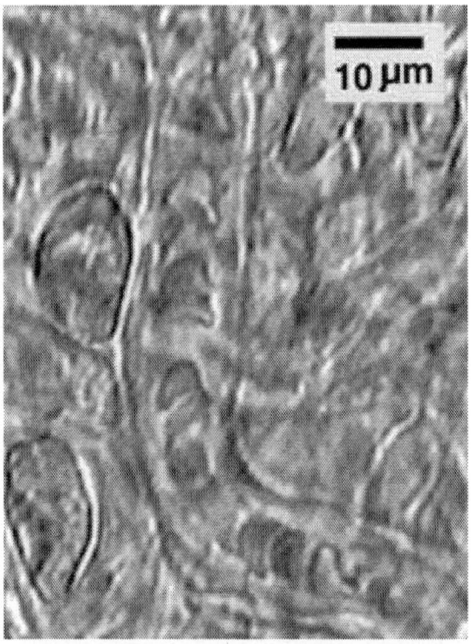

Fig. 6. RBCs deformation *in vivo* capillary (Minamiyama, 2000).

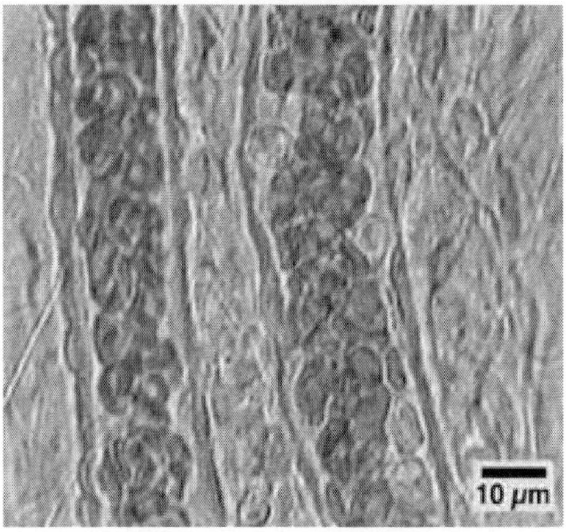

Fig. 7. Rolling of WBCs (yellow colour) in arterioles (Minamiyama, 2000).

Platelets are cells with no nuclei, round or oval discoid shape, in general, and with diameters from about 1 to 2 μm (see Figure 5). The number of platelets is usually less than the WBCs and they may have little effect on the blood flow behaviour. Although platelets play an important role in blood coagulation and thrombus formation, this topic is beyond the scope of the present review. Plasma is a yellowish fluid which contains 90% of water by volume and 10% of proteins, inorganic substances, vitamins, dissolved gases, etc. The proteins within the plasma flow, due to their large molecular size, usually do not pass through the capillary wall, thus generating an osmotic pressure. In *in vitro* experiments the osmotic pressure is an important parameter that needs special attention (Lima et al., 2012).

4. In vitro blood flow behaviour in straight microchannels

4.1 Fahraeus effect and Fahraeus-Lindqvist effect

In large arteries, where the diameter of the blood vessels is large enough compared to individual cells, it has been proved adequate to consider blood as a single-phase fluid (Caro et al., 1978). Accordingly, blood in large arteries may be treated as a homogeneous fluid where its particulate nature is ignored. Moreover, due to the large Reynolds number (Re) in arteries, blood flow is governed by inertial forces. However, arteries divide into successive smaller arteries and consequently the cross-sectional area of the vascular bed increases. As a result both pressure and velocity decrease as the blood flows into the smaller vessels. When the blood reaches the arterioles and capillaries the Re became less than 1, where viscous force dominates over inertial forces. At this microscale it is fundamental to take into account the effects of the multiphase properties of the blood on its flow behaviour (Caro et al., 1978). A clear example of the multiphase nature of the blood is the formation of a plasma layer at microvessels less than 300 μm, known as Fahraeus-Lindqvist effect (Fahraeus & Lindqvist, 1931).

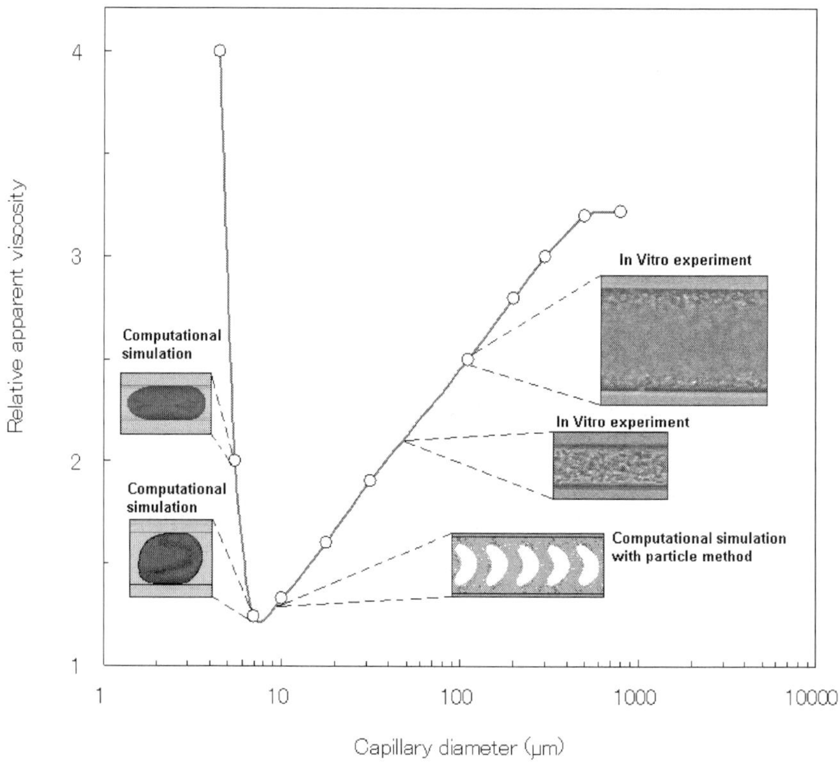

Fig. 8. Relative apparent viscosity of *in vitro* blood through glass capillaries (adapted from Pries et al., 1992; Wada & Kobayashi, 2002; Tsubota et al., 2006).

In the classical work of Robin Fahraeus, he observed that blood flow behaviour and its hematocrit are strongly affected by microtubes diameters less than 300 μm. The Fahraeus effect indicates that the Hct in the glass capillaries (< 300 μm) is lower than the feed Hct, which suggests that the Hct decreases as the blood proceeds through narrower microvessels. This phenomenon results from the axial migration of the RBCs to the centre of the microtube and consequent faster motion of the cells when compared with the suspending medium, such as plasma or dextran (Fahraeus & Lindqvist, 1931). The Fahraeus-Lindqvist effect is somehow related to the above phenomenon. Again for microtubes diameters less than 300 μm, Fahraeus and Lindqvist observed that the apparent blood viscosity decreases as the microtube diameter became smaller (Fahraeus & Lindqvist, 1931). After them, several works have extended their experiment down to diameters of about 3 μm and they have observed that the decrease of the apparent viscosity continues down to diameters of about 10 μm. However, the Fahraeus-Lindqvist effect is reversed at diameters 5 to 7 μm (see Figure 8) (Pries et al., 1992).

4.2 Particles and RBCs in diluted suspensions

In Poiseuille flow, the behaviour of suspended particles depends on several factors such as shear rate, particle deformability, size and shape. Generally, at low shear rates and diluted suspensions, rigid spherical particles and hardened RBCs (HRBCs) tend to move axially without any radial migration. On the other hand, deformable bodies, such as healthy RBCs tend to migrate towards the tube axis due to a radial hydrodynamic force. For higher (>1) particle Reynolds number (Re_p) where the inertial forces become important, both deformable bodies and rigid spheres have axial migration, however the spheres not always migrate toward the centre. The spheres near the wall moves towards the centre whereas the ones in the centre moves towards the wall. At the end they reach an equilibrium radial position of 0.6R, where R is the tube radius. This effect is known as tubular pinch effect (see Figure 9) (Caro et al., 1978).

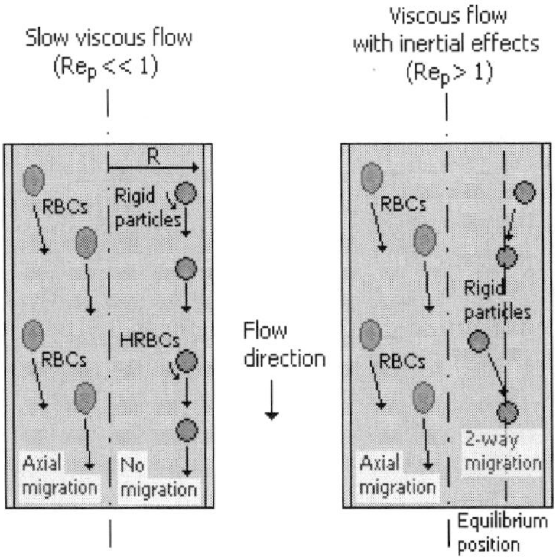

Fig. 9. Schematic representation of migration differences of rigid, healthy RBCs and hardened RBCs (HRBCs) in the centre of a capillary. Re_p corresponds to the particle Reynolds number (adapted from Goldsmith, 1971a, 1971b).

4.3 RBCs in concentrated suspensions

Although the flow properties of RBCs in diluted suspensions were extensively studied for many the years, such is not the case when the RBCs flow within a crowded environment. The reason is mainly related to technical limitations of optical systems to obtain reliable measurements at Hct bigger than 10%. However, Goldsmith and coworkers (Goldsmith & Turitto, 1986) have overcome this technical difficulty by using transparent RBCs (known as ghost cells) as the suspension medium. By using ghost cells they were able to study the behaviour of individual RBC flowing in concentrated suspension of RBC ghosts. The motion of RBCs in concentrated suspensions is appreciably different from those observed in very diluted suspensions (Hct < 1 %). At concentrated suspensions the motion of RBCs is disturbed not only by the collisions with neighbouring cells but also by the plasma layer near the wall. In this way, the cell paths exhibit continuous erratic displacements with the largest ones occurring in the region between 0.5 and 0.8 of the tube radius from the axis. At a given microtube, the magnitude of radial displacements tends to increase with the concentration of RBC ghost cells. However, at concentrations bigger than 50%, the displacement decreases. At Hct > 50%, although the crowded environment leads to an increase of the cell deformation, it also limits the magnitude of the RBC radial dispersion (Goldsmith & Turitto, 1986).

Recently, Lima et al. demonstrated the ability of confocal micro-PIV not only to measure both pure water and suspensions of RBCs through a square glass microchannel (Lima et al., 2006) but also to measure the velocity profiles of both physiological saline (PS) and in vitro blood (20% Hct) in a rectangular polydimethysiloxane (PDMS) microchannel (Lima et al., 2008). Good agreement between the measured velocity profiles of pure water and an established analytical solution was obtained for both studies. Further work was also performed by the Lima et al. but this time to measure both ensemble and instantaneous velocity profiles for *in vitro* blood with Hcts up to 17% (Lima et al., 2007). Although the ensemble velocity profiles were markedly parabolic, some fluctuations in the instantaneous velocity profiles were found to be closely related to the Hct increase. Hence, those results have suggested that the presence of RBCs within the plasma flow influences the measurements of the instantaneous velocity fields (see Figure 10).

Lima and his colleagues have also observed that by using a confocal micro-PIV system (see Figure 2) it was possible to measure with good accuracy blood plasma containing trace particles with Hct up to 9%. For Hct bigger than 9%, the light absorbed by the RBCs has contributed significantly to diminish the concentration of fluorescent tracer particles in the acquired confocal images. This low density images become evident for Hct bigger than 20 %, which generates errors in the velocity fields. Hence, Lima et al. (Lima et al., 2008, 2009) have developed a new approach to track individual tracer cells at high concentration suspensions of RBCs. The confocal micro-PTV system (see Figure 4) was employed, for the first time, in an effort to obtain detailed quantitative measurements on the motion of blood cells at both diluted and high suspensions of RBCs in simple straight microchannels. Lima et al. have successfully labelled both RBCs and WBCs and have measured their motions through microchannels. The ability of the confocal system to generate thin in-focus planes has allowed measurements in flowing blood at concentrated suspensions of: cell-cell hydrodynamic interaction, RBC orientation and RBC radial dispersion at different depths (Lima et al., 2008, 2009). To analyse the ability of the confocal micro-PTV system to track RBCs, the motions of labelled RBCs were followed at several Hcts (3% to 37%).

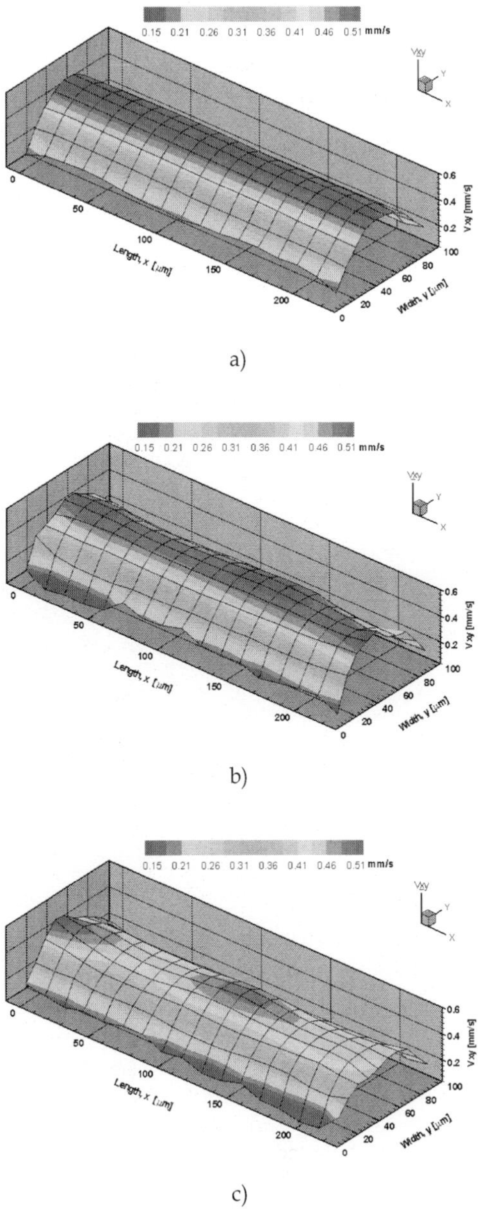

Fig. 10. Time series of the instantaneous velocity profiles of (a) pure water (b) *in vitro* blood with a 9% Hct and (c) *in vitro* blood with a 17% Hct, in the central plane of the microchannel with a $\Delta t = 10$ ms (adapted from Lima et al., 2007).

For the calculation of the radial dispersion coefficient (D_{yy}), measurements were performed at middle plane of the microchannels. However to investigate complex microrhelogical events in flowing blood (such as interaction and orientation of blood cells) all measurements were performed near the wall of the microchannel (z = 20 μm) with Hct ~ 20% and Re ~ 0.007. Figure 11 shows the trajectories of two-RBC interactions near the wall and within the plasma layer. This figure shows the radial disturbance effect enhanced by the collision of a neighbouring RBC. The hemodynamic interaction effect of WBC on the motion of RBCs was also possible to be measured. Figure 12a shows a RBC interacting with a WBC. In Figure 12a it is possible to observe that the transversal displacement increases due to the collision with a flowing WBC. An interesting measurement of both RBC translational and rotational motion was also possible by adjusting the image contrast (see Figure 12b). The translational motion was measured at the centre of the RBC whereas the rotational was measured along the RBC membrane.

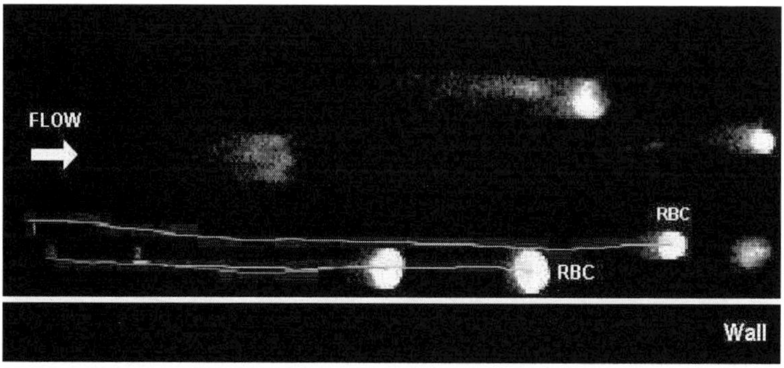

Fig. 11. Two-RBC interactions in a straight microchannel.

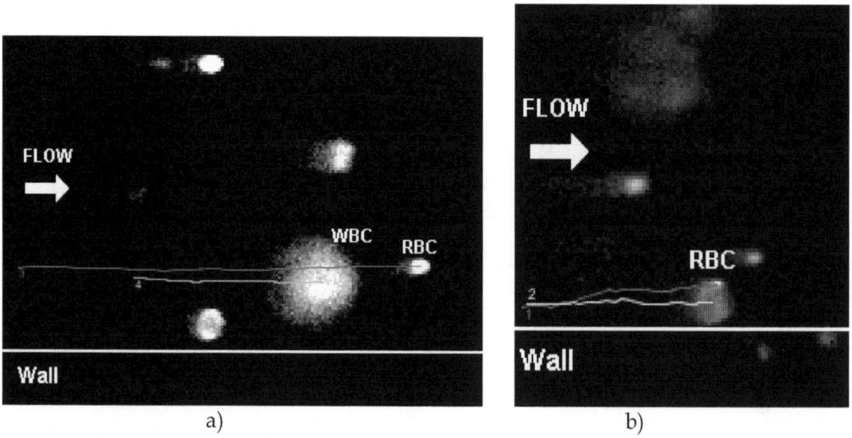

Fig. 12. (a) RBC-WBC interaction in a straight microchannel; (b) Translational and rotational motion of a RBC.

Further research was carried by using in vitro blood with several Hcts and low Reynolds numbers (Re ~ 0.005). The paths of hundreds labeled RBCs were measured in the centre plane of both straight glass and PDMS circular microchannel (Lima et al., 2008, 2009, 2009). The RBC dispersion coefficient (D_{yy}) for two different diameters (75µm and 100µm) and for several Hcts is shown in Figure 13. The results show that RBC D_{yy} rises with the increase of the Hct and that RBC D_{yy} tends to decrease with the diameter.

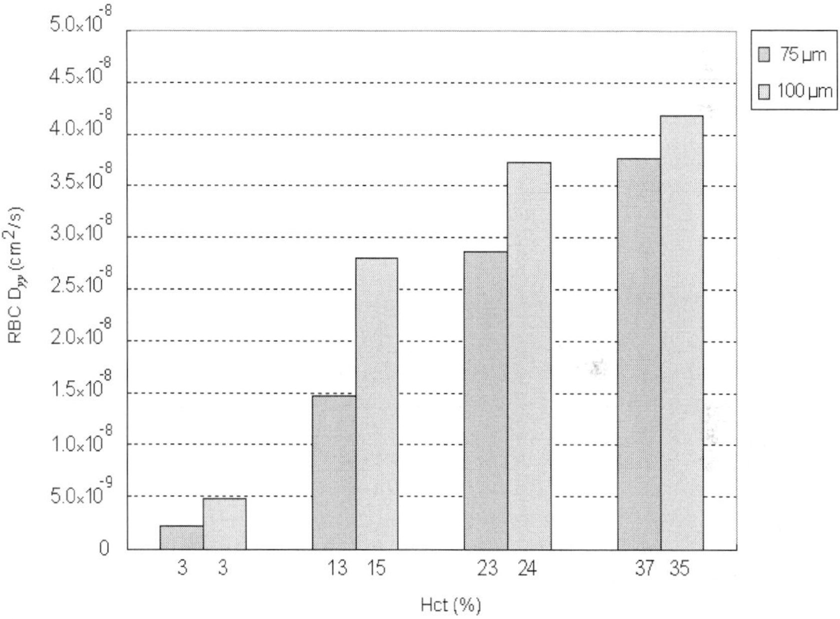

Fig. 13. Effect of the Hct on the RBC D_{yy} at 75µm PDMS microchannel and 100 µm glass capillary (adapted from Lima et al., 2008, 2009).

4.4 Cell-free layer (CFL)

In microcirculation the cell-free layer is believed to reduce the friction between red blood cells (RBCs) and endothelial cells and consequently reduce blood flow resistance. However, the complex formation of the cell-free layer has not yet been convincingly described mainly due to multi-physical and hemorheological factors that affect this phenomenon. Recent studies have measured the effect of hematocrit (Hct) on the thickness of the cell-free layer in straight circular polydimethylsiloxane (PDMS) microchannels. The formation of a cell-free layer is clearly visible in the images captured (see Figure 14) and by using a combination of image analysis techniques we are able to detect an increase in the cell-free layer thickness as Hct decreases.

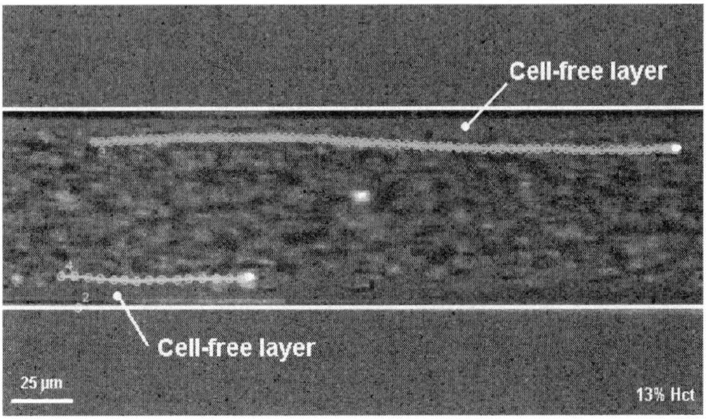

Fig. 14. Labelled RBCs flowing around the boundary region of the cell-free layer (Lima et al., 2009).

Labelled RBCs flowing around the boundary region of the cell-free layer were able to track manually by using the MtrackJ plugin from Image J. Figure 14 shows an example of the trajectories of two labelled RBCs flowing close to the boundary of the cell-free layer. The radial position of the tracked RBCs is then determined and the corresponding thickness of the cell-free layer is calculated. Finally, the data is time-averaged. When the number of labelled RBCs flowing close to the boundary region is not significant, additional analysis is performed by manually measuring the distance from the boundary region to the wall for several points along the microchannel (Lima et al., 2009; Lima et al., 2009). Examination of Figure 15 shows an overall reduction of the thickness of the cell-free layer as Hct is increased. In particular, the thickness decreases almost four fold as Hct is increased from 3% to 37% (Lima et al., 2009; Lima et al., 2009).

4.5 Sedimentation effects

Recently Garcia and his colleagues (Garcia et al., 2010, 2011) have investigated the flow behaviour of two different physiological fluids frequently used in biomedical microdevices. The working fluids used in this study were physiological saline (PS) and dextran 40 (Dx40) containing about 6% of sheep red blood cells (RBCs), respectively. By using a syringe pump and a video camera it was possible to measure qualitatively the flow behaviour within a horizontal capillary. To analyze the dynamic sedimentation of PS and Dx40 containing RBCs they decided to use flow rates close to the one observed in vivo, i.e., 10 µl/min. During the experiment we made flow qualitative visualizations measurements in glass capillaries with diameters of about 1,2 mm. The visualizations were captured by a camera for about 15 minutes. Figure 16 shows the flow qualitative measurements for 0 minutes and 15 minutes. This image shows clearly that for a period of 15 minutes the RBC tend to settle down in the fluid with PS whereas using Dx40 we did not observe any RBC sedimentation. Although not shown in Figure 16, for the case of PS fluid we did not observe any RBC sedimentation for the first 10 minutes. According to our visualization the RBC tend to settle down for period of time superior to 10 minutes.

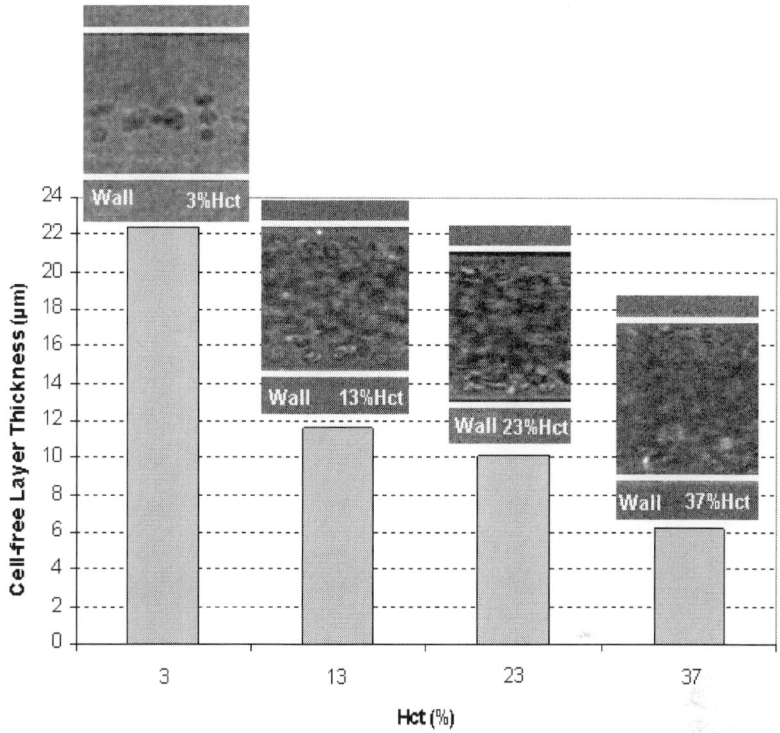

Fig. 15. Average thickness of the cell-free layer at several Hcts layer (Lima et al., 2009; Lima et al., 2009).

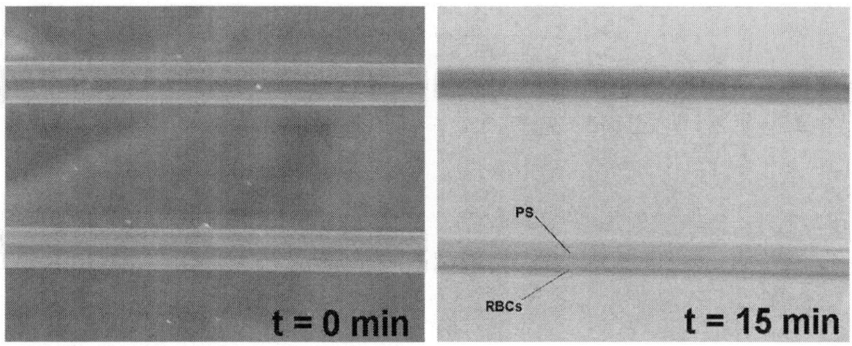

Fig. 16. Dynamic sedimentation measurements for two different time periods of PS and Dx40 containing RBCs, with a flow rate of 10 µl/min (Garcia et al., 2010, 2011).

Additionally, flow visualization measurements were also performed in glass microchannels (see Fig.17) and compared with *in vivo* blood flow (see Fig.17c). Figure 17 shows that for the case of Dx40 there is a clear formation of cell-free layer adjacent to the walls of microchannels. However, in the fluid with PS the RBCs do not exhibit a clear tendency to migrate into the microtube axis. The *in vivo* visualization measurements (Fig. 17c) have shown a clear tendency for the formation of a plasma layer in microvessels (Kim et al., 2006; Minamiyama, 2000). These results indicate that *in vitro* blood containing Dx40 has a flow behaviour closer to the one observed *in vivo* microvessels.

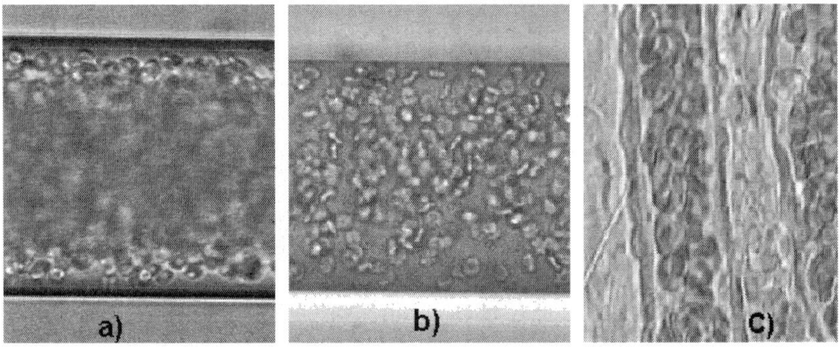

Fig. 17. *In vitro* flow visualization in glass microchannels for a period time bigger than 10 minutes a) Dx40 containing RBCs; b) PS containing RBCs. c) *In vivo* flow visualization in a microvessel (Lima et al., 2009a, 2009b; Minamiyama, 2000).

5. In vitro blood flow behaviour in microchannels with complex geometries

5.1 Bifurcation and confluence

By using a soft lithographic technique it is possible to fabricate polydimethysiloxane (PDMS) microchannels with complex geometries similar to human blood arterioles and capillary networks (Lima et al., 2011). In this section we show the application of a confocal micro-PTV system to track RBCs through a rectangular polydimethysiloxane (PDMS) microchannel with a diverging bifurcation and a confluence (see Figure 18).

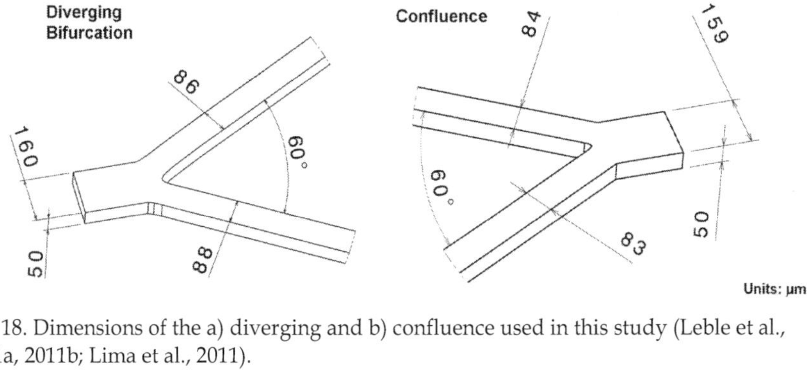

Fig. 18. Dimensions of the a) diverging and b) confluence used in this study (Leble et al., 2011a, 2011b; Lima et al., 2011).

By using a confocal system, we have measured the effect of both bifurcation and confluence on the flow behaviour of both fluorescent particles suspended in pure water (PW) and RBCs in concentrated suspensions. For the case of trace particles in PW we have observed that the trajectories were almost symmetric and do not present so many fluctuations for both geometries. These results are consistent with the Stokes flow regime. In contrast, for the case of labelled RBCs the trajectories are more asymmetric when compared with PW trajectories. Additionally, we can also observe several fluctuations on their trajectories possibly due to cell interactions enhanced by the high local Hct originated at this region (Lima et al., 2011a, 2011b).

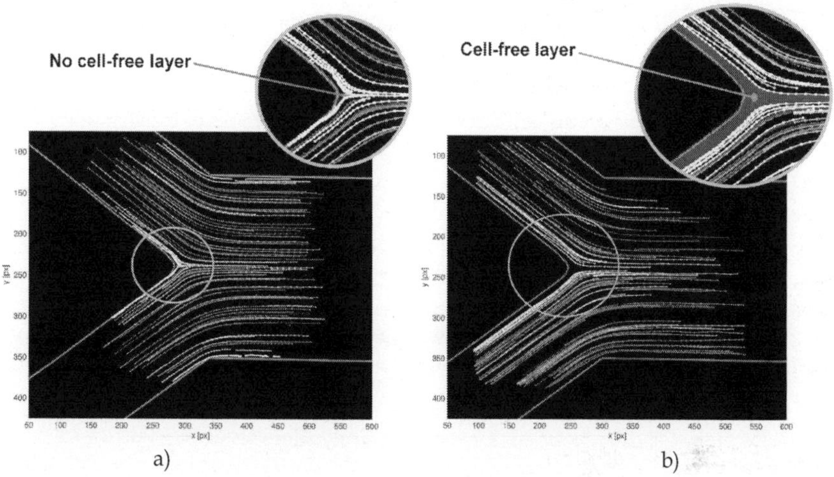

Fig. 19. Trajectories in a confluence of a) fluorescent particles in PW and b) labelled RBCs in Dx40 (Leble et al., 2011a, 2011b; Lima et al., 2011).

In the confluence, it is possible to observe that the trace particles tend to flow very close to the inner walls and as a result they tend to flow in the centre of the microchannel, just downstream of the confluence apex (see Fig.19a). However, for the case of labelled RBCs we could not measure any trajectory passing in this centre region (see Fig.19b). This is due to the existence of a cell-free layer (CFL) in both inner walls and a consequent formation of a triangular CFL in the region of the confluence apex (see Fig.19b) (Leble et al., 2011a, 2011b; Lima et al., 2011). As this triangular CFL seems to play an important role on the *in vitro* blood flow characteristics, a detailed quantitative study, to clarify the CFL effect in the velocity profiles, is currently under way and it will be published in due time (Leble et al., 2011).

5.2 Stenosis

The behaviour of RBCs in a microchannel with stenosis was also investigated using a confocal micro-PTV system. Individual trajectories of RBCs in a concentrated suspension of 10% hematocrit (Hct) were measured successfully. Results indicated that the trajectories of healthy RBCs became asymmetric before and after the stenosis, while the trajectories of tracer particles in pure water were almost symmetric. The effect of deformability of RBCs on the cell-free layer thickness, by hardening RBCs using a glutaraldehyde treatment, was also investigated.

Fujiwara et al. have found that deformability has a considerable effect on the asymmetry of the cell-free layer thickness and as result they concluded that the motions of RBCs are influenced strongly by the Hct, the deformability, and the channel geometry (Fujiwara et al., 2009).

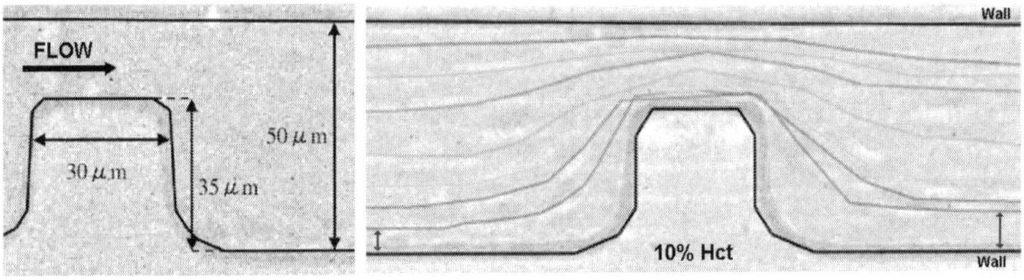

Fig. 20. Geometry of the stenosis and Flow of blood with. trajectories of labelled RBCs with 10% Hct (Fujiwara et al., 2008, 2009).

5.3 Capillary networks

The flow of red blood cells through a column packed with soda lime glass spheres was recently studied by Couto and her colleagues (Couto et al., 2011). Since the diameter of the glass spheres was 337.5 μm and the packing porosity 0.4 it was easy to determine (Dias et al., 2006, 2007, 2008; Dias, 2007) that the average capillary diameter of the porous network was 150 μm, this diameter being within the range of the typical dimensions observed in human blood arterioles.

The samples used in the referred study (Couto et al., 2011) were suspensions of sheep RBCs (with major diameter close to 6.5 μm) in physiological saline (PS) containing 0.1 to 1% Hct and the experimental apparatus was that shown in Fig. 21 and contains: a pump (1); injector (2); a chromatographic column packed with the above mentioned glass spheres (3); refractive index detector (4) and data acquisition system (5a and 5b). The mobile phase was PS and the flow rates varied between 0.2 ml/min and 1 ml/min.

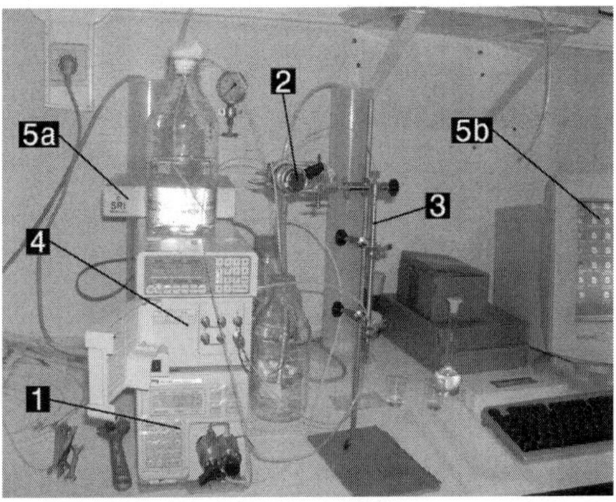

Fig. 21. Chromatographic apparatus (Couto et al., 2011).

An infinite small sized marker (sucrose) dissolved in PS was used in order to know the velocity of the carrier fluid (PS). The different experiments (different flow rates and Hcts) have shown that the RBCs migrate faster through the capillary network than the fluid (PS) that suspends the RBCs, as can be seen in Fig. 22. The authors (Couto et al., 2011) suggested that this behaviour can be explained by the theory that supports the hydrodynamic fractionation (Tijssen et al., 1986; Stegeman et al., 1993; Dias et al., 2008; Dias, 2007, 2008) and by the formation of a cell-free layer adjacent to the walls of the capillaries.

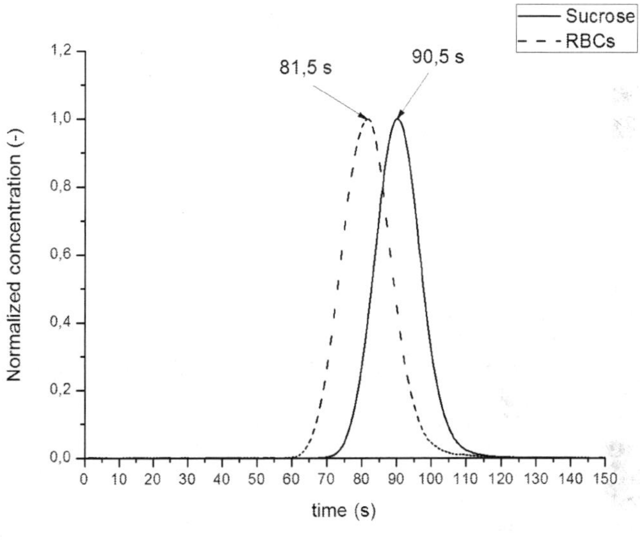

Fig. 22. Chromatogram for 1ml/min.

6. Conclusions

Advances in computers, image analysis, and optics have made it possible to combine both particle image velocimetry (PIV) and particle tracking velocimetry (PTV) system with a spinning disk confocal microscope. This revision summarise the most relevant studies of *in vitro* blood flow, through simple and complex microchannels, by means of a confocal micro-PIV/PTV system.

In vitro blood studies showed that the confocal micro-PIV system is able to measure with good accuracy blood plasma with Hct up to 9%, in a 100-μm square microchannel. However, for Hct bigger than 9%, the light absorbed by the RBCs contributes to diminish the concentration fluorescent particles in the acquired confocal images. This low density images become more evident for Hct bigger than 20%, which generates spurious errors in the velocity profiles. Hence, a Langragian approach was proposed to the confocal system in order to track individual blood cells at high Hcts. Owing to its optical sectioning ability and consequent improvement of the image contrast and definition, the proposed confocal micro-PTV system eliminates several problems and concerns of the microvisualization systems used in the past and provides additional detailed description on the RBC motion. Hence, the proposed confocal system has shown detailed RBC trajectories of RBC-RBC interaction at moderate and high Htcs (Hcts up to 35%) never obtainable by other conventional methods. As a result, by measuring hundreds of RBC trajectories, it was possible to conclude that RBC paths are strongly dependent on the Hct and as a result the RBC dispersion coefficient tends to increase with the Hct. Another unique measurement was the possibility to obtain both translational and rotational motion of RBCs flowing in highly concentrated suspensions. Hence, it was possible to compare in detail the motion of a RBC without any kind of interaction (rolling on the wall of the microchannel) with a RBC interacting with neighbouring blood cells. These remarkable results, have shown for the first time, that RBC rolling on the wall and without interaction tends to rotate in regular and periodically way whereas RBCs that interact with neighbouring cells tend to rotate in a rather erratic way. Very recently, our confocal system have shown also for the first time, a very astonishing blood flow phenomenon happening downstream of a confluence. Our results show the formation of a triangular cell-free layer (CFL) in the region of the confluence apex which consequently promotes a development of thin CFL in the middle of the microchannel. This finding suggests that in our microcirculatory system we may have CFLs not only on the walls but also in the middle of the microvessels. Additionally, the confocal system have also proved to be powerful tool to obtain further insight onto the flow behaviour of blood through other kinds of complex geometries such as diverging bifurcations, and stenosis.

The net of capillaries obtained by packing chromatographic columns with glass spheres may be used as a simple model in order to further understand the blood flow in complex microvascular networks.

7. Future directions

Past *in vitro* research performed with classical glass microchannels has revealed several amazing phenomena happening in microcirculation. However, recently several studies on the blood flow behaviour have shown quantitative difference between the results in microvessels and in glass microchannels. The reason for these differences still remains unclear mainly because glass microchannels differ from microvessels in several aspects, such as elasticity and geometry and biological effect by the endothelial inner surface. These limitations encountered in glass microchannels can be overcome by using PDMS microchannels. Hence, in the near future we are planning to develop a biochip to mimic the *in vivo* environment. By using an innovative cellular micropatterning technique based on electrochemical method, we expect to culture living cells on their surfaces and consequently to provide experimental evidence on several microcirculation mysteries, such as the role of the glycocalyx on the flow behaviour of blood and the thrombogenesis process.

Computational modelling is a powerful way to obtain detailed information on the mechanical behaviours of multiple RBCs. Recently, several numerical methods have been proposed to analyse microscale blood flows in microvessels such as the particle method and the elastic RBC flow model. We expect in the near future to compare the reported experimental results with the numerical methods mentioned above. This collaborative work between experimental and computational methods will contribute not only to improve the modelling of cell behaviour but also to provide better understanding on several microcirculation phenomena

Another area for further research is the improvement of the current particle tracking methods. In this work a manual tracking method was used due to the inability of the automatic methods to track RBCs when they experienced collisions. Hence, a more reliable automatic tracking method needs to be developed to reduce the time-consuming and also to avoid the tedious work performed during the post-processing procedure.

8. Acknowledgment

The authors acknowledge the financial support provided by: PTDC/SAU-BEB/108728/2008, PTDC/SAU-BEB/105650/2008 and PTDC/EME-MFE/099109/2008 from the FCT (Science and Technology Foundation) and COMPETE, Portugal. The authors would like also to thank all the colleagues and students for their valuable comments, suggestions and technical assistance throughout this research work.

9. References

Adrian, R. (1991). Particle-imaging techniques for experimental fluid mechanics. *Annual Review of Fluid Mechanics.*, 23, pp. 261-304

Bitsch, L., Olesen, L., Westergaard, C., Bruus, H., Klank, H., & Kutter, J. (2005). Micro particle-image velocimetry of bead suspensions and blood flows. *Experiments in Fluids*, 39 (3), pp. 505-511.

Caro, C., Pedley, T., Schroter, R., & Seed, W. (1978). *The mechanics of the circulation*, Oxford University Press, Oxford, England.

Chiu, J., Chen, C., Lee, P., Yang, C., Chuang, H., Chien, S., & Usami, S. (2003). Analysis of the effect of distributed flow on monocytic adhesion to endothelial cells. *Journal of Biomechanics*, 36, pp. 1883-1895.

Couto, A., Teixeira, L., Leble, V., Lima, R., Ribeiro, A., & Dias, R. (2011). Flow of red blood cells in capillary networks ", in T Yamaguchi, Y. Imai, MSN Oliveira, R Lima (ed.), *Japan-Portugal Nano-BME Symposium: proceedings of the 2011 conference*, Porto/Braganca, Portugal, pp. 35-38, 2011.

Dias, R. (2007). Transport phenomena in polydisperse porous media (in Portuguese). P.hD. Dissertation, Minho University, Braga, Portugal.

Dias, R. (2008). Size fractionation by slalom chromatography and hydrodynamic chromatography, *Recent Patents on Engineering*, 2, pp. 95-103

Dias, R., Teixeira, J., Mota, M., & Yelshin, A. (2006). Tortuosity variation in low density binary particulate bed. *Separation and Purification Technology*, 51, pp. 180-184

Dias, R., Fernandes, C., Teixeira, J., Mota, M., & Yelshin, A. (2007). Permeability and effective thermal conductivity of bisized porous media. *International Journal of Heat and Mass Transfer*, 50, pp. 1295-1301

Dias, R., Fernandes, C., Teixeira, J., Mota, M., & Yelshin, A. (2008). Starch analysis using hydrodynamic chromatography with a mixed-bed particle column, *Carbohydrate Polymers*, 74, pp. 852-857

Dias, R., Fernandes, C., Teixeira, J., Mota, M., & Yelshin, A. (2008). Permeability analysis in bisized porous media: Wall effect between particles of different size, *Journal of Hydrology* 349 470-474

Electron Microscopy Facility at The National Cancer Institute at Frederick (NCI-Frederick). A three-dimensional ultra structural image analysis of a T-lymphocyte (right), a platelet (center) and a red blood cell (left), using a Hitachi S-570 scanning electron microscope (SEM) equipped with a GW Backscatter Detector. 2005. Available from: http://en.wikipedia.org/wiki/File:Red_White_Blood_cells.jpg

Fahraeus, R., & Lindqvist, T. (1931). The viscosity of the blood in narrow capillary tubes. *American Journal of Physiology.*, Vol. 96, n°3, pp. 562-568

Fujiwara, H., Ishikawa, T., Lima, R., Marsuki, N., Imai, Y., Kaji, H., Nishizawa, M., & Yamaguchi, T. (2008). Motion of Red Blood Cells and Cell Free Layer Distribution in a Stenosed Microchannel, *Proceedings of 16th Congress of the European Society of Biomechanics*, pp. 14-17, Lucerne, Switzerland, May 17-22

Fujiwara, H., Ishikawa T., Lima, R., Marsuki, N., Imai, Y., Kaji, H., Nishizawa, M., & Yamaguchi, T. (2009). Red blood cell motions in a high hematocrit blood flowing through a stenosed micro-channel. *Journal of Biomechanics*, 42, pp. 838-843

Garcia, V., Correia, T., Dias, R., & Lima, R. (2010). Flow of physiological fluids in microchannels: the sedimentation effect, *Proceedings of 6th World Congress of Biomechanics*, pp. 1071-1074, Singapore, Singapore, August 1-6, 2010

Garcia, V., Correia T., Dias R., & Lima R. (2011). Dynamic Sedimentation Measurements of Physiological Fluids in Biomedical Devices", in T Yamaguchi, Y. Imai, MSN Oliveira, R Lima (ed.), *Japan-Portugal Nano-BME Symposium: proceedings of the 2011 conference*, Porto/Bragança, Portugal, pp.47-48, 2011

Goldsmith, H. (1971a). Red cell motions and wall interactions in tube flow, *Federation Proceedings 30* (5), 1578-1588

Goldsmith, H. (1971b). Deformation of human red cells in tube flow. *Biorheology*, 7, pp. 235-242.

Goldsmith, H. & Turitto, V. (1986). Rheological aspects of thrombosis and haemostasis: basic principles and applications. ICTH-Report-Subcommittee on Rheology of the International Committee on Thrombosis and Haemostasis. *Thrombosis and Haemostasis.*, Vol.55, No.3, pp. 415–435

Kim, S., Kong, R., Popel, A., Intaglietta, M., & Johnson, P. (2006). A computer-based method for determination of the cell-free layer with in microcirculation. *Microcirculation*, 13 (3), pp. 199-207

Kim, G., & Lee, S. (2006). X-ray PIV measurements of blood flows without tracer particles. *Experiments in Fluids*, 41, pp. 195-200

Koutsiaris, A., Mathioulakis, D., & Tsangaris, S. (1999). Microscope PIV for velocity-field measurement of particle suspensions flowing inside glass capillaries. *Measurement Science and Technology*, 10, pp. 1037-1046

Leble, V., Dias, R., Lima, R., Fernandes, C., Ishikawa, T., Imai, Y., & Yamaguchi, T., (2011) "Motions of trace particles and red blood cells in a PDMS microchannel with a converging bifurcation", in T Yamaguchi, Y. Imai, MSN Oliveira, R Lima (ed.), *Japan-Portugal Nano-BME Symposium: proceedings of the 2011 conference*, Porto/Braganca, Portugal, pp. 29-30

Leble, V., Lima, R., Fernandes, C., Dias, R. (2011). Flow of red blood cells through a microchannel with a confluence", *Proceedings of the Congresso de Métodos Numéricos em Engenharia 2011*, CD-ROM paper ID267.pdf, Coimbra, Portugal, 2011.

Leble, V., Lima, R., Ricardo, D., Fernandes, C., Ishikawa, T., Imai, Y., &Yamaguchi, T. (2011). Asymmetry of red blood cell motions in a microchannel with a diverging and converging bifurcation ", *Biomicrofluidics*, 5 (4), 044120 (15 pages).

Lima, R., Wada, S., Tsubota, K., & Yamaguchi, T. (2006). Confocal micro-PIV measurements of three dimensional profiles of cell suspension flow in a square microchannel. *Measurement Science and Technology,* Vol. 17, n° 4, pp. 797-808

Lima, R. (2007). Analysis of the blood flow behavior through microchannels by a confocal micro-PIV/PTV system, PhD (Eng.), Bioengineering and Robotics Department, Tohoku University, Sendai, Japan, 2007.

Lima, R., Wada, S., Takeda, M., Tsubota, K., & Yamaguchi, T. (2007). In vitro confocal micro-PIV measurements of blood flow in a square microchannel: the effect of the haematocrit on instantaneous velocity profiles. *Journal of Biomechanics,* 40, pp. 2752-2757

Lima, R., Ishikawa, T., Imai, Y., Takeda, M., Wada, S., & Yamaguchi, T. (2008). Radial dispersion of red blood cells in blood flowing through glass capillaries: role of heamatocrit and geometry, *Journal of Biomechanics,* 41, pp. 2188-2196

Lima, R., Wada, S., Tanaka, S., Takeda, M., Ishikawa T., Tsubota, K., Imai, Y., & Yamaguchi, T. (2008). In vitro blood flow in a rectangular PDMS microchannel: experimental observations using a confocal micro-PIV system. *Biomedical Microdevices,* Vol. 10, n° 2, pp. 153-167

Lima, R., Nakamura, M., Omori, Y., Ishikawa T., Wada, S., & Yamaguchi T. (2009). Microscale flow dynamics of red blood cells in microchannels: an experimental and numerical analysis, In: Tavares and Jorge (Eds), *Advances in Computational Vision and Medical Image Processing: Methods and Applications,* Springer, Vol.13, 203-220

Lima, R., Ishikawa, T., Imai, Y., Takeda, M., Wada, S., & Yamaguchi, T. (2009). Measurement of individual red blood cell motions under high hematocrit conditions using a confocal micro-PTV system. *Annals of Biomedical Engineering,* Vol.37, n° 8, pp. 1546-1559

Lima R., Oliveira, M., Ishikawa, T., Kaji, H., Tanaka, S., Nishizawa, M., & Yamaguchi, T. (2009). Axisymmetric PDMS microchannels for in vitro haemodynamics studies. *Biofabrication,* Vol.1, n° 3, pp. 035005.

Lima, R., Oliveira, M., Cerdeira, T., Monteiro, F., Ishikawa, T., Imai,Y., & Yamaguchi, T. (2009). Determination of the cell-free layer in circular PDMS microchannels, *ECCOMAS Thematic Conference on Computational Vision and Medical Image Processing,* Porto, Portugal.

Lima, R., Fernandes, C., Dias, R., Ishikawa, T., Imai, Y., Yamaguchi, T. (2011). Microscale flow dynamics of red blood cells in microchannels: an experimental and numerical analysis, In: Tavares and Jorge (Eds), *Computational Vision and Medical Image Processing: Recent Trends,* Springer, Vol.19, pp. 297-309.

Lima, R., Dias, R., Leble, V., Fernandes, C., Ishikawa, T., Imai, Y., Yamaguchi, T. (2012). Flow visualization of trace particles and red blood cells in a microchannel with a diverging and converging bifurcation, *ECCOMAS Thematic Conference on Computational Vision and Medical Image Processing,* Olhão, Portugal, pp. 209-211.

Lima, R., Ishikawa, T., Imai, Y., & Yamaguchi, T. (2012). Blood flow behavior in microchannels: advances and future trends, In: Dias et al. (Eds), *Single and two-Phase Flows on Chemical and Biomedical Engineering,* Bentham Science Publishers Springer, (in press).

Meinhart, C., Wereley, S., & Gray, H. (2000). Volume illumination for two-dimensional particle image velocimetry. *Measurement Science and Technology,* 11, pp. 809-814

Minamiyama, M. (2000). In Vivo Microcirculatory Studies: In Vivo Video Images of Microcirculation Part 2, Available from: http://www.ne.jp/asahi/minamiya/medicine/

Nash, G. & Meiselman, H. (1983). Red cell and ghost viscoelasticity. Effects of hemoglobin concentration and in vivo aging. *Biophysical Journal,* 43. pp. 63-73

Park, J., Choi, C., & Kihm, K. (2004). Optically sliced micro-PIV using confocal laser scanning microscopy (CLSM). *Experiments in Fluids,* 37, pp. 105-119.

Park, J., & Kihm, K. (2006). Use of confocal laser scanning microscopy (CLSM) for depthwise resolved microscale-particle image velocimetry (μ-PIV). Optics and Lasers in Engineering, 44, pp. 208-223.

Parthasarathi, A., Japee, S. & Pittman, R. (1999). Determination of red blood cell velocity by video shuttering and image analysis. *Annals of Biomedical Engineering,* 27, pp. 313-325

Pries, A., Neuhaus, D. & Gaehtgens, P. (1992). Blood viscosity in tube flow: dependence on diameter and hematocrit. *Am. J. Physiol.*, Vol. 263, nº 6, pp. 1770-1778

Santiago, J., Wereley, S., Meinhart C., Beebe, D., & Adrian, R. (1998). A particle image velocimetry system for microfluidics. *Experiments in Fluids,* 25, pp. 316-319.

Stegeman, G., Kraak, J., & Poppe, H. (1993). Hydrodynamic chromatography of polymers in packed columns. *Journal of Chromatography A,* 657(2), pp. 283-303

Sugii, Y., Nishio, S., & Okamoto, K. (2002). In vivo PIV measurement of red blood cell velocity field in microvessels considering mesentery motion. *Physiological Measurement,* 23(2), pp. 403-416

Sugii, Y., Okuda, R., Okamoto, K., & Madarame, H. (2005). Velocity measurement of both red blood cells and plasma of in vitro blood flow using high-speed micro PIV technique. *Measurement Science and Technology,* 16, pp. 1126-1130

Tanaani, T., Otsuki, S., Tomosada, N., Kosugi, Y., Shimizu, M., & Ishida, H. (2002). High-speed 1-frame/ms scanning confocal microscope with a microlens and Nipkow disks. *Applied Optics,* 41 (22), pp. 4704-4708

Tijssen, R., Bos, J., & Kreveld, M. (1986). Hydrodynamic Chromatography in Open Microcapillary Tubes. *Anal. Chem.*, 58, pp 3036-3034

Tsubota, K., Wada, S., & Yamaguchi, T. (2006). Simulation study on effects of hematocrit on blood flow properties using particle method. *Journal of Biomechanical Science and Enginneering,* 1, pp. 159-170

Uijttewaal, W., Nijhof, E. & Heethaar, R. (1994). Lateral migration of blood cells and microspheres in two-dimensional Poiseuille flow: a laser Doppler study. *Journal of Biomechanics,* 27, pp. 35-42

Vennemann, P., Kiger, K., Lindken, R., Groenendijk, B., Stekelenburg-de Vos, S., Hagen, T., Ursem, N., Poelmann, R., Westerweel, J., & Hierk, B. (2006). In vivo micro particle image velocimetry measurements of blood-plasma in the embryonic avian heart. *Journal of Biomechanics,* 39, pp. 1191-1200

Wada, S., & Kobayashi, R. (2002). Simulation of the shape change of a red blood cell at the entrance of a capillary, *Proceedings of the 4th World Congress of Biomechanics,* Calgary, Canada.

18

Electroporation of *Kluyveromyces marxianus* and β-D-galactosidase Extraction

Airton Ramos[1] and Andrea Lima Schneider[2]
[1]*State University of Santa Catarina*
[2]*University of Joinville*
Brazil

1. Introduction

Nowadays electroporation is well established as a method for increasing the permeability of biological membranes aiming to include some kind of molecule inside cells (anticancer drugs, for example) or to extract molecules from cells (enzymes, DNA, etc.). The permeabilized cells show a distribution of hydrophilic pores with diameters of several nanometers in the regions where the induced transmembrane potential rises above a threshold value from 200 mV to 1 V (Hibino *et al*, 1993; Teissie & Rols, 1993). The pore density and their diameters are dependent on the stimulation conditions: field strength, waveform and duration of stimulus (Weaver & Chizmadzhev, 1996; Teissié *et al*, 2005; Miklavčič & Puc, 2006; Chen *et al*, 2006)

Some previous studies have demonstrated experimentally the possibility of enzyme extraction from yeast by electroporation. Galutzov and Ganev (Galutzov & Ganev, 1999) investigated the extraction of glutathione reductase, 3-phosphoglicerate kinase e alcohol dehydrogenase from *Saccharomyces Cerevisiae* by electroporation. They used sequences of electric field pulses with strength 275 kV/m and duration of 1 ms. They observed increase in concentration of enzymes in the supernatant to about 8 hours after exposure to the field. The extraction efficiency was higher compared to other methods with mechanical or chemical lyses. Treatment with dithiothreitol before exposure to the field accelerated the extraction of glutathione reductase and alcohol dehydrogenase. This effect was considered to be related to the increased porosity of the cell wall due to the break of disulfide bonds in the layers of mannoproteins.

Ganev *et al* (Ganev *et al*, 2003) developed and used an electroporation system to stimulate a flow of yeast suspension up to 60 mL/min. They obtained the extraction of hexokinase, 3-phosphoglicerate kinase and 3-glyceraldehyde phosphate dehydrogenase from *Saccharomyces Cerevisiae*. They found that the maximum extraction is obtained after 4 hours with 15 pulses of frequency 6 Hz, but similar results were obtained for different combinations of field strength between 270 and 430 kV/m and pulse duration between 1 and 3 ms, so that stronger fields require shorter pulse to produce the same result in the extraction. The activity of enzymes extracted by electroporation was about double of those extracted by enzymatic and mechanical lysis of cells.

The extraction of β-D-galactosidase has a great interest due to its use in food and pharmaceutical industries. This enzyme is responsible for hydrolysis of lactose, disaccharide of low sweetness present on milk, resulting in its monosaccharide glucose and galactose. Its industrial importance is the application in dairy products for the production of foods with low lactose content, ideal for lactose intolerant consumers by improving the digestibility of milk and dairy. This is an important issue since lactase deficiency is present in about two thirds of the adult population worldwide, mainly in developing countries (Swagerty *et al*, 2002). In addition, lactase allows getting better technological characteristics and improves sensory and rheological properties of dairy products. Increase the power and sweetness that reduces the addition of sucrose, reducing the calorie content of foods. The formation of monosaccharides in dairy products helps in the metabolism of yeast fermented products. Lactase also reduces the probability of occurrence of the Maillard reaction, as galacto-oligosaccharides obtained did not act as reducing sugars.

The enzyme extraction method based on cell membrane permeabilization by electric field pulses applied to a suspension of yeast has advantages over chemical and mechanical methods due to its simplicity, efficiency in the extraction and preservation of enzyme activity and the cell itself, depending on the stimulation conditions. This study aims to evaluate the relationship between the change in membrane conductance during electrical stimulation of the cells and the enzyme β-D-galactosidase activity released by cells and to determine the stimulation conditions that maximize the extraction of this enzyme from *Kluyveromyces marxianus* yeasts.

The electroporation dynamics (opening and closing pores) is not completely understood. Part of this problem is because the electroporation is evaluated by indirect measurements (Kinosita & Tsong, 1979; He *et al*, 2008; Saulis *et al*, 2007). A number of methods have been used in the study of electroporation based on electrical measurements (Kinosita & Tsong, 1979; Huang & Rubinsky, 1999; Kotnik *et al*, 2003; Pavlin *et al*, 2005; Pliquett *et al*, 2004; Ivorra & Rubinsky, 2007; Suzuki *et al*, 2011). Electrical measurements and modeling were used to evaluate the effectiveness of electroporation in individual cells (Koester *et al*, 2010; Haque *et al*, 2009), cell suspensions (Kinosita & Tsong, 1979; Pavlin *et al*, 2005; Suzuki *et al*, 2011) and tissues (Grafström *et al*, 2006; Ivorra & Rubinsky, 2007; Laufer *et al*, 2010).

The membrane conductance after electroporation is related to electrical conductivity of cell suspension. Models are developed for isolated spherical or spheroidal cells using proposed membrane conductance distributions (Kinosita & Tsong, 1979; Pavlin & Miklavcic, 2003) and are obtained from the static solution to Laplace's equation using the simplest possible structure of a cell with a nonconductive thin membrane filled internally by a homogeneous medium. More complex situations in which the interaction between cells is not neglected or when the membrane conductance is calculated based on dynamic models of electroporation can be solved by numerical methods (Neu & Krassowska, 1999; Ramos *et al*, 2004; Ramos, 2010).

Conductivity measurement have been used in previous studies in order to determine the variation of the membrane conductance during electroporation (Kinosita & Tsong, 1979; Pavlin *et al*, 2005; Suzuki *et al*, 2011). But, caution is needed when using this approach. The impedance of the electrode interface with the suspension has strong dispersion of reactance and resistance at low frequencies, up to about 1 kHz (McAdams *et al*, 1995). Ionic diffusion inside double layer of cells also results in low-frequency dielectric dispersion. Additionally, interfacial polarization shows strong dispersion with relaxation times of less than 1 μs for cells of a few microns in diameter (Foster & Schwan, 1995). Due to the reactive and dispersive effects, the precise determination of the suspension conductivity cannot be done using instantaneous values of voltage and current with pulsed waveform, since the spectral content of these signals is very wide.

The heating of the electrolyte during the pulse application also affects the relationship of conductivity with the membrane conductance. The variation of conductivity due to power dissipation in an aqueous electrolyte can be estimated by $\Delta\sigma/\sigma=\alpha\sigma_o E^2\Delta t/\rho c$, where α is the temperature coefficient, ρ and c are respectively the density and specific heat of water, E is the electric field strength applied and Δt is the time length of the pulse. For an aqueous NaCl electrolyte with initial conductivity of 20 mS/m and field of 400 V/m (typical values in our experiments) the variation of conductivity is 1.53% per millisecond. Thus, for a time of 10 ms, we can estimate a contribution of about 15% of variation in the suspension conductivity due only to heating of the sample. The conductivity of the external medium can also vary due to the efflux of ions through the hydrophilic pores created in the cell membrane. The external conductivity increases while the internal conductivity decreases, changing the relationship between suspension conductivity and membrane conductance.

Simple estimates of conductivity by measuring the instantaneous current and voltage during the pulse application are not reliable for a correct evaluation of the membrane conductance. In order to accomplish this goal in this study we measure the electrical impedance of the sample in a wide range of frequencies before and after the pulse application. Using a delay of 60 seconds to measure the impedance after the pulse, the generated heat is allowed to dissipate through the metal electrodes into the air. Once the volume of the suspension is small (about 300 μL), we can predict that thermal effects are negligible after 60 seconds.

The analysis of the impedance spectra enables us to identify and separate the effects of dispersion at low frequencies. In addition, one can adjust the parameters of a dielectric dispersion model for interfacial polarization of cell suspensions to obtain estimates of cell concentration, internal and external conductivities and membrane conductance for both intact cells and electroporated cells.

2. Methods

2.1 Experimental method

Cells of yeast *Kluyveromyces marxianus* CBS 6556 were used in the electroporation experiments. The cells were grown in stirred flasks containing 0.5 L with 150 mL of Bacto peptone (2%), yeast extract (1%) and lactose (2%) at 30 °C for 12 hours and 150 rpm. The colonies in the stationary phase were then washed three times in distilled water and centrifuged each time for six minutes at 12,000 rpm in an Eppendorf centrifuge and finally re-suspended in distilled water.

Samples in the final suspension were observed and photographed under a Olympus CX31 microscope with attached camera Moticam 1000 and software Motic Images Plus 2.0. 120 cell diameter measurements were performed in six different colonies used in the enzyme activity and electrical impedance assays. The average radius obtained was 4.87 μm with a standard deviation of 1.07 μm.

The electroporator used in the experiments consists of a differential power amplifier with a gain of 50 V/V and an arbitrary waveform generator implemented in LabView™ (National Instruments) triggering a PCI 6251 card (National Instruments). Figure 1 shows a schematic representation of the electroporator. A current meter probe using a LTSP 25-NP sensor (LEM Components) and a voltage probe using resistive dividers and an INA 111 amplifier (Burr Brown) was implemented and used to measure current and voltage applied to the sample. The signals from the probes were acquired by the program through the PCI 6251 card using 16-bit resolution and 500 kHz of sampling rate simultaneously with the generation of the applied voltage. The sample holder is made of a cylindrical tube of nylon covering two steel electrodes 0.02 m in diameter and 0.001 m in spacing. The sample of the yeast suspension is injected and removed from the space between electrodes using syringes. The volume stimulated in each pulse application is 311 μL. All experiments were performed at room temperature of 25 °C. For each experiment, the electroporator was configured to generate an output voltage pulse from 100 to 400 Volts with duration from 1 to 10 ms.

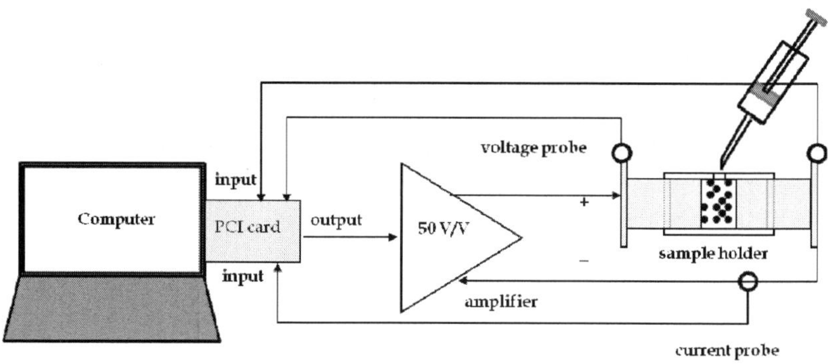

Fig. 1. Schematic of the electroporator

The enzyme activity assays were made 4 hours after pulsation. The cells were centrifugated for six minutes at 12,000 rpm in an Eppendorf centrifuge. To the supernatant was assigned the fraction of enzyme suspended outside the cells; to the pellets were assigned the enzyme associated to the cell walls. The cromogen ONPG, described by Lederberg (Lederberg, 1950) was used as a substrate. The assay mixture contained 780 μL sodium/phosphate buffer with pH 7.6 (containing 47 mM 2-mercaptoethanol and 1mM $MgCl_2$), 110 μL 35 mM ONPG and 110 μL of the enzyme solution. After one minute of incubation in a Thermomixer (Eppendorf) at 30° C, the reaction was stopped by 0.22 mL 1M Na_2CO_3. One unit (U) of β-galactosidase is defined as the amount of enzyme that releases 1 μmol of orto-nitrophenolate per minute under the assay conditions. This can be evaluated by means of measuring the increase of absorbance at 405 nm in a LKB spectrophotometer, using 1 cm optic path glass cuvettes. The molar extinction coefficient used was 3.1 μmol^{-1} cm^2 (Furlan *et al*, 2000).

The electrical impedance of the sample was measured before and after electroporation pulsation. We used a 4294A impedance analyzer (Agilent Technologies) in the range 40 Hz to 40 MHz. The time interval between the pulse application and the second measurement was kept in 60 seconds for all samples. This time is needed to allow disconnecting the sample holder from electroporator and connecting to the impedance analyzer as well as to allow the impedance reading to stabilize.

2.2 Mathematical method

The dispersion model for interfacial polarization in suspensions of spherical cells is obtained from Maxwell-Wagner theory of dispersion. For spherical particles of complex conductivity γ_c suspended in a medium of complex conductivity γ_o and occupying a volume fraction p, the following relationship applies between these quantities and the complex conductivity of the suspension γ_s (Foster & Schwan, 1995):

$$\frac{\gamma_s - \gamma_o}{\gamma_s + 2\gamma_o} = p\frac{\gamma_c - \gamma_o}{\gamma_c + 2\gamma_o} \tag{1}$$

Where $\gamma_c = \sigma_c + j\omega\varepsilon_c\varepsilon_o$, $\gamma_o = \sigma_o + j\omega\varepsilon_w\varepsilon_o$ and $\gamma_s = \sigma_s + j\omega\varepsilon_s\varepsilon_o$. In these equations ω is the angular frequency, ε_o is the vacuum permittivity, σ_c, σ_o and σ_s are the conductivities of cells, external medium and suspension, respectively, and ε_c, ε_w and ε_s are the dielectric constant of cells, water and suspension, respectively. The complex conductivity of cells can be estimated using the simple model consisting of a homogeneous internal medium with conductivity $\gamma_i = \sigma_i + j\omega\varepsilon_w\varepsilon_o$ surrounded by a spherical membrane of thickness h much smaller than the radius R and with complex conductivity $\gamma_m = h(G_m + j\omega C_m)$, where G_m and C_m are the conductance and capacitance per unit area of membrane, respectively. The result obtained after making approximations that keeps only terms of first order in (h/R) is the following (Foster & Schwan, 1995):

$$\gamma_c \cong \frac{\gamma_i + (2h/R)\gamma_m}{1 + (h/R)(\gamma_i - \gamma_m)/\gamma_m} \tag{2}$$

Substituting (2) in (1), the resulting expression can be separated into first order dispersion equations for the process of interfacial polarization at the cell membrane surface. The general expressions for the conductivity and dielectric constant of the suspension are written below:

$$\sigma_s = \sigma_{so} + \frac{\omega^2\tau_m^2\Delta\sigma_s}{1 + \omega^2\tau_m^2} \tag{3}$$

$$\varepsilon_s = \varepsilon_\infty + \frac{\Delta\varepsilon_s}{1 + \omega^2\tau_m^2} \tag{4}$$

$$\Delta\sigma_s = \frac{\varepsilon_o\Delta\varepsilon_s}{\tau_m} \tag{5}$$

In these equations, σ_{so} and ε_∞ are respectively the low frequency conductivity and high frequency dielectric constant of the suspension. $\Delta\sigma_s$ and $\Delta\varepsilon_s$ are the dispersion amplitudes of conductivity and dielectric constant, respectively, and τ_m is the relaxation time for interfacial polarization. Based on the model described by equations (1) and (2), the dispersion parameters of the first order equations (3) and (4) are presented below (Foster & Schwan, 1995):

$$\Delta\varepsilon_s = \frac{9pRC_m}{4\varepsilon_o\left[1+\frac{p}{2}+\frac{RG_m}{\sigma_i\sigma_o}(2\sigma_o+\sigma_i+p(\sigma_o-\sigma_i))\right]^2} \tag{6}$$

$$\sigma_{so} = \sigma_o\left[\frac{1-p+\frac{RG_m}{\sigma_i\sigma_o}\left(\sigma_o+\frac{\sigma_i}{2}+p(\sigma_i-\sigma_o)\right)}{1+\frac{p}{2}+\frac{RG_m}{\sigma_i\sigma_o}\left(\sigma_o+\frac{\sigma_i}{2}-\frac{p}{2}(\sigma_i-\sigma_o)\right)}\right] \tag{7}$$

$$\tau_m = RC_m\frac{\sigma_i+2\sigma_o-p(\sigma_i-\sigma_o)}{2\sigma_i\sigma_o(1+p)+RG_m\left[(\sigma_i+2\sigma_o)-p(\sigma_i-\sigma_o))\right]} \tag{8}$$

The numerical method is initially applied to the parameterization of the impedance model of the sample. By considering the geometry of the electrodes with parallel faces and with radius much larger than the spacing, the following expression adequately represents the sample impedance:

$$Z_m = \frac{R_{ct}}{1+(j\omega\tau_e)^\beta}+\frac{d/A}{\sigma_s+j\omega\varepsilon_s\varepsilon_o} \tag{9}$$

Where A and d are the area and spacing of the electrodes, respectively. The first term in the second member represents the impedance of the electrode-electrolyte interface (McAdams *et al*, 1995). The second term is the impedance of the suspension. The parameters of the interface impedance model are: the charge transfer resistance R_{ct}, the surface relaxation time τ_e and the constant β. In the suspension impedance model the parameters to be obtained are shown in equations (3) and (4): σ_{so}, ε_∞, $\Delta\sigma_s$ or $\Delta\varepsilon_s$ and τ_m.

The parameterization algorithm used is based on successive approximations. Initially, each parameter is assigned a range of search. The parameters are stored in integer variables with 16 bits of resolution. Each interval is divided into 2^{16}-1 = 65,535 subintervals. The approximation process is performed by calculating all the answers of the equation (9) for a given parameter that varies throughout its subintervals, keeping the other parameters fixed at initial values. The value that minimizes the mean square error between the model and the measured impedance spectrum is selected. The process is repeated for all parameters, while maintaining the selected values of the parameters already adjusted. After several cycles of this procedure, the parameters of the model specified in equation (9) converge to the desired response. The convergence with mean square error less than 1% of the mean square value of the impedance magnitude was achieved on average with 10 cycles of calculation. Figure 2 shows the result of the parameterization for an assay with applied field of 200 kV/m and time length of 10 ms. The obtained parameters are shown in the figure.

Using the values of σ_{so}, $\Delta\sigma_s$, $\Delta\varepsilon_s$ e τ_m obtained from the impedance spectrum measured before electroporation, the volume fraction p and membrane capacitance were calculated. In this case, the membrane conductance is very small, usually between 1 and 10 S/m^2 (Foster & Schwan, 1995) and the terms containing G_m in equations (6) to (8) can be neglected. Accordingly, these equations can be rewritten in the approximate forms:

$$\Delta\varepsilon_s = \frac{9pRC_m}{\varepsilon_o(2+p)^2} \tag{10}$$

$$\sigma_{so} = 2\sigma_o\frac{(1-p)}{2+p} \tag{11}$$

$$\tau_m = \frac{RC_m}{2\sigma_o}\frac{(1-p)}{(1+p)} \tag{12}$$

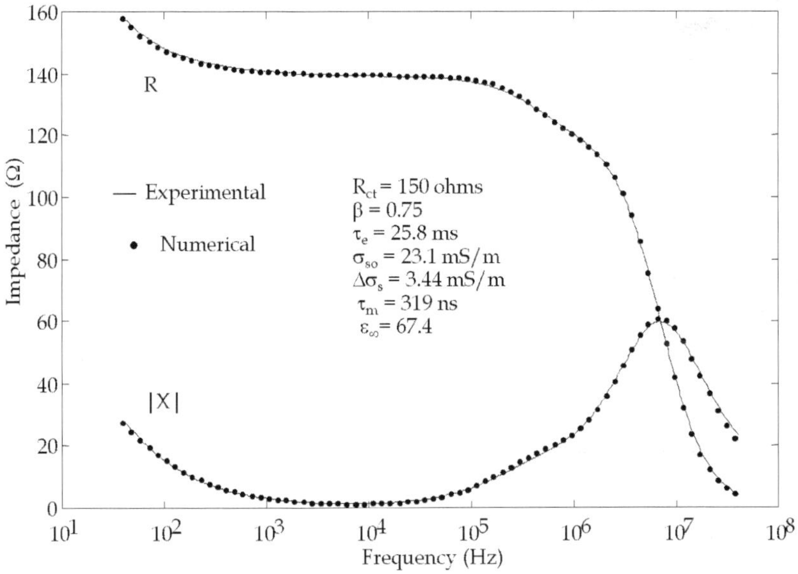

Fig. 2. Experimental and Theoretical impedance spectra to an assay with 200 kV/m and 10 ms. R - resistance; |X| modulus of reactance.

For the equation (12) it was assumed that $\sigma_i >> \sigma_o$, since the final suspension is obtained by diluting the cells in distilled water. Combining these equations with equation (5), we obtain an equation for calculating the volume fraction from σ_{so} e $\Delta\sigma_s$:

$$\frac{\Delta\sigma_s}{\sigma_{so}} = 9\frac{p(1+p)}{(2+p)(1-p)^2} \tag{13}$$

With the value of p in equation (10) yields the membrane capacitance C_m. Using the values of σ_{so}, $\Delta\sigma_s$, $\Delta\varepsilon_s$ and τ_m obtained from the impedance spectrum measured after electroporation, the membrane conductance and internal and external conductivities were calculated. Newton's method was used for this purpose. Defining the following variables: $x_1=RG_m$, $x_2=1/\sigma_i$ e $x_2=1/\sigma_o$, equations (6), (7) and (8) can be written in the respective forms:

$$F_1 = a_1 + 2a_1x_1x_2 + 2a_1a_2x_1x_3 - 1 = 0 \tag{14}$$

$$F_2 = b_1x_3 + b_1x_1x_2x_3 + b_1b_3x_1x_3^2 - x_1x_2 - b_2x_1x_3 - 1 = 0 \tag{15}$$

$$F_3 = c_1 + c_1c_2x_1x_3 + c_1c_3x_1x_2 - c_2x_3 - c_3x_2 = 0 \tag{16}$$

Where the coefficients are given in the Table 1 below.

$a_1 = \sqrt{\frac{\varepsilon_0\Delta\varepsilon_s(2+p)}{9pRC_m}}$	$a_2 = \frac{1-p}{2+p}$	——
$b_1 = \sigma_s\frac{(2+p)}{2(1-p)}$	$b_2 = \frac{(1+2p)}{2(1-p)}$	$b_3 = a_2$
$c_1 = \frac{\tau_m}{RC_m}$	$c_2 = \frac{(1-p)}{2(1+p)}$	$c_3 = \frac{(2+p)}{2(1+p)}$

Table 1. Coefficients of the dispersion equations for applying Newton's method.

Applying Newton's method the convergence was obtained in five steps with $\left\|[F_1F_2F_3]\right\|_\infty < 10^{-10}$ using the initial values: G_m = 1000 S/m², σ_i = 500 mS/m e σ_o = 20 mS/m.

3. Results and discussion

3.1 Impedance measurement

Each electroporation experiment was performed by applying a single pulse of electric field with strength 100, 200, 300 and 400 kV/m and time length from 1 to 10 ms. Figure 3 shows the typical behavior of the apparent conductance of the sample during electrical stimulation. These curves were obtained as the ratio between the voltage and current measured in the sample during the pulse application. This ratio is named apparent conductance because the sample actually has complex impedance with frequency dependent resistance and reactance. Since the applied pulse has a wide range of spectral components, it is not possible to obtain the conductance of the medium simply by dividing the instantaneous voltage and current in the sample. In any case, the initial apparent conductance increases with the applied field, indicating the occurrence of electroporation. The slope of each curve also indicates that electroporation increases during the pulse. For more intense pulses the conductance shows greater variation. For intense fields, however, the heating of the sample is appreciable and this contributes to increase the sample conductance. Some authors, in previous studies, used instantaneous measurements of voltage and current for conductivity calculation and deduced the membrane conductance from these measurements (Kinosita & Tsong, 1979, Pavlin et al, 2005; Suzuki et al, 2011). It may indeed have a special interest in this approach since it would allow an assessment of the electroporation dynamics (pore opening rate) during application of the pulse. However, without an adequate measurement technique, the results may be adversely affected by other effects, such as the surface impedance of the electrodes and dielectric dispersion due to ion diffusion and accumulation on cell surface.

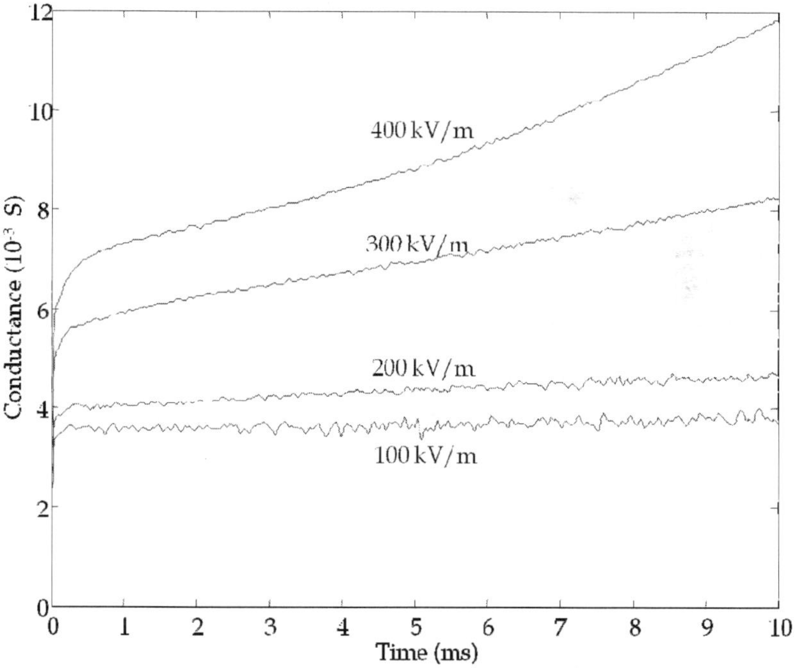

Fig. 3. Apparent sample conductance during the electroporation pulse with strength from 100 to 400 kV/m and time length of 10 ms.

A measurement technique that can be used to compensate for the reactive effects is the technique of small signals. In this case, one can use a small amplitude sinusoidal signal added to the electroporation pulse. This signal can be used to measure the change in conductance of the sample during the pulse. If the small-signal frequency is sufficiently far from the dispersion band of the medium, the sample behaves like a real conductance and the conductivity obtained can be properly related to the variation of the membrane conductance. According to the impedance spectrum shown in Figure 2, the frequency of 10 kHz is adequate for this purpose. Another aspect to consider is the heating that results in increased conductivity of the electrolyte in the suspension. This effect seems to happen in the increase of the curve inclination for 400 kV/m in Figure 3 for pulse length higher than 5 ms. To avoid the interference of heating is necessary to limit the intensity of the applied field or the time length of the pulse.

Figure 4 shows the impedance spectra obtained before and after pulse application with 10 ms and field strengths of 100, 200, 300 and 400 kV/m. There is a strong reduction of the resistance through the frequency range up to 10 MHz and a significant reduction of the reactance at high frequencies for fields greater than 100 kV/m. One can assign both variations to the increase in membrane conductance. However, another effect that decreases the electrical impedance is the efflux of ions from the cytoplasm through the pores created in the cell membrane. This process has little effect on the apparent sample conductance shown in Figure 3, because its time constant is of the order of several seconds (Pavlin et al, 2005), but significantly affects the sample impedance measured after 60 seconds from pulse application. Another process that can have an effect is the cell swelling due to water influx through the pores due to the osmotic pressure difference. This process has time constant of tens of seconds to mouse melanoma cells (Pavlin et al, 2005). In yeast the effect of osmotic pressure is possibly reduced by the presence of the cell wall. Furthermore, in the experiments conducted in this study due to the small volume fraction of the suspension (about 3%) and low conductivity of the external medium (about 20 mS/m), the effects of cell swelling in the impedance are small. The field of 100 kV/m possibly lies just above the threshold of electroporation for yeast. The effects are relatively small as can be seen in Figure 4. There was also a tendency of saturation in the sample impedance for intense fields, suggesting that a maximum permeation can be achieved for fields of the order 400 kV/m.

3.2 Suspension conductivity and membrane conductance

Electroporation assays were repeated three times in all conditions of stimulation with samples prepared using the same procedure described above. The mathematical method used allowed to obtain the volume fraction, the membrane capacitance and conductivity of the external medium before electroporation. The range of values obtained for the set of 72 samples showed small standard deviation. The results obtained are: $p = 0.0332 \pm 0.0011$, $C_m = 3.5 \times 10^{-3} \pm 2.8 \times 10^{-4}$ F/m^2 and $\sigma_o = 24.6 \pm 2.7$ mS/m. The low membrane capacitance over the typically reported value for animal cells (of the order of 10^{-2} F/m^2) probably is due to the effect of the ionic distribution in the cell wall on the outer surface of the cell membrane. The cell wall of yeasts consists of two main types of macromolecules, polysaccharides glucan and mannan-type and several proteins, forming a reticulated structure with a thickness much larger than the cell membrane. The electrostatic interactions between these molecules and ions carried to the membrane by an applied electric field determine the spatial distribution of charge different from that seen in cells devoid of cell wall. The cell wall can also act as a filter for the efflux of macromolecules through the pores of the cell membrane as will be seen in relation to enzyme activity in this study.

The mathematical method applied to electroporated suspensions allowed to determine the change in conductivity of the external medium and membrane conductance. Figure 5 shows the variation of conductivity obtained with the impedance measurement before and after 60 seconds of pulse application as a function of field strength and pulse length. Figure 6 shows the distribution of membrane conductance obtained in the same analysis. The two sets of values are very similar. The correlation between them is mainly due to the fact that both depend on the number and size of pores in the cell membrane created by the applied field. Ions leaving the cells through these pores increase the conductivity of the external medium. This increase is small for 100 kV/m because this field is only slightly above the electroporation threshold. But as the applied field increases, the efflux of ions is increased and also shows a dependence on the pulse length. The conductivity measurement of the external medium can be used as a reliable indicator of the permeation state, provided that the reactive and dispersive effects in the sample are properly compensated.

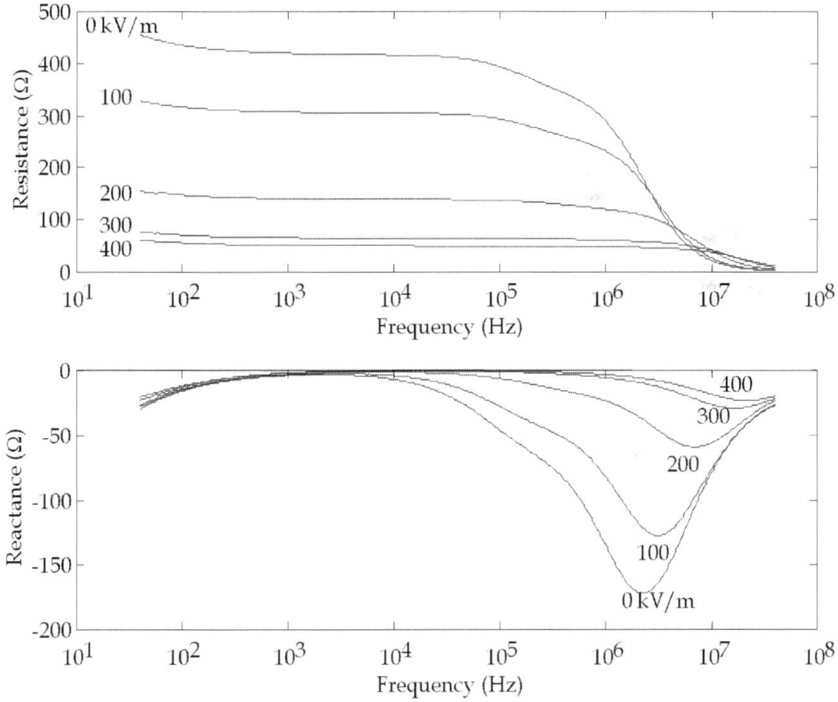

Fig. 4. Resistance and reactance obtained from the impedance spectra measured before (0 kV/m) and after (60 s) electroporation pulse with 10 ms and strength from 100 to 400 kV/m.

In Figure 6 the conductance increases rapidly with increasing applied field. The pulse length has increasing influence on membrane conductance as the applied field increases, but shows saturation for field of 400 kV/m and time length higher than 2 ms. The proposed models of pore creation in electroporation are based on the Boltzmann statistical distribution that depends on the energy stored in the pores of the membrane (Glaser et al, 1988; Krassowska & Neu, 1999; Ramos, 2010). So these models have terms that depend exponentially on the squared transmembrane potential. It is expected therefore that the strength of the applied field has great influence on the change in membrane conductance, as shown in this figure. However, saturation of the conductance for intense fields means that the permeation state does not allow the transmembrane potential to grow indefinitely.

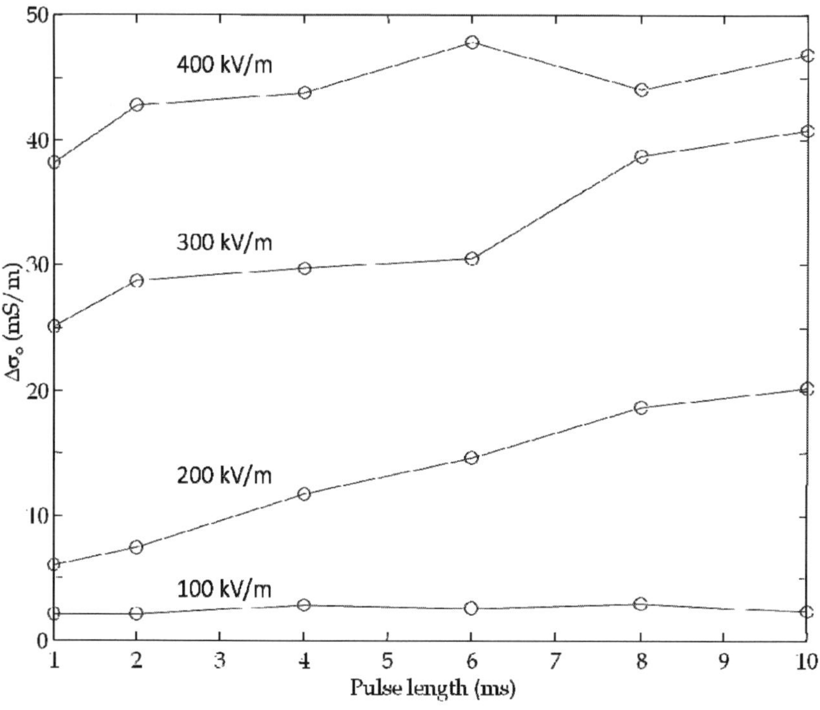

Fig. 5. Increase of external medium conductivity as a function of applied field strength and pulse duration.

Some previous studies with electroporation of animal cells resulted in very different membrane conductance values. Kinosita and Tsong (Kinosita & Tsong, 1979) used human red blood cells suspensions stimulated with single pulses of amplitude between 100 and 600 kV/m and duration up to 80 μs. They calculated the conductivity using instantaneous values and modeled the conductivity from a static solution to the electric potential internal and external to the cells. By fitting the model with the experimental results, they obtained conductance values of 10^5 and 10^6 S/m^2 to a field of 400 kV/m with duration of 2 and 80 μs, respectively. Human erythrocytes and the yeasts used in this study have different shapes but about the same size. However, the difference in the conductance obtained is big compared to the results in Fig. 6. Possibly, there are significant influences of the conductivity measurement procedures and modeling method used. In addition, the cells in question are very different. As the erythrocyte has an oblate spheroid shape with axial ratio 0.28, the yeast is approximately spherical and the cell wall can play a role in reducing the transmembrane potential and membrane conductance. In the study by Pavlin *et al.* (Pavlin *et al*, 2005) mouse melanoma cells were electroporated with 8 pulses of electric field of the same amplitude and duration 100 μs each. The suspension conductivity was calculated using instantaneous values of voltage and current. They estimated the cell conductivity and membrane conductivity from numerical methods Membrane conductivity values obtained with a field of 84 kV/m were $3.5x10^{-5}$ S/m and $1.4x10^{-5}$ S/m for two medium conductivity, 1.58 S/m and 127 mS/m, respectively. Considering a membrane thickness of 5 nm, the membrane conductance is $7x10^{3}$ and $2.8x10^{3}$ S/m^2 respectively. The critical field for electroporation is probably lower for melanoma cells than for yeast, since the former are larger and do not have cell wall. The conductance values are within the order of magnitude as were obtained in this study.

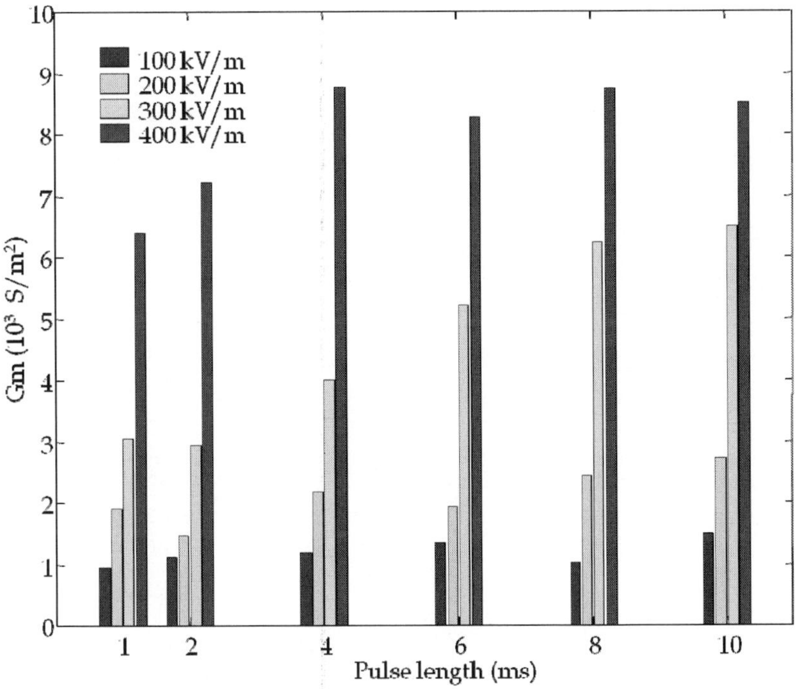

Fig. 6. Membrane conductance as a function of applied field strength and pulse duration.

3.3 Enzyme activity

Figure 7 shows the results of the β-D-galactosidase activity assays in suspensions electroporated with field strength from 100 to 400 kV/m and pulse length from 2 to 10 ms.

The fraction of enzyme activity found in the supernatant was very low in all trials. The values marked supernatant in the figure were obtained with field of 400 kV/m. The highest activity was detected in the cells themselves after centrifugation, indicating that although the enzyme is available outside the cell, it is not diluted in the supernatant. The enzyme is possibly trapped in the molecular network of the cell wall. Note that there is high correlation between the distributions of membrane conductance and enzymatic activity, especially above 200 kV/m. The enzymatic activity in the cell fraction for 400 kV/m is located just above 1 U for all pulse lengths in the same way that the conductance of the membrane shows saturation just above 8,000 S/m^2 for this field. Since the enzyme molecules must pass through the pores of the membrane to reach the cell wall, it can be predicted that the conditions that maximize the conductance of the membrane also maximize the extraction of the enzyme. The fact of the enzyme to be attached to the cell wall suggests an important application of the technique by means of immobilization. Cell immobilization consists in confinement of cells maintaining their catalytic activities. The enzyme β-D-galactosidase is not excreted naturally by the microorganism *Kluyveromyces marxianus*, but by electroporation it is possible to get it on the cell wall. Combining electroporation and cell immobilization is possible to obtain high catalytic activity in small volumes, provided that the cells remain viable after electrical stimulation and confinement.

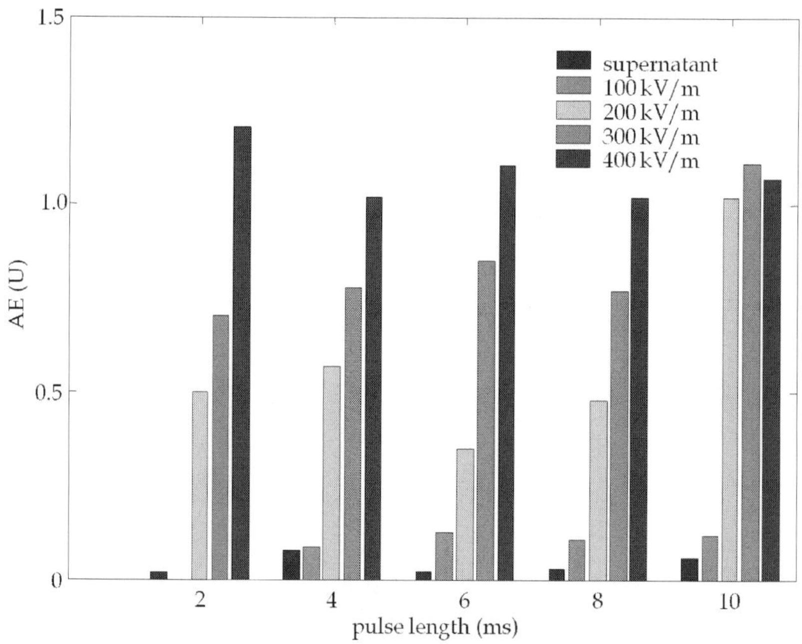

Fig. 7. Enzymatic activity for β-D-galactosidase in electroporated suspensions with fields strength from 100 to 400 kV/m and pulse length from 2 to 10 ms. The activity in the supernatant corresponds to the assay with 400 kV/m.

4. Conclusion

In this work it was studied the influence of the applied field strength and pulse duration on the increase in membrane conductance and activity of the enzyme β-D-galactosidase released by yeasts *Kluyveromyces marxianus* in suspension as a result of electroporation. The numerical technique for analyzing the electrical impedance spectra of the suspension has advantages over other modeling cited in the text because it allows properly compensate the reactive and dispersive effects caused by the impedance surface of the electrodes and ion accumulation on the cell membrane. It was found that membrane conductance and electrolyte conductivity measured after electroporation are strongly correlated, since both depend on the number and size of pores in the membrane. The protocol used with only a single pulse was able to produce large changes in membrane conductance for fields greater than 100 kV/m. The enzyme activity is also correlated to the membrane conductance. The membrane conductance increased between 8,000 and 9,000 S/m^2 for 400 kV/m. The enzyme activity was slightly greater than 1 U for all pulse duration. Both the membrane conductance and enzyme activity showed saturation for field of 400 kV/m, that is, the result is about independent on pulse length for pulses longer than 2 ms. The enzyme molecules after going through the pores in the cell membrane possibly get stuck in the molecular network of the cell wall. This was concluded based in the verification that the enzyme activity in the supernatant was very low in all assay conditions. Impedance measurement can allow the assessment of the permeation state of the membrane after pulse application, provided that the reactive and dispersive effects are properly modeled. This can be used as a probe for electroporation effectiveness evaluation aiming to control the enzyme extraction.

5. Future directions

Comparative studies with other methods of enzyme extraction, by chemical or mechanical process, should be conducted to determine the efficiency of electroporation compared to traditional techniques. The cell viability after electroporation also should be studied under different stimulation conditions, because it is an important factor to consider in certain applications. Another important study to conduct refers to the obtaining and using of immobilized enzymes on the cell wall of yeasts from electroporation process. The possibility of combining the technique of electroporation with the immobilization of enzymes appears promising but needs to be carefully tested and characterized.

6. References

Chen, C.; Smye, S.W.; Robinson, M.P. & Evans, J.A., (2006) Membrane Electroporation theories: a review, *Med. Biol. Eng. Comput.*, vol. 44, pp. 4-14

Foster, K.R. & Schwan, H.P. (1995) Dielectric properties of tissues, in: Handbook of Biological Effects of Electromagnetic Fields, Polk, C. & Postow, E. (Ed), 2ª Ed., pp. 25-102, CRC, New York

Furlan, S.A.; Schneider, A.L.S.; Merkle, R.; Carvalho, J.M.F. & Jonas R. (2000) Formulation of a lactose-free, low cost culture medium for the production of β–D-galactosidase by *Kluyveromyces marxianus*, *Biotechnology Letters*, vol. 22, pp. 589-593

Ganeva, V. & Galutzov, B. (1999) Electropulsation as an alternative method for protein extraction from yeast, *FEMS Microbiology Letters*, vol. 174, pp. 279-284

Ganeva, V.; Galutzov, B. & Teissie, J. (2003) High yield electroextraction of proteins from yeast by a flow process, *Analytical Biochemistry*, vol. 315, pp. 77-84

Glaser, R.W.; Leikin, S. L.; Chernomordik, L. V.; Pastushenko, V. F. & Sokirko, A. I. (1988) Reversible electrical breakdown of lipid bilayers: formation and evolution of pores, *Biochim. Biophys. Acta*, vol. 940, pp. 275-287

Grafström, G., Engström, P., Salford, L. G. & Persson, B. R. (2006) 99mTc-DTPA uptake and electrical impedance measurements in verification of *in vivo* electropermeabilization efficiency in rat muscle, *Cancer Biother.Radiopharm.*, vol. 21, pp. 623–635

Haque, A., Zuberi, M., Diaz-Rivera, R. E. & Porterfield, D. M. (2009) Electrical characterization of a single cell electroporation biochip with the 2-D scanning vibrating electrode technology, *Biomed Microdevices*, vol. 11, pp. 1239–1250

He, H., Chang, D. C. & Lee, Y. K. (2008) Nonlinear current response of micro electroporation and resealing dynamics for human cancer cells, *Bioelectrochemistry*, vol. 72, pp. 161-168.

Hibino, M.; Itoh, H. & Kinosita, Jr. K. (1993) Time courses of cell electroporation as reveled by submicrosecond imaging of transmembrane potential, *Biophysical Journal*, v. 64, pp. 1798-1800

Huang, Y. & Rubinsky, B. (1999) Micro-electroporation: improving the efficiency and understanding of electrical permeabilization of cells, *Biomed. Microdevices*, vol. 2, pp. 145–150

Ivorra, A. & Rubinsky, B. (2007) In vivo electrical impedance measurements during and after electroporation of rat liver, *Bioelectrochemistry*, v. 70, pp. 287–295

Kinosita, K. & Tsong, T.Y. (1979) Voltage-induced conductance in human erythrocyte membranes, *Bioch. Bioph. Acta*, vol. 554, pp. 479-497

Kotnik, T., Pucihar, G., Rebersek, M., Miklavcic, D. & Mir, L. M. (2003) Role of pulse shape in cell membrane electropermeabilization, *Biochimica et Biophysica Acta*, vol. 1614, pp. 193-200

Koester, P. J., Tautorat, C., Beikirch, H., Gimsa, J. & Baumann, W. (2010) Recording electric potentials from single adherent cells with 3D microelectrode arrays after local electroporation, *Biosensors and Bioelectronics*, vol. 26, pp. 1731-1735

Laufer, S., Ivorra, A., Reuter, V. E., Rubinsky, B. & Solomon, S. B. (2010) Electrical impedance characterization of normal and cancerous human hepatic tissue, Physiol. Meas., vol. 31, pp. 995-1009

Lederberg, J. (1950) The β-D-galactosidase of *Escherichia coli* strain K-12, *J. Bacteriol.* , vol. 60, pp. 381-392

McAdams, E.T.; Lackermeier, A.; McLaughlin, J.A.; Macken, D. & Jossinet, J. (1995) The linear and non-linear electrical properties of the electrode-electrolyte interface, *Biosensors & Bioelectronics*, vol. 10, pp. 67-74

Miklavčič, D. & Puc M. (2006) Electroporation, in: *Wiley Encyclopedia of Biomedical Engineering*, Akay M. (Ed), pp. 1-11, John Wiley & Sons Inc., New York

Neu, J.C. & Krassowska, W. (1999) Asymptotic model of electroporation, *Phys. Review E.*, vol. 59, pp. 3471-3482

Pavlin, M.; Kanduser, M.; Rebersek, M.; Pucihar, G.; Hart, F. X.; Magjarevic, R. & Miklavcic, D. (2005) Effect of cell electroporation on the conductivity of a cell suspension, *Biophysical Journal*, vol. 88, pp. 4378-4390

Pavlin, M. & Miklavcic, D. (2003) Effective conductivity of a suspension of permeabilized cells: A theoretical analysis, *Biophys. J.*, vol. 85, pp. 719-729

Pliquett, U., Elez, R., Piiper, A. & Neumann, E. (2004) Electroporation of subcutaneous mouse tumors by rectangular and trapezium high voltage pulses, *Bioelectrochemistry*, vol. 62, pp. 83–93

Ramos, A. (2010) Improved numerical approach for electrical modeling of biological cell clusters, *Med. Biol. Eng. Comput.*, vol. 48, pp. 311-319

Ramos, A., Suzuki D.O.H. & Marques J.L.B. (2004) Numerical simulation of electroporation in spherical cells, *Artificial Organs*, v. 28, pp. 357-361

Reed, S. D. & Li, S. (2009) Electroporation Advances in Large Animals, *Curr Gene Ther.*, vol. 9, pp. 316–326

Rice, J., Ottensmeier, C. H. & Stevenson, F. K. (2008) DNA vaccines: precision tools for activating effective immunity against cancer, *Nature Reviews Cancer*, vol. 8, pp. 108-120

Saulis, G., Satkauskas, S. & Praneviciute, R. (2007) Determination of cell electroporation from the release of intracellular potassium ions, *Analytical Biochemistry*, vol. 360, pp. 273-281

Sersa, G., Miklavcic, D., Cemazar, M., Rudolf, Z., Pucihar, G. & Snoj, M. (2008) Electrochemotherapy in treatment of tumours, *EJSO*, vol. 34, pp. 232-240

Suzuki, D. O. H.; Ramos, A.; Ribeiro, M. C. M.; Cazarolli, L. H.; Silva, F. R. M. B.; Leite, L. D. & Marques, J. L. B. (2011) Theoretical and Experimental Analysis of Electroporated Membrane Conductance in Cell Suspension, *IEEE Transactions on Biomedical Engineering, In press*

Swagerty, D.L.; Walling, A.D. & Klein, R.M. (2002) Lactose Intolerance, *Am Fam Physician*, vol. 65 (9), (Mai 1), pp. 1845-1851

Teissié, J.; Golzio, M.; & Rols M. P. (2005). Mechanisms of cell membrane electropermeabilization: A minireview of our present (lack of ?) knowledge, *Biochim. Biophys. Acta.*, vol. 1724, (Aug. 2005), pp. 270-280

Teissie, J. & Rols, M.P. (1993) An experimental evaluation of the critical potential inducing cell membrane electropermeabilization, *Biophysical Journal*, vol. 65, pp. 409-413

Weaver, J.C. & Chizmadzhev, Y. A. (1996) Theory of electroporation: a review, *Bioelectrochemistry*, vol. 41: pp. 135-160

19

Physiological Analysis of Yeast Cell by Intelligent Signal Processing

Andrei Doncescu[1], Sebastien Regis[1], Katsumi Inoue[2] and Nathalie Goma[3]
[1]*University of Toulouse, LAAS CNRS UPR 8001*
[2]*National Institute of Informatics*
[3]*IPBS CNRS*
[1,3]*France*
[2]*Japan*

1. Introduction

Before getting into the details of this chapter, let us make some light upon the abiotic/biotic debate. The issue could be summarized as two main differences between biotic and abiotic: the first one is the internal regulation of biotic systems and what is generally called by some researchers "cellular intelligence" related to the possibility of communication between cells. More precisely, in both types of systems it is possible to identify mass and energy exchanges (thermodynamic laws control), but within the biotic systems only one can find a certain project capability, using an ascending informational system (genome towards metabolic networks and environment adaptation systems) and a descending one (inverse).

The living organisms science gave birth to two main research areas: biomimetics and systemic biology. Biomimetics is a new discipline based not on what could be extracted from nature but on what could be learned from it, through the biologic systems or biosystems. Many attempts on defining systems in general exist. The classic one is the definition given by Bertalanffy: the system is an "organized complex", delimited by the existence of "strong interactions or non trivial interactions", *i.e.* non linear interactions. A biologic system is supposed to replicate itself and develop a system of reactions to exterior perturbations. This replication is done on the basis of a non-systemic, not organized or less organized exploitation of the surrounding environment. As the biologic system "works" as an algorithm, it is quite normal that since the first days of the molecular biology (1959) the engineers intensified and diversified their references to biology, even before the general acceptance in the scientific community of the term nanotechnology. The convergence between biotechnology and nanotechnology is due to the conceptual statement "bio is nano". Many examples of biomimetics achievements may be recalled: the artificial pancreas, the artificial retina, biomaterials. The latter is very interesting because biomaterials are not homogeneous. Biosystems are also used to develop innovating methods allowing measuring physiologic parameters, to find diagnostics for diseases, and to evaluate the effectiveness of new therapeutic compounds. Encouraging activities take place in the biomedical field: the cancer, brain/heart vascular diseases, infectious diseases.

The biologic systems, as a result of billions of years of evolution, are complex and degenerated systems and this double characteristic makes their understanding extremely difficult. In general, for a biologic system, the cyclic issues are related to the measure redundancy, to variables pertinence and to the significant correlation between the parameters and the type of the model that has to be used. The difficulty of these models is the intrinsic nature of some of the constituting elements and their phenomenological reductionism. By giving a few examples their limited character will better understood: the phenomenological modeling does not take into account the metabolic capabilities of the system, the stoechiometrical modeling does not take into account the dynamics of the system, thus a "time-space" analysis is not possible, etc. Such observations drive us to envisage a new approach of biologic problems: passing from the analytic paradigm to the complexity paradigm, via the so called approach of biology of systems or biosystemics or systemic biology.

The systemic biology is, as a simple definition, the integration of mathematics, biology, physics and computer science for creating new models for the biologic systems. Kitano, one of the fathers of Biology of Systems defines the biosystemic strategy (13) as:

1. Defining and analysing the structure of these systems;
2. Studying their behaviour and characteristics under different conditions;
3. Studying the regulation processes through which the systems control their equilibrium states and manage their variations;
4. Identifying the processes that allow building systems that are adapted to a given function

From a purely biologic standpoint, there exist complex groups of interacting proteins, performing:

1. the metabolism;
2. the synthesis of DNA;
3. information processing;

These interactions are network-like organized. The purpose of this biochemical diagram where each node represents a specific protein, which regulates the biochemical conversions, is to explain the cellular physiology starting from the dynamics of the net, in a cells population context. We can now understand that, in this context, the biologic systems are uncertain and subordered to viability constraints. From a qualitative dynamics standpoint, the viability constraints induct two states: the homeostasis and the chaos. The homeostasis defined by C. Bernard and W. Cannon is the capability of a living system to preserve its vital functions, by maintaining, in a certain structural stability range, its parameters and, in a certain viability range, its internal variables. The longevity of this living is a function of this stability. The chaos, in its common definition, is more opposed the concept of order than to those of stability and viability. It is possible to continuously pass from order to chaos, by increasing the complexity of the studied system, and this can be done by simple variations of some of its bifurcation parameters, variations that might provoke a change in the nature of the systemÕs dynamics attractors by overriding critical bifurcation values. The two notions are derived from the notion of attractor of a dynamic system in the context of a wide regulation network. We can give as an example the nature of biologic regulation: direct, indirect, or causal, governing the response of these systems. As the evolution of these systems is still rather unknown due to the continuous or discrete way of evolution we can suppose the existence of response thresholds. Biology inspires an analysis of the non-linear dynamics in terms of feedback loops (positive or negative). A positive feedback loop within the interaction graph of a differential system is a necessary condition of multistationarity which becomes, in biology, the cellular differentiation. A negative feedback loop within the interaction graph is a necessary condition for a periodic stable behaviour, very important in biology. It is quite possible that the oscillators coupling and multiple feedback loops interaction could lead to better oscillations coherence. The biologic regulation networks allow, among other things, to model genes interactions within a cell. Consequence to genome sequency, including the humain genome sequence, the postgenomics field has the goal to characterize the genes, the functions and the intercations beetween genes. The network of regulation takes an important and difficult role to assume the analysis at different scales, which means: "setup of new models using the biologic data and predicts the behavior of biologic systems from information extracted from genome sequence". But how Monod had enhanced: "everything which exists in universe is the result of hazard and necessity which it is not in contradiction with Occam principle to do not introduce supplementary clauses when it is not necessary. It is important to mention that the hazard presented in biology is not stochastic which means "to drive" the hazard but tychastic which describes some phenomenaÕs which escape to all statistic regularity. Therefore it is impossible to speak about the predictive capacity of the model which is the final goal of theoretical biology. From a realist view point we have made the hypothesis that the DNA could not include the finest maps of the organism but only some information about the iterative process of bifurcation and growth. If the approaches proposed before are in-silico, in the case of the in vitro the extraction of correct information is primordial. Basically, the information obtained is realized by direct observation and also by the interpretation of the response of the system. To be more accurate in this explication this approach is based on the perturbation of the analyzed system, supposed in a steady state, by a pulse of metabolite which belongs to the non linear differential model which described the biological system. Using the response of the system it is possible to deduce the relations between this variable and some variables of the model. For the complex models the analysis of the picks and the slope of the response directly link to the concentration of the metabolite it is not possible. The extraction of the information from responses supposes the cooperation of two parties :

1. the development of a model able to observe the dynamic of the system with a lot of precision
2. using of the mathematical tools allowing to tune the model to experimental observations

which means to solve a regression problem. If the model is linear the regression is linear therefore without any theoretical interest. Comparing with linear models the non-linear models offer infinity of possibility without the difficulties enclosed in the resolution of this kind of approach. One strategy is the Lotka-Voltera modelling. This method has been applied in ecology and focuses on the interaction between two species of type predator Ð prey. The inconvenient of this method in study of metabolic pathway or fermentation is that he metabolite depends of many compounds. The deduction of a non linear model from experimental data is an inverse problem which could be solved by a regression method or genetic algorithms which minimize the error between the model and the data. In practice the local minima which stop the convergence of the algorithms. One smart solution is the utilisation of Bayesian Methods or Simulated Annealing when the systems are small size, no noise and we use a PC cluster. Another approach is the non linear estimation by NARMAX but these methods did not work with strong non linearties. The challenge in the case of the modeling of biological systems is the elucidation of the optimal evolution of the equations system when initial conditions are incomplete or missing. In this case, the analysis of the trajectories of the system is the central point to make the difference between regular trajectories (periodical or quasi periodic) and chaotic paths in the space of phases. The change of trajectories is directly related to the parameters of the model. Periodic trajectories will be identified by Poincaré sections and by using the Harmonic Wavelet Transform we will be able to make the difference between quasi-periodical theoretical and the chaos. The interest of the analysis by wavelet is the linearization of the model to find the steady states stationary of the biological system excited by a non-stationary process. The original system will be decomposed into linear subsystems, each having the response in a frequency band of well defined. The final response is calculated by the addition of each subsystem response. This type of analysis allows the studying of the influence of modes of regulation on the time of relaxation of the cell and to find out the stationary states of the cellular cycle.

Today, the pace of progress in fermentation is fast and furious, particularly since the advent of genetic engineering and the recent advances in computer sciences and process control. The high cost associated with many fermentation processes makes optimization of bioreactor performance trough command control very desirable. Clearly, control of fermentation is recognized as a vital component in the operation and successful production of many industries. Despite the complexity of biotechnological processes, biotechnologists are capable of identifying normal and abnormal situations, undertaking suitable actions accordingly. Process experts are able to draw such conclusions by analysing a set of measured signals collected from the plant. The inexistence of satisfactory mathematical models impedes model-based approaches to be used in supervisory tasks, thus involving other strategies to be applied. That suggests that, despite the lack of process models, measured data can be used instead in the supervisory system development. The advances in measurement, data acquisition and handling technologies provide a wealth of new data which can be used to improve existing models.

In general, for a biologic system, the cyclic issues are related to the measure redundancy, to variables pertinence and to the significant correlation between the parameters and the type of the model that has to be used. The difficulty of these models is the intrinsic nature of some of the constituting elements and their phenomenological reductionism. Moreover, the dynamic nature and the inherent non-linearity of bio-processes make system identification difficult. The majority of kinetic models in biology are described by coupled differential equations and simulators implement the appropriate methods to solve these systems. Particularly, analysis of states occuring during experiences is a key point for optimization and control of these bioprocesses. Thus, model-based approaches using differential equations (26), expert system (31), fuzzy sets and systems (23), (9), neural networks (8) have been developed. However, although model-based approaches give more and more accurate results close to real outputs (10), these methods using simulation techniques can lead to wrong conclusions, because of lack of description parameters or during an unexpected situation. Non-model-based methods have an increasing success and are based on the analysis of the process biochemical signals. The detection and the characterization of the physiological states of the bioprocess are based on signal processing and statistical analysis of signals. For example, methods based on covariance (21) and moving averages (4) have been proposed, but they do not take account of the changes occurring in the signals. Wavelet transform is a powerful tool for non-stationary signal analysis due to its good localization in time and frequency domains. Wavelets are thus sensitive to changes in signals. Bakshi and Stephanopoulos (3), then Jiang et al. (12) have successfully used wavelets to analyze and detect states during bioprocesses.

One of the main contribution of Artificial Intelligence to biological or chemical processes turns out to be the classification of an increasing amount of data. Can we do more than that and can an AI program contribute to help in discovery of hidden rules in some such complex process. In fact, even if we can predict, for instance, mutagenicity of a given molecule or the secondary structure of proteins, with high degree of accuracy, this is not sufficient to give a deep insight of the observed behavior. In this paper we present a method using Maximum of Modulus of Wavelets Transform, Hölder exponent evaluation and correlation product for the detection and the characterization of physiological states during a fermentation fed-batch bioprocess. Therefore, we consider the estimation of nonoscillating and isolated Lipschitz singularities of a signal.

2. Yeast biotechnology

The main process we are concerned is a bio-reaction, namely the dynamical behavior of yeast during chemostat cultivation. Starting from the observation of a set of evolutive parameters, our final aim is to extract logical rules to infer the physiological state of the yeast. Doing so, we obtain not only a better understanding of the system's evolution but also the possibility to integrate the inferred rules in a full on-line control process. The first thing we have to do is to capture and analyze the parameters given by the sensors. These signals must be treated to be finally given to the logic machine. Thus, two things have to be done : first, to denoise the signals, secondly to compute the local maximum values of the given curves. In fact, we are more interested in the variations of the signals than in their pure instantaneous values. We use a method issued from wavelets theory (1) and which tends to replace classical Fourier analysis. At the end of this purely analytic treatment, we dispose of a set of clean values for each critical parameter. Now, our idea is to apply Inductive Logic Programming to exhibit, starting from a finite sample set of numerical observations, a number of logical formulae which organize the knowledge using causal relationships. Inductive logic programming is a sub-field of machine learning based upon a first-order logic framework. So instead of giving a mathematical formula (for instance a differential equation) or a statistical prediction involving the different parameters, we provide a set of implicative logical formulae. A part of these formulae can generally be inferred by a human expert, so it a a way to partially validate the mechanism. But its remains some new formulae which express an unknown causality relation : in that sense, this is a kind of knowledge discovery. As far as we know, one of the novelties of our work is the introduction of a time dimension to simulate the dynamic process. In logic, this time variable is in general not considered except with some specific modal logics. So, we modelize the time with an integer-valued variable.

The methodology has been applied to a biotechnological process. Saccharomyces Cerevisiae is studied under oxidative regime (i.e., no ethanol production) to produce yeast under a laboratory environment in a bioreactor. Two different procedures are applied: a batch procedure that is followed by a continuous procedure. The batch procedure is composed by a sequence of biological stages. This phase can be thought as a start-up procedure. Biotechnologists state that the behaviour in the batch procedure influences later in induced phenomena in the continuous phase. So complete knowledge of the batch phase is of great importance for the biotechnologist. The traditional way to get acquainted of such knowledge is at present carried out through offline measurements and analysis which most of the time produce results when the batch procedure has ended, thus lacking of real time performance. Instead, the proposed methodology allows for real time implementation. This example deals with the batch procedure. Among the set of available on-line signals the expert chooses the subset of signals which, according to the expert knowledge contain the most relevant information to determine the physiological state:

1. DOT : partial oxygen pressure in the medium.
2. O2 : oxygen percent in the output gas
3. CO2 : carbon dioxide percent in the output gas
4. pH.
5. OH- ion consumption : derived from control action of the pH regulator and the index of reflectivity.

The consumption of negative OH ions is evaluated from the control signal of the pH regulator. The actuator is a pump, switched by an hysteresis relay, that inoculates a basic solution (NaOH). The reflectivity, which is measured by the luminance, seems to follow the biomass density. Nevertheless its calibration is not constant and depends on the run. Yeasts are a very well-studied micro-organisms and today, such micro-organism like *Saccharomyces cerevisiae* which make the object of this study, are largely used in various sectors of the biomedical and biotechnology industrial processes. So, this is a critical point to control such processes. Two directions have been explored:

1. the *on-line* analysis : it does not allow to identify in an instantaneous manner and with certainty the physiological state of the yeast.
2. the *off-line* analysis : it allows to soundly characterize the current state, but generally too late to take into account this information and to adjust the process on the fly by actions of regulators allowing to adjust some critical parameters such that pH, temperature (addition of basis, heats, cooling).

To remedy these drawbacks, computer scientists in collaboration with micro-biologists develop tools for supervised control of the bioprocess. They use the totality of informations provided by the sensors during a set of sample processes to infer some general rules to which the biological process obeys. These rules can be used to control the next processes. This is exactly the problem we tackle in this paper. To sum up, our application focus on the evolutive behavior of a *bio-reactor* (namely yeast fermentation) that is to say an evolutive biological system whose interaction with physical world, described with pH, pressure, temperature, etc..., generates an observable reaction. This reaction is studied by the way of a set of sensors providing a large amount of (generally) numerical data, but, thanks to the logical framework, symbolic data could also be integrated in the future. For an approach based upon classification and fuzzy logic, one can see (24) : this work is devoted to discover the different states of the bio-reactor but not to predict its behavior.

In a yeast culture, measures result of biology phenomena and physical mechanisms. That is why to bring the culture, it is always decisional between biology and physico-chemical. The biological reaction is function of the environment and an environmental modification will improve two types of biological responses. The first one is a quasi steady-state response, the micro-organism is in equilibrium with the environment. The biological translation of this state is kinetics of consummation, production and this phenomenon is immediate. The second biological response is a metabolic one, which can be an oxidative or fermentative mode, or a secondary metabolism. The characteristic of this response is that the time constants are relatively long. For cultures, in term of production, the essential parameters are metabolism control and performance (productivity and substrate conversion in biomass yield). With this goal, the process must be conducted by a permanent intervention in order to bring the culture to an initial point to a final point. This control can be done from acquired measures on process, which are generally gases. Indirect measures show the environmental dynamic, which is shown by gas balance, with respiratory quotient (RQ) and pH corrector liquid (see figure 1).

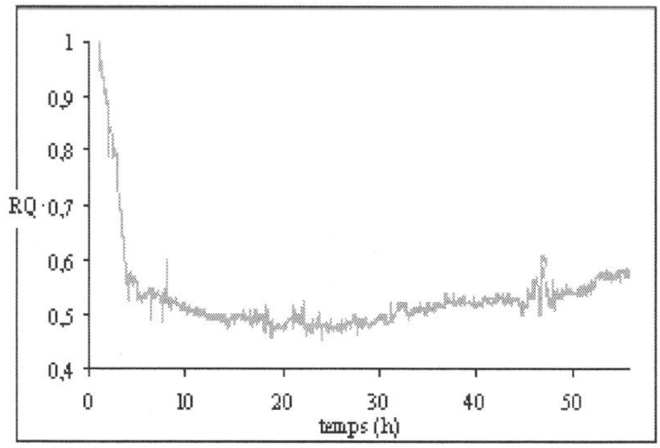

Fig. 1. An example of respiratory quotient evolution during a culture. x-axis is the time of the experience, y-axis is the amplitude of the signal.

Then, there are physical phenomenon, which are associated to real reactors. These mechanisms can be decomposed in many categories : transfer phenomenon (mass, thermal and movement quantity), regulation (realised by an operator), introduction of products, and mixing. These mechanisms interfere with biology and it is significant to notice that relaxation times of these phenomena are of size order of response time of biological response. With all these phenomena, a variable can be described by the following equation (see (26)) :

$$\frac{dV}{dt} = \Delta.(\frac{V_{equilibrium} - V(t)}{\tau_{physical}}) + r_{V(t)} + \Phi_{V(t)} \quad (1)$$

where:

- $\frac{dV}{dt}$ corresponds to the dynamic of the system.

- $\Delta.(\frac{V_{equilibrium}-V(t)}{\tau_{physical}})$ is variable variation between biological and physical parameters. $\tau_{physical}$ is the time constant of physical phenomena; this constant can not be characterised because it depends on reaction progress.
- $r_{V(t)}$ is the volumic density of reaction of the variable V, it is a biological term.
- $\Phi_{V(t)}$ corresponds to an external intervention which results of a voluntary action.

Moreover, it is essential to observe that there is a regulation loop between biology and physic (see figure 2). The problematic is, from measures, to isolate or eliminate perturbations. These responses depend on physical phenomena or human interventions (process regulation). It is to quantify biological kinetics and by this way to optimise biological kinetics and control that is to say identify modifications of the biological behaviour. For example, in the case of yeast production, it is important to maintain an oxidative metabolism by the control of glucose residual concentration, fermentative metabolism is prejudicial to the yield. The aim is to maintain an optimal production to avoid the diminution of substrate conversion yield, that is to say to remark the biological change between oxidative and fermentative metabolism.

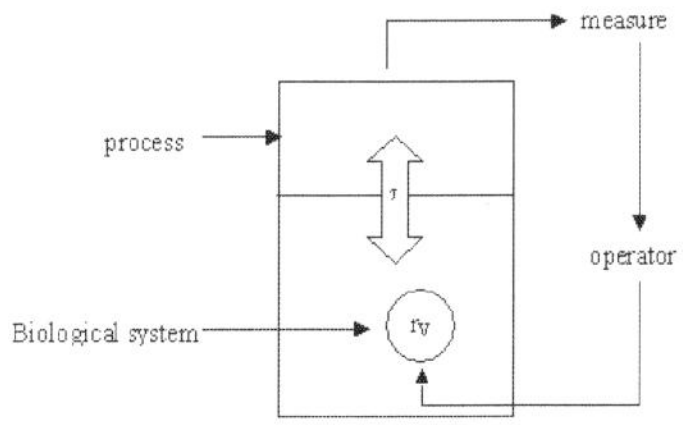

Fig. 2. Interactions between the biological system, the process and the operator.

3. Knowledge based methodology

In learning there is a constant interaction between the creation and the recognition of concepts. The goal of the methodology is to obtain a model of the process, which can be used in a supervisory system for condition monitoring. The complexity of this model imposes the co-operation of data mining techniques along with the expert knowledge. When only expert knowledge is used to identify process situations or states, any of these situations can arise: Ø the expert can express only a partial knowledge from process, Ø he does know the existence of several states but he ignores how to recognise them from on-line data, or/and Ø he doesn't have a clear idea on which states to recognise. For example, in the yeast production batch phase, biotechnologists apply expert rules when recognising some of the physiological states from on-line data. Nevertheless those rules usually don't take into account other phenomena that can change the evolution of signals without any influence in the physiological state. This leads to wrong conclusions. It is mainly due to the fact that the expert is not able to draw conclusions from the analysis of multiple signals between which there exist true relationships. Nevertheless, a classification tool copes well with this drawback. This proves the need of an iterative methodology to identify the biological states, which refines the expert knowledge with the analysis of past data sets.

Initialize : $E' = E$ (initial set of examples)
$H = \emptyset$ (initial hypothesis)
While $E' \neq \emptyset$ do
Choose $e \in E'$
Compute a covering clause C for e
$H = H \cup \{C\}$
Compute $Cov = \{e' \mid e' \in E, B \cup H \models e'\}$ $E' = E' \setminus Cov$ End while

Fig. 3. General Progol scheme

3.1 Standard ILP task

We stay within the pure setting i.e. where programs do not involve negation. In that case, the meaning of a logic program is just its least Herbrand model, which is a subset of the Herbrand universe i.e. the full set of ground atoms. In that setting, a concept C is just a subset of the Herbrand base. As shortly explained in our introduction, an ILP machine takes as input :

- a finite proper subset $E =< E^+, E^- >$ (the training set in Instance Based Learning terminology) where E^+ can be considered as the positive examples i.e. the things known as being true and is a subset of C, E^- as the negative examples and is a subset of $\overline{C}$.
- a logic program usually denoted B (as background knowledge) representing a basic knowledge we have concerning the concept to approximate. This knowledge satisfies two natural conditions : it does not explained the positive examples : $B \not\models E^+$ and it does not contradict the negative ones : $B \cup E^- \not\models \bot$

So the ILP task consists in finding a program H such that $H \cup B \models C$. One of the most popular method is to find H such that $H \cup B \models E^+$ and $H \cup B \cup E^- \not\models \bot$. In the field of classification, it is known that this approach, minimizing the error rate over the sample set (here we have zero default on the sample set) does not always guaranty the best result for the whole concept C.

Nevertheless, as far as we know, no alternative induction principle is used for ILP. Of course, as explained in the previous section, an ILP machine could behave as a classifier. Back to the introduction, the sample set $S = \{(x_1, y_1), \ldots, (x_i, y_i), \ldots, (x_n, y_n)\}$ is represented as a finite set of Prolog facts $class(x_i, y_i)$ constituting the set E^+. The ILP machine will provide an hypothesis H. Consulting H with a Prolog interpreter, for a given element x, we get the class y of x by giving the query $class(x, Y)$? to the interpreter.

3.2 Progol machinery

Back to the standard ILP process, instead of searching for consequences, we search for premises : it is thus rather natural to reverse standard deductive inference mechanisms. That is te case for Progol which uses the so-called inverse entailment mechanism ((20)). Progol is a rather complex machine and we only try to give a simplified algorithm schematizing its behavior in figure 3. One can read the tutorial introduction of CProgol4.4[1] from which we take our inspiration.

The main point we want to update is the choice of the relevant clause C for a given training example e. Let us precise here how this clause is chosen.

[1] available on **http://www.cs.york.ac.uk/mlg/progol.html** where a full and clear description is given.

3.3 The choice of the covering clause

It is clear that there is an infinite number of clauses covering e, and so Progol need to restrict the search in this set. The idea is thus to compute a clause C_e such that if C covers e, then necessarily $C \models C_e$. Since, in theory, C_e could have an infinite cardinality, Progol restricts the construction of C_e using mode declarations and some other settings (like number of resolution inferences allowed, etc...). Mode declarations imply that some variables are considered as input variables and other ones as output variables : this is a standard way to restrict the search tree for a Prolog interpreter.

At last, when we have a suitable C_e, it suffices to search for clauses C which θ-subsume C_e since this is a particular case which validates $C \models C_e$. Thus, Progol begins to build a finite set of θ-subsuming clauses, $C_1, \ldots, C_n$. For each of these clauses, Progol computes a natural number $f(C_i)$ which expresses the *quality* of C_i : this number measures in some sense how well the clause explains the examples and is combined with some compression requirement. Given a clause C_i extracted to cover e, we have :

$$f(C_i) = p(C_i) - (c(C_i) + h(C_i) + n(C_i))$$

where :

- $p(C_i) = \#(\{e \mid e \in E, B \cup \{C_i\} \models e\})$ i.e. the number of covered examples
- $n(C_i) = \#(\{e \mid e \in E, B \cup \{C_i\} \cup \{e\} \models \bot\})$ i.e. the number of incorrectly covered examples
- $c(C_i)$ is the length of the body of the clause C_i
- $h(C_i)$ is the minimal number of atoms of the body of C_e we have to add to the body of C_i to insure output variables have been instantiated.

The evaluation of $h(C_i)$ is done by static analysis of C_e. Then, Progol chooses a clause $C = C_{i_0} \equiv \arg\max_{C_i} f(C_i)$ (i.e. such that $f(C_{i_0}) = max\{f(C_j) \mid j \in [1,n]\}$). We may notice that, in the formula computing the number $f(C_i)$ for a given clause C_i covering e, there is no distinction between the covered positive examples. So $p(C_i)$ is just the number of covered positive examples. The same computation is valuable for the computation of $n(C_i)$ and so success and failure could be considered as equally weighted.

To abbreviate, we shall denote $Progol(B,E,f)$ the output program P currently given by the Progol machine with input B as background knowledge, E as sample set and using function f to chose the relevant clauses. In the next section, we shall explain how we introduce weights to distinguish between examples.

4. A boosting-like mechanism for Progol

As explained in our introduction, a Progol machine is a consistent learner i.e. it renders only hypothesis with no error on the training set : so the sample error at the end of a learning loop, $\epsilon^t = \Sigma_{\{i|x_i \text{ misclassified}\}} w_t(i)$, is 0 since each example is necessarily correctly classified. So we cannot base our solution over the computation of such an error since the nullity of this error is a halting condition for a standard boosting algorithm. So we introduce a new way to adjust the weights. Given an example e_i, since it is covered we have $B \cup H_t \vdash e$. Given an other problem instance e, we claim that the longer the proof for $B \cup H_t \vdash e$, the riskier the prediction for e.

5. Inductive logic programming : basic concepts

Mathematical logic has always been a powerful representation tool for declarative knowledge and Logic Programming is a way to consider mathematical logic as a programming language. A set of first order formulae restricted to a clausal form, constitutes a logic program and as such, becomes executable by using standard mechanisms of theorem proving field, namely unification and resolution. Prolog is the most widely distributed language of this class. In this context, the data and their properties, i.e. the observations, are represented as a finite set of logical facts E. E could generally been discomposed into the positive examples E^+ and the negative ones E^-. In case of background knowledge, it is described as a set of Horn clauses B. This background knowledge is supposed to be insufficient to explain the positive observations and the logical translation of this fact is : $B \not\models E^+$ but there is no contradiction with the negative knowledge: $B \cup E^- \not\models \perp$. So an ILP machinery ((20)), with input E and B, will output a program H such that $B \cup H \models E$. So H constitutes a kind of explanation of our observations E. Expressed as a set of logical implications (Horn clauses) $c \rightarrow o$, c becomes a possible cause for the observation $o \in E$. We give here a simple scheme giving a functional view of an ILP machine.

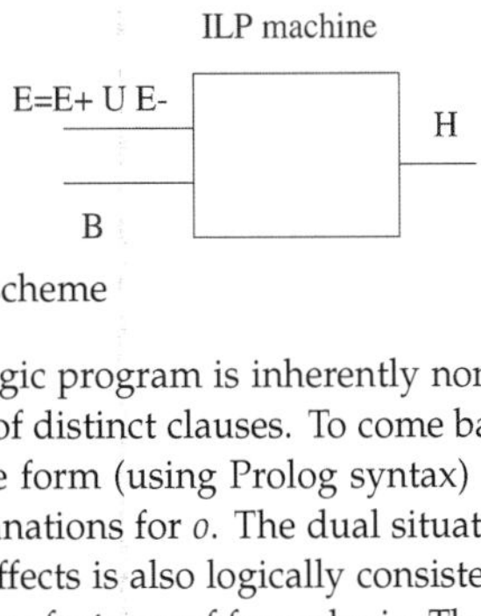

Fig. 4. ILP machine functional scheme

It is important to note that a logic program is inherently non deterministic since a predicate is generally defined with a set of distinct clauses. To come back to our introductive notation, we can have two clauses of the form (using Prolog syntax) $o \leftarrow c$ and $o \leftarrow c'$: this means that c and c' are potential explanations for o. The dual situation $o \leftarrow c$ and $o' \leftarrow c$ where the same cause produces distinct effects is also logically consistent. So this is a way to deal with uncertainty and to combine some features of fuzzy logic. The main difference is that we have a sound and complete operational inference system and this is not the case for fuzzy logic.

6. Formalization of our problem

We have 4 potential states for the bio-reactor : we shall denote e_1, e_2, e_3 and e_4 these states to avoid unusefull technical words. e_4 will be considered as a terminal state where the bio-reactor is stable because of the complete combustion of the available ethanol. We add a specific state e_5 corresponding to a stationary situation where the process is going on without perturbation. The transition between two states is a critical section where the chosen observable parameters (bio-mass, pH and O_2 rate) give rise to great variations.

The predicate to learn with our ILP machine is :

$$\textbf{to-state}(E_i, E_t, P_1, P_2, P_3, T)$$

meaning that the bio-reactor is going into state E_t knowing that at step T, the current bio-reactor parameters are the P_i's and the current state E_i. It is thus clear that we can deal with as many parameters as we want, but we restrict to 3 in this experiment. As explained in our introduction, we introduce the variable T to simulate the dynamic behavior of our process. As far as we know, previous experiments using inductive logic programming generally compute causal relationship between parameters which do not involve time. So we have to learn a transition system where we do not know what are the basic actions activating a transition. Our informations about the system are given by sensors providing numerical signals for p_1 (bio-mass), p_2 (pH value) and p_3 (O_2 rate),. These signals are analyzed using a wawelet-based system, we visualize the curve of the different functions and we extract the values of the differential for each given function. These values constitutes the input of our learning system. So, we want to obtain a causal relationship between the transitions of the system and the values of the differentials of the curve describing the evolution of our parameters.

So, we add a predicate **derive**$(P, T, P1)$ which expresses the fact that, for the curve of the parameter P,

at time T, the value of the differential is $P1$. It is thus easy to describe what is a pike for the curve describing P : this is included in our background knowledge. These pikes correspond to

local minima/maxima for the given parameter. So, we are also interested in the sign of

the derivative and we include specific predicates (**positive/2**, **negative/2**)

to compute and test this sign.

As background knowledge (corresponding to the B input of our scheme 4), we have the definitions of predicates **derive/3**,

positive/2, **negative/2**, **pike/2**. Here is an overview of the mode declaration

to describe the potential causes of a state transition.

```
:- modeb(*,pike(+parameter,-float))?
:- modeb(3,pike(-parameter,+float))?
:- modeb(1,positive(+parameter,+float))?
:- modeb(1,negative(+parameter,+float))?
:- modeb(1,between(+float,+float,+float))?
:- modeb(1,between(-float,+float,+float))?
% a (very little) part of

% our background knowledge.
pike(P,T) :- derive(P,T, P1),P2 is P1, between(P2,-0.001,0.001).
```

The results in this paper are obtained using the last implementation of Progol, namely **CProgol4.4** freely available on the following site **http://www.cs.york.ac.uk/mlg/progol.html**. Of course, we get a lot of rules, depending on the quantity of introduced examples. Some of them are not really interesting : they only generalize one or two examples. But we get, for instance, the next one (among the simplest ones to explain) :

```
to_state(E,E,A,B,C,T) :- derive(p1,A,T),
        derive(p2,B,T), derive(p3,C,T),
        positive(p1,T), positive(p2,T),
        positive(p3,T).
```

This rule indicates that there is no evolution of the metabolism state (the bio-reactor remains in the same state) when the parameters have an increasing slope but that we do not encounter maxima or minima. In general, the obtained rules are long except those ones generalizing only one or two examples. Nevertheless, there are some observations where this rule could be overcame : this means that we need (at least) an other parameter $p4$ to better understand the behaviour of the machinery.

7. Detection and characterization of physiological states

In microbiology, a physiological state (or more simply, a state) is, qualitatively, the set of potential functionalities of a micro-organism, and, quantitatively, the level of expression of theses functionalities. The environment has a strong influence on the activity of the micro-organism due, on one hand, to its chemical composition (nature of substrate, pH...) and, on the other hand to its physical properties (temperature, pression...). Yeast can react on the availability of substrates such as carbon and nitrogen sources, or oxygen, by a flexible choice of different metabolic pathway. It is possible to analyze the global metabolism by genetical analysis, biochemical or biophysical analysis but the complexity of the biological system requires a simplification of the characterization by the analysis of some functionalities of some known mechanisms. The quantification of materials and energy interactions flows between the micro-organism and the environment enables to have a macroscopic characterization of several intrinsic metabolism of yeast population which, by correlation, enables to differentiate several physiological states even if the biological characterization is unknown. Thus the detection, as far as we know, is based on the analysis of biochemical signals measured during the bioprocess. A bioprocess is the set up of the fermentors protocol. Fermentors are composed of a number of different components which can be grouped by their functions, i.e. temperature control, speed control, continuous culture accessories. In this context the ultimate aim of bioprocess analysis therefore is a detailed monitoring of biological system, the chemical and physical environment and how these interact. However, no reliable technique exist to carry out real-time measurement of non-volatile substrates and metabolites in the fermentor. Several works using various approaches, lead to the conclusion that the limits of a state are linked to the singularities of biochemical signals: Steyer et al. (31) (using expert system and fuzzy logic), Bakshi and Stephanopoulos (3) (using expert system and wavelets) and Doncescu et al. (6) (using inductive logic) show that the beginning and the end of a state correspond to singularities of the biochemical signals measured during the process. In a fed-batch bioprocess, a physiological state can occur several times during the experience. After the detection of states, it is then necessary to characterize these states. The characterization is often based on the statistical properties of the biochemical signals. Experts in microbiology characterize the states by analysing and comparing the variations and the values of different biochemical signals and by a deductive reasoning using " if-then" rules. These approaches can be linked to mathematical methods based on correlation. Classification methods based on Principal Components Analysis (PCA) (27), adaptive PCA (15), and kernel

PCA (14) enable to distinguish and characterize the different states. However, these methods (except the adaptive PCA) do not take into account the temporal variation of the signals. The adaptive PCA is a PCA applied directly on wavelet coefficients in order to take into account the variations of the biological system. It has been shown that it can characterize the Lipschitz singularities of a signal by following the propagation across scales of the modulus maxima of its continuous wavelet transform. For identifying the boundaries of states, we propose to use the Maximum of Modulus of Wavelets Transform (17)(16) to detect the signals singularities. The singularities are selected according to their Hölder exponent evaluation between -1 and 1. The characterization of the states is based on the correlation product between the signals on intervals whose boundaries are the selected singularities.

8. Detection and selection of singularities by wavelets and Hölder exponent

The singularities of the biochemical signal correspond to the boundaries of the states. These signals are non-stationary and non-symmetrical; they are not chirps and have no infinite oscillations (see figure 5).
Several authors have proposed to use wavelets to detect the singularities of the signals for the detection of states: Bakshi and Stephanopoulos (3) and more recently Jiang et al. (12). Besides singularities correspond to maxima of modulus of wavelets coefficients. Bakshi and Stephanopoulos (3) propose to detect the maxima by analysing the variation of the wavelet coefficients through a multi-scale analysis but they don't explicitly characterize the nature of detected singularities. Jiang et al. (12) propose to select meaningful singularities by using a threshold on the finest scale, but the determination of the threshold remains empirical. After the detection of singularities by the Maxima of Modulus of Wavelet Transform, we propose to use the evaluation of Hölder exponent to characterize the type of singularities and eventually select meaningful singularities.

The wavelets are a powerful mathematical tool of non-stationary signal analysis, signals whose frequencies change with time. Contrarily to the Fourier Transform, Wavelet Transform can provide the time-scale localization. The performance of the Wavelet Transform is better than of the windowed Fourier Transform. Because of these characteristics, Wavelet Transform can be used for analyzing the non-stationary signals such as transient signals. Wavelets Transformation (WT) is a rather simple mechanism used to decompose a function into a set of coefficients depending on scale and location. The definition of the Wavelets Transform is:

$$W_{s,u}f(x) = (f \star \psi_{s,u})(x) = \int f(x)\psi(\frac{x-u}{s})dx \tag{2}$$

where ψ is the wavelet, f is the signal, $s \in R^{+*}$ is the scale (or resolution) parameter, and $u \in R$ is the translation parameter. The scale plays the role of frequency. The choice of the wavelet ψ is often a complicated task. We assume that we are working with an admissible real-valued wavelet ψ with r vanishing moments ($r \in N^*$).

The wavelet is translated and dilated as in the next relation :

$$\psi_{u,s} = \frac{1}{\sqrt{s}}\psi(\frac{t-u}{s}) \tag{3}$$

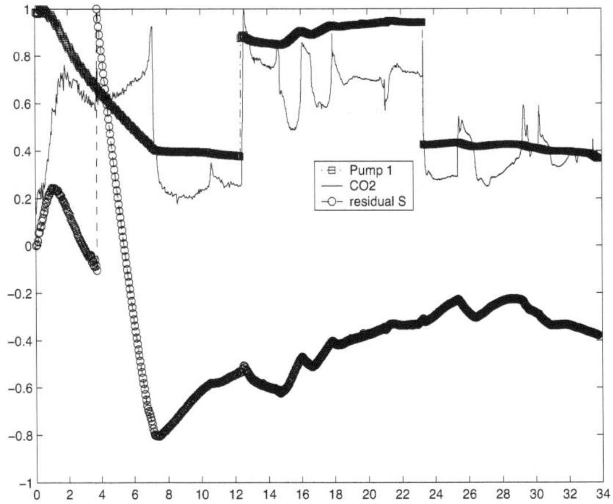

Fig. 5. Example of biochemical signals measured during the bioprocess. Pump 1 is a pump providing substance in the process, CO2 is the measured carbon dioxid and residual S is the residual substrate of the micro-organisms of the bioprocess. The signals have been normalized.

The dilation allows the convolution of the analyzed signal which different sizes of "window" wavelet function. For the detection of the singularities and of the inflexion points of the biochemical signal, we use the Maxima of Modulus of Wavelets Transform (16). The idea is to follow the local maxima at different scales and to propagate from low frequencies to high frequencies. These maxima correspond to singularities, particularly when the wavelet is the derivative of a smooth function:

$$\psi(x) = \frac{d\theta(x)}{dx}$$

$$W_{s,u}f(x) = f * \psi_{s,u} = f(x) * \frac{d\theta(x/s)}{dx}$$

Yuille and Poggio (35) have shown that if the wavelet is derivative of the Gaussian, then the maxima belong to connected curves which are continuous from a scale to another. The detection of the singularities of the signal is thus possible by using the wavelets (see for example figure 6).

The discretization form of Continuous Wavelet Transform is based on the next form of the Mother Wavelet :

$$\psi^{m,n}(t) = a_0^{-m/2}\psi(\frac{t - nb_0a_0^m}{a_0^m}) \tag{4}$$

By selecting a_0 and b_0 properly, the dilated mother wavelet constitutes an orthonormal basis of $L^2(R)$. For example, the selection of $a_0 = 2$ and $b_0 = 1$ provides a dyadic-orthonormal Wavelet Transform (DWT). The decomposed signals by DWT will have no redundant information thanks to the orthonormal basis.

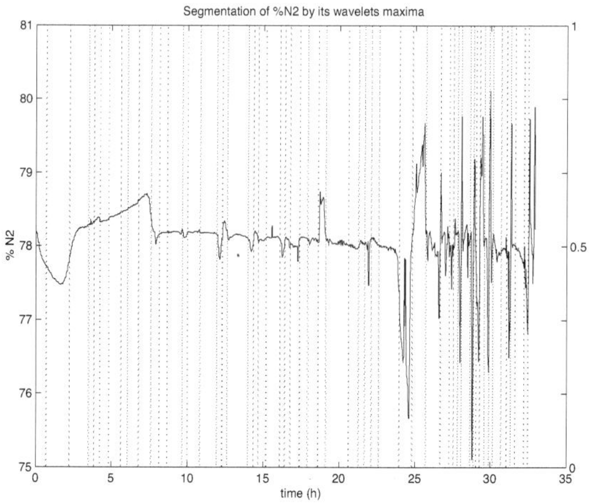

Fig. 6. Segmentation of N2 (nitrogen). Each vertical dotted line correspond to a singularity of the signal detected by wavelets. The wavelet is a DOG (first derivative of Gaussian) and the scales go from 2^0 to 2^3.

Jiang et al. (12) have proposed to select the maxima by using thresholding. Besides, all the singularities are not relevant only some of them are meaningful. However, as stated above, the thresholds proposed by Jiang et al. are chosen empirically. To select the meaningful singularities, we proposed using the Hölder exponent. The Hölder exponent is a mathematical value allowing characterization singularities. The fractal dimension could also be used but only the Hölder exponent can characterize locally each singularity. A singularity in a point x_0 is characterized by the Hölder exponent (also called Hölder coefficient or Lipschitz exponent). This exponent is defined like the most important exponent α allowing to verify the next inequality:

$$|f(x) - P_n(x - x_0)| \leq C|x - x_0|^{\alpha(x_0)} \tag{5}$$

We must remark that $P_n(x - x_0)$ is the Taylor Development and basically $n \leq \alpha(x_0) < n + 1$. Hölder exponent measures the remainder of a Taylor expansion and more of this measures the local differentiability:

1. $\alpha \geq 1$, $f(t)$ is continuous and differentiable.
2. $0 < \alpha < 1$, $f(t)$ is continuous but non-differentiable.
3. $-1 < \alpha \leq 0$, $f(t)$ is discontinuous and non-differentiable.
4. $\alpha \leq -1$, $f(t)$ is not longer locally integrable.

Therefore Hölder exponent could be extended to the distribution. For example the Hölder exponent of a Dirac is equal to -1. A simple computation leads to a very interesting result of the Wavelets Transform (11):

$$|W_{s,u}f(x)| \simeq s^{\alpha(x_0)} \tag{6}$$

This relation is remarkable because it allows to measure the Hölder exponent using the behavior of the Wavelets Transform. Therefore, at a given scale $a = 2^N$ the $W_{a,b}f(x)$ will be maximum in the neighborhood of the signal singularities. The detection of the Hölder coefficient is linked to the vanishing moment of the wavelet: if n is the vanishing moment of the wavelet, then it can detect Hölder coefficients less than n (16). We use a *DOG* wavelet (DOG: first derivative of Gaussian) with a vanishing moment equal to 1; consequently we can only detect Hölder coefficients smaller than 1. This is not a real problem because we are interested (*in this application*[2] by the singularities as step or dirac and the Hölder coefficient of these singularities are smaller than 1. Moreover, the meaningful singularities of the fed-batch bioprocess have Hölder exponents smaller than 1 which correspond to sharp singularities. This type of variations are meaningful for the fed-batch bioprocess fermentation because of many external regulations of the process. Moreover, for Hölder coefficients greater than 1 particularly for integer values, there are difficulties to interpret the Hölder coefficient (see (19) cited in (17)). To evaluate the Hölder coefficient using the wavelets, there are two main ways:

(1) the graphical method which consists in finding the maximum line i.e. the maximum which propagates through the scales, and computes the slopes of this maximum line (often using a log-log representation). The computed slope corresponds to the Hölder coefficient (16).
(2) the minimization method which consists in minimizing a function which has one of the parameters the Hölder coefficient (17). The function is the following:

$$\sum_j \left(ln_2(|s_j|) - ln_2(C) - j - \frac{\alpha(x_0) - 1}{2} ln_2(\sigma^2 + 2^{2j}) \right)^2 \tag{7}$$

where s_j represents the maximum at scale j, C is a constant depending on the singularity localized in x_0, σ is the standard deviation of a Gaussian approximation (see (17)), and $\alpha(x_0)$ the Hölder exponent.

In (17), a gradient descent algorithm is proposed to solve the minimization, but this technique is very sensitive to local minima. Recently, a minimization using Genetical Algorithms has been proposed (18) and used in bioprocess. More precisely it uses Differential Evolutionary (DE) algorithms. The DE algorithms was introduced by Rainer Storn and Kenneth Price (33).

9. Differential evolution

Differential Evolution (DE)(33) is one of Evolutionary Algorithms (EA) which are a class of stochastic search and optimization methods including Genetic Algorithms (GA), evolutionary programming, evolution strategies, genetic programming and all methods based on genetics and evolution. Through its fast convergence and robustness properties, it seems to be a promising method for optimizing real-valued multi-modal objective functions. Compared to traditional search and optimization methods, the EAs are more robust and straightforward to use in complex problems : they are able to work with minimum assumptions about the objective functions. These methods are slower because due to the generation of the population

[2] However it is always possible to use other wavelets with greater vanishing moment for others applications in bioprocesses

and the selection of individuals for crossing. The goal is to obtain the trade-off between accuracy and computing time.

The generation of the vectors containing the parameters of the model is made by applying an independent procedure :

$$X_{i,G} = X_{1,i}.....X_{D,i} \tag{8}$$

with $i = 1...NP$, is the index of one individual of the population; D is the number of parameters which have to be estimated; NP is the number of individuals in one population; G is the index of the current population; i is one individual of the population and $X_{j,i}$ is the parameter j of the individual i in the population G.

As Genetic Algorithms are stochastic processes, the initial population has been chosen randomly, but the initialization of the parameters is based on experts knowledge. Trial parameter vectors are evaluated by the objective function. Several objective functions are tested to produce results on Hölder coefficient detection. For simple GA algorithms the new vectors are the result of the difference between two population vectors and the result is added to a new one. It's a simple crossing operation. The objective function determines if the new vector is more efficient than a candidate population member and replace it if this simple relation is true. In the case of the DE the generation of the new vectors are realized by the difference between the "old vectors" given an weight to each one.

We have tested and compared different schemes of individual generations :

- $DE/rand/1$: For each vector $X_{i,G}$ a perturbed vector $V_{i,G+1}$ is generated according to :

  $$V_{i,G+1} = X_{R1,G} + F * (X_{R2,G} - X_{R3,G})$$

  $R1, R2, R3 \in [1, NP]$: individuals of population, chosen randomly, $F \in [0, 1]$: controls the amplification $(X_{R2,G} - X_{R3,G})$
  $X_{R1,G}$: the perturbed vector. There is no relation between $V_{i,G+1}$ and $X_{i,G}$. The objective function must evaluate the quality of this new trial parameter with respect to the old member. If $V_{i,G+1}$ yields a lower objective function value, $V_{i,G+1}$ is set to $X_{i,G+1}$ in the next generation or there is no effect.

- $DE/best/1$: It is like $DE/rand/1$ but is generating $V_{i,G+1}$ by integrating the most performante vector :

  $$V_{i,G+1} = X_{best,G} + F * (X_{R1,G} - X_{R2,G})$$

  $X_{best,G}$: best vector of population G, $R1, R2 \in [1, NP]$: individuals of population, chosen randomly. As $DE/rand/1$, the objective function compares the quality of $V_{i,G+1}$ and $X_{i,G}$; the smallest of the two is kept in the next population.

- Hydrid Differential evolution algorithms: As DE algorithms, a perturbed vector is generated, but the weight F is a stochastic parameter.

To increase the diversity potential of the population, a crossover operation is introduced. $X_{i,G+1} = (X_{1i,G+1}, X_{2i,G+1}.....X_{Di,G+1})$ becomes :

$$V_{ji,G+1} \begin{cases} j = (n)_D, (n+1)_D, (n+L-1)_D \\ X_{ij,G} \text{ otherwise} \end{cases}$$

$n \in [1, D]$: starting index, chosen randomly
$(n)_D$ = n mod D
$L \in [1, D]$: number of parameters which are going to be exchanged

10. Use of GA for Hölder's coefficients detection

10.1 Implementation

The cost function we have to minimize is the following (17):

$$\sum_j \left(log_2(|a_j|) - log_2(C) - j - \frac{h(x_0) - 1}{2} log_2(\sigma^2 + 2^{2j}) \right)^2 \tag{9}$$

In the Holder objective function three parameters have to be estimated : $h(x_0)$, C and σ. Thus, one individual X in GA's population is represented by the vector X_h, X_C, X_σ. In our case, the size of population equals 30.

Using the graphical method and the DE, the Hölder coefficient found is quite close to -1, whereas the value computed by gradient descent is not correct. Moreover, if we consider the Hölder coefficient of the Step function, only DE provides quite good results while the graphical method and the values of the gradient descent are too far from the theoretical value. The last median square is not so accurate as DE's. The results obtained indicate that the *DE* can be used for the analyzed data .

For this simulation, the results are summarized in the following table :

Singularity	Dirac	Step 1	Step 2
Theoritical Hölder Coef.	-1	0	0
Hölder Coef. by Graph. Method	-0.5	0.51	0.51
Hölder Coef. by Grad. Descent	0.26	0.89	0.89
Least Median Square	-0.5	0.802301	0.802301
Hölder Coef. by AG	-0.5	-0.03	-0.04

We note that the graphical method is the fastest and used method, but the evaluation of the Hölder coefficient is sometimes imprecise as noted in (34), (22).

On a simple signal (see figure 7), this new method using DE provides better results than those of existing methods as shown in table 1.

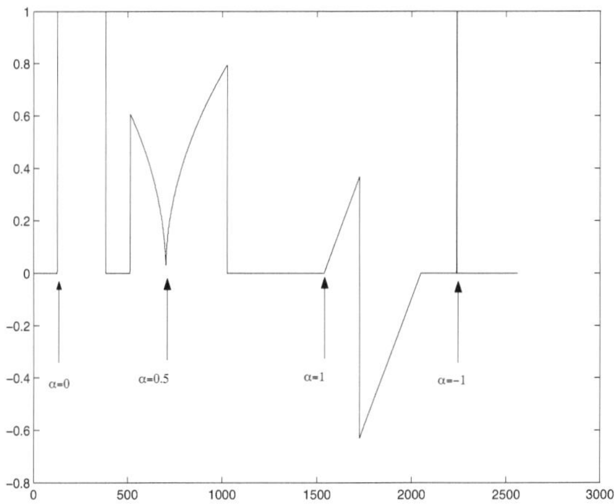

Fig. 7. Simple signal with singularity (step, cups, ramp and dirac) whose Hölder exponents α are known .

Singularity	Dirac	Step	cups	Ramp
theoritical Hölder coef.	-1	0	0,5	1
Hölder exponent by graphical method	-1,13	0,16	0,61	0,84
Hölder exponent by gradient descent	-0,24	0,39	0,74	1,20
Hölder exponent by DE	-1,02	0,02	0,52	1,0007

Table 1. Results of Hölder exponent evaluation by several methods. The wavelet used here is a LOG (second derivative of Gaussian).

11. Characterization by correlation product and classification

Once the states are bounded by the detected and selected singularities using the wavelets, they are characterized by the analysis of the correlations between the biochemical signals. On each interval defined by the singularities, a product of correlation is computed between all pairs of signals. The correlation coefficient (also called Bravais-Pearson coefficient, see (30)) is given by the equation:

$$\frac{\frac{1}{n}\sum_{i=1}^{n}(x_i-\overline{x})(y_i-\overline{y})}{\sigma_x\sigma_y} \tag{10}$$

where x_i represent the values of one parameter (in a given interval), y_i the values of the second parameter (in the same interval), n the number of elements, $\overline{x}$ the average of the elements x_i (of the first biochemical signal), $\overline{y}$ the average of the elements y_i (of the second biochemical signal), et σ_x et σ_y the standard deviation of each of the two signals.
The correlation coefficient is equivalent to the cosine of the scalar product between two

biochemical signals projected in the correlation circle of a PCA realized between the two biochemical signals. On each interval, the sign of each correlation coefficient between two signals is kept. Each interval is thus characterized by a set of positive of negative signs. The intervals with the same set of signs are put in the same class as illustrated in the figure 8.

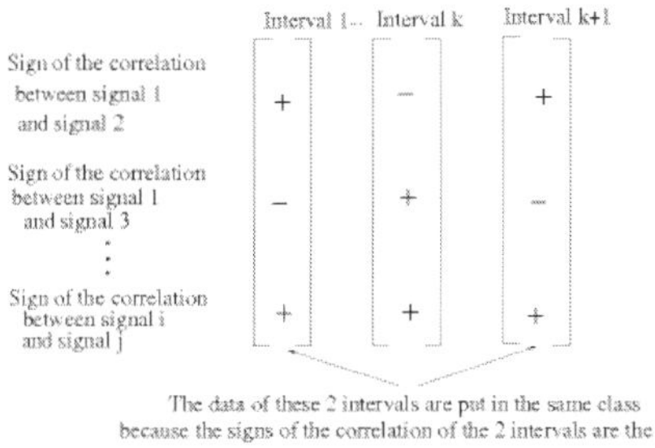

Fig. 8. Principle of the classification method based on wavelets, Hölder exponent and correlation coefficient

Ruiz et al. (27) propose a classification method based on PCA for a neighboring application (wastewater treatment): the data are projected in the space generated by the two first principal components. The method enables to reduce the size of the data space and to take account of the correlation of the signals. However the PCA doesn't take account of the time: the temporal evolution of the process is not taken into account. Ruiz et al. propose to use time analysis window of fixed size. But as the window has a fixed size, it doesn't really take account of the changes occurring during the bioprocess. So the method proposed in this article seems to be more adapted if it is necessary to take account of the variation of the process.

12. Experimental results

Tests have been done on two fed-batch fermentation bioprocesses and the first results have been presented in (25). The two bioprocesses are biotechnological processes using yeast called *Saccharomyces Cerevisiae*. In the first bioprocess we have applied the method to differentiate intrinsic biological phenomena from reactions of micro-organism to extern actions (changes in the environment). In the second bioprocess we directly use the method to detect and classify the states of the bioprocess. For the two fed-batch, the maximum scale is chosen empirically. Mallat and Zhong (17) propose to use as maximal scale $log_2(N) + 1$ where N is the number of measured samples of the signals. However if we use this maximal scale, several singularities would be removed. The empirical value which has been found it is 12. Concerning the Hölder exponent we are interested by the singularities between -1 and 1. For the evaluation of Hölder exponent using Genetical Algorithms, tests have shown that 100 iterations are sufficient for an acurate evaluation (18).

12.1 Differentiation between biophysical and biological phenomena

The first bioprocess is a bioprocess lasting about 25 hours. 12 biochemical signals have been measured during the bioprocess.
In a fed-batch bioprocess, there are two kinds of signals: the signals given by parameters

regulated by an extern action (expert in microbiology or control system) and the signals given by non regulated parameters. An example of regulated parameter is the agitation which is the speed of the rotor of the bioreactor and an example of non regulated parameter is the N2 (nitrogen). The actions on regulated parameters induce modifications of the physiology of the micro-organisms and physical changes in the bioreactor: there are *biophysical* phenomena. On the other hand, during the bioprocess, the micro-organisms have intrinsic physiological behavior: there are *biological* phenomena.
Is it possible to distinguish biophysical phenomena and biological phenomena?
To answer this question, we propose the following steps:

1. search the variations of the regulated signals. These variations are sharp variations which correspond to singularities as Dirac or step.
2. compare the sign of correlation product between regulated signals and non regulated signals before and after each detected singularity of the regulated signals. If the sign is the same before and after, there is no influence: it is a biological phenomenon. If the sign changes before and after, there is an influence: it is a biophysical phenomena.

We must note that:

- only the singularities of the regulated signal are detected and selected,
- to compare the sign of correlation product before and after each singularity, me must choose a reference temporal interval. Besides, the first temporal interval (delimited by the detected singularities) is considered as a biological interval as the bioprocess begins and the initial conditions are considered as biological.

An example of comparison between the agitation and the nitrogen is given in figures 9 and ??.

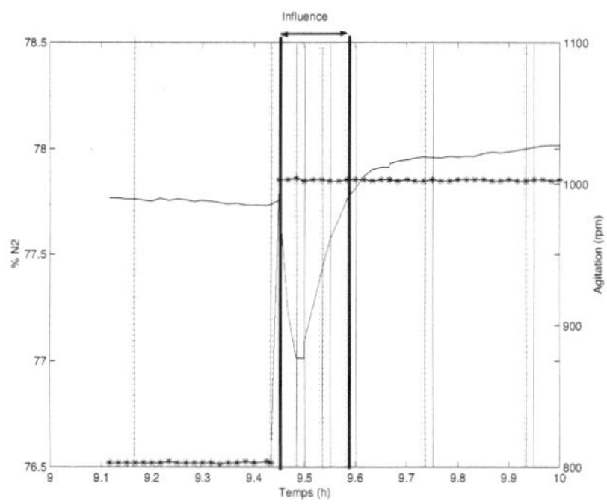

Fig. 9. An example of intervals (horizontal lines are singularities and correspond to boundaries of the temporal interval) with the segmentation given by the detection of regulated signals. This example has a duration of one hour (from 9 hours to 10 hours) taken from the first fed-batch. There are 14 intervals. Signals are agitation (stars) expressed in rotation per minute (rpm) and the percentage of nitrogen N2 (solid line).

Results confirm the observations of the expert. All the intervals considered as biological by the proposed method are considered as biological by the expert. Particularly, the last interval is considered as a biological phenomenon, which is well known by experts, as at the end of a bioprocess, regulated signals are not modified. Another example is given by biological intervals located in the middle of the bioprocess which correspond to spontaneous oscillations.

12.2 Detection and classification of states

We have studied Saccharomyces cerevisiae dynamical behaviour during fed-batch aerated cultivation in oxidative metabolism. The maximal growth rate of this yeast was calculated to 0,45 h-1. The aim of our work was to determine by on line analysis, different physiological states of the yeast behavior only with the available sensors (pH, temperature, oxygen Ě). Off-line metabolites and intracellular carbohydrate reserve analysis help in a first approach to identify the physiological states. State recognition is performed by signal processing technics. The second bioprocess is a bioprocess lasting about 34 hours. 11 biochemical signals have been measued during the bioprocess.
We recall the used method for the characterization of intervals for the classification is given in section 4 and summarised in figure 8. The classification provided by the method gives interesting results shown in the figure 10. Once again, results obtained correspond to the experts observations. Particularly, the most interesting result concerns the detection and the characterization of a state resulting of an external action. Besides, the class number 8 corresponds to the addition of an acid[3] (the acid is not a regulated parameter as in the first example, but is directly introduced by the expert during the experience) in the bioprocess. All apparition of class 8 correspond exactly to an acid addition. These results were confirmed and validated. As far as we know, it is the first time that this kind of non-model-based approach can find and characterize automatically the addition of acid in a fed-bacth process. The results are promising and further analysis of the classification is necessary.

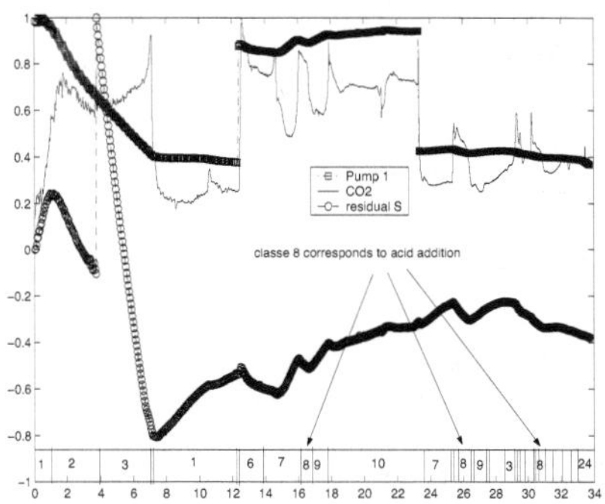

Fig. 10. Classification provided by the method. The wavelet is a DOG and the scales go from 2^0 to 2^{10}.

13. Discussion and conclusion

We apply logical tools to get explanation rules concerning the behavior of a bio-reactor. The ability to incorporate background knowledge and re-use past experiences marks out ILP as a

[3] because of industrial confidentiality, we are not allowed to gives more information

very effective solution for our problem. Instead of simply giving classification results, we get some logical rules establishing a causality relationship between different parameters of the bio-machinery. Among these rules, some ones are validated by expert knowledge, but some new ones have been provided. It yet appears that some previous rules have to be removed or modified to fit with new observations.

One of the main interest of this kind of approach is the fact that the resulting theory is easy to understand, even for a non specialist : the first order logic is, from a syntactic viewpoint, close to the natural language.

Intelligibility of resulting explanations is an other argument in favor of the ILP tools. A drawback of standard logic is the difficulty to deal with the time dimension : in some sense, standard logic is static and thus, not well suited to described dynamic process. One could hope that modal logic would be of some help, but it remains to design an inductive machine dealing with the temporal modalities, i.e. a way to reverse temporal logic inference system.

14. References

[1] Arneodo A. and al. Ondelettes, multifractales et turbulence de l'ADN aux croissances cristallines. *DIDEROT EDITEUR*, Paris, 1995.

[2] J. Aguilar-Martin, J. Waissman-Vilanova, R. Sarrate-Estruch, and B. Dahou. Knowledge based measurement fusion in bio-reactors. In *IEEE EMTECH*, May 1999.

[3] Bakshi, B. and Stephanopoulos, G. (1994). Representation of process trends-III. multiscale extraction of trends from process data. *Computer and Chemical Engineering*, 18(4):267–302.

[4] Cao, S. and Rhinehart, R. (1995). An efficient method for on-line identification of steady state. *Journal of Process Control*, 5(6):363–374.

[5] Domingo P. and Pazzani M.. On the optimality of the simple bayesian classifier under zero-one loss. *Machine Learning*, 29,103-130, 1998.

[6] Doncescu, A., Waissman, J., Richard, G., and Roux, G. (2002). Characterization of bio-chemical signals by inductive logic programming. *Knowledge-Based Systems*, 15(1-2):129–137.

[7] Edelman, G. M. and Gally, J. A. (2001). Degeneracy and complexity in biological systems. In *Proc Nat Acad Science USA*.

[8] Gadkar, K., Mehra, S., and Gomes, J. (2005). On-line adaptation of neural networks for bioprocess control. *Computer and Chemical Engineering*, 29:1047–1057.

[9] Guillaume, S. and Charnomordic, B. (2004). Generating an interpretable family of fuzzy partitions from data. *IEEE Transactions on Fuzzy Systems*.

[10] Hvala, N., Strmcnik, S., Sel, D., Milanic, S., and Banko, B. (2005). Influence of model validation on proper selection of process models-an industrial case study. *Computer and Chemical Engineering*.

[11] Jaffard, S. (1997). Multifractal formalism for functions part 1 and 2. *SIAM J. of Math. Analysis*, 28(4):944–998.

[12] Jiang, T., Chen, B., He, X., and Stuart, P. (2003). Application of steady-state detection method based on wavelet transform. *Computer and Chemical Engineering*, 27(4):569–578.

[13] Kitano, H. (2002). Computational systems biology. In *Nature 6912, 206*.

[14] Lee, J.-M., Yoo, C., Lee, I.-B., and Vanrolleghem, P. (2004). Multivariate statistical monitoring of nonlinear biological processes using kernel PCA. In *IFAC CAB'9*, Nancy, France.

[15] Lennox, J. and Rosen, C. (2002). Adaptative multiscale principal components analysis for online monitoring of wastewater treatment. *Water Science and Technology*, 45(4-5):227–235.

[16] Mallat, S. and Hwang, W.-L. (1992). Singularity detection and processing with wavelets. *IEEE Trans. on Information Theory*, 38(2):617–643.

[17] Mallat, S. and Zhong, S. (1992). Characterization of signals from multiscale edges. *IEEE Trans. on PAMI*, 14(7):710–732.

[18] Manyri, L., Regis, S., Doncescu, A., Desachy, J., and Urribelarea, J. (2003). Holder coefficient estimation by differential evolutionary algorithms for saccharomyces cerivisiae physiological states characterisation. In *ICPP-HPSECA*, Kaohsiung, Taiwan.

[19] Meyer, Y. (1990). *Ondelettes et Opérateurs*, volume I. Hermann.

[20] S. Muggleton. Inverse entailement and Progol. New Gen. Comput.,13:245-2,1998.

[21] Narasimhan, S., Mah, R., Tamhane, A., Woodward, J., and Hale, J. (1986). A composite statistical test for detecting changes in steady state. *American Institute of Chemical Engineering Journal*, 32(9):1409–1418.

[22] Nugraha, H. B. and Langi, A. Z. R. (2002). A wavelet-based measurement of fractal dimensions of a 1-d signal. In *IEEE APCCAS*, Bali, Indonesia.

[23] Polit, M., Estaben, M., and Labat, P. (2002). A fuzzy model for an anaerobic digester, comparison with experimental results. *Engineering Applications of Artificial Intelligence*, 15(5):385–390.

[24] Rocca J.. Technical report of Laboratoire d'automatisme et architecture des sytemes. 1998.

[25] Régis, S., Doncescu, A., Faure, L., and Urribelarea, J.-L. (2005). Détection et caractérisation d'un bioprocédé par l'analyse de l'exposant de hölder. In *GRETSI 2005*, Louvain-la-Neuve, Belgium.

[26] Roels, J. (1983). *Energetics and kinetics in biotechnology*. Elsevier Biomedical Press.

[27] Ruiz, G., Castellano, M., Gonzàlez, W., Roca, E., and Lema, J. (2004). Algorithm for steady states detection of multivariate process: application to wastewater anaerobic digestion process. In *AutMoNet 2004*, pages 181–188.

[28] S. Régis. *Segmentation, classification, et fusion d'informations de séries temporelles multi-sources: application à des signaux dans un bioprocédé*. Thèse de Doctorat (PhD thesis), Université des Antilles et de la Guyane, Novembre 2004.

[29] S. Régis, L. Faure, A. Doncescu, J.-L. Uribelarrea, L. Manyri, and J. Aguilar-Martin. Adaptive physiological states classification in fed-batch fermentation process. In *IFAC CAB'9*, Nancy, France, March 2004.

[30] Saporta, G. (1990). *Probabilités, et Analyse des données et Statistique*. Technip.

[31] Steyer, J., Pourciel, J., Simoes, D., and Uribelarrea, J. (1991). Qualitative knowledge modeling used in a real time expert system for biotechnological process control. In *IMACS International Workshop "Decision Support Systems and Qualitative Reasoning"*.

[32] J.P. Steyer. *Sur une approche qualitative des systèmes physiques : aide en temps rèel à la conduite des procédés fermentaires*. Thèse de Doctorat, Université Paul Sabatier, Toulouse France, Décembre 1991.

[33] Storn, R. and Price, K. (1996). Minimizing the real functions of the icec'96 contest by differential evolution. In *Proc. of the 1996 IEEE International Conference on Evolutionary Computation*.

[34] Struzik, Z. R. (1999). *Fractals: Theory and Application in Engineering*, pages 93–112. Springer Verlag.

[35] Yuille, A. and Poggio, T. (1986). Scaling theorems for zero-crossing. *IEEE Transaction for zero-crossing*, 8(1):15–25.

20

Protocol of a Seamless Recombination with Specific Selection Cassette in PCR-Based Site-Directed Mutagenesis

Qiyi Tang[1,*,#], Benjamin Silver[2,*] and Hua Zhu[2,#]
[1]*Department of Microbiology/AIDS Research Program, Ponce School of Medicine, Ponce, PR,*
[2]*Department of Microbiology and Molecular Genetics, New Jersey Medical School, Newark, NJ, USA*

1. Introduction

Genetic mutation has made great contributions to determining protein structure and function, viral pathogenesis, biological engineering, and vaccine development [1-9]. In order to alter genetic information, gene mutation (also called mutagenesis) can be achieved by many different methods. The process of mutagenesis can occur naturally, as the root of evolution; by mutagens, such as chemicals or radiation; and experimentally, by laboratory techniques [10-13]. Current experimental mutagenesis methods can be generally classified into random and directed mutation.

Experimentally directed mutagenesis methods include: insertional mutagenesis [14], PCR mutagenesis [15, 16], signature tagged mutagenesis [17], site-directed mutagenesis [18, 19] and transposon mutagenesis [20-22]. Different procedures are involved in traditional mutagenesis, including molecular cloning that depends on preparations of vector and inserted DNA fragments and ligations. This traditional mutagenesis method is not only time-consuming, but also labor intensive, and modern advancements in mutagenesis have overcome these obstacles. The development of the Bacterial Artificial Chromosome (BAC) clone of large DNA viruses was a breakthrough in the viral mutagenesis field. The BAC clone of a virus can be maintained stably and propagated inside a bacterial cell, which allows for easy manipulation of the viral genome. Any required mutation can be easily and rapidly achieved inside the *E. coli* cell and this mutation can be verified before making recombinant virus [23-27]. Since the development of this novel method for construction of recombinant viruses, detailed functional study of virus genome has been done using this specific BAC recombinatory mutagenesis approach [23-27].

Recombination is an important procedure in experimental mutagenesis. There are two recombination systems that are often used: DNA sequence-specific recombinase-driven recombination and homologous recombination. The DNA sequence-specific recombinase-driven recombination includes Cre-Lox and FLP-FRT recombination systems [28-36]. Cre-

---

* These authors contributed equally
\# Corresponding Authors

Lox system depends on Cre recombinase that specifically recognizes lox P (locus of X-over bacteriophage P1) sites, 34-basepair (bp) specific sequences and results in recombination by the excision of intervening DNA sequence and joining of site-specific ends. FLP-FRT involves the recombination of sequences between short flippase recognition target (FRT) sites (also a 34-bp DNA sequence) by the flippase recombination enzyme (FLP or Flp) derived from *Saccharomyces cerevisiae* yeast. After recombination, one copy of the specific DNA sequence will remain in the vector, which will cause potential problems for further mutagenesis, DNA stability and, therefore, is not suitable for some applications, such as vaccine development. In addition, BAC sequence excision methods should be carefully considered, depending upon the design of the BAC. For example, it will become problematic if both the BAC vector and gene-specific antibiotic marker contain the same flanking excision sequences (such as loxP) because this is likely to cause the removal of a much larger sequence of genomic DNA than originally intended.

Homologous recombination is a type of genetic recombination in which nucleotide sequences are exchanged between two identical sequences of DNA [37, 38]. Wild-type *E. coli* is ineffective at inducing homologous recombination in foreign DNA because linear DNA is commonly degraded by RecBCD exonuclease. In order to circumvent this problem, SW102 strains were developed that contain a temperature-sensitive λ prophage encoding one gene to temporarily repress RecBCD (*gam*), as well as two genes (*exo* and *beta*) utilized for homologous recombination via double-strand break repair [38]. More specifically, exonuclease degrades DNA from the 5′ end of double-strand break sites, while Beta binds to and protects the 3′ from further degradation [39, 40]. These overhangs from double-strand breaks allow recombination between viral and plasmid DNA. Because the λ phage is temperature sensitive (due to the expression of a temperature-sensitive λ *cI*-repressor), linear DNA uptake and recombination can occur within a few minutes when the cell-culture temperature is increased from 32 to 42°C [38]. This allows the bacterial cells to function normally when grown at 32°C. *E. coli* also require thousands of homologous base pairs in order for recombination to occur. Addition of the modified temperature-sensitive λ phage is important because this allows homologous recombination to occur within a relatively small region of the homologous sequence, which is important because BAC mutants are usually created using PCR-amplified gene sequences with about 40 base pairs of flanking sequences that are homologous to the viral BAC [37].

PCR-based preparation for insertion of DNA provided convenience in performing mutagenesis studies. Differential PCR techniques enable researchers to make any mutation, as needed: large deletion, point mutation, substitution, insertion, non-sense mutation and shift-mutation. Allowing for the use of a positive and negative selection system is another advancement in the area of mutagenesis, especially when applied to site-directed mutagenesis when accuracy and precision are of high priority. There are multiple ways to carry out site-directed mutagenesis of a viral BAC. For example, selectable markers are necessary to isolate the successful mutation of a viral BAC, and selectable markers can be an antibiotic resistant gene (such as kanamycin or zeocin resistant genes) or a foreign metabolic gene (such as *galK*). In the case of a gene knockout, the foreign DNA usually contains a selectable marker flanked by a DNA sequence homologous to the flanking regions for the gene of interest. Around 40 bp of a flanking sequence are typically used for homologous recombination. The viral BAC and the marker with homologous sequences are then inserted into *E. coli* via electroporation. Colonies with the BAC recombinant virus can be selected based upon selection markers and verified by PCR [27].

This protocol describes the use of the *galK* positive- and counter- selection schemes to make gene mutations (*e.g.* point mutations, deletions, and insertions) within viral BACs. This system includes only two steps of recombination within a modified bacterial strain, SW102 [41], using selection and counter-selection media, and easily designed PCR. The SW102 strain, derived from DY380 *E. coli* [38, 42, 43], differs from DY380 only in that the galactokinase (*galK*) gene of the galactose operon is defective in SW102 strain. When SW102 bacteria are incubated on minimal media with galactose as the sole source of carbon, the bacteria cannot grow without *galK* supplied *in trans* [41]. When the *galK* gene is provided *in trans*, in this case it replaces a gene of interest, it can complement the defective *galK* gene in the bacteria and the bacteria can grow in minimal media with galactose, therefore, the first step is a positive selection. Later in the protocol, when *galK* is removed from the viral BAC and replaced with a mutated version of the original gene, a counterselection takes place in that clones containing *galK* will be negatively selected for by growing the bacteria on medium with a substance that produces a toxic intermediate only when a functional *galK* is present.

This protocol explains in detail how to use the *galK* positive and counterselection strategies to make any desired mutations (*e.g.* point mutations, deletions, and insertions) based on plasmid or BAC. The modified plasmid or BAC will not contain any extra DNA sequence; therefore, it is referred to as a "seamless" mutation.

2. Materials and methods

Bacterium: *E. coli* SW102 strain (free reagents from Biological Resources Branch of NCI-Frederick) [41]
Plasmid: p*galK* (free reagents from Biological Resources Branch of NCI-Frederick) [41]
Luria-Broth (LB) medium

Tryptone	10 g
Yeast Extract	5 g
NaCl	10 g

Dissolve components in distilled and deionized water (ddH_2O) and adjust the total volume up to 1 liter.
For LB agar: add agar to a final concentration of 1.5%.

Heat the mixture to boiling to dissolve agar and sterilize by autoclaving at 15 psi, from 121-124°C for 15 minutes.

1X M9 medium (1 liter)
6 g Na_2HPO_4
3 g KH_2PO_4
1 g NH_4Cl
0.5 g NaCl

Dissolve components in ddH_2O and make the total volume up to 1 liter. Autoclave

M63 minimal plates

1L 5X M63
10 g $(NH_4)_2SO_4$
68 g KH_2PO_4
2.5 mg $FeSO_4 \cdot 7H_2O$
Dissolve components in ddH_2O and make the total volume up to 1 liter. Adjust to pH 7 with KOH.
Autoclave

Other Reagents

0.2 mg/ml D-biotin (sterile filtered) (1:5000)
20% galactose (autoclaved) (1:100)
20% 2-deoxy-galactose (autoclaved) (1:100)
20% glycerol (autoclaved) (1:100)
10 mg/ml L-leucine (1%, heated, then cooled down and sterile filtered)
25 mg/ml chloramphenicol in Ethanol (1:2000)
1 M $MgSO_4 \cdot 7H_2O$ (1:1000)

Procedure of making the M63 minimal plates:

1. Autoclave 15 g agar in 800 ml H_2O in a 2-liter flask.
2. Add 200 ml autoclaved 5X M63 medium and 1 ml 1 M $MgSO_4 \cdot 7\ H_2O$.
3. Adjust volume to 1 liter with H_2O if necessary.
4. Let cool down to 50°C ("hand touchable hot"), add 10 ml carbon source (final concentration 0.2%), 5 ml biotin (1 mg), 4.5 ml leucine (45 mg), and 500 µl chloramphenicol (final concentration 12.5 mg/ml) or other appropriate antibiotics. Pour the plates, 33-40 plates per liter.

MacConkey indicator plates:

Prepare MacConkey agar plus galactose according to manufacturer's instructions. After autoclaving and cooling to 50°C, to one liter, add 500 µl chloramphenicol (final concentration 12.5 mg/ml) or other appropriate antibiotics, and pour the plates, 33-40 plates per liter.

3. Protocol

3.1 Preparing SW102 that harbors plasmid or BAC

Select the plasmid or BAC that contains the target gene and will be used as a vector for making mutations. Information about the vector, including antibiotic-resistance and the targeted gene, needs to be known. For example, to make any mutation of a gene in murine cytomegalovirus (MCMV), the BAC of SM3fr [46] is usually used. SM3fr contains whole genome of MCMV with chloramphenicol resistance. The DNA sequence and gene structure of SM3fr have been published and can be accessed in public gene bank.

3.1.1 Preparation of electrocompetent cells (Fig. 1. 1a)

1. A 5-ml overnight culture of *E. coli* SW102 in LB medium will be prepared either from the frozen stock or from a single colony at 32°C or lower. The SW102 strain is resistant

to tetracycline (12.5 μg/ml), it is not necessary, but safe to include tetracycline in this step in order to exclude any possible contamination.

2. The overnight LB culture of SW102 will be diluted by 1:50 by adding 0.5 ml of the overnight culture to an autoclaved 50 ml Erlenmeyer baffled flask with 25 ml LB, but first save 1 ml LB that will be used as a reference for measuring the OD_{600nm}. The diluted SW102 in the flask will be incubated for 3-5 hrs with appropriate antibiotic selection in a 32°C shaking incubator until the density reaches an OD_{600nm} of 0.6. At this point, a bottle of ice-cold 10% glycerol or autoclaved ddH_2O needs to be prepared. (If the competent cells are to be used right away, use autoclaved ddH_2O). The competent cells can be used right away or stored at -70°C for later use.
3. When the OD_{600nm} is 0.6, the flasks containing the bacteria will be cooled down in the ice water bath slurry for a minute or two and subsequently transferred into pre-cooled 15 ml Falcon tubes.
4. The bacteria will be centrifuged in a cold centrifuge (4°C) for 5 min at 5000 RPM (standard Beckman or Eppendorf centrifuge).
5. All supernatant will be poured off and the centrifuge tubes will be briefly inverted on a paper towel, and 1 ml ice-cold ddH_2O or 10% glycerol will be added to resuspend the pellet. And the tube will be kept in the ice. The pellet will be resuspended in the ddH_2O or 10% glycerol by gently shaking the tube in the ice-water bath (gently move the tubes around in circles while keeping them in the ice water slurry, this can take a while for the first time). When the cells are completely resuspended, another 9 ml ice-cold ddH_2O or 10% glycerol will be added, the tube will be inverted for a couple of times, and centrifuged again for 5 minutes.
6. The supernatant will be poured off and the pellet will be resuspended with 10 ml ice-cold ddH_2O or 10% glycerol, as in Step 5, resuspension should be much faster this time).
7. The resuspended cells will be centrifuged once more, as in Step 5.
8. The supernatant will be completely removed by inverting the tube on a paper towel (be careful that you do not lose the pellet). The pellet will be resuspended in 250 μl ice-cold 10% glycerol. The competent cells can be used immediately for transformation or aliquoted and stored at -80°C (volume should be around 50 μl).

3.1.2 Transformation by electroporation (Fig. 1. 1b)

1. Plasmid or BAC DNA will be transformed into the SW102 competent cells made in Step 1.1. The freshly made or stored electrocompetent cells will be mixed with 1-5 μg DNA. The mixture of cells and DNA will be transferred to a pre-cooled 0.1 cm cuvette. It is important that the DNA solution contains low salt because high salt can cause electric shock during electroporation.
2. The cuvette will be placed into the electroporator power source and cuvette holder (Bio-Rad). The conditions for transformation are set according to the strain. For SW102 cells, use 25 mFD, 200 W, and 1.8 kV. The time constant (tau value) should be 3-4 msec. After the electroporation, the bacteria will be transferred immediately to a tube with 1 ml LB medium and incubated at 32°C in a shaking water bath for 1 hr.
3. The incubated bacteria will be smeared onto LB agar plates that contain appropriate antibiotics. The transformed bacteria on selective LB agar will grow as colonies after incubation at 32°C for 18-24 hrs.

4. The generated SW102 harboring plasmid or BAC will be verified by picking up a colony, isolating the DNA by BAC Minipreparation (see Step 1.3.) and detecting the DNA with PCR analysis of the BAC (Fig. 3) and/or restriction enzyme digestion (Fig. 4). This plasmid- or BAC-harboring SW102 will be given a name and used to make desired mutation of the target gene. For example, if the SW102 harbors MCMV BAC SM3fr, it will be called SW102_SM3fr.

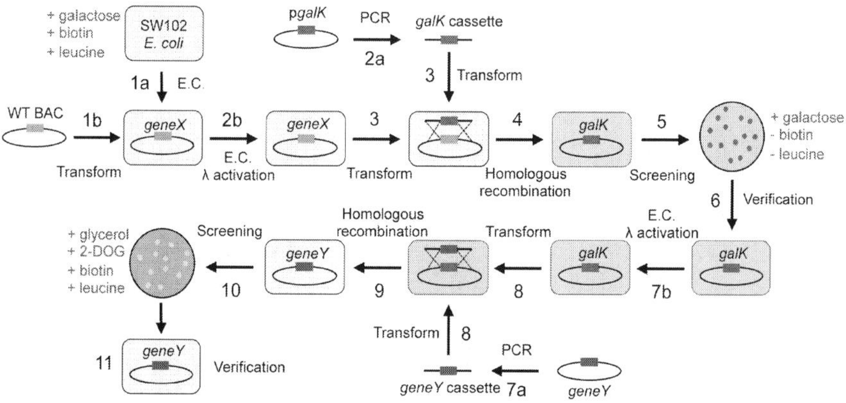

Fig. 1. **Summary of the *galK*-based mutagenesis in *E. coli* SW102. 1a.** Prepare electrocompetent (E.C.) SW102 *E. coli*. **1b.** Electroporate WT virus BAC into electrocompetent SW102. **2a.** Prepare *galK* cassette by PCR with a set of primers conferring sequence homology to the viral BAC sequences flanking *geneX*. **2b.** Prepare electrocompetent SW102 *E. coli* harboring WT viral BAC and activate defective λ phage recombination system by shaking in a 42°C water bath for 15 minutes. **3.** Electroporate the *galK*-expressing cassette into recombination-activated electrocompetent SW102 strain harboring WT BAC. **4.** Upon homologous recombination, *geneX* is replaced by *galK*. **5.** Confirm presence of *galK* by growing bacteria on M63 plates with galactose as the sole source of carbon and antibiotic, selecting colonies to screen on MacConkey agar with galactose as the sole source of carbon. The *galK*-containing recombinant clones will produce red colonies on MacConkey agar with galactose. **6.** Select red colony from screening process to verify by PCR and continue. **7a.** Prepare *geneY* cassette (PCR cassette containing desired mutation in *geneX*, referred to as *geneY*). **7b.** From red colony selected in Step 5, prepare electrocompetent SW102 harboring *galK* mutant BAC and activate defective λ phage recombination system, as in 2b. **8.** Electroporate *geneY* cassette into electrocompetent and recombination-activated SW102 containing *galK* mutant clone. **9.** Upon homologous recombination, *galK* is replaced by *geneY*. **10.** Grow bacteria on M63 with glycerol, DOG and antibiotic agar plates. **11.** Select colony and verify for production of virus.

3.1.3 BAC minipreparation

The following protocol is usually used and works very well for generating BAC DNA for initial analysis:

1. 5 ml overnight LB culture with chloramphenicol (almost all known BACs are chloramphenicol resistant) in a 15-ml Falcon tube is pelleted, and the supernatant is removed.
2. Then the pellet is dissolved in 250 µl buffer P1 (Miniprep kit, Qiagen, CA) and transferred to an Eppendorf tube.
3. The bacteria are lysed in 250 µl P2 buffer with gently mixing and incubating for 5 min at room temperature.
4. The lysate is neutralized with 250 µl buffer P3 (also called N3 buffer), followed by mixing and incubating on ice for 5 min.
5. The supernatant is cleared by two rounds of centrifugation at 13,200 RPM for 5 min in a small Eppendorf centrifuge (or other model tabletop centrifuge). Each time the supernatant is transferred to a new tube.
6. The DNA is precipitated by adding 750 µl isopropanol, mixing and incubating on ice for 10 min, and centrifugation for 10 min at 13,200 RPM in a small Eppendorf centrifuge (or other model tabletop centrifuge).
7. The pellet is washed once in 70% ethanol and the air-dried pellet is dissolved in 50-100 µl TE buffer. The isolated BAC DNA can be used for 1) restriction analysis, 2) PCR analysis and 3) DNA sequencing analysis.

3.2 Positive selection to replace the targeted DNA with *galK* gene

3.2.1 PCR to generate the *galK* cassette (Fig. 1. 2a)

1. Design primers with 50 bp homology flanking the desired site to be modified. The 3′ end of these primers will bind to the *galK* cassette. For example, if a single base pair (bp) mutation will be generated, the homology arms should extend 50 bp on either side of the target bp. If the target bp is not included in the arms, it will result in a deletion of that base pair in the first step. If the target bp was changed into another bp in the arm, it will result in single bp mutation. If a small or a large deletion will be made, design the *galK* primers so that the deletion is made already in the first step. The primers should be as follows:

Forward: 5′ 50bp homology: CCTGTTGACAATTAATCATCGGCA-3′
Reverse: 5′ 50bp homology complementary strand: TCAGCACTGTCCTGCTCCTT-3′

2. Plasmid p*galK* will be used for PCR to amplify the *galK* gene using the primers designed as above and a proofreading DNA polymerase. It is important to use this type of DNA polymerase because the two-step substitution in the procedure will use PCR products and accuracy is a high priority. DNA template for PCR is the p*galK* plasmid. PCR can be started at 94°C for 4 min to denature the template, followed with 30 cycles of three temperatures: 94°C, 15 sec; 60°C, 30 sec; 72°C, 1 min; and the PCR will be extended for 7 min at 72°C.
3. When the PCR is finished, 1-2 µl DpnI (New England Biolabs, MA) should be added into each 25 µl reaction that is mixed and incubated at 37°C for 1 hour. This step serves to remove any plasmid template; plasmid is methylated so that DpnI can degrade it, PCR products are not methylated so DpnI cannot degrade it. Finally, the DpnI-digested PCR product will be separated in agarsoe gel and purified from gel. The PCR product will be eluted with 50 µl ddH_2O, 10-30 ng will be used for transformation.

3.2.2 Preparation of electrocompetent cells harboring BAC

SW102 *E. coli* strain has a defective λ prophage that, when activated, can produce recombinase. These activated and electrocompetent SW102 harboring plasmid or BAC DNA (*e.g.* SW102_SM3fr) (Fig. 1. 2b) will be prepared from the electrocompetent SW102 harboring plasmid or BAC DNA prepared in Step 1.2 of the protocol. The procedure is as follows:

1. Inoculate an overnight culture of SW102 cells containing the BAC in 5 ml LB with appropriate antibiotics (*e.g.* SW102_SM3fr in LB with chloramphenicol) at 32°C.
2. Next day, add 0.5 ml of the overnight SW102 harboring plasmid or BAC DNA in 25 ml LB with antibiotics in a 50-ml baffled conical flask and incubate at 32°C in a shaking water bath to an OD_{600nm} of approximately 0.6 (0.55-0.6). This usually takes 3-4 hrs. During this time, turn on two shaking water baths: one at 32°C, the other at 42°C. Make ice/water slurry and pre-chill 50 ml of ddH_2O.
3. When the OD_{600nm} of SW102 harboring plasmid or BAC DNA culture reaches 0.6, transfer 10 ml of the culture to another baffled 50-ml conical flask and heat-shock at 42°C for exactly 15 min in a shaking water bath. This step is to induce SW102 to produce recombinase. The remaining culture is left at 32°C as the un-induced control.
4. After 15 min induction, the SW102 in two flasks (10 ml induced and 10 ml un-induced) are briefly cooled in ice-water bath and then transferred to two 15-ml Falcon tubes and centrifuged at 4°C. It is important to keep the bacteria as close to 0°C as possible in order to get high efficiency competent cells.
5. Pour off all of the supernatant and resuspend the pellet in 1 ml ice-cold autoclaved ddH_2O by gently swirling the tubes in the ice-water bath slurry (no pipetting). This step may take a while. When the cells are resuspended, add another 9 ml ice-cold autoclaved ddH_2O. Pellet the samples again as in Step 1.4.
6. Resuspend the pellet again with I ml of ice-cold autoclaved ddH_2O by gently swirling and then add 9 ml ddH2O. The bacteria are centrifuged again, as above.
7. After the second washing and centrifugation step, all supernatant must be removed by inverting the tubes on a paper towel, and the pellet is resuspended in approximately 50 µl of ice-cold ddH_2O and is kept on ice until electroporated with PCR product. If the electrocompetent cells are prepared with 10% glycerol, the aliquots can be made and saved at -80°C for later use.

3.2.3 Electroporation of *galK* cassette

1. 25 µl of electrocompetent SW102 cells harboring plasmid or BAC DNA and 10-30 ng of PCR amplified *galK* cassette will be added to a 0.1 cm cuvette (BioRad). Electroporation will be carried out at 25 mF, 1.75 kV, and 200 ohms (Fig. 1. 3). After reaction, 1 ml LB will be immediately added to the cells, and the cells will be cultured at 32°C for 1 hour in a shaking water bath.
2. After the recovery incubation, the bacteria are washed twice with M9 buffer as follows: 1 ml of the culture is centrifuged in an Eppendorf tube at 13,200 RPM for 15 sec. Then the supernatant is removed with a pipette. The pellet is resuspended with 1 ml M9 buffer, and pelleted again. This washing step will be performed once more. After the second wash, the supernatant will be removed and the pellet will be resuspended in 1 ml M9 buffer. A serial of dilutions in M9 buffer will be made (100 µl, 100 µl of a 1:10 dilution, and 100 µl 1:100) and plated onto M63 minimal media plates with galactose,

leucine, biotin, and appropriate antibiotics (Fig. 1. 5). It is important to remove any rich media from the culture prior to selection on minimal media by washing the bacteria in M9 buffer. The uninduced SW102 will be plated as a control.

3. The plates will be incubated for 3 days at 32°C in a cabinet-type incubator. Colonies will be visible at the beginning of third day and be able to be picked up at the end of that day.
4. Pick up a few colonies and streak the colonies onto MacConkey agar plates with galactose, indicator and appropriate antibiotics to obtain single colonies (Fig. 1. 5). The colonies appearing after the 3 days of incubation should be *galK* positive, but in order to get rid of any *galK* negative contaminants (usually called hitch-hikers), it is important to obtain single, bright red colonies before proceeding to next step (Fig. 1. 6). *galK* negative colonies will be white or colorless and the *galK* positive bacteria will be bright red or pink due to a pH change resulting from fermented galactose after an overnight incubation at 32°C (Fig. 2).
5. Pick up a few bright red (*galK* positive) colonies and inoculate in 5 ml LB + antibiotics and incubate overnight at 32°C. There is normally no need to further characterize the clones. But the *galK* positive clones can be Miniprepared (Step 1.3) and verified by PCR using primers that flank the site of the *galK* gene (Fig. 3):

Forward: 5′ CTGTTGACAATTAATCATCGGCA-3′
Reverse: 5′ TCAGCACTGTCCTGCTCCTT-3′

The recombinant *galK* clones should be named for storage. Take MCMV BAC as an example: SW102_SM3fr_X*galK* is the name of the bacteria and SM3fr_X*galK* is the name of the BAC. "X" stands for the site of the *galK* in the BAC.

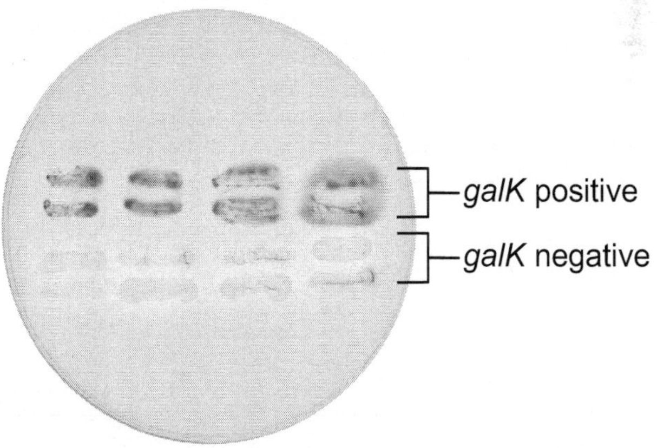

Fig. 2. **Positive selection for *galK* mutant clones and negative selection for WT/mutant/rescue clones.** SW102 bacteria with WT, *galK* mutant (*geneX* replaced by *galK* gene), *geneY* mutant (*galK* replaced by mutated *geneX*), or rescue (*geneX* restored) BACs were plated on MacConkey agar with galactose as the sole source of carbon and antibiotic. Recombinant BAC clones containing *galK* appear as red colonies; clones with WT BAC, *geneY* mutant BAC, or rescue BAC appear as white/colorless colonies.

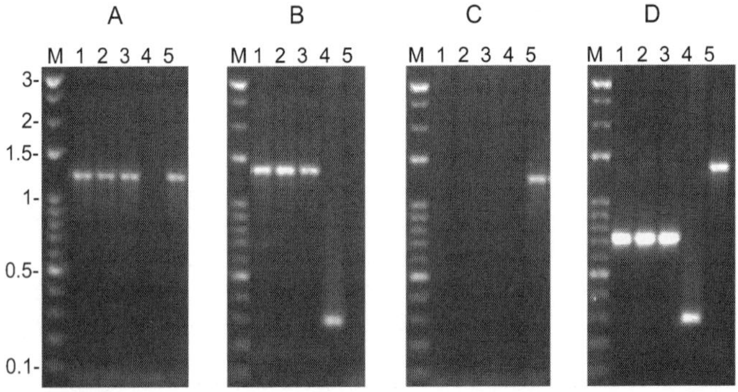

Fig. 3. **PCR verification. A.** PCR using *galK* primers with *galK* mutant clones (*geneX* replaced by *galK* – clones produced from Fig. 1. 4) as template. 1.3kb band indicates presence of *galK* gene: Lanes 1-3 are *galK* mutant clones #1-3, respectively; Lane 4 is original BAC (negative control); Lane 5 is p*galK* (positive control). **B.** PCR using primers that override the homologous sequences with *galK* mutant clones as template. 1.4kb band indicates presence of *galK*+BAC sequence, 300 bp band indicates BAC sequence only: Lanes 1-3 are *galK* mutant clones #1-3, respectively; Lane 4 is original BAC (positive control); Lane 5 is p*galK* (negative control). **C.** PCR using *galK* primers with mutant clones (*galK* replaced by *geneY*) as template (mutant clones #1-3 were created, respectively, from *galK* mutant clones #1-3 in Panels 1+2). 1.4kb band indicates presence of *galK*+BAC sequence: Lanes 1-3 are mutant clones #1-3, respectively; Lane 4 is original BAC (negative control); Lane 5 is a *galK* mutant clone used to derive a mutant clone (i.e. *galK* mutant clone #1 from Panels 1+2) (positive control). **D.** PCR using primers that override the homologous sequences with mutant clones as template. 700 bp band indicates presence of mutant gene (*geneY*), 300 bp band indicates WT BAC sequence, 1.4kb band indicates presence of *galK*+BAC sequence: Lanes 1-3 are mutant clones #1-3, respectively; Lane 4 is original BAC (positive control); Lane 5 is a *galK* mutant clone used to derive a mutant clone (positive control). All gel electrophoreses were on 1% agarose gels. M = 1 kb-Opti DNA Marker (ABM, Canada). Marker units are kilobases.

3.3 Counterselection to replace the *galK* gene for desired mutant generation

3.3.1 PCR to generate the DNA fragment to substitute *galK* gene (Fig. 1. 7a)

Design primers with 50 bp homology flanking the desired site to be modified. This 50 bp homology is usually the same as that in making *galK* gene. Usually the mutations are contained in the templates. The DNA template is a WT BAC or plasmid with the gene of interest mutated in the required fashion. The PCR product should therefore contain the desired mutations.

Forward: 5′ 50bp homology target gene (18-20 bp)
Reverse: 5′ 50bp homology complementary strand target gene (18-20 bp)

3.3.2 Electroporation of DNA fragment (same conditions as in Step 2.2)

1. Both the preparation of electrocompetent cells from the SW102 harboring plasmid or BAC with *galK* gene and the activation of defective λ prophage recombinase are

necessary (Fig. 1. 7b), and the procedure is a repetition of the prepration and activation of electrocompetent SW102 harboring WT BAC or plasmid in Step 2.2.

2. Transform the PCR product into electrocompetent SW102 harboring *galK* mutant plasmid or BAC by electroporation with 0.2-1 μg of PCR product that contains the desired mutation and with homology to the area flanking the *galK* gene (Fig. 1. 8). After electroporation, the bacteria will be recovered in 10 ml LB in a 50 ml baffled conical flask by incubating at 32°C in a shaking water bath for 4.5 hrs. This long recovery period serves to obtain bacteria that only contain the desired recombined BAC or plasmid, and thus have lost any BAC still containing the *galK* cassette.
3. 1 ml of the recovery culture will be centrifuged and the pellet will be resuspended with M9 buffer and washed twice with M9 buffer. After second washing, the pellet will be resuspended in 1 ml of M9 buffer and the bacteria will be plated in a serial dilution (100 μl, 100 μl of a 1:10 dilution and 100 μl 1:100) onto M63 minimal media plates that contain glycerol, leucine, biotin, 2-deoxygalactose (DOG), and appropriate antibiotics (Fig. 1. 10).
4. Incubate at 32°C for three days. Further verification can be accomplished by PCR and/or DNA sequencing (Fig. 1. 11). A name is required for any mutation. For MCMV BAC, we name the bacterial strain SW102_SM3fr_XY and the BAC SM3fr_XY. "X" stands for the site of the mutation in the BAC genome, and "Y" stands for the mutations (deletion, insertion, point mutation or other). For BAC mutagenesis, especially for making any mutation on viruses, a rescue BAC for each mutation is very important.

3.4 Generation of rescue clone of each mutation

The mutagenesis protocol, for some purposes, does not need to progress to this step. However, for some studies, especially for viral mutagenesis, it is necessary to make rescue viruses so that the observed phenotype can be compared and confirmed. The same *galK* method will be used to make a rescue clone that was used to generate the original mutation, except for starting with the mutant BAC and working backwards.

1. The SW102_XY will be used to make electrocompetent cells, using the same procedure as in Step 2.2.
2. The competent cells will be electroporated with the PCR product of *galK* cassette (exactly the same cassette as the one produced in Step 2.1), which will result in SW102_X*galK*.
3. After growth and verification, SW102_X*galK* will undergo electrocompetent cell preparation, as before, and electroporated with a DNA fragment that will be made using the same primers, but with a template that contains no mutation.
4. Therefore the rescue clone is made using the backwards steps. We can also give a name such as SW102_XYRes for the bacteria.

3.5 Maxipreparation of BAC DNA (all recombinant clones)

Now, all of the plasmids or BAC DNA can be isolated for any purpose, *e.g.* in the case of herpesviruses, the BAC DNA needs to be isolated and purified for making viruses. Since BAC is usually a large DNA vector, its isolation and identification are different from that of regular plasmid protocol. Fortunately, several high quality kits have been commercially available for preparation of BAC DNA on a large-scale. In this case, the BAC DNA needs to be extracted from the SW102_XY (or SW102_X as a control) for transfection and production of virus.

1. Select a colony to inoculate 5 ml LB with chloramphenicol (final concentration 12.5 mg/ml) and shake overnight in an incubator at 32°C.

2. The following day, save 200-500 µl of culture to make a stock (see below), and add the remainder of the 5 ml culture to 500 ml LB with chloramphenicol (final concentration 12.5 mg/ml) and shake overnight in an incubator at 32°C. To make a bacterial stock, add 100% glycerol to the saved culture to a final concentration of 15% glycerol and store at -80°C.
3. Use the Nucleobond Maxiprep BAC DNA isolation kit (Clontech Laboratories Inc., CA) to extract BAC DNA from the culture. Because of their large size, BAC DNAs need to be handled in a way that avoids any harsh physical shearing force, including vortexing or passing quickly through fine pipette tips. Freeze-and-thaw should also be avoided.
4. The final DNA products are resuspended in 250 µl sterile ddH_2O and quantified by spectroscopy.
5. BAC DNA solutions should always be stored at 4°C.

3.6 Verification of BAC DNA integrity [Varicella zoster virus (VZV) is used as an example in the following sections]

1. Digest 3 µg of mutant BAC DNA, with WT digestion in parallel as control, with 20 U of restriction enzyme. Example: 3 µl of 1 µg/µl VZV WT BAC DNA, 20 U (1 µl) HindIII restriction enzyme (New England Biolabs, MA), 1 µl 10X NEBuffer 2 (New England Biolabs, MA), 5 µl ddH_2O.
2. Incubate overnight at 37°C and run gel electrophoresis on 0.5% agarose gel. Fig. 4 highlights the pattern observed when digesting WT VZV BAC, ORF7 Deletion VZV BAC, and ORF7 Rescue VZV BAC, respectively.

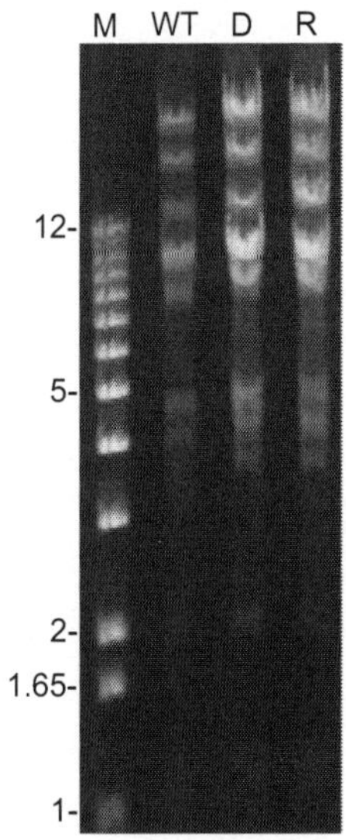

Fig. 4. **Verification of BAC DNA integrity.** For all BACs, 3 µg BAC DNA was digested with 20 U HindIII restriction enzyme overnight at 37°C and ran electrophoretically on 0.5% agarose gel. M: 1 kb Plus DNA Ladder (Invitrogen, CA), units are kb; WT: VZV WT BAC DNA; D: VZV ORF7 Deletion BAC DNA; R: VZV ORF7 Rescued BAC DNA.

3.7 Transfection of BAC DNA for virus production

BAC DNA from Maxi-preparations is transfected into human cells (*e.g.* MeWo, ARPE-19) using the FuGene 6 transfection kit (Roche, Indianapolis, IN), according to manufacturer's standard protocol. 1.5 µg of BAC DNA and 6 µl of transfection reagent are used for a single reaction in one well of 6-well tissue culture plates. Highly concentrated (>250 µg/µl) BAC DNA solutions are viscous, and BAC DNA molecules easily precipitate out of the solution when added to transfection reagent solutions. When such precipitation becomes visible, it is irreversible; predictably, the results of the transfection assays are often poor. Therefore, pre-dilute each BAC DNA before gently mixing it with the transfection reagent.

1. For each reaction, 1.5 µg of BAC DNA is diluted in serum-free medium, and the volume of DNA solution is adjusted to 50 µl with the serum-free medium.
2. For each reaction, 6 µl of transfection reagent is combined with 94 µl of medium.
3. Using pipettor tips, gently stir the DNA solution into the transfection reagent.
4. Incubate mixture for 25 minutes at room temperature.
5. Add DNA-transfection reagent solution to culture plate.

3.8 Infected cell culture

1. Transfected cells are grown in a 6-well tissue culture plate in 2 ml DMEM supplemented with 10% fetal calf serum, 100U of penicillin-streptomycin/ml, and 2.5 ug of amphotericin B/ml [47, 48].
2. Upon visualization of infection, Usually viral plaques will be developed and visualized under microscopy as shown in Fig. 5.

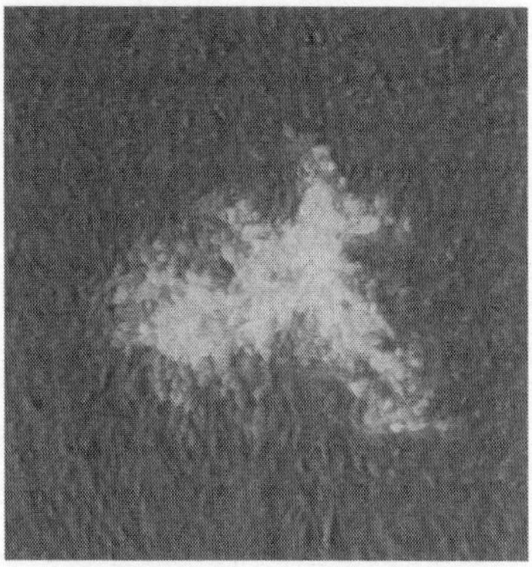

Fig. 5. **Generation of VZV by transfection of viral BAC DNA.** Human ARPE-19 cells were chemically transfected with WT VZV BAC DNA. Infected cells expressing EGFP (inserted into BAC vector) and form green plaques. One plaque is visualized by fluorescent microscope.

3.9 Summary of the protocol

The protocol of the seamless recombination with specific selection cassette in PCR-based site-directed mutagenesis is summarized in Fig. 1, using BAC as an example. Firstly, SW102 *E. coli* is made to be electrocompetent (E.C.) (Fig. 1. 1a). Then, the WT BAC is electroporated into the electrocompetent SW102 (Fig. 1. 1b). The *galK* cassette is prepared by PCR with a set of primers conferring sequence homology to the viral BAC sequences flanking *geneX* (Fig. 1. 2a). Electrocompetent SW102 *E. coli* harboring WT viral BAC is prepared, and the defective λ phage recombination system is activated by shaking in a 42°C water bath for 15 minutes (Fig. 1. 2b). The *galK*-expressing cassette is electroporated into recombination-activated SW102 strain harboring WT BAC (Fig. 1. 3). Upon homologous recombination, *geneX* is replaced by *galK* (Fig. 1. 4). The presence of *galK* in the recombinant clones is selected by growing bacteria on M63 plates with galactose as the sole source of carbon and the proper antibiotic. Colonies are then selected to screen on MacConkey agar with galactose as the sole source of carbon. The *galK*-containing recombinant clones will produce red colonies on MacConkey agar with galactose (Fig. 1. 5). Fig. 2 highlights the easily perceived selection model of the *galK* mutagenesis approach, as red colonies are indicative of *galK* presence, whereas the colorless colonies do not express *galK*. A red colony from the screening process is chosen to verify by PCR and continue on with the rest of the protocol (Fig. 1. 6). A *geneY* cassette (PCR cassette containing desired mutation in *geneX*, referred to as *geneY*, or other gene) is prepared by PCR with primers conferring homologous sequences to the *galK* region in the mutant BAC (Fig. 1. 7a). From the red colony, SW102 harboring *galK* mutant BAC, selected in Step 5, are prepared to be electrocompetent and recombination-activated as in Fig. 1. 2b (Fig. 1. 7b). The *geneY* cassette is electroporated into the electrocompetent and recombination-activated SW102 strain harboring *galK* mutant clone (Fig. 1. 8). Upon homologous recombination, *galK* is replaced by *geneY* (Fig. 1. 9). Bacteria are grown on M63 with glycerol, DOG and antibiotic agar plates to counterselect for recombinant mutant BACs (Fig. 1. 10). Since the recombinants will now lack *galK*, selection takes place against the *galK* cassette by resistance to 2-deoxy-galactose (DOG) on minimal plates with glycerol as the carbon source (Fig. 1. 10) [27]. DOG is harmless, unless phosphorylated by functional *galK*. Phosphorylation by *galK* turns DOG into 2-deoxy-galactose-1-phosphate, a toxic intermediate [44]. From the resulting DOG-resistant colonies, some will be background colonies, where the bacteria have lost the *galK* cassette by a deletion, and the rest will be truly recombinant clones. Therefore, recombinant colonies containing the modified gene sequence can be quickly selected due to the negative or counterselection of colonies with *galK*, which makes this timesaving system also highly efficient. The resulting recombinant clones will be verified by PCF (Fig. 3) and restriction enzyme digestion (Fig. 4). Transfection of the mutated viral BAC into mammalian cells then produces an infectious virus (Fig. 5) [43].

4. Discussion

Molecular cloning vectors were once plasmids that could only carry and replicate small-sized DNA and have been developed to yeast artificial chromosome (YAC), bacterial artificial chromosome (BAC) and bacteriophage P1-derived artificial chromosome (PAC) that can carry and replicate large DNA molecules. Based on these vectors, recombineering techniques have contributed profoundly to investigating protein structure, function, and to elucidate viral pathogenesis, among others. However, the methods for BAC mutagenesis we use today were not easily attained as the large size of BACs posed a serious obstacle for their exact manipulation, as is required for viral research. To overcome these obstacles, techniques were developed that utilized the power of homologous recombination in order to create recombinant viruses, with the ability to safeguard every step in the process. We can now replace, and therefore delete, large DNA fragments with selectable marker cassettes, and within the described *galK* mutagenesis system there is also a counterselection model as well, using new systems that circumvent the problems associated with conventional genetic engineering as there is no longer a size restriction as seen when using restriction enzymes or other previous methods [37,44].

As previously mentioned, the generation of both the mutant and rescued BACs within the *galK* system take advantage of counterselection. For all such counterselection schemes, any event that leads to the loss of the counterselectable marker during negative selection will mean the survival of unwanted bacteria, leading to trace amounts of background. In the *galK* system, BAC replication appears to be the epicenter of background formation [41]. Despite the reliable stability of BACs, rare deletions do occur during counterselection, leading to background. Although there is spontaneous deletion background, it is insignificant relative to the great percentage of correct recombinants due to the high frequency of recombination from the λ prophage system. Furthermore, increasing the length of homology arms used for recombination can increase specific homologous recombination efficient and reduce the number of background deletions relative to the increased number of correct recombinants.

So far, most mutagenesis studies using the BAC system require generation of a rescue clone of the mutation to assure that no mutations occur anywhere other than the target site. The procedure of making rescue BAC DNA requires an original DNA fragment to be inserted back into the viral genome. This can be achieved by PCR amplification of the DNA fragment along with homology arms flanking the mutated region and insertion of the amplified fragment back into the mutant genome by homologous recombination. This method is analogous to procedure for generating recombinant mutants, as the only difference lies in the fact that there is no designed point mutation or deletion achieved via PCR. Antibiotic-resistance selection systems are the most extensively used method, however, removal of the antibiotic-resistance gene is not only necessary for functional analysis of a viral gene, but also required for preparing viral vaccine strains. The *galK* mutagenesis protocol outlined above is a seamless mutagenesis model because there is no requirement for further excision of the flanking homologous sequences that contain LoxP or FRT that might cause the loss of viral DNA during the process of making viruses in mammalian cells, as there is in antibiotic-resistance based mutagenesis. Thus, the process of making mutants by the above-mentioned protocol is considered to be accurate as there are no unintended mutations that could occur as a result, and even if there are, the strong counterselection strategy and troubleshooting strategies help to clear any background mutants.

5. Conclusion

These and other various advantages are responsible for the increased efficacy of the homologous recombination-based method for the construction of recombinant viruses. Outdated procedures for traditional mutagenesis, including molecular cloning that depends on preparations of vector and inserted DNA fragments and ligations, are laboring and time-intensive. The development of the Bacterial Artificial Chromosome (BAC) clone of large DNA viruses was an innovation that advanced the viral mutagenesis field to a new peak for global mutation and pathogenesis studies as any required mutation can be easily and rapidly achieved by the novel recombineering method for construction of recombinant viruses by homologous recombination. This mutagenesis method has led to a great expansion in the field of molecular research, whereas *galK* mutagenesis takes this recombineering strategy to a heightened level of accuracy and, therefore, results.

6. Future directions

The amount of biomedical research utilizing plasmids and BACs has grown rapidly during the past decade, resulting in invaluable knowledge about protein structure and function, viral pathogenesis, vaccine development and gene therapy. Since the construction of the first herpesvirus BAC 12 years ago, BACs have been generated for all major human and animal herpesviruses, and this technology has greatly facilitated genetic and functional studies of herpesviruses, because recombinant viruses, especially herpesviruses, were previously difficult to produce due to their large size. Soon, we may have BACs for not only all herpesviruses [27], but all DNA viruses, as well as novel global mutational studies for several virus BACs thanks to accurate and seamless mutagenesis procedures such as the *galK* recombineering protocol. Global and local studies of virus pathogenesis should help identify new antiviral targets and produce more effective and safe vaccines. In short, future virus BAC-based mutagenesis studies achieved by the seamless *galK* mutagenesis protocol should help provide exciting new discoveries about viral pathogenesis, protein structure and function, as well as therapeutics for both viral and non-viral diseases.

7. References

[1] Ahmed, R., et al., *Genetic analysis of in vivo-selected viral variants causing chronic infection: importance of mutation in the L RNA segment of lymphocytic choriomeningitis virus.* J Virol, 1988. 62(9): p. 3301-8.

[2] Chow, L.H., *Studies of virus-induced myocardial injury in mice: value of the scid mutation on different genetic backgrounds and combined with other mutations.* Lab Anim Sci, 1993. 43(2): p. 133-5.

[3] Cutter, J.L., *All that was needed for a pandemic to occur was a genetic mutation in the H5N1 virus that would enable efficient human-to-human transmission. Afterword.* Ann Acad Med Singapore, 2011. 39(4): p. 343-2.

[4] Figlerowicz, M., P.D. Nagy, and J.J. Bujarski, *A mutation in the putative RNA polymerase gene inhibits nonhomologous, but not homologous, genetic recombination in an RNA virus.* Proc Natl Acad Sci U S A, 1997. 94(5): p. 2073-8.

[5] Garcia-Lerma, J.G., et al., *A novel genetic pathway of human immunodeficiency virus type 1 resistance to stavudine mediated by the K65R mutation.* J Virol, 2003. 77(10): p. 5685-93.

[6] Taddie, J.A. and P. Traktman, *Genetic characterization of the vaccinia virus DNA polymerase: cytosine arabinoside resistance requires a variable lesion conferring phosphonoacetate resistance in conjunction with an invariant mutation localized to the 3'-5' exonuclease domain.* J Virol, 1993. 67(7): p. 4323-36.

[7] Treanor, J., et al., *Evaluation of the genetic stability of the temperature-sensitive PB2 gene mutation of the influenza A/Ann Arbor/6/60 cold-adapted vaccine virus.* J Virol, 1994. 68(12): p. 7684-8.

[8] Chavali, S., et al., *Protein molecular function influences mutation rates in human genetic diseases with allelic heterogeneity.* Biochem Biophys Res Commun, 2011. 412(4): p. 716-22.

[9] Liu, Z., et al., *Beyond the rotamer library: genetic algorithm combined with the disturbing mutation process for upbuilding protein side-chains.* Proteins, 2003. 50(1): p. 49-62.

[10] Mason, A.B., et al., *Evolution reversed: the ability to bind iron restored to the N-lobe of the murine inhibitor of carbonic anhydrase by strategic mutagenesis.* Biochemistry, 2008. 47(37): p. 9847-55.

[11] Mohan, U. and U.C. Banerjee, *Molecular evolution of a defined DNA sequence with accumulation of mutations in a single round by a dual approach to random chemical mutagenesis (DuARCheM).* Chembiochem, 2008. 9(14): p. 2238-43.

[12] Symonds, N., *Evolution. Anticipatory mutagenesis.* Nature, 1989. 337(6203): p. 119-20.

[13] van Duin, M., et al., *Evolution and mutagenesis of the mammalian excision repair gene ERCC-1.* Nucleic Acids Res, 1988. 16(12): p. 5305-22.

[14] Bessereau, J.L., *Insertional mutagenesis in C. elegans using the Drosophila transposon Mos1: a method for the rapid identification of mutated genes.* Methods Mol Biol, 2006. 351: p. 59-73.

[15] Vallejo, A.N., R.J. Pogulis, and L.R. Pease, *PCR Mutagenesis by Overlap Extension and Gene SOE.* CSH Protoc, 2008. 2008: p. pdb prot4861.

[16] Yang, Y.X., et al., *PCR-based site-specific mutagenesis of peptide antibiotics FALL-39 and its biologic activities.* Acta Pharmacol Sin, 2004. 25(2): p. 239-45.

[17] Lehoux, D.E. and R.C. Levesque, *PCR screening in signature-tagged mutagenesis of essential genes.* Methods Mol Biol, 2002. 192: p. 225-34.

[18] Luo, S., et al., *Site-directed mutagenesis of gentisate 1,2-dioxygenases from Klebsiella pneumoniae M5a1 and Ralstonia sp. strain U2.* Microbiol Res, 2006. 161(2): p. 138-44.

[19] Balliet, J.W., et al., *Site-directed mutagenesis of large DNA palindromes: construction and in vitro characterization of herpes simplex virus type 1 mutants containing point mutations that eliminate the oriL or oriS initiation function.* J Virol, 2005. 79(20): p. 12783-97.

[20] Largaespada, D.A., *Transposon-mediated mutagenesis of somatic cells in the mouse for cancer gene identification.* Methods, 2009. 49(3): p. 282-6.

[21] Kim, Y.C., et al., *Transposon-directed base-exchange mutagenesis (TDEM): a novel method for multiple-nucleotide substitutions within a target gene.* Biotechniques, 2009. 46(7): p. 534-42.

[22] Largaespada, D.A., *Transposon mutagenesis in mice.* Methods Mol Biol, 2009. 530: p. 379-90.

[23] Dunn, W., et al., *Functional profiling of a human cytomegalovirus genome.* Proc Natl Acad Sci U S A, 2003. 100(24): p. 14223-8.

[24] Murphy, E., et al., *Coding potential of laboratory and clinical strains of human cytomegalovirus.* Proc Natl Acad Sci U S A, 2003. 100(25): p. 14976-81.

[25] Yu, D., M.C. Silva, and T. Shenk, *Functional map of human cytomegalovirus AD169 defined by global mutational analysis.* Proc Natl Acad Sci U S A, 2003. 100(21): p. 12396-401.

[26] Dolan, A., et al., *Genetic content of wild-type human cytomegalovirus.* J Gen Virol, 2004. 85(Pt 5): p. 1301-12.

[27] Warden, C., Q. Tang, and H. Zhu, *Herpesvirus BACs: past, present, and future.* Journal of biomedicine & biotechnology, 2011. 2011: p. 124595.

[28] Sauer, B., *Functional expression of the cre-lox site-specific recombination system in the yeast Saccharomyces cerevisiae.* Mol Cell Biol, 1987. 7(6): p. 2087-96.

[29] Sauer, B. and N. Henderson, *Site-specific DNA recombination in mammalian cells by the Cre recombinase of bacteriophage P1.* Proc Natl Acad Sci U S A, 1988. 85(14): p. 5166-70.

[30] Orban, P.C., D. Chui, and J.D. Marth, *Tissue- and site-specific DNA recombination in transgenic mice.* Proc Natl Acad Sci U S A, 1992. 89(15): p. 6861-5.

[31] Zhu, X.D. and P.D. Sadowski, *Cleavage-dependent ligation by the FLP recombinase. Characterization of a mutant FLP protein with an alteration in a catalytic amino acid.* J Biol Chem, 1995. 270(39): p. 23044-54.

[32] Dixon, J.E., A.C. Shaikh, and P.D. Sadowski, *The Flp recombinase cleaves Holliday junctions in trans.* Mol Microbiol, 1995. 18(3): p. 449-58.

[33] Schlake, T. and J. Bode, *Use of mutated FLP recognition target (FRT) sites for the exchange of expression cassettes at defined chromosomal loci.* Biochemistry, 1994. 33(43): p. 12746-51.

[34] Jayaram, M., *Phosphoryl transfer in Flp recombination: a template for strand transfer mechanisms.* Trends Biochem Sci, 1994. 19(2): p. 78-82.

[35] Xu, T. and S.D. Harrison, *Mosaic analysis using FLP recombinase.* Methods Cell Biol, 1994. 44: p. 655-81.

[36] Stricklett, P.K., R.D. Nelson, and D.E. Kohan, *The Cre/loxP system and gene targeting in the kidney.* The American journal of physiology, 1999. 276(5 Pt 2): p. F651-7.

[37] Lee, E.C., et al., *A highly efficient Escherichia coli-based chromosome engineering system adapted for recombinogenic targeting and subcloning of BAC DNA.* Genomics, 2001. 73(1): p. 56-65.

[38] Yu, D.G., et al., *An efficient recombination system for chromosome engineering in Escherichia coli.* Proceedings of the National Academy of Sciences of the United States of America, 2000. 97(11): p. 5978-5983.

[39] Carter, D.M. and C.M. Radding, *The role of exonuclease and beta protein of phage lambda in genetic recombination. II. Substrate specificity and the mode of action of lambda exonuclease.* J Biol Chem., 1971. 246(8): p. 2502-12.

[40] Little, J.W., *An exonuclease induced by bacteriophage lambda. II. Nature of the enzymatic reaction.* J Biol Chem. , 1967. 242(4): p. 679-86.

[41] Warming, S., et al., *Simple and highly efficient BAC recombineering using galK selection.* Nucleic Acids Res, 2005. 33(4): p. e36.

[42] Zhang, Y., et al., *DNA cloning by homologous recombination in Escherichia coli.* Nature biotechnology, 2000. 18(12): p. 1314-7.

[43] Zhang, Z., Y. Huang, and H. Zhu, *A highly efficient protocol of generating and analyzing VZV ORF deletion mutants based on a newly developed luciferase VZV BAC system.* Journal of virological methods, 2008. 148(1-2): p. 197-204.

[44] Dulal, K., Z. Zhang, and H. Zhu, *Development of a gene capture method to rescue a large deletion mutant of human cytomegalovirus.* Journal of virological methods, 2009. 157(2): p. 180-7.

[45] Sharan, S.K., et al., *Recombineering: a homologous recombination-based method of genetic engineering.* Nature protocols, 2009. 4(2): p. 206-23.

[46] Borst, E.M., et al., *Cloning of the human cytomegalovirus (HCMV) genome as an infectious bacterial artificial chromosome in Escherichia coli: a new approach for construction of HCMV mutants.* J Virol, 1999. 73(10): p. 8320-9.

[47] Marchini, A., H. Liu, and H. Zhu, *Human cytomegalovirus with IE-2 (UL122) deleted fails to express early lytic genes.* Journal of virology, 2001. 75(4): p. 1870-8.

[48] Moffat, J.F., et al., *Tropism of varicella-zoster virus for human CD4+ and CD8+ T lymphocytes and epidermal cells in SCID-hu mice.* Journal of virology, 1995. 69(9): p. 5236-42.

21

Extraction of Drug from the Biological Matrix: A Review

S. Lakshmana Prabu[1] and T. N. K. Suriyaprakash[2]
[1]*Anna University of Technology, Tiruchirappalli, Tamil Nadu,*
[2]*Periyar College of Pharmaceutical Sciences,*
The Tamil Nadu Dr. M.G.R. Medical University, Chennai, Tamil Nadu,
India

1. Introduction

The assessment of therapeutic compliance is commonly done by either indirect method or direct method. In indirect method, the assessments are done by indirect measurement of parameters such as discussion with patients and pill counts at intervals during the treatment which don't measure the drug concentration in a matrix such as blood or urine. In direct method, the assessments which rely upon evidence provided by the patients or care giver on the presumptive compliance based upon electronic medical event monitoring system and this is based upon either the qualitative or quantitative measurement of the drug under investigation in a biological matrix provided by the system.

A more objective assessment of patient compliance has its own limitations. The most widely used matrix is plasma, but the major limitation with this approach is that it provides the clinician with the concentration of drug within the systematic circulation at the time of sample collection. This concentration is primarily related to the time interval between the administration of the last dose and the sample collection time although other pharmacokinetic parameters can also influence the concentration. Plasma samples should be collected prior to the administration of the next dose. Plasma monitoring is a useful adjunct for the assessment of therapeutic compliance (Williams, 1999).

Bioanalysis is a sub-discipline of analytical chemistry covering the quantitative measurement drugs and their metabolites in biological systems. Bioanalysis in the pharmaceutical industry is to provide a quantitative measure of the active drug and/or its metabolite(s) for the purpose of pharmacokinetics, toxicokinetics, bioequivalence and exposure–response (pharmacokinetics /pharmacodynamics studies). Bioanalysis also applies to drugs used for illicit purposes, forensic investigations, anti-doping testing in sports, and environmental concerns. Bioanalytical assays to accurately and reliably determine these drugs at lower concentrations. This has driven improvements in technology and analytical methods.

Some techniques commonly used in bioanalytical studies include:

- Hyphenated techniques
    - LC–MS (liquid chromatography–mass spectrometry)
    - GC–MS (gas chromatography–mass spectrometry)

  - LC-DAD (liquid chromatography-diode array detection)
  - CE-MS (capillary electrophoresis-mass spectrometry)
- Chromatographic methods
  - HPLC (high performance liquid chromatography)
  - GC (gas chromatography)
  - UPLC (ultra performance liquid chromatography)
  - Supercritical fluid chromatography

The area of bioanalysis can encompass a very broad range of assays which support the clinical and nonclinical studies. Many factors influence the development of robust bioanalytical methods for analyzing samples from clinical and nonclinical studies which includes the matrices of interest, the range over which analytes need to be measured, the number and structures of the analytes, the physicochemical properties of the analytes, and their stability in the biological matrices from the time of sample draw to analysis also needs to be measured.

Because biological samples are extremely complex matrices comprised of many components that can interfere with good separations and or good mass spectrometer signals, sample preparation is an important aspect of bioanalytical estimation. This is important whether samples originate as tissue extracts, plasma, serum or urine. The question sometimes arises as to whether serum or plasma should be collected for analysis. In general, from a bioanalytical perspective, there are few advantages to choosing serum over plasma except where chemical interferences in a given assay might require processing blood all the way to serum.

Nearly all bioanalytical assays involve the use of an internal standard processed along with the sample. The area ratio of analyte to internal standard is used in conjunction with a standard curve to back calculate the concentration of analyte in the sample. The internal standard is expected to behave similarly to the analyte with respect to extraction efficiency across the range of concentration, which helps compensate for sample to sample differences in sample preparation. Often, an analogue or similarly behaving compound is used as an internal standard.

To produce adequate and precise results, certain criteria like minimal loss or degradation of sample during blood collection, the appropriate sample cleanup and internal standard, chromatographic conditions that minimize the interference and ion suppression, and sufficient signal to noise to allow for reproducible peak integration.

However, an examination of the individual plasma samples could show one or more with an unacceptable interference that is effectively washed out when the samples are pooled. Thus, it is important to use several individual matrix samples when evaluating matrix effects. If unacceptable matrix interferences are observed, it is necessary to further clean up the sample to eliminate the interference.

A key component of the sample preparation is the emphasis on analyte stability which needs to be carefully assessed from the time of sample drawn till the analysis is complete. It is important to study the analytes stability in blood at the appropriate temperatures from the time the sample is drawn until after centrifugation when plasma or serum are separated and stored in a new vial. It is also important to ensure that the anticoagulant or other components of the blood collection do not interfere with the sample preparation (Destefano & Takigiku, 2004).

Blood is the transporter of many vital substances and nutrients for the entire body and thus contains many endogenous and exogenous compounds in different concentrations. Drug determination in human plasma is often complicated by low concentrations (0.1 - 10ng mL^{-1} level). An extra problem posed by blood sample is the complex sample matrix due to proteins, which can lead to protein binding of the analyte and by limited sample volumes normally 0.5 - 1ml will be available for the determination. The magnitude of the challenge of protein purification becomes clearer when one considers the mixture of macromolecules present in the biological matrices. Hence, sample preparation is crucial in drug analysis which includes both analyte pre-concentration and sample cleanup (Ho *et al.*, 2002).

To produce meaningful information, an analysis must be performed on a sample whose composition faithfully reflects that of the bulk of material from which it was taken. Biological samples cannot normally be injected directly into the analyzing system without sample preparation. Sample pretreatment is thus of utmost importance for the adequate analysis of drugs. However, as sample pretreatment can be a time consuming process, this can limit the sample throughput. The proper selectivity can be obtained during the sample preparation, the separation and the detection. A major differentiation between the analyte of interest and the other compounds is often made during the first step. Sensitivity is to a large extent obtained by the detector. Thus, sample pretreatment is required for achieving sufficient sensitivity and selectivity, whereas the time should be kept to a minimum in order to obtain adequate speed. Therefore, there is a clear trend towards integration of sample pretreatment with the separation and the detection. Numerous sample preparation techniques have been developed for bioanalytical purpose. Sample preparation is a difficult step, especially in clinical and environmental chemistry and generally involves filtration, solid phase extraction with disposable cartridges, protein precipitation and desalting. Sample preparation prior to chromatographic separation is performed to dissolve or dilute the analyte in a suitable solvent, removing the interfering compounds and pre-concentrating the analyte.

The principle objectives of sample preparation from biological matrix are;

a. Isolation of the analytes of interest from the interfering compounds
b. Dissolution of the analytes in a suitable solvent and pre-concentration.

In an analytical method sample preparation is followed by a separation and detection procedure. In spite of the fact that sample preparation, in most of the analytical procedures, takes 50-75% of the total time of the analysis, most technical innovations of the last 5 years are related to separation and detection.

Extraction is one of humankind's oldest chemical operations. Extraction is the withdrawing of an active agent or a waste substance from a solid or liquid mixture with a liquid solvent. The solvent is not or only partially miscible with the solid or the liquid. By intensive contact between analyte and the extraction medium this leads the analyte transfers from the solid or liquid mixture into the extraction medium (extract). After thorough mixing the two phases can be separated either by gravity or centrifugal forces (Gy, 1982; Arthur & Pawliszyn, 1990; Zief & Kiser, 1990).

2. Sampling

The sampling and sample preparation process begins at the point of collection and extends to the measurement step. The proper collection of sample during the sample process (called primary sampling), the transport of this representative sample from the point of collection to the analytical laboratory, the proper selection of the laboratory sample itself (called secondary sampling), and the sample preparation method used to convert the sample into a form suitable for the measurement step can have a greater effect on the overall accuracy and reliability of the results than the measurement itself.

Primary sampling is the process of selecting and collecting the sample to be analyzed. The objective of sampling is a mass or volume reduction from the parent batch, which itself can be homogeneous or heterogeneous. If the wrong sample is collected or the sample is not collected properly, then all the further stages in the analysis become meaningless and the resulting data are worthless. Unfortunately, sampling is sometimes left to people unskilled in sampling methodology and is largely ignored in the education process, especially for non-analytical chemists (Smith & James, 1981). Once the primary sample is taken, it must be transported to the analytical laboratory without a physical or chemical change in its characteristics. Even if a representative primary sample is taken, changes that can occur during transport can present difficulties in the secondary sampling process. Preservation techniques can be used to minimize changes between collection and analysis. Physical changes such as adsorption, diffusion and volatilization as well as chemical changes such as oxidation and microbiological degradation are minimized by proper preservation.

Common preservation techniques used between the point of collection and the point of sample preparation in the laboratory are

- Choice of appropriate sampling container
- Addition of chemical stabilizers such as antioxidants and antibacterial agents
- Freezing the sample to avoid thermal degradation
- Adsorption on a solid phase

In secondary sampling, if the sample has made it to the laboratory, a representative subsample must be taken. Statistical appropriate sampling procedures are applied to avoid discrimination, which can further degrade analytical data. Clearly speeding up or automating the sample preparation step will reduce analysis time and improve sample throughput (Keith, 1990).

Before sample preparation, solid or semisolid substances must be put into a finely divided state. Procedures to perform this operation are usually physical methods, not chemical methods. The reasons for putting the sample into a finely divided state are that finely divided samples are more homogeneous, so secondary sampling may be carried out with greater precision and accuracy, and they are more easily dissolved or extracted because of their large surface-to-volume ratio.

2.1 Sample preparation

Sample preparation is necessary for at least two reasons:

a. To remove as many of the endogenous interferences from the analyte as possible
b. To enrich the sample with respect to the analyte, thus maximizing the sensitivity of the system.

It also serves to ensure that the injection matrix is compatible with the selected column and mobile phase.

2.2 Goal and objectives of sample preparation

Two of the major goals of any sample pretreatment procedure are

- Quantitative recovery
- A minimum number of steps.

Successful sample preparation has a threefold objective.

- In solution
- Free from interfering matrix elements
- At a concentration appropriate for detection and measurement

The most common approach in analyte separation involves a two phase system where the analyte and interferences are distributed between the two phases. Distribution is an equilibrium process and is reversible. If the sample is distributed between two immiscible liquid phase, the techniques is called liquid-liquid extraction. If the sample is distributed between a solid and a liquid phase, the technique is called liquid-solid adsorption.

Often, when analysis involves the measurement of trace amounts of a substance, it is desirable to increase the concentration of the analyte to a level where it can be measured more easily. Concentration of an analyte can be accomplished by transferring it from a large volume of phase to a smaller volume of phase. Separation can be carried out in a single batch, in multiple batches or by continuous operation.

2.3 Types of samples

Sample matrices can be classified as organic and inorganic. Biological samples are a subset of organic samples but often require different sample preparation procedures in order to preserve biological integrity and activity. Compared to volatile compounds or solid, liquid samples are much easier to prepare for analytical measurement because a dissolution or an extraction step many not be involved. The major consideration for liquid samples is the matrix interferences, the concentration of analyte, and compatibility with the analytical techniques. When a sample is a solid, the sample pretreatment process can be more complex. There are two specific cases: the entire sample is of interest and must be solubilized or only a part of the solids is of interest and the analytes must be selectively removed. If the solid is a soluble salt or drug tablet formulation, the only sample preparation that may be required is finding a suitable solvent that will totally dissolve the sample and the components of interest. If the sample matrix is insoluble in commonly solvents but the analytes of interest can be removed or leached out, then sample preparation can also be rather straightforward. In these cases, techniques such as filtration, Soxhlet extraction, supercritical fluid extraction, ultrasonication or solid-liquid extraction may be useful. If both the sample matrix and the sample analytes are not soluble in common solvents, then more drastic measures may be needed.

3. Physicochemical properties of drug and their extraction from biological material (Chang 1977; Moore 1972; Barrow 1996; Wiltshire 2000)

3.1 Molecular phenomena for solubility and miscibility

To dissolve a drug, a solvent must break the bonds like ionic bond, hydrogen bond and Van der Waals forces which inter links the compound to its neighbors and must not break substantial intermolecular bonds of the solvent without replacing them with drug solvent interaction. Because breaking of bonds is an endothermic process, requires energy and causing an increasing in enthalpy. Similarly, if the gain in entropy from the dissolution of two solvents in each other is insufficient to counteract any reduced amount of intermolecular bonding, they will not be completely miscible.

3.2 Water miscibility and water immiscibility

Commonly alcohols can have hydrogen bonding with water and also dipole-dipole interactions will aid miscibility. On the other hand, presence of alkyl groups will reduce the solubility with water and the interaction may be by means of dispersive force. Hydrocarbons are hydrophobic in nature, which dissolves the compounds by dispersive forces. Whereas halogenated hydrocarbons are more polar and dissolve the compounds by dispersive forces and dipolar interactions.

Hydrophilic groups, which are polar in nature, will encourage the solubility in water, whereas C-C, C-H and C-X bonds are hydrophobic in nature will encourage the solubility in organic solvents. Drug with several aromatic rings will have poor solubility in water due to lack of hydrogen bonding with water and the strong intermolecular dispersive forces of the solid drug will encourage the ready solubility in organic solvents.

3.3 Distribution coefficient

Drug which are in ionised forms are hydrophilic in nature than the unionized form because of the hydration of the ions, therefore the ionized forms are difficulty to extract into organic solvents whereas the unionized forms will dissolve in the organic solvents which can be extracted into organic solvents.

3.4 Choice of solvent

Several factors are to be considered while choosing a solvent to extract a drug from the matrix in addition to its powder to dissolve the required compounds which includes selectivity, density, toxicity, volatility, reactivity, physical hazards and miscibility with aqueous media.

- Ethyl acetate is a powerful solvent for many organic compounds and will therefore extract a considerable amount of endogenous material with the required drug.
- If the drug is relatively non-polar, a more selective extraction could be obtained by using a hydrocarbon solvent.
- Halogenated hydrocarbons like chloroform and dichloromethane are excellent, volatile solvents. However they are denser than water which makes them difficult to use for analysis.

- Benzene is a useful solvent, reasonably volatile, inert and immiscible with water, but its toxicity precludes its use.
- Toluene has similar properties as a solvent to benzene is not particularly toxic, however its boiling point is 111°C and it is not really sufficient volatile for use as a solvent in bio-analysis.
- Chloroform is an excellent solvent but reactivity with bases reduces its uses with basic drugs that need to be extracted at high pH.
- Di-isopropyl ether is less miscible with water than di-ethyl ether but is much more likely to form explosive peroxides and is best avoided.
- Diethyl ether is a good, volatile solvent but it is quite soluble (~4%) in water and difficult to blow to complete dryness.

3.5 Mixed solvents

In some cases pure solvents will not be satisfactory for the extraction of the compound of interest. Alcohols are excellent solvent but those with lower boiling points are too soluble in water whereas less miscible one are having high boiling points, but the use of mixed solvents containing alcohols can solve the problem. A 1:1 mixture of tetrahydrofuran and dichloromethane is a powerful solvent for the extraction of polar compounds from aqueous solutions.

3.6 Plasma proteins and emulsions

Presence of proteins can cause difficulties in extracting the drug from plasma. Emulsions are often formed and partial precipitation can unclear the interface between the two layers. The proteins can be precipitated by addition of 10-20% trichloroacetic acid or five volumes of a water-miscible solvent like acetonitrile.

3.7 Role of pH for solvent extraction

Organic acids and bases are usually much less soluble in water than its salts. As a general rule, extraction of bases into an organic solvent should be carried out at high pH usually about 2 pH units above the pKa and extraction of acids carried out at low pH. If the drug is reasonably non-polar base, it could be back extracted from the organic solvent into acid, basified and re-extracted into the organic solvent and vice versa for the acidic drugs.

4. Sample pretreatment in different biological matrices (Horne, 1985; Christians & Sewing, 1989; McDowall *et al.*, 1989; Ingwersen, 1993; Krishnan & Ibraham 1994; Simmonds *et al.*, 1994; Allanson *et al.*, 1996; Plumb *et al.*, 1997)

4.1 General concern with biological samples

Extraction of biological samples before injection into an HPLC system serves a number of objectives.

- Concentration
- Clean-up
- Prevention of clogging of analytical columns

- Elimination of protein binding
- Elimination of enzymatic degradation of the analyte

4.2 Serum, plasma, and whole blood

Serum and plasma samples may not need to be pretreated for SPE. In many cases, however, analytes such as drugs may be protein-bound, which reduces SPE recoveries. To disrupt protein binding in these biological fluids, use of one of the following methods for reversed phase or ion exchange SPE procedures.

- Shift pH of the sample to extremes (pH<3 or pH>9) with acids or bases in the concentration range of 0.1M or greater. Use the resulting supernatant as the sample for SPE
- Precipitate the proteins using a polar solvent such as acetonitrile, methanol, or acetone (two parts solvent per one part biological fluid is typical). After mixing and centrifugation, remove the supernatant and dilute with water or an aqueous buffer for the SPE procedure
- To precipitate proteins, treat the biological fluid with acids or inorganic salts, such as formic acid, perchloric acid, trichloroacetic acid, ammonium sulfate, sodium sulfate, or zinc sulfate. The pH of the resulting supernatant may be adjusted prior to use for the SPE procedure
- Sonicate the biological fluid for 15 minutes, add water or buffer, centrifuge, and use the supernatant for the SPE procedure

4.3 Urine

Urine samples may not require pretreatment for reversed phase or ion exchange SPE, but often is diluted with water or a buffer of the appropriate pH prior to sample addition. In some cases, acid hydrolysis (for basic compounds) or base hydrolysis (for acidic compounds) is used to ensure that the compounds of interest are freely solvated in the urine sample. Usually a strong acid (e.g. concentrated HCl) or base (e.g. 10M KOH) is added to the urine. The urine is heated for 15- 20 minutes, then cooled and diluted with a buffer, and the pH adjusted appropriately for the SPE procedure. Enzymatic hydrolysis that frees bound compounds or drugs also may be used.

4.4 Solid samples

Solid samples ex. tissues, faeces are normally homogenized with a buffer or an organic solvent, then remaining solids removed by centrifugation, and the diluted sample applied to the cartridge.

5. Methods of extraction

The aim of the sample preparation process is to provide a suitable sample, usually for chromatographic analysis, which will not contaminate the instrumentation and where the concentration in the prepared sample is reflective of that found in the original. The method of sample preparation selected is generally dictated by the analytical technique available and the physical characteristics of the analytes under investigation (Watt *et al.*, 2000). The two main sample preparation methods are matrix cleanup or direct injection. In a matrix cleanup procedure, the aim is to remove as much endogenous material as possible from the drug sample.

Sample preparation is traditionally carried out (a) by liquid-liquid extraction, (b) solid-phase extraction or (c) by precipitation of the plasma proteins, while the final analysis in most cases is accomplished by liquid chromatography interfaced with mass spectrometry or tandem mass spectrometry or capillary gas chromatography.

5.1 Liquid-Liquid Extraction (LLE) (Christian & O'Reilly, 1986; Harris, 1994; Majors & Fogelman, 1993; Wells, 2003)

One of the most useful techniques for isolating desired components from a mixture is liquid-liquid extraction (LLE). LLE is a method used for the separation of a mixture using two immiscible solvents. In most LLEs, one of the phases is aqueous and the other is an immiscible organic solvent. The concept "like dissolves like" works well in LLE. The ability to separate compounds in a mixture using the technique of LLE depends upon how differently the compounds of the sample mixture partition themselves between the two immiscible solvents. Selective partitioning of the compound of interest into one of two immiscible or partially miscible phases occurs by the proper choice of extraction of solvent. In this technique sample is distributed in two phases in which one phase is immiscible to other. LLE separates analytes from interferences by partitioning the sample between two immiscible liquids or phases. First, the component mixture is dissolved in a suitable solvent and a second solvent that is immiscible with the first solvent is added. Next, the contents are thoroughly mixed (shaking) and the two immiscible solvents allowed separating into layers. The less dense solvent will be the upper layer, while the more dense solvent will be the lower layer. The components of the initial mixture will be distributed amongst the two immiscible solvents as determined by their partition coefficient. The relative solubility that a compound has in two given solvents can provide an estimation of the extent to which a compound will be partitioned between them. A compound that is more soluble in the less dense solvent will preferentially reside in the upper layer. Conversely, a compound more soluble in the more dense solvent will preferentially reside in the lower layer. Lastly, the two immiscible layers are separated, transferred and the component in that solvent is isolated. Generally after extraction hydrophilic compounds are seen in the polar aqueous phase and hydrophobic compounds are found mainly in the organic solvents. Analyte is extracted into the organic phase are easily recovered by evaporation of the solvent, the residue reconstituted with a small volume of an appropriate solvent preferably mobile phase while analyte extracted in to the aqueous phase can be directly injected into a RP column. LLE technique is simple, rapid is relative cost effective per sample as compared to other techniques and near quantitative recoveries (90%) of most drugs can be obtained by multiple continuous extraction (Fig.1).

Several useful equations can help illustrate the extraction process. The Nernst distribution law states that any neutral species will distribute between two immiscible solvents so that the ratio of the concentration remains constant.

$$K_D = C_o / C_{aq}$$

Where K_D is the distribution constant, C_o is the concentration of the analyte in the organic phase, and C_{aq} is the concentration of the analyte in the aqueous phase.

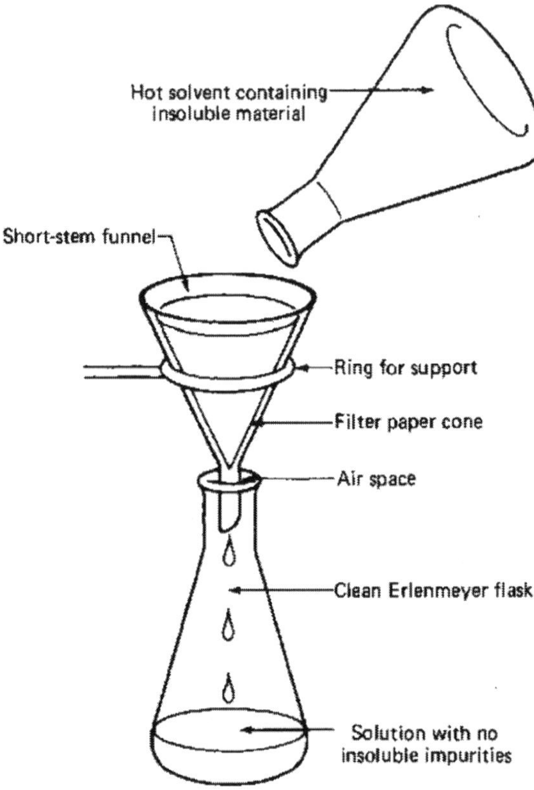

Fig. 1. Gravity Filtration Setup

To increase the value of K_D, several approaches may be used:

- The organic solvent can be changed to increase solubility of the analyte
- If the analyte is ionic or ionizable, its K_D may be increased by suppressing its ionization to make it more soluble in the organic phase. It can also be extracted into the organic phase by the formation of an ion pair through the addition of a hydrophobic counter-ion.
- Metal ions can form a complex with hydrophobic complexing agents.
- The salting out effect can be used to decrease analytes concentration in the aqueous phase.

If the K_D value is unfavorable, addition extraction may be required for better solute recovery. In this case, a fresh portion of immiscible solvent is added to extract additional solute. Normally, the two extracts are combined. Generally, for a given volume of solvent, multiple extractions are more efficient in removing a solute quantitatively than a single extraction. Sometimes, back extractions can be used to achieve a more complete sample cleanup.

If K_D is very low or the sample volume is high, it becomes nearly impossible to carryout multiple simple extractions in a reasonable volume. Also, if the extraction rate is slow, it may take a long time for equilibrium to be established. In these cases, continuous liquid-liquid extraction is used, where pure solvent is recycled through the aqueous phase.

Benefit of this technique is that, with a judicious choice of solvents and pH, very clean extracts can be obtained with good selectivity for the targeted analyte. The drug is extracted from the aqueous phase to the organic phase. One point of note is that LLE system unlike solid-phase systems, are more likely to give consistent results year after years, as there is usually less batch to batch variation with solvents.

The extraction of drug from the aqueous phase is mainly depends on the following factors:

- Solubility of analyte in the organic solvent
- Polarity of the organic solvent
- pH of the aqueous phase

In some cases there is a possibility that interferences may present in the extracted sample. In that case back liquid-liquid extraction can be performed, this gives a clear extracts. Here two times organic solvent is used for the extraction of analyte from the matrix. Often, however, it is not possible to find the optimum condition that provides both high recovery and purity of the analyte in one extraction step. Low recoveries may require further extraction to achieve acceptable value. About the purity it may require second extraction procedure with different solvent or pH of the aqueous phase. Each successive extraction increase the analytical time, also the resulting large volume of extraction solvent must be evaporated to recover the product. If extraction requires many steps, techniques such as Craig Counter Current distribution can be used to increase recovery and purity. However this technique increases the cost and time of the analysis.

5.1.1 Selection of the solvent

There are also practical concerns when choosing extraction solvents. As mentioned previously, the two solvents must be immiscible. The properties of an ideal solvent is that it should withdraw the active agent from a mixture by liquid-liquid extraction are

- Selectivity: Only the active agent has to be extracted and no further substances which mean that a high selectivity is required.
- Capacity: To reduce the amount of necessary solvent, the capacity of the solvent has to be high.
- Miscibility: To achieve simple regeneration of the solvent the miscibility of solvent and primary solvent has to be low.
- Difference in density: After extraction, the two phases have to be separated in a separator and for this a high positive difference in density is required.
- Optimal surface tension: σ low → low amount of energy for dispersing required; if surface tension < 1 mN/m stable emulsions are produced; $\sigma > 50$ mN/m → high amount of energy for dispersing and high tendency to coalesce.
- Recovery: The solvent has to be separated from the extract phase easily to produce solvent free active agents.

- Corrosion: If the solvent is corrosive prices for construction increases.
- Low price
- No or low toxicity and not highly flammable
- Flame temperature: 25°C higher than operating temperature
- Vapour pressure: To prevent loss of solvent by evaporation a low vapour pressure at operating temperature is required.
- Viscosity: A low viscosity of the solvent leads to low pressure drop and good heat and mass transfer.
- Chemical and thermal stability
- Environmentally acceptable or easily recoverable
- Convenient specific gravity
- Suitable volatility
- High chemical stability and inertness
- Not prone to form an emulsion
- Dissolves the neutral but not the ionized form of the analyte

The stoichiometric ratio of the analyte in the organic phase compared to that in the aqueous phase is known as the distribution ratio D. Ideally, this ratio should approach 100% in order to minimize the losses through the effects of small changes in sample composition, temperature and pH. Reproducibility also increases with increasing extraction efficiency, although a consistent low recovery may be acceptable if an internal standard is used to compensate for changes in efficiency.

5.1.2 Extraction under basic and acidic conditions

As mentioned above, the ability to separate compounds of a mixture using liquid-liquid extraction procedures depends upon the relative solubility that each compound has in the two immiscible solvents. A change in the pH of the solvent (the addition of acid or base) can change the solubility of an organic compound in a solvent considerably.

Liquid/liquid extraction is the most common technique used to separate a desired organic product from a biological matrix. The technique works well if your target compound is more soluble in one of two immiscible solvents. Extraction usually involves shaking a solution that contains the target with an immiscible solvent in which the desired substance is more soluble than it is in the starting solution. Upon standing, the solvents form two layers that can be separated. The extraction may have to be repeated several times to effect complete separation.

In general liquid-liquid extractions can separate four different classes of compounds:

a. **Organic bases:** Any organic amine can be extracted from an organic solvent with a strong acid such as 1M hydrochloric acid
b. **Strong acids:** Carboxylic acids can be extracted from an organic solvent with a weak base such as 1M sodium bicarbonate
c. **Weak acids:** Phenols can be extracted from an organic solvent with a strong base such as 1M sodium hydroxide
d. **Non-polar compounds** stay in the organic layer

5.1.3 Disadvantages

- Large solvent consumption is needed for extraction of drug.
- LLE is time consuming process when compare to other methods.
- LLE require an evaporation step prior to analysis to remove excess of organic solvent.
- LLE technique is not a suitable one for the estimation of several analytes.
- Emulsion formation may be possible when two immiscible phases were used in the extraction procedure.

5.2 Solid Phase Extraction (Zwir Ferenc & Biziuk, 2006; James, 2000; Krishnan & Abraham, 1994; Moors *et al.*, 1994; Plumb *et al.*, 1997; Arthur & Pawliszyn, 1990; Zief & Kiser, 1990; MacDonald & Bouvier, 1995; Wells, 2003: Scheurer & Moore, 1992)

Since the 70's SPE has become a common and effective technique for extracting analytes from complex samples. Solid phase extraction is the very popular technique currently available for rapid and selective sample preparation. Many sample preparation methods today rely on solid-phase extractions, an advantage being that SPE is amenable to automation and parallel processing. SPE evolved to be a powerful tool for isolation and concentration of trace analysis in a variety of sample matrices. The versatility of SPE allows use of this technique for many purposes, such as purification and trace enrichment (Rawa *et al.*, 2003).

The objectives of SPE are to reduce the level of interferences, minimize the final sample volume to maximize analyte sensitivity and provide the analyte fraction in a solvent that is compatible with the analytical measurement techniques. As an added benefit, SPE serves as a filter to remove sample particulates.

The degree of enrichment achievable for a particular sample is dependent upon:

a. The selectivity of the bonded phase for the analyte
b. The relative strength of that interaction

SPE prepares multiple samples in parallel (typically 12-24) and uses relatively low quantities of solvents and the procedures can be readily automated. As the name implies the principle of SPE is an extraction technique similar to that of LLE, involving a partitioning of solutes between two phases. However, instead of two immiscible liquid phases, as in LLE, SPE involves partitioning between a liquid (sample matrix or solvent with analytes) and a solid (sorbent) phase (Table 1).

SPE is a more efficient separation process than LLE, easily obtains a higher recovery of analyte by employing a small plastic disposable column or cartridge, often the barrel of a medical syringe packed with 0.1 to 0.5 g of sorbent which is commonly RP material (C_{18}-silica). The components of interest may either preferentially adsorbed to the solid, or they may remain in the second non-solid phase. Once equilibrium has been reached, the two phases are physically separated by decanting, filtration, centrifugation or a similar process. If the desired analyte is adsorbed on the solid phase, they can be selectively desorbed by washing with an appropriate solvent. If the component of interest remains in a liquid phase, they can be recovered via concentration, evaporation and or recrystallization. When SPE is performed in this single step equilibrium batch mode, it will be similar to LLE, where the solid sorbent simply replaces one of the immiscible liquids. By passing a liquid or gas through the uniform solid bed, the liquid solid phase extraction technique becomes a form of column chromatography, now commonly called phase extraction that is governed by liquid chromatographic principle.

Polarity			Solvent	Miscible in Water?
Non-polar	Strong Reversed Phase	Weak Normal Phase	Hexane	No
			Isooctane	No
			Carbon tetrachloride	No
			Chloroform	No
			Methylene Chloride	No
			Tetrahydrofuran	Yes
			Diethly ether	No
			Ethyl acetate	Poorly
			Acetone	Yes
			Acetonitrile Yes	Yes
			Isopropanol	Yes
			Methanol	Yes
			Water	Yes
Polar	Weak Reversed Phase	Strong Normal Phase	Acetic Acid	Yes

Table 1. Characteristics of Solvents Commonly Used in SPE

Liquid samples are added to the cartridge and wash solvent is selected to either strongly retain or un-retain the analyte. Interferences are eluted or washed from the cartridge, even as the analyte is strongly retained, so as to minimize the presence of interferences in the final analyte fraction, the analyte is then eluted with a strong elution solvent, collected and either injected directly or evaporated to dryness followed by dilution with the HPLC mobile phase. Conversely, when interferences are strongly held in the cartridge, the analyte can be collected for the further treatment. Advantages of SPE over LLE include a more complete extraction of the analyte, more efficient separation of interferences from analyte, reduced organic solvent consumption, easier collection of the total analyte fraction, more convenient manual procedures, better removal of particulates and more easy automation.

5.2.1 Mechanism of Solid Phase Extraction process (Font *et al.*, 1993; Sabik *et al.*, 2000)

The ideal process is to create a digital chromatography system on the SPE cartridge such that the analyte is at first fully bound, then the interferences are completely eluted, and then the analyte is entirely eluted; it is either all on or all off the cartridge. The separation mechanism is the function due to the intermolecular interactions between analyte and the functional groups of the sorbent.

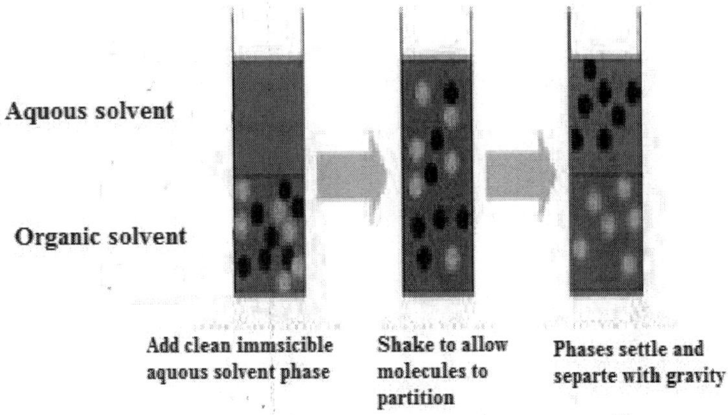

Fig. 2. Partitioning of drugs towards aqueous and organic solvent

The selection of an appropriate SPE extraction sorbent depends on understanding the mechanism(s) of interaction between the sorbent and analyte of interest. That understanding in turn depends on knowledge of the hydrophobic, polar and inorganic properties of both the solute and the sorbent. The most common retention mechanisms in SPE are based on van der Waals forces ("non-polar interactions"), hydrogen bonding, dipole-dipole forces ("polar" interactions) and cation-anion interactions ("ionic" interactions).

Each sorbent offers a unique mix of these properties which can be applied to a wide variety of extraction problems (Fig 2). Four general theory interactions exist (Yu *et al.*, 2004):

a. **Reversed phase** involves a polar or moderately polar sample matrix (mobile phase) and a non-polar stationary phase. The analyte of interest is typically mid- to non- polar.

Retention occurs via non-polar interaction between carbon-hydrogen bonds of the analyte and carbon-hydrogen bonds of the sorbent function groups due to Van der Waals or dispersion forces.

The materials that are used as reversed phases are carbon-based media, polymer-based media, polymer-coated and bonded silica media.

Carbon-based media consist of graphitic, non-porous carbon with a high attraction for organic polar and non-polar compounds from both polar and non-polar matrices. Retention of analytes is based primarily on the analyte's structure, rather than on interactions of functional groups on the analyte with the sorbent surface.

Polymer-based sorbents are styrene/divivinylbenzene materials. It is used for retaining hydrophobic compounds which contain some hydrophilic functionality, especially aromatics.

Polymer-coated and bonded silica media is hydrophobic-bonded silica that is coated with a hydrophilic polymer. The pores in the polymer allow small, hydrophobic organic compounds of interest (e.g. drugs) to reach the bonded silica surface, while large interfering compounds (e.g. proteins) are shielded from the bonded silica by the polymer and are flushed through the SPE tube.

Several SPE materials, such as the alkyl- or aryl-bonded silicas (LC-18, ENVI-18, LC-8, ENVI-8, LC-4, and LC-Ph) are in the reversed phase category.

b. **Normal phase** involve a polar analyte, a mid- to non-polar matrix (e.g. acetone, chlorinated solvents and hexane) and a polar stationary phase. Retention of an analyte under normal phase conditions is primarily due to interactions between polar functional groups of the analyte and polar groups on the sorbent surface. Ex. Hydrogen bonding, dipole-dipole, induced dipole-dipole and pi-pi.

These phases can offer a highly selective extraction procedure capable of separating molecules with very similar structures. The main drawback is that the analyte must be loaded onto the sorbent in a relatively non-polar organic solvent such as hexane.

Polar-functionalized bonded silicas (e.g. LC-CN, LC-NH2, and LC-Diol), and polar adsorption media (LC-Si, LC-Florisil, ENVI-Florisil, and LC-Alumina) typically are used under normal phase conditions.

c. The **bonded silicas** have short alkyl chains with polar functional groups bonded to the surface. These silicas, because of their polar functional groups, are much more hydrophilic relatively to the bonded reversed phase silicas.

The bonded silicas LC-CN, LC-NH2, and LC-Diol - have short alkyl chains with polar functional groups bonded to the surface.

d. **Ion exchange SPE** can be used for compounds that are in a solution. Anionic (negatively charged) compounds can be isolated on an aliphatic quaternary amine group that is bonded to the silica surface. Cationic (positively charged) compounds are isolated by using the silica with aliphatic sulfonic acid groups that are bonded to the surface.

Biofluids can usually be applied directly to ion-exchange sorbents following dilution of the sample with water or a buffer, and possibly adjustment of pH. However, elution from strong ion-exchange sorbents can be a problem as high ionic strength or extremes of pH, may be required which may affect analyte stability or further processing of sample.

Anionic (negatively charged) compounds can be isolated on **LC-SAX** or **LC-NH2** bonded silica cartridges. Cationic (positively charged) compounds are isolated by using **LC-SCX** or **LC-WCX** bonded silica cartridges.

5.2.2 General properties of bonded silica sorbents

Although other materials are available ex. polymeric resins and alumina, the vast majority of SPE extractions are carried out by using bonded silica materials similar to those used in HPLC columns except the particle size and diameter. Bonded silica materials are rigid and do not shrink or swell like polystyrene-based resins in different solvents. Use of too high flow rate when processing cartridges may affect retention of analytes, particularly during the sample loading and elution steps. Potentially the capacity of the cartridge will be affected by all the components from the sample not only the analytes of interest.

5.2.3 Steps of Solid Phase Extraction

Generally following steps are followed for developing the method for extracting the analyte from plasma (Fig 3).

a. Pretreatment of sample - which includes dilution of sample or pH adjustment, filtration to avoid the blocking of the SPE cartridge and for better adsorption.
b. Conditioning of the cartridge - which is the main step in case of reverse phase SPE cartridges. Preconditioning is mainly done by solvent such as methanol, acetonitrile, isopropyl alcohol or tetrahydrofuran which is necessary to obtain reproducible result. Without this step, a highly aqueous solvent cannot penetrate the pores and wet the surface. Thus, only a small fraction of the surface area is available for interaction with the analyte. For the same reason, it is important not to let the cartridge dry out between the salvation step and addition of the sample.
c. Loading the sample - Sample size must be scaled to suit the size of the cartridge bed. A typical reverse phase cartridge may have capacity for up to 100 mg of very strongly retained substances.
d. Wash - very important step in case of the sample treatment by SPE. In this step a suitable solvent or water mixture is passed through SPE bed to remove the contaminants.
e. Elution of fraction - in this a suitable solvent or buffer is used to elute the analyte from the SPE bed for analysis.

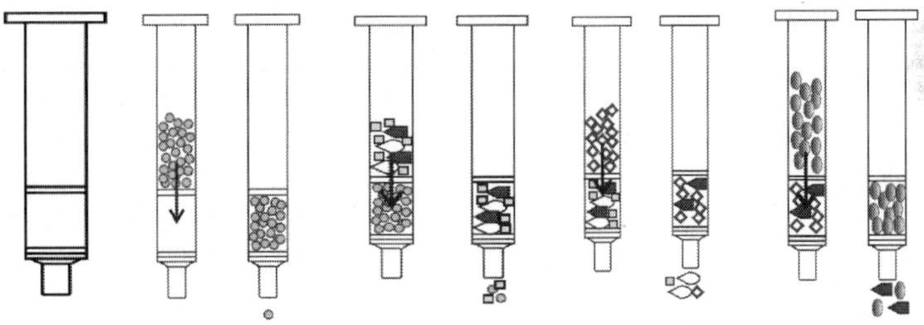

(a) (b) (c) (d) (e)

Fig. 3. Five steps of SPE: (a) selection of tube, (b) conditioning of tube, (c) addition of sample, (d) washing and (e) elution

5.2.4 A strategy for method development for plasma samples

- Rationale
- Practical consideration
- Pretreatment of samples and cartridges
- Screening sorbents and pH values
- Optimizing the washing procedure
- Optimizing the elution procedure
- Final optimization and simplification
- Strategies for removing persistent interferences

5.2.5 Developing SPE methods

In developing a SPE method, the properties of the isolate, sorbent and the matrix should be considered. The mechanisms of retention and the various secondary interactions may occur, and that a selective extraction from biofluid also requires the sorbent not to extract a large number of unknown compounds from the matrix. The best conditions are not easily predicted and the method needs to be developed experimentally in combination with the analytical method being used.

The following stages are recommended for method development.

a. Consider physic-chemical properties of analyte, nature of matrix and known chromatographic properties of analytes and the possible interaction with SPE sorbents.
b. Screen a range of cartridges (ex. C_{18}, C_8, C_2, Ph, CBA, SCX, SAX, PRS, NH_2, DEA, CH, Si and polymeric sorbent) under simple conditions (ex. from aqueous buffer solutions) looking for good retention of the analyte. If radiolabelled analyte is available this can conveniently be used to track analyte in such screening experiments. This experiment should not only identify likely cartridges for use in the assay, but should be used to try to confirm possible mechanism of interaction between the analyte and sorbent.
c. Select a more limited number of sorbents and examine conditions for loading/wash/elution (consider if pH control is needed, possible strength (% organic solvent) of wash solvents). Try the extraction from bio-fluid and select sorbent for final development.
d. Final development of extraction conditions and chromatographic analysis. Consider the robustness of the assay when finalizing extraction conditions. Ex. Do not select a wash solvent where a small change in composition could lead to elution of analyte from the cartridge.

The choice of different cartridges, manufactures and formats is becoming so extensive that it can appear almost overwhelming. It is generally better to build experience with a more limited set of sorbents, perhaps concentrating on cartridges from only one manufacturer. Also concentrate on investigating the use of cartridges with different functional groups (i.e. test C_{18}, C_8, C_2, Ph, CBA, SCX, SAX, PRS, NH_2, DEA, CH, Si, etc.), and those that use a contrasting mechanism to the analytical separation.

5.2.6 Characteristic features of SPE

- Complete flexibility
- Longer column lifetimes
- Powerful contaminant removal
- Greater recovery
- Better reproducibility
- More sensitivity

5.2.7 Advantages of SPE over LLE

- In SPE by choosing selective adsorbent analyte can be driven completely by adsorption and desorption
- In single stage LLE each extraction step equivalent to one chromatographic plate on the other hand by SPE in single step one can generate 10-50 plates

- Higher plate numbers in SPE leads to higher recoveries and purer of the analyte as compared to LLE
- For extracting more than one component from a mixture of component of different desorption solvent are required in case of SPE. To achieve similar results with LLE, one must perform several liquid extractions
- SPE is less time consuming and not tedious as compare to LLE

5.2.8 Limitation

- Depending on the nature of the analyte, SPE may not always be the method of choice, and liquid-liquid extraction may be a more viable solution.

6. Protein precipitation method (Backes, 2000; Wells, 2003)

This method is least one in bioanalytical. This is a very simple technique for extraction of the analyte from the matrix. If protein binding is suspected, then protein precipitation prior to sample extraction may be considered. Reagents to evaluate include perchloric, trichloroacetic and tungstic acids, and organic solvents such as acetonitrile or methanol. With all of these it is necessary to bear in mind the ability of the analytes and the matrix requirements of the extraction procedures. If protein binding is believed to be through a covalent linkage, then there is very little change of breaking it since this is the strongest of the intermolecular forces.

The main requirement for this technique is that the analyte should be freely soluble into reconstituting solvent. Preparation of sample through protein precipitation achieves separation by conversion of soluble proteins to an insoluble state by salting out or by addition of water miscible precipitation solvent or organic solvents such as acetone, ethanol, acetonitrile or methanol. Ideally, precipitation results in both concentration and purification, and is often used early in the sequence of downstream purification, reducing the volume and increasing the purity of the protein prior to any chromatography steps. In addition, precipitating agents can be chosen that provide a more stable product than found in the soluble form.

Proteins might stick to each other through one of three forces: electrostatic, hydrophobic, and van der Waals. The last one is difficult to distinguish from hydrophobic and operates over only in a very short range. Electrostatic forces operate at long range, but between like molecules are repulsive rather than attractive, so molecules have the same charge and repel each other.

Proteins are made insoluble by altering their surface properties, charge characteristics or changing the solvent characteristics; but changing the solvent characteristics being preferred. Greater the initial concentration of the desired protein, greater is the efficiency of precipitation; proteins are least soluble as its isoelectric point (pI) ranges from 4 - 10. The selection of a buffer at or near the pI of the protein is recommended. However some proteins may denature at their pI and above the pI. The solubility of a protein increases with the addition of salt and reaches a maximum after which there is a rapid linear decrease in solubility. There are several methods to reduce the solubility of proteins, which are ionic precipitation ex. ammonium sulphate, sodium chloride; metal ions ex. Cu^{+2}, Zn^{+2} and Fe^{+2};

non-ionic polymers ex. polyethylene glycol; organic solvents ex. ethanol, acetone; tannic acids, heparin, dextran sulphates, cationic polyelectrolytes ex. protamines; short chain fatty acids ex. caprylic acid; trichloroacetic, lecithins ex. concanavalin A and group specific dyes ex. procion blue. The use of temperature, pH or organic solvents can lead to denaturation and should be performed with care to minimize any decrease in yield or activity.

6.1 Type of protein precipitation

Salting out: Ammonium sulphate is the salt usually used for salting out, because of its high solubility and high ionic strength (which is proportional to the square of the charge on the ion, so that the ionic strength of 1M $(NH_4)_2SO_4$ is 3 times that of 1M NaCl). Neither ion associates much with proteins, which is good since such association usually destabilizes proteins. Its solubility changes little with temperature, it is cheap, and the density of even a concentrated solution is less than that of protein, so that protein can be centrifuged down from concentrated solutions.

Solvent Precipitation: When large amounts of a water-miscible solvent such as ethanol or acetone are added to a protein solution, proteins precipitate out. The conventional wisdom is that this is due to decrease of the dielectric constant, which would make interactions between charged groups on the surface of proteins stronger. Water miscible solvents associates with water much more strongly than do proteins, so that its real effect is to dehydrate protein surfaces, which then associate by van der Waals forces, at least if they are isoelectric or reasonably close to it. Removal of water molecules from around charged groups would also deshield them and allow charge interactions to occur more strongly, if there are areas of opposite charge on the surfaces of two proteins.

In practice, solvent precipitation is usually performed at low temperature. The condition for the protein is at 0°C and the solvent colder, -20°C in an ice-salt bath, because proteins tend to denature at higher temperatures though if sufficient control can be achieved and your protein is more stable than others, this can be selective and achieve greater purification.

Solvent precipitation can be done with polyethylene glycol at concentrations between 5 and 15%. It probably works the same way, by competing with the protein for water, but is less likely to inactivate the protein and does not require such low temperatures, but it tends to give an oily precipitate.

Commonly the sample is centrifuged at high speed for sufficient time, all the precipitated components of plasma will be settled at the bottom and clear supernatant liquid will be separated out. The obtained supernatant liquid can be injected directly into the HPLC or it can be evaporated and reconstituted with the mobile phase and further clean up of the sample can be carried out by using micro centrifuge at very high speed.

6.2 Advantage

- Now protein precipitation plates are available, able to remove the unwanted plasma proteins from plasma fluid samples prior to analysis
- Protein precipitation plates can be used in a wide range of aqueous and organic sample preparation including total drug analysis and sample preparation prior to HPLC or LC-MS/MS

- Protein precipitation plates are compatible with small volume of solvent
- Protein precipitation plate contains hydrophobic PTFE membrane as a prefilter removes the unwanted precipitated proteins prior to analysis
- Traditionally in this method plasma is mixed with protein precipitating agent and diluting solvent then the whole mixture is vertex, mixed, centrifuge and filter
- By using the new protein precipitate filter plate, precipitating solvent is added first followed by the plasma sample. This method does not require any mixing. Generally these plates are fitted to 96 well extraction plates. This new process showed 90% removal of plasma proteins when compare to the old method 60-65%

6.3 Disadvantage

- May increase the back pressure of the HPLC system
- Some components of plasma which are soluble in diluting solvent that bound to stationary phase permanently that will affect the column performance.

7. Solid Phase Microextraction (SPME) (Pawliszyn *et al.*, 1997; Pawliszyn, 1995, 1998, 1999, 2003; Wercinski 1999)

Miniaturization of sorbent technology and the concomitant decrease in solvent purchase, exposure and disposal has also taken a further giant step with the development of SPME. Solid-Phase Microextraction (SPME) is a very simple and efficient, solventless sample preparation method. SPME integrates sampling, extraction, concentration and sample introduction into a single solvent-free step. In this technique a fused silica fiber coated with polyacrylate, polydimethylsiloxane, carbowax or other modified bonded phase is placed in contact with a sample, exposed to the vapour above a sample (solid, liquid) or placed in the stream of a gaseous sample to isolate the analyte and concentrate analytes into a range of coating materials. After extraction, the fibers are transferred with the help of syringe like handling device to analytical instrument like gas chromatography (GC) and GC/mass spectrometry (GC/MS) for separation and quantification of the target analyte. In such a manner SPME has been used frequently to analyze volatile and semi-volatile compounds and may be used to purge and trap procedures. The method saves preparation time and disposal costs and can improve detection limits. The most interesting aspect of this technology involves the ability to use the exposed fiber as extraction and sample delivery device. Phases for SPME are available in a range of polarities and properties for analyses of volatile and semi-volatile compounds as well as application to extraction of analytes from liquid samples. One of the limitations of SPME is the low capacity of the fiber and the perturbation of equilibria that can occur in the presence of sample components or analytes at very high concentration versus those of lesser concentration. Dilution of the sample can overcome some of these problems but not all, as limits of detetion for trace analytes are compromised. Formaldehyde, Trition X-100, Phenylurea, pesticides and amphetamines are some of the analytes which are successfully extracted using SPME.

7.1 SPME basics (Vas & Vekey, 2004)

The concept of SPME may have been derived from the idea of an immersed GC capillary column. The SPME apparatus looks like modified syringe containing a fiber holder and a fiber assembly, the latter containing a 1–2 cm long retractable SPME fiber. The SPME fiber itself is a thin fused-silica optical fiber, coated with a thin polymer film conventionally used as a coating material in chromatography. In SPME the amount of extraction solvent is very small compared to the sample volume. As a result, exhaustive removal of analytes to the extracting phase does not occur; rather equilibrium is reached between the sample matrix and the extracting phase. In practical, the extracting phase is a polymeric organic phase commonly poly(dimethylsiloxane) and polyacrylate which is permanently attached to rod. The rod consists of an optical fiber made of fused silica, which is chemically inert. A polymer layer is used to protect the fiber against breakage. Poly(dimethylsiloxane) behaves as a liquid, which results in rapid extraction compared to polyacrylate, which is a solid. When the coated fiber is placed into an aqueous matrix the analyte is transferred from the matrix into the coating. The extraction is considered to be complete when the analyte has reached an equilibrium distribution between the matrix and fiber coating. The amount of extracted analyte is independent of the volume of the sample. Therefore, there is no need to collect a defined amount of sample prior to analysis. Thus, the fiber can be exposed directly to the ambient air, water, production stream, etc., and the amount of extracted analyte will correspond directly to its concentration in the matrix.

7.2 Principle modes of SPME

7.2.1 Direct extraction

In the direct-extraction mode, the coated fiber is inserted directly into the sample, and analytes are extracted directly from the sample matrix to the extraction phase. For gaseous samples, natural air convections and high diffusion coefficients are typically sufficient to facilitate rapid equilibration. For aqueous matrices, more efficient agitation techniques are required, such as forced flow, rapid fiber or vial movement, stirring or sonication.

7.2.2 Headspace configuration

In the headspace mode, the vapor above the bulk matrix is sampled. Thus, analytes must be relatively volatile in order to be transported from the bulk matrix to the fiber coating.

7.2.3 Advantages

Sampling of the headspace protects the fiber coating from damage by hostile matrices, such as those at very high or low pH, or those with large molecules, such as proteins which tend to foul the coating.

7.2.4 Types of extraction in SPME

- Fiber extraction
- In-tube extraction
- Stir BAR sorptive extraction (SBSE)

7.2.5 Advantage of SPME

- In SPME volatile, semi-volatile and non-volatile organic and inorganic analytes can be used for analyzed

- During desorbtion of the analyte, the polymeric phase is cleaned and therefore ready for reuse. The absence of solvent in SPME is an important feature, as it is not only environmentally friendly but makes the separation faster
- Important feature of SPME is its small size, which is convenient for designing portable devices for field work
- Solvent free environment, fast extraction, convenient automation and easy hyphenation with analytical instrument

8. Matrix Solid-Phase Dispersion (MSPD) (Barker *et al.*, 1989, 1993; Walker *et al.*, 1993)

Matrix solid phase dispersion is a sample preparation technique for use with solid sample matrices. MSPD is a microscale extraction technique, typically using less than 1g of sample and low volumes of solvents. It has been estimated to reduce solvent use by up to 98% and sample turnaround time by 90%.

Conventional extraction of organic analytes from tissue usually begins with a homogenization of a small amount of sample tissue with bulk bonded silica based sorbent in a pestle and mortar. The mechanical shearing forces produced by the grinding process disrupt the structure of the tissue, dispersing the sample over the surface of the support sorbent by hydrophilic and hydrophobic interaction which produces the mixture to become semi-dry and free-flowing, and a homogenous blend of sample. The bound solvent in the sorbent will aid complete sample disruption during the sample blending process and the sample disperses over the surface of the bonded phase-support material to provide a new mixed phase for isolating analytes from various sample matrices. The blend is then transferred into a pre-fitted SPE cartridge and elution of interference compounds and analytes of interest. This technique has recently been applied, using acid alumina, to extract the organic analyte. However, MSPD procedure needs longer analytical time generally and its limit of determination (LOD) is limited.

In method development using MSPD sorbents, the following points are to be considered

- Sample pre-treatment
- Interference elution
- Analyte elution
- Sample clean up

9. Supercritical fluid extraction (Mohamed & Mansorri, 2002; Antero, 2000)

Supercritical fluid extraction is becoming a very popular technique for the removal of non-polar to moderately polar analytes from solid matrices. Supercritical fluids (SCFs) are increasingly replacing the organic solvents that are used in industrial purification and recrystallization operations because of regulatory and environmental pressures on hydrocarbon and ozone-depleting emissions. SCF processes eliminate the use of organic solvents, so it has attracted much attention in the industrial sectors like pharmaceuticals, medical products and nutraceuticals. Pharmaceutical chemists have found SCFs useful for extraction of drug materials from tablet formulation and tissue samples.

Supercritical fluids exhibit a liquid-like density, while their viscosity and diffusivity remain between gas and liquid values. The recovery of a supercritical solvent after extraction can be carried out relatively simply by reducing the pressure and evaporating the solvent. Above the critical temperature the liquid phase will not appear even the pressure is increased. The compressibility of a supercritical fluid just above the critical temperature is large compared to the compressibility of ordinary liquids. A small change in the pressure or temperature of a supercritical fluid generally causes a large change in its density. The unique property of a supercritical fluid is that its solvating power can be tuned by changing either its temperature or pressure. The density of a supercritical fluid increases with pressure and becomes liquid-like, the viscosity and diffusivity remain between liquid-like and gas-like values. Additionally, supercritical fluids exhibit almost zero surface tension, which allows facile penetration into microporous materials leads to more efficient extraction of the analyte than the organic solvents. Carbon dioxide is a relatively good supercritical solvent will dissolve many relatively volatile polar compounds. In the presence of small amounts of polar co-solvents like water and short-chain alcohols to the bulk, the carbon dioxide gas can enhance the solubility of polar, non-volatile solutes in supercritical carbon dioxide. Supercritical fluids can be used to extract analytes from samples.

The main advantages of using supercritical fluids for extractions is that they are inexpensive, extract the analytes faster and more environmental friendly than organic solvents. For these reasons supercritical fluid CO_2 is the reagent widely used as the supercritical solvent.

9.1 Advantages

- SCFs have solvating powers similar to organic solvents, with higher diffusivity, lower viscosity and lower surface tension
- The solvating power can be changed by changing the pressure or temperature for effective extraction
- Separation of analytes from solvent is fast and easy
- Polarity can be changed by using co-solvent leads to have more selective separation of the analyte
- Products are free from residual solvents
- SCFs are generally cheap, simple and safe
- Disposal costs are less
- SCF fluids can be recycled

10. Column switching (Falco *et al.*, 1993, 1994; Henion *et al.*, 1998; Lee & Kim 2011)

Column switching techniques afford an interesting and creative form of sample preparation. This approach depends on the selectivity of appropriately chosen HPLC stationary phase to retain and separate the analyte of interest while allowing unretained components to be eliminated from the column. The benefits of this technique include total automation and quantitative transfer of targeted compounds within the column switching system. In the heart cut mode a narrow retention time region containing a desired components is cut from the chromatogram and transferred onto another HPLC column for further separation. In this instance, quantitative transfer of the components without adsorptive or degradative losses can be assured.

10.1 Advantages

It is capable of having increased selectivity by the judicious choice of two or more HPLC stationary phases. A limitation of column switching system is that sample throughout will likely not be as high as for other sample clean up methods. A second limitation of the column switching approaches includes restricted sample enrichment because of the limited amount of original, untreated, crude sample that can be loaded onto the first column of the HPLC separation. These limitations can be overcome by combining online SPE and a column switching system. In this method the recovery is more but very expensive one.

11. Future directions

Bio-equivalency is an important one for the Pharmaceutical Formulations especially in the Pharmaceutical Regulatory Market. The availability of methodology for the extraction procedure of the interested analyte coupled along with the analytical method for the quantification of the interested analyte in GC-MS/MS or LC-MS/MS will greatly facilitate future studies to rigorously establish a bio-equivalency of the Pharmaceutical formulations in the Pharmaceutical regulatory market.

12. Conclusion

The subject area of bioanalysis is a sub-discipline of analytical chemistry which covers a very broad range of assays like quantitative measurement of drugs and their metabolites in various biological systems like whole blood, plasma, serum, urine, faeces and tissues. The biological samples cannot be analyzed directly into the analytical system for the quantification of the interested analyte. Estimation of the analyte in the biological matrix can be done after the isolation of the interested analyte from the interferences in the biological sample. Isolation and estimation of the analyte is based on the sample preparation and extraction of the analyte from the biological matrix. The process adopted for the isolation of the interested analyte like sample preparation procedure and isolation steps must ensure the stability of the analyte until the completion of the analytical estimation. Bioanalysis in the pharmaceutical industry is to provide a quantitative measure of the active drug and/or its metabolite(s) for the purpose of pharmacokinetics, toxicokinetics, bioequivalence and exposure-response (pharmacokinetics/pharmacodynamics) studies. In this chapter, various extraction methods of the analyte from the biological matrix have been described with its advantages and disadvantages.

13. References

Allanson J.P. Biddlecombe RA, Jones AE, Pleasance S. (1996). The use of automated solid phase extraction in the "96 well" format for high throughput bioanalysis using liquid chromatography coupled to tandem mass spectroscopy. *Rapid Communications in Mass Spectroscopy*, 10, 811-816.

Antero L. (2000). *Supercritical fluid extraction of organic compounds from solids and aqueous solution.* Ph.D. Dissertation, Helsinki University of Technology, (Espoo, Finland).

Arthur CL, Pawliszyn J. (1990). Solid phase microextraction with thermal desorption using fused silica optical fibers. *Analytical Chemistry,* 62, 2145-2148.

Backes D. (2000) Strategy for the development of quantitative analytical procedures, In: *Principles and Practice of Bioanalysis,* Venn RF, 342-358, Taylor & Francis, NY.

Barker S A, Long AR, Short CR. (1989). Isolation of drug residues from tissues by solid phase dispersion, *Journal of Chromatography,* 475, 353–361.

Barker SA, Long AR, Hines ME. (1993). Disruption and fractionation of biological materials by matrix solid phase dispersion. *Journal of chromatography,* 629, 23-24.

Barrow GM. (1996). *Physical Chemistry,* 6th Ed. NY, McGraw-Hill (ISE).

Chang R. (1977). *Physical chemistry with applications to biological systems,* Macmillan Publishing, NY.

Christian GD., O'Reilly JE. (1986). *Instrumental Analysis,* 2nd Ed. Newton, MA: Allyn & Bacon.

Christians U, Sewing KF. (1989). Whole Blood Sample Clean-Up for Chromatographic Analysis, In: *Selective sample handling and detection in high performance liquid chromatography,* Volume 39, part 2, Frei RW, Zech K, 82-132, Elsevier, Amsterdam.

Destefano AJ, Takigiku R. (2004). Bioanlaysis in a regulated environment, In: *Pharmacokinetics in Drug development: regulatory and Development Paradigms, Volume* 2, Bonate PL, Howard DR, 105-125, AAPS, Arlington, VA.

Falco PC, Hernadez RH, Cabezav AS. (1993). Column-switching techniques for high-performance liquid chromatography of drugs in biological samples. *Journal of Chromatography: Biomedical Applications,* 619(2), 177-190.

Falco PC, Hernandez RH, Cabeza AS. (1994). Column-switching techniques for screening of diuretics and probenecid in urine samples. *Analytical Chemistry, 66* (2), 244–248.

Font G, Manes J, Moltoj C. (1993). Solid-phase extraction in multi-residue pesticide analysis of water. *Journal of Chromatography A,* 642, 135-161.

Fried K, Wainer IW. (1997). Column-Switching techniques in the biomedical analsis if stereoisomeric drugs: why, how and when. *Journal of Chromatography B: Biomedical Sciences and Applications,* 689(1), 91-104.

Gy PM. (1982). *Sampling of particulate materials Theory and Practice,* Elsevier, Amsterdam.

Harris DC. (1994). *Quantitative chemical Analysis,* 4th Ed. NY, WH. Freeman.

Henion J, Brewer E, Rule G. (1998). Sample Preparation for LC/MS/MS: Analyzing Biological and Environmental Samples. *Analytical Chemistry News & Features,* 650A-656 A.

Ho TS, Bjergaard SP, Rasmussen KE. (2002). Liquid-phase microextraction of protein bound drugs under non-equilibrium conditions. *Analyst,* 127, 608-13.

Horne KC. (1985). Analytichem International Sorbent Extraction Technology Handbook, Analytichem International Inc. January 14-15, 24201 Frampton Avenue, Harbor City, CA 90710 USA.

Ingwersen SH. (1993). Combined reverse phase and anion exchange solid phase extraction for the assay of the neuroprotectant NBQX in human plasma and Urine. *Biomedical Chromatography,* 7(3), 166-171.

James C. (2000). Solid-Phase Extraction, In: *Principles and Practice of Bioanalysis,* Venn RF, 28-43, Taylor & Francis, NY.

Keith LH. (1990). Environmental sampling: a summary, *Environmental Science and Technology*, 24 (5), 610–617.

Krishnan TR, Ibraham I. (1994). Solid phase extraction technique for the analysis of biological samples. *Journal of Pharmaceutical and Biomedical Analysis*, 12, 287-94.

Lee HJ, Kim KB. (2011). Application of Column-Switching Methods in HPLC for Evaluating Pharmacokinetic Parameters, In: *Advances in Chromatography*, Volume 49, Grushka E, Grinberg N, 291-340. CRC Press, USA.

MacDonald PD, Bouvier ESP. (1995). *Solid phase extraction application guide and bibliography*, Milford, MA, Water.

Majors RE, Fogelman KD. (1993).The Integration of Automated Sample Preparation with Analysis in Gas Chromatography, *American Laboratory*, 25(2): 40W-40GG.

McDowall RD, Doyle E, Murkitt GS, Picot VS. (1989). Sample preparation for the HPLC analysis of drugs in biological fluids. *Journal of Pharmaceutical and Biomedical Analysis*, 7(9), 1087-1096.

Mohamed RS, Mansoori G. (2002). *The use of supercritical fluid extraction technology in food processing*. The World Market Research Centre, London, UK.

Moore WJ. (1972). *Physical Chemistry*, 5th Ed. Harlow, Longman.

Moors M, Steenssens B, Tielemans I, Massart DL. (1994). Solid phase extraction of small drugs on apolar and ion exchange silica bonded phases: towards the development of a general strategy. *Journal of Pharmaceutical and Biomedical Analysis*, 12: 463-81.

Pawliszyn J. (1995). New directions in sample preparation for analysis of organic compounds. *Trends in Analytical Chemistry*, 14, 113-122.

Pawliszyn J, Pawliszyn B, Pawliszyn M. (1997). Solid Phase microextraction. *The chemical Educator*, 2(4), DOI 10.1333/s00897970137a.

Pawliszyn J. (1998). Solid phase microextraction Theory and Practice, Wiley-VCH. Inc. NY.

Pawliszyn J. (1999). Applications of solid phase microextraction. Royal Society of Chemistry, Cambridge.

Pawliszyn J. (2003). Sample Preparation: Quo Vadis?. *Analytical Chemistry*, 75, 2543-2558.

Plumb RS, Gray RD, Jones CM. (1997). Use of reduced sorbent bed and disk membrane solid phase extraction for the analysis of pharmaceutical compounds in biological fluids, with applications in the 96-well format. *Journal of Chromatography B: Biomedical Application*, 694, 123-133.

Sabikh, Jeannot R, Rondeaub. (2000). Multiresidue methods using solid phase extraction techniques for monitoring priority pesticides, including triazines and degradation products, in ground water. *Journal of Chromatography A*, 885, 217-236.

Scheurer J, Moore CM. (1992). Solid Phase extraction of drugs form biological tissue. A Review. *Journal of Analytical Toxicology*, 16, 264-269.

Simmonds RJ, James CA, Wood SA. (1994). A rational approach to the development of solid phase extraction methods for drugs in biological matrices, In: *Sample preparation for biomedical and environmental analysis*, Stevenson D, Wilson ID, 79, Plenum Press, NY.

Smith R, James GV. (1981). *The sampling of bulk materials*, The royal society of chemistry, London.

Vas G, Vekey K. (2004). Solid-phase microextraction: a powerful sample preparation tool prior to mass spectrometric analysis. *Journal of Mass Spectrometry*, 39, 233-254.

Walker CC, Lott HM, Barker SA. (1993). Matrix solid-phase dispersion extraction and the analysis of drugs and environmental pollutants in aquatic species. *Journal of chromatography*, 642, 225-242.

Watt AP, Morrison D, Evans DC. (2000). Approaches to higher throughput pharmacokinetics in drug discovery. *Drug Discovery Today*, 5(1), 17-24.

Wells DA. (2003). Protein precipitation: High throughput techniques and strategies for method development, In: *High Throughput Bioanalytical Sample Preparation - Methods and Automation Strategies,* Wells DA, 199-254, Elsevier, Amsterdam.

Wells DA. (2003). Protein precipitation: Automation strategies, In: *High Throughput Bioanalytical Sample Preparation - Methods and Automation Strategies,* Wells DA, 255-276, Elsevier, Amsterdam.

Wells DA. (2003). Liquid Liquid Extraction: High throughput techniques, In: *High Throughput Bioanalytical Sample Preparation - Methods and Automation Strategies,* Wells DA, 277-306, Elsevier, Amsterdam.

Wells DA. (2003). Liquid Liquid Extraction: Strategies for method development and optimization, In: *High Throughput Bioanalytical Sample Preparation - Methods and Automation Strategies,* Wells DA, 307-326, Elsevier, Amsterdam.

Wells DA. (2003). Liquid Liquid Extraction: Automation strategies, In: *High Throughput Bioanalytical Sample Preparation - Methods and Automation Strategies,* Wells DA, 327-360, Elsevier, Amsterdam.

Wells DA. (2003). Solid Phase Extraction: High throughput techniques, In: *High Throughput Bioanalytical Sample Preparation - Methods and Automation Strategies,* Wells DA, 361-432, Elsevier, Amsterdam.

Wells DA. (2003). Solid Phase Extraction: Strategies for method development and optimization, In: *High Throughput Bioanalytical Sample Preparation - Methods and Automation Strategies,* Wells DA, 433-484, Elsevier, Amsterdam.

Wells DA. (2003). Solid Phase Extraction: Automation strategies, In: *High Throughput Bioanalytical Sample Preparation - Methods and Automation Strategies,* Wells DA, 485-504, Elsevier, Amsterdam.

Wercinski SCS. (1999). *Solid Phase microextraction-A Practical guide.* Marcel Dekker: NY.

Williams J. (1999). The assessment of therapeutic compliance based upon the analysis of drug concentration in hair, In: *Drug Testing Technology Assessment of field application,* Mieczkowski T, 1-32, CRC Press, Boca Raton, London, NY, Washington DC.

Wiltshire H. (2000). Strategy for the development of quantitative analytical procedures. In: *Principles and Practice of Bioanalysis,* Venn RF, 1-27, Taylor & Francis, NY.

Yu J, Wu C, Xing J. (2004). Development of new solid-phase microextraction fibers by sol-gel technology for the determination of organophosphorus pesticide multiresidues in food. *Journal of Chromatography A,* 1036, 101-111.

Zief M, Kiser R. (1990). An overview of solid phase extraction for sample preparation. *American Laboratory*, 22(1), 70-83.

Zwir Ferenc A, Biziuk M. (2006). Solid Phase extraction technique Trends, opportunities and Applications. *Polish Journal of Environmental Studies,* 15(5), 677-690.

Part 4

E-Health and Educational Aspects of Bioengineering

22

Quality Assessment of E-Health Solutions in Primary Health Care – Approach Based on User Experience

Damir Kralj
Ministry of the Interior, PD Karlovac
Croatia

1. Introduction

The significance of primary health care (PHC) within the overall health care system of the each country is tremendous. PHC provides the first contact between patients and health care system, and keeps the most complete medical records of particular patient which could be used later for different medical secondary purposes. Well organized and computerized PHC significantly improves both the quality of care and contributes to significant savings in treatment. In order to improve the quality of such information systems, it is necessary to introduce a methodology for measuring their actual quality. Our research focuses on the creation of models for assessing the quality of IT solutions, based on users' (doctors') experiences, within the newly introduced primary health care information system in the Republic of Croatia.

The process of implementation of the national e-Health infrastructure in the Croatian public health care system started in 2006 by introduction of the Croatian primary health care information system (PHCIS or CEZIH in Croatian language) (Croatian Institute for Health Insurance [CIHI], 2010). The first areas of the system implementation includes the integration of family doctor's offices (FDO) into a comprehensive system, that includes the integration of various types of FDO specialized solutions with national infrastructure, Croatian Institute for Health Insurance and Public Health Authority. The system is generally tested "in vivo" i.e. in real production conditions and with real patients' data collected in FDO. The central part of the information system was designed by the renowned company, specialized in area of those projects, as a very stable and quality system based on well-defined business processes, legal and semantic rules, and communication and messaging standards such as EN13606 and HL7v3 (Končar & Gvozdanović, 2006). Design of the applications for managing of the electronic healthcare records (EHR) in FDO was left to a number of small IT companies competing on the Croatian market. These applications had to undergo certification process defined by the Ministry of Health and Social Welfare (MHSW). Certification included only the area of communication and basic data exchange with the central part of the system. The concept and functionality of these applications has been left to the manufacturers of these applications (Kralj & Tonković, 2009). With such situation in place, it seems very difficult to measure the quality and effectiveness of an information system which is in the early stage of development. For these reasons, our motivation was to establish a methodology to quantify and qualify overall quality criteria.

2. Methods used in the project

For the purposes of this study, we defined a methodology that consists of eight steps showed on Fig. 1. As we can see, our methodology is based on overview and analysis of domestic papers and foreign projects, studies, standards, initiatives and certification criteria. On these foundations, we constructed our assessment and built assessment tool i.e. questionnaire.

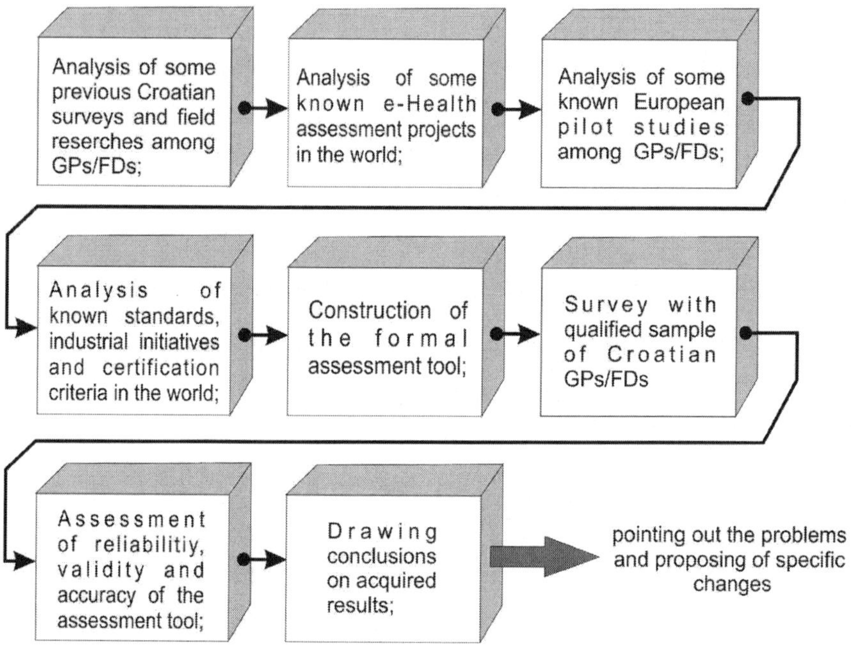

Fig. 1. Preview of used methodology

3. Overview of the relevant documents and projects

The basic idea of the formation of such a methodology arises from so-called frameworks for assessing of community readiness for the introduction of e-Health. One of the earliest references is the "Framework for rural and remote readiness in telehealth" that was conducted in 2002 by Canada's advanced research and innovation network CANARIE (CANARIE, 2002). This paper describes the basic assumptions that derive from the theory of change and stages of change. Readiness is defined as a cognitive indicator of actual conditions, with determining the factors that contribute to success and factors affecting the failure of some innovations. The next interesting example can be found in association of the

Aga Khan University in Pakistan and the University of Calgary in Canada (Khoja et al., 2007a). The subject of the project was development of tools for e-Health readiness assessment in developing countries. In this project were proposed methods for validation and reliability testing of the tool for e-Health readiness assessment. The assessment is based on a quantitative presentation of qualitative data. In order to verify the reliability of the tool and to avoid multiple control testing, there was introduced a calculation of the Cronbach's Alpha (α) coefficient of correlation for each category of readiness and for all categories combined. A third interesting example is found in the study "e-Health Readiness Framework from Electronic Health Records Perspective" (Li, 2008) conducted on the University of New South Wales in Australia. Research contribution of this study consists of three essential elements: a model of framework, methodology of assessment and evaluation of framework based on criteria and case studies. Our work is taking good reference in some basic analysis from these models. However, some early results have shown that they are not sufficient in Croatian example. More precisely, all the models referenced above are based on an analysis of isolated cases ("in vitro") by gathering the elements to assess the readiness of a small part of health system for the introduction of e-Health concept, while our framework requires experiences assessment in real production ("in vivo") and large scale deployment, which leaves us with highly challenging environment that requires careful assessment and offers less change manoeuvre space. Analysis of the Croatian papers drew our attention to specific problems before (Kern & Polašek, 2007) and shortly after (Kralj & Tonković, 2009) the beginning of implementation of e-health concept. Analysis of worldwide standards such as HL7, EN13606 and DICOM, and initiatives such as Integrating the Healthcare Enterprise (IHE) and EHR-implement, is simply unavoidable. In addition, when creating our methodology, we have also taken into account latest recommendations from European Institute for Health Records (EuroRec) EHR-Q TN project, criteria of The EuroRec EHR Quality Seal Level 1 and Level 2 (EuroRec, 2010), projects and recommendations of the American Office of the National Coordinator for Health Information Technology (ONC) and certification criteria of the Certification Commission for Health Information Technology (CCHIT) (Centers for Medicare and Medicaid Services, 2010), which has lead us to the final readiness assessment model. It should be noted that these American recommendations and criteria resulted in mid-2010 with a set of certification criteria called Meaningful Use of EHR Stage 1, which is a direct consequence of the American Recovery and Reinvestment Act (ARRA) of 2009. The contents of European studies that were conducted by research agencies Empirica (Dobrev et al., 2008) and Health Consumer Powerhouse (Björnberg et al., 2009) were also of great help in the making process of the assessment tool.

4. Construction of the assessment tool

Based on previously mentioned foundations we made a framework for the assessment tool i.e. questionnaire. The framework consists of seven main units. While the first unit contains general questions about the doctor and his/her office, the remaining six units measure major dimensions i.e. categories of experience which our work has identified as needed. As we see in Table 1, these six categories are: basic experience, technological experience, engagement, domain experience, organizational experience and societal experience. Each of these categories is a key performance indicator (KPI) of the current state of implementation of the e-Health concept in the health system as a whole. When designing this framework, we tried to include the key factors that can describe doctors' problems and attitudes, doctors' involvement in the process of adopting of new technologies, the impact of new technologies on the domain workflow, changes in communication with other health organizations and offices, and, of course, the impact on communication between doctor and patient. In addition, we have tried as much as possible to reduce any overlap between categories i.e. to ensure unambiguity of the categories.

A) BASIC	B) TECHNOLOGICAL	C) ENGAGEMENT
• Attitude about use of computers in FDO; • Organization of work on computer support; • Impact assessment of use of computers to work process; • Attitude about basic elements of e-Health.	• Problems with hardware and network support in FDO; • Quality and reliability of EHR applications in FDO; • Readiness of diagnostic equipment for use in e-Health; • Data protection and patient safety.	• Self-assessment of the IT and medical domain knowledge; • FD engagement in process of new system implementation; • Use of EHR for evaluation of doctor's work and research; • Care about the safety and security of the EHR.
D) DOMAIN	**E) ORGANIZATIONAL**	**F) SOCIETAL**
• Domain usability and functi-onality of EHR applications; • Structuring and encoding of information in EHR application; • Implementation of advanced decision support systems; • Monitoring and quality of work assessment according to working guidelines; • Overall satisfaction with the EHR applications from the domain view.	• Use of e-mail communication with other health institutions; • Possibilities of migration to a paperless business; • Elements of e-business integrated into EHR application; • Forms of electronic reporting built in existing application support; • Interoperability and compa-tibility of EHR applications with current diagnostic systems.	• The impact of use of computers and EHR applications on patients' satisfaction; • The impact of health contents available on the Internet on behaviour of patients in FDO; • Forms of electronic communication between doctors and patients.

Table 1. Structure of the framework with general description of its categories

Based on previously described framework we made a rather comprehensive questionnaire. In total there are 118 questions of which 103 issues have been defined for assessment. These 103 questions for the assessment consist of 32 multiple choice questions in a Likert scale of 1-5, 54 questions with dichotomous answers (YES-NO i.e. 1 or 0), and 17 questions with offered answers that should be marked. General questions about the doctor and his/her office are very important for assessing the quality of the population sample. In addition, based on information about the structure of the measured population we can perform comparison of the results depending on the specific groups within the population (e.g. gender, specialization, age, years of service, etc.). The time allocated for completing the questionnaire was estimated at 20 minutes. The questionnaire therefore is rather straightforward and easy to use and populate.

Given that the questionnaires as this are very cumbersome to display on the site of small format, Table 2 shows the part of the questionnaire form with general questions about the doctor and his/her office, while Table 3 shows the main part of the questionnaire form for all six categories for assessment broken on multiple pages. Each category i.e. part of the questionnaire with each other is separated by a space line. For easier orientation in the questionnaire, all items i.e. questions are numbered. Questions are marked with a combination of the ordinal number of subcategories within the main category and the ordinal number of questions within the subcategories.

<table>
<tr><td rowspan="6">Dana about FDO</td><td>County:</td><td></td></tr>
<tr><td>Municipal:</td><td></td></tr>
<tr><td>City:</td><td></td></tr>
<tr><td>FD office type:</td><td>a) urban
b) rural
c) insular</td></tr>
<tr><td>FD office autonomy:</td><td>a) in a health center
b) under lease
c) private</td></tr>
<tr><td>Practice organization:</td><td>a) standalone
b) group practice</td></tr>
<tr><td rowspan="6">Data about FD</td><td>Age:</td><td></td></tr>
<tr><td>Years of working:</td><td></td></tr>
<tr><td>Gender:</td><td>M - F</td></tr>
<tr><td>Specialization?</td><td>Yes - No</td></tr>
<tr><td>Do you use in your work the computer and the application for managing of EHR?</td><td>Yes - No</td></tr>
<tr><td>Name of the EHR application (program) that you use:</td><td></td></tr>
</table>

Table 2. Part of the questionnaire form with general questions about the doctor and his office

A	Question	Answer		
1.1	How long have you been using the computer in your practice? (years, months)			
1.2	Do you use a computer to record administrative data about patients?	Yes - No		
2.1	Who performs an update of administrative patient data?	a) doctor b) nurse c) doctor and nurse d) administrator		
2.2	Do you use your computer for recording of patients' medical data?	Yes - No		
2.3	Who performs an update of medical information about patients?	a) doctor b) nurse c) doctor and nurse d) administrator		
2.4	Do you use your computer during the examination and interview with the patient?	Yes - No		
3.1	Evaluate the impact of using of the computer on the quality of your work in the office.	significantly reduces the efficiency	1 - 2 - 3 - 4 - 5	significantly increases the efficiency
3.2	Evaluate the impact of computers due to the dynamics of your practice.	significantly slows	1 - 2 - 3 - 4 - 5	significantly accelerates
4.1	Express your opinion on the impact of the degree of integration of health information systems on the efficiency of the entire health system.	significantly reduces the efficiency	1 - 2 - 3 - 4 - 5	significantly increases the efficiency
4.2	Express your opinion on electronic prescribing of drugs (e-Prescription).	I do not support at all	1 - 2 - 3 - 4 - 5	I fully support
4.3	Express your opinion on electronic referral of patients (e-Referral).	I do not support at all	1 - 2 - 3 - 4 - 5	I fully support
4.4	Express your attitude about the secondary use of medical records of patients for the purpose of development and progress of the entire health care system.	I do not support at all	1 - 2 - 3 - 4 - 5	I fully support
4.5	Express your attitude about the creation of a central registry of electronic health records for all patients ("central EHR").	I do not support at all	1 - 2 - 3 - 4 - 5	I fully support

B	Question	Answer		
1.1	Does the nurse use a separate computer that is networked with your computer?	Yes - No		
1.2	Who performed the installation of your computer and network support in the office?	a) equipment supplier b) software vendor	c) friends or acquaintances d) yourself	
1.3	Which operating system are you using on your computer?	a)MS Windows XP b)MS Windows Vista c)MS Windows 7	d)MacOS c)Linux	
1.4	On which way are you connecting to the Internet?	a) modem (PSTN) b)ISDN c)ADSL	d)GSM or similar e)through the proxy of the greater network	
1.5	Does your nurse have access to the Internet?	Yes - No		
1.6	Rate the size of the cost of the hardware and network support in your practice.	very small	1 - 2 - 3 - 4 - 5	very large
1.7	Rate the size of your office communication costs.	very small	1 - 2 - 3 - 4 - 5	very large
2.1	How many of the EHR applications you changed so far? (number)			
2.2	Is your current HER application certified to work on the central HIS (CEZIH)?	Yes - No		
2.3	Rate the quality and availability of contextual help system in your EHR application (e.g. press the F1 key for the current problem)?	very poor or there is no	1 - 2 - 3 - 4 - 5	high quality and accessible
2.4	Rate telephone support system (helpdesk), if it is ensured by the vendor of your EHR application?	very poor or there is no	1 - 2 - 3 - 4 - 5	high quality and accessible
2.5	Rate the remote administration and troubleshooting, if it is ensured by the vendor of your EHR application?	very poor or there is no	1 - 2 - 3 - 4 - 5	high quality and accessible
2.6	Rate the remote version update, if it is ensured by the vendor of your EHR application?	very poor or there is no	1 - 2 - 3 - 4 - 5	high quality and accessible
2.7	Rate the remote update of prescribed nomenclatures, if it is ensured by the vendor of your EHR application?	very poor or there is no	1 - 2 - 3 - 4 - 5	high quality and accessible
2.8	Rate the size of the cost of the software support in your practice.	very small	1 - 2 - 3 - 4 - 5	very large
3.1	Do you use any kind of equipment that provides computer-readable results (ECG, spirometry, ultrasound, holter, etc.)?	Yes - No		

3.2	Mark a letter before the name of the equipment that you use, and which can be connected to your computer. (multiple answers possible)	a) ECG b) spirometer c) blood pressure gauge	d) ultrasound e) ECG holter f) RR holter
4.1	Which of the following actions require, in your opinion, a greater degree of security and data protection?	a) transactions between bank accounts b) transmission of electronic health records c) both equally	
4.2	Which of the following categories, in your opinion, is more important for patient safety in health care system?	a) protection against of unauthorized access to patient data b) timely access to patient's data c) both equally	
4.3	Which are the safety and privacy protection elements that you use in your practice? (multiple answers possible)	a) physical access limitation (locking) b) password on the PC startup c) password on the entrance of the EHR application d) encrypting the entire contents of the hard disk c) none of the above	
4.4	Which are the elements of protection against data loss that you use in your office? (multiple answers possible)	a) regular data backup included in EHR application b) making of additional backup copies which are stored separately c) use of the devices for uninterruptible power supply (UPS)	
5.1	Do you know what the IHE certification is? (short explanation - full name)	Yes - No	
5.2	Do you know what the HL7 standard is? (short explanation - purpose)	Yes - No	
5.3	Do you know what the EN13606 standard is? (short explanation - purpose)	Yes - No	
5.4	Do you know what the DICOM standard is? (short explanation - purpose)	Yes - No	
5.5	Should the doctors be, at least roughly, familiar with the above standards and recommendations?	Yes - No	

C	Question	Answer		
1.1	Did you attend any kind of informatics schools or courses in the past five years?	Yes - No		
1.2	Rate your level of IT knowledge.	very low	1 - 2 - 3 - 4 - 5	very high
1.3	Rate the doctors' overload with necessary level of ICT knowledge.	very low	1 - 2 - 3 - 4 - 5	very high
1.4	Rate your level of domain (medical) knowledge.	very low	1 - 2 - 3 - 4 - 5	very high

2.1	Rate the frequency of your visits to bibliographic databases on the Internet.	rarely (or never)	1 - 2 - 3 - 4 - 5	often
2.2	Rate the frequency of your visits to health portals on the Internet.	rarely (or never)	1 - 2 - 3 - 4 - 5	often
2.3	Rate the frequency of your visits to e-journals on the Internet.	rarely (or never)	1 - 2 - 3 - 4 - 5	often
2.4	Rate the intensity of use of e-mail in the life and work.	rarely (or never)	1 - 2 - 3 - 4 - 5	often
2.5	Do you know what HON certificate is? (brief description - purpose)	Yes - No		
3.1	Have you been engaged in developing and testing some of the CEZIH certified EHR applications?	Yes - No		
3.2	Are you a member of an informal group of doctors who help each other in their work with purpose of better understanding and use of EHR applications?	Yes - No		
3.3	Do you have the role of "leader" in such a group?	Yes - No		
4.1	Do you use the information from your computer application for the professional evaluation of your work?	Yes - No		
4.2	Do you use the information from your computer application for administrative and financial evaluation of your work?	Yes - No		
4.3	Do you use the information from your computer application for your research work?	Yes - No		
5.1	How often do you change the password for entry into the EHR application?	a) daily b) weekly c) monthly	d) sometimes (not too often) e) still use the first one f) I do not use a password	
5.2	How the doctors, who replace you in your absence, realize access to your EHR application?	a) use my account b) I open new user account for every replacement c) I have opened a special account for replacement regardless of the physician		
5.3	How often do you make EHR data backup?	a) daily b) weekly c) monthly	d) sometimes e) after each change f) I do not perform backup	

D	Question	Answer		
1.1	Rate how your EHR application follows the domain workflow i.e. organization of the work (SOAP).	very bad	1 - 2 - 3 - 4 - 5	very well
1.2	Evaluate the usability of the user interface of your application (ease of handling and intuitiveness).	very difficult and confusing	1 - 2 - 3 - 4 - 5	very easy and intuitive
1.3	Is in your EHR application visible reason and the content of previous patient's visit(s), prior to entering data of a new visit?	Yes - No		
2.1	Mark the letter before the name of the disease classification which your application supports. (multiple answers possible)	a) ICD10 b) ICPC-2	c) Read d) SNOMED	
2.2	Is your EHR application capable for structured and atomized input of patient's vital parameters?	Yes - No		
2.3	Is your EHR application capable for menu oriented input of previously defined items (instead of typing a free text)?	Yes - No		
2.4	Does your EHR application contains regularly updated list of drugs prescribed by the Ministry of Health and Social Welfare?	Yes - No		
2.5	Does your EHR application contains regularly updated nomenclatures of diagnostic procedures prescribed by the Ministry of Health and Social Welfare?	Yes - No		
2.6	Does your EHR application contains regularly updated sets of working guidelines prescribed by the Ministry of Health and Social Welfare?	a) Yes, on the computer b) No, but, if necessary, it connects me with MHSW Internet portal	c) No, nor it connects me on external sources d) I don't know	
2.7	Does your EHR application contain regularly updated nomenclature of medical institutions as prescribed by the Ministry of Health and Social Welfare?	Yes - No		

!!!	NOTE: The set of questions 3.x refers to a systems which based on the described state of the patient helps the doctor by offering a closest solution (or several solutions) as assistance for a final decision. These systems can be part of the application and / or built in diagnostic equipment (e.g. ECG with auto-diagnostic). In the case of drug prescribing, these systems are based on possible drug interactions and side effects, etc.			
3.1	Does your EHR application have inbuilt functionalities for diagnosis decision support?	Yes - No		
3.2	If your previous answer is "Yes", rate the quality and usability of the system.	completely useless	1 - 2 - 3 - 4 - 5	fully usable
3.3	Are you using an advanced decision support system for determining a diagnosis independent of your EHR application (software or equipment with inbuilt functionalities)?	Yes - No		
3.4	Does your EHR application has inbuilt advanced helping functionalities for drug prescribing?	Yes - No		
3.5	If your answer is "Yes", rate the quality and usability of the system.	completely useless	1 - 2 - 3 - 4 - 5	fully usable
3.6	Does your EHR application has inbuilt advanced helping functionalities to assist physicians to refer patients for further treatment?	Yes - No		
3.7	If your previous answer is "Yes", rate the quality and usability of the system.	completely useless	1 - 2 - 3 - 4 - 5	fully usable
3.8	Rate how your EHR application monitors chronic diseases?	very poor or not at all	1 - 2 - 3 - 4 - 5	very good
3.9	Rate how your EHR application monitors allergies?	very poor or not at all	1 - 2 - 3 - 4 - 5	very good
4.1	Does your EHR application has some visible indicators (gauges, visual indicators) that alerts you to the current efficiency and the quality of your work (rates and coefficients)?	Yes - No		
4.2	Does your EHR application has any form of an advanced system for short-term and long-term evaluation of the quality of your work?	Yes - No		
5.1	From domain point of view, rate the overall satisfaction with your EHR application.	very unsatisfied	1 - 2 - 3 - 4 - 5	very satisfied
5.2	From domain point of view, compare your CEZIH compatible application with the application you were using before CEZIH system.	significantly worse	1 - 2 - 3 - 4 - 5	much better

E	Question	Answer
1.1	Do you use e-mail to communicate with your colleagues in primary health care?	Yes - No
1.2	Do you use e-mail for communication with specialists in clinics?	Yes - No
1.3	Do you use e-mail for receiving of laboratory results of your patients?	Yes - No
1.4	Do you use e-mail for receiving of specialist medical examination of your patients?	Yes - No
1.5	Do you use web-services or e-mail for ordering patients to specialists in clinics (e-ordering)?	Yes - No
2.1	Do you store medical documents received by e-mail in the particular folders inside of your EHR application?	Yes - No
2.2	Do you scan medical paper documentation of your patients and store them in electronic form to particular folders of your EHR application?	Yes - No
3.1	Can you perform e-ordering directly from your EHR application?	Yes - No
3.2	Does your EHR application support an electronic referral (e-referral)?	Yes - No
3.3	Does your EHR application support electronic drug prescribing (e-prescription)?	Yes - No
4.1	What is the form of the reports that you submit to the Croatian Institute for Health Insurance?	a) paper form b) paper form and floppy disk c) electronically through the web portal CEZIH d) electronically directly from the application
4.2	Does your application support electronically reporting to the Croatian Institute for Health Insurance?	Yes - No
4.3	Does your application support electronically reporting to Public Health?	Yes - No
4.4	Is your application ready for exchange (synchronization) of medical data with a central registry of EHRs?	Yes - No

4.5	Can you from your EHR application directly check the status of the insured patient in the Croatian Institute for Health Insurance?	Yes - No		
5.1	What do you do when foreign and, increasingly, domestic insured, bring you the results of diagnostic procedures (X-ray, CT, MRI, etc.) made on CD or DVD?	a) I browse the pictures on the computer, and store the medium with patient's paper documents b) I browse the pictures on the computer, and store them in the particular folders of my EHR application c) I do not browse the pictures, but I ask the patient to bring me a hardcopy of findings (film or paper)		
5.2	Does your application allow direct preview and storage of these digital records?	Yes - No		

F	Question	Answer		
1.1	Rate the satisfaction of the patients with using of the EHR application in your practice.	very unsatisfied	1 - 2 - 3 - 4 - 5	very satisfied
1.2	Do you grant to your patients, on their request, insight into their medical history on your computer?	Yes - No		
1.3	Do you issue to your patients a complete history of his/her illness in electronic form (CD, floppy, etc.), for the purpose of the transfer to another physician and to ease work to the newly elected physician and, also, to contribute to patient's safety?	Yes - No		
2.1	Do your patients use available health contents on the Internet to be further informed about their condition?	Yes - No		
2.2	Do your patients comment with you the information about their problems that they have been collected on the Internet?	Yes - No		
3.1	Do you use e-mail to communicate with your patients?	Yes - No		
3.2	Do you use some form of electronic ordering patients for examination in your practice?	Yes - No		
3.3	Do your patients use e-mail for delivering of information about their medical condition (e.g. monitoring of chronic disease)?	Yes - No		
3.4	If your office has its own web page, which contents are available on it? (multiple answers possible)	a) advertising b) health advices c) e-ordering system d) useful links to other health contents	e) subsystem for acquisition of data for monitoring of chronic diseases f) I have no web page	

Table 3. The main part of the questionnaire form with questions for assessment purpose

5. Analysis of survey process and data collected

The survey was conducted during the period from mid-December 2009 until the end of January 2010. Questionnaire was made in electronic PDF/FDF form with the ability to automatically return to the sender via e-mail, and in the classical paper form. The questionnaires in electronic form were offered via dedicated mailing list, which has approximately 1100 formal users (assuming that the number of active users is much smaller), while about 70 questionnaires were distributed in paper form at the professional meetings and collected on spot or received by post. Random sample selection depended on FDs' free will to fill the questionnaire.

A total of 115 complete and correctly filled questionnaire forms were collected (87 or 75.7% of 115 in electronic and 28 or 24.3% of 115 in paper form). Therefore, we included approximately 4.7% of total 2450 Croatian FDs. By analysis of general data about the respondents and their offices, we got the structure of the analysed sample, which is showed in Table 4.

Category	Characteristics		
Age	Median: 49	Interquartile range: 44 - 51	
Years of working	Median: 23	Interquartile range: 18 - 26	
Gender	Male: 23,6 %	Female: 76,4 %	
Specialization	Yes: 66 %	No: 34 %	
FD office autonomy	Health center: 18.9 %	Under lease: 69,8 %	Private: 11,3 %
FD office type	Urban: 64,1 %	Rural: 32,1 %	Insular: 3,8 %

Table 4. Characteristics of tested sample of the Croatian family doctors and their offices

By comparison of data from well-known official Croatian health statistical publications (Baklaić et al., 2007), and data known from some previous analysed works (Kern & Polašek, 2007; Kralj & Tonković, 2009) with data showed in Table 4, it can be concluded that analysed sample is representative enough to draw conclusions from the study.

For the purposes of the upcoming numerical and statistical analysis, a quantification of the collected responses was performed. In addition to quantitative analysis, we performed a qualitative analysis of collected data that can assess the actual state of e-Health concept implementation, and point on the existing problems and shortcomings of the current model of e-Health concept implementation.

6. Results analysis and discussion

The results of qualitative and quantitative analysis of the categories and total experience are shown in Table 5. Due to limited space, the qualitative ratings are summarized for the most important elements, while the quantitative rates provide fairly realistic overall scores on a scale from 0 to 1. Prior to conducting of the survey, we hypothesized that actual state of the implementation of e-Health concept in the Croatian primary health care corresponds to the descriptive assessment: "somewhere halfway". The presented overall quantitative result to some extent confirms this assessment.

<table>
<tr><th>Category</th><th>Results</th></tr>
<tr><td rowspan="2">A</td><td>-40% of FDs believe that the new system and EHR applications slow down their work;
-In 4.3% of FDOs nurses write medical information in the EHR, while in 10.4% of FDOs the doctor updates the administrative and demographic data of patients;
-34% of FDs do not support e-prescribing, while 35% do not support e-referral;
-50% of FDs are mainly against the secondary use of medical data;
-66% of FDs do not believe in the security and confidentiality of data in a central EHR;</td></tr>
<tr><td>Mean rate: 0.696 Items: 12 Cronbach α: 0.667</td></tr>
<tr><td rowspan="2">B</td><td>-All contracting FDOs are equipped with the necessary ICT equipment;
-Automatic remote software update is provided for all EHR applications;
-All EHR applications use the same formal structured and coded lists of health registers and nomenclatures that are automatically updated on a regular basis;
-All EHR applications have authorized access and role specific access rights;
-41% of FDs have some diagnostic devices that provides results in an electronic format suitable for inserting in EHR;
-Transfer to another EHR application is rather difficult due to portability and "data lock" issues (including basic demographic data, prescriptions, referrals, and several types of reports)=> EHR is not longitudinal in its most important part;</td></tr>
<tr><td>Mean rate: 0.555 Items: 24 Cronbach α: 0.694</td></tr>
<tr><td rowspan="2">C</td><td>-13% of FDs believed to be overloaded with unnecessary knowledge of IT technologies;
-50% of FDs considered that they should have at least roughly knowledge of the norms and recommendations upon which is based the e-Health concept;
-26% FDs attended IT schools or courses in the past 5 years;
-17% of FDs assess their IT knowledge as very high;
-24% of FDs are members of some informal groups for helping in better understanding of functionalities of their EHR applications;
-57% of FDs use the data from their EHR applications for quality evaluation of their work;
-75% FDs give to their replacement doctors to work on their user account (security risk);
-Only 60% of FDs make daily backup their data (EHR);</td></tr>
<tr><td>Mean rate: 0.427 Items: 18 Cronbach α: 0.722</td></tr>
<tr><td rowspan="2">D</td><td>-In only 34% cases FDs considered that EHR applications very well follow domain work flow, while in 49.6% of the cases considered that the user interface is user friendly and intuitive;
-All applications support atomized entry of demographic and administrative data for uniquely identified patient, which are available from all parts of his EHR;
-In 61% of EHR applications is possible atomized (structured) input of the physical status;
-All applications contain ICD-10 classification of diseases, and equal central updated nomenclatures of procedures, medication and health care institutions;
-In 72.6% and 75.4% cases EHR applications offer support for chronic disease and allergies monitoring, respectively
-Decision support systems are in their beginnings as a simpler forms of work assistance;
-In 41.5% cases EHR applications have built-in clinical and pharmacological guidelines;
-In 51.9% cases EHR applications have built-in visual indicators for the financial indexes for diagnostic-therapeutic procedures, drug prescribing and the rate of sick leave;
-35.7% of FDs are very satisfied with the overall domain properties of their EHR application;</td></tr>
<tr><td>Mean rate: 0.430 Items: 23 Cronbach α: 0.822</td></tr>
</table>

Category	Results		
E	-All EHR applications are capable for e-prescribing and e-referral (not in function in testing time); -All EHR applications have the ability to add scanned paper-based diagnostic test results into the EHR, but only 22.6% of FDs use this feature; -EHR applications support some forms of electronic reporting (not all yet fully implemented in the central system); -82.6% FDs communicate by email with their colleagues in primary health care, while only 18.3% with doctors in clinics and hospitals; -All EHR applications are capable to remotely check the patient's health insurance status;		
	Mean rate: 0.324	Items: 17	Cronbach α: 0.689
F	-In 23.5% cases patients are satisfied with the implementation of the new information system; -EHR applications currently do not provide patients with reports on their health status in electronic human readable format; -Only 27% of FDs communicate with patients via e-mail and other electronic media; -Only 9.6% FDs collect information about chronic diseases of their patients via e-mail.		
	Mean rate: 0.446	Items: 9	Cronbach α: 0.541
Overall	Mean rate: 0.48	Items: 103	Cronbach α: 0.886

Table 5. Major qualitative results, average quantitative results and reliability coefficients of experiences assessment presented by categories

To determine and prove the reliability of our measurement tool, we used a calculation of the Cronbach α coefficient of correlation for each of categories (Cronbach, 1951). The recommended amount of this coefficient for a high degree of reliability, i.e. internal consistency of questionnaire, is ≥0.7. Before calculating the Cronbach α coefficient, we conducted verification of the required sample size with Bonett's formula (Bonett, 2002) using null hypothesis of Cronbach α coefficient equal to 0.7, against a two-sided alternative at α=0.05 and power (1-β)=0.8. For total number of 103 items and estimated coefficient to approximately 0.8, we calculated a minimum sample size of 41, which is significantly less than our 115. Cronbach α calculation was performed with SPSS Statistics 17.0.

Our population sample was not previously prepared for the testing. For this type of testing are common slightly smaller amounts of the Cronbach α than in controlled or clinical conditions. As we see from Table 5, the lowest Cronbach α has a category of social experience (0.541), however, it is a common occurrence in the questionnaires that have fewer than ten questions. So called face validity and content validity (Khoja, 2007b) of our measurement tool were confirmed through interviews and commentaries of the doctors. Comments were positive, and confirm the relevance of all categories in over 75% of cases. To determine the detailed structural validity we should apply factor analysis. To determine accuracy, it would be necessary to carry out additional field researches and calculations of correlations. The reliability and validity do not automatically withdraw the accuracy of the collected data. Although it is theoretically possible to achieve higher reliability and internal consistency of the questionnaire with incorrect data, sufficient reliability is a prerequisite for accuracy. We see this as the subject of further research.

As we see from the results presented in Table 5, categories A, C and partly F reflect the doctors' views about essential objectives of the e-Health concepts and doctors' engagement in achieving these goals. From the results of all other categories we can see how EHR applications meet the current worldwide certification criteria. Based on identified system performance, and current Croatian certification criteria (CIHI, 2010), we can conclude that Croatian EHR applications would be able to almost entirely meet the criteria of EuroRec EHR-Q Seal 1 and in some parts even the Seal 2 criteria, which is subject to more detailed analysis. However, in domain functionality, which is better covered by American ONC Meaningful Use of HER Stage 1, is still necessary to significantly improve the functionality. Here we primarily mean the introduction of full electronic data (clinical and administrative) interchange with all health care organizations, insurers and, of course, patients. Furthermore, we see some encouraging first results in applying of the working guidelines, guideline-based decision support systems and monitoring of chronic diseases and allergies. A similar situation is with monitoring and indication of the quality of doctor's work. These are definitely significant areas of further improvement.

7. Possible directions for future research

Continued research in order to improve our measurement methodology i.e. our measurement tool, is more than essential. It is necessary to continuously align our measurement methodology with best international practices. We expect that assessment of doctors' attitudes and their engagement in acquiring of the ICT knowledge will be of minor importance in the coming period, because, as the information system evolves, awareness and ICT knowledge of medical population becomes larger, and the focus of interest becomes the functionalities of applied software solutions. Judging by the latest global trends, the greater importance will have functionalities that contribute to the e-Health privacy and security, use of decision support systems in order to increase the quality of treatment, and, of course, functionalities that will allow patients to monitor phases of their own treatment and to more easily achieve their rights. References for that have to be drawn from the European projects and thematic networks such as epSOS (Smart Open Services for European Patients) (epSOS, 2011) and CALLIOPE (Call for Interoperability) (CALLIOPE, 2011). Objective of these projects is the harmonization of functionalities of the EHR applications and legislations among the current and future EU Member States in order to achieve cross-border interoperability. As we pointed out previously in the discussion, another important area of further research is the application of appropriate statistical methods to determine the reliability and accuracy of the measurement. In addition, development of appropriate statistical methods is essential for comparison of the measurement results between different stages of development of the applied EHR systems.

8. Conclusion

In this article, we have presented some preliminary results of what is envisioned to be a comprehensive methodology and criteria to measure quality of EHR system implementations in primary health care. Lord Kelvin once said: "If you can not measure it, you can not improve it." So, the focus of this article was on a measuring tool which is the basis for data analysis that serves to identify some key areas of quality to measure. From the amount of collected survey data and results of their analysis, we can conclude that in the practical implementation of this assessment method exist certain problems. The form of the questionnaire is very complex since it is necessary to perform testing of measured population across all categories simultaneously and in one pass. This can result in a weaker survey response of the tested population. However, with a simple questionnaire we could not manage to collect enough of useful information. Furthermore, one can say that our methodology is limited because the assessment of the functionalities of EHR applications is reduced only to the functionalities that are visible to doctors and can be expressed as an experience. However, we must be aware that in the quality EHR application, all the key features must be visible, or at least well-documented in the user guide and contextual help system. Analysis of data collected by our measurement tool can be held within six basic categories, but it is possible to evaluate the categories i.e. functionalities that are derived from a combination of basic categories. For example, by combining data from several basic categories, we can analyse functionalities such as the implementation of working guidelines and decision support systems (Kralj et al., 2010), or patients' privacy and safety protection (Kralj et al., 2011). We entered in the designing process of our measurement tool with the main idea to construct and implement an open type methodology. That means that we have decided to continuously align our measurement methodology with best international practices. Croatian certification criteria are still mainly based on the local requirements and needs of current developments, and do not draw direct reference to some of the internationally recognized quality indicators and frameworks, or take into account clinical protocols, experts practice and expectations on readiness and experience by users. Since the certification of EHR applications is performed by successive stages of development, we expect to be relatively easy to fully comply with worldwide technical criteria, however it remains to be seen what additional requirements we will identify as important, or how would international certification processes apply to localized environments and large scale deployment. The preliminary results give us confidence that our assessment methodology could be used as the potential tool for monitoring of further improvements of Croatian certification criteria, also in respect to forthcoming development phases of the Croatian healthcare information system.

9. Acknowledgment

I would like to express my gratitude to prof. dr. Stanko Tonković, from the Faculty of Electrical Engineering and Computing, University of Zagreb, Croatia, and also dr. Miroslav Končar, from the ORACLE Croatia, Zagreb, Croatia, for their guidance and support during the making of this work. I also want to thank all the Croatian family doctors who responded and participated in the survey.

10. References

Baklaić, Ž.; Dečković-Vukres, V. & Kuzman M. (2008). *Croatian Health Service Yearbook 2007,* Croatian National Institute of Public Health, Zagreb, Croatia

Björnberg, A.; Garrofé, B.C. & Lindblad, S. (2009). *Euro Health Cosumer Index 2009 – Report,* Health Consumer Powerhouse, Brussels, Belgium

Bonett, D. G. (2002). Sample size requirement for testing and estimating coefficient alpha. *Journal of Educational and Behavioral statistics,* Vol.4, No.27, (2002), pp. 335-340

CALLIOPE. (2011). A European thematic network for e-Health interoperability. 10.10.2011, Available from: http://www.calliope-network.eu

CANARIE. (2002). Final report: Framework for rural and remote readiness in telehealth. Written by the alliance of building capacity, June 2002, 10.05.2010, Available from: http://www.fp.ucalgary.ca/.../Projects-Canarie-final%20Report,%20June%202002.htm

Centers for Medicare and Medicaid Services: ONC Meaningful Use of EHR. (2010). 02.11.2010, Available from: https://www.cms.gov/EHRIncentivePrograms

Croatian Institute for Health Insurance. (2010). CEZIH PZZ. 02.11.2010, Available from: http://www.cezih.hr

Cronbach, L. J. (1951). Coefficient alpha and the internal structure of tests. *Psychometrika,*Vol.3, No.16, (1951), pp. 297-334

Dobrev, A.; Haesner, M.; Hüsing. T. et al. (2008). *Benchmarking ICT use among General Practitioners in Europe – Final Report,* Empirica, Bonn, Germany

epSOS. (2011). Smart open services for european patients. 10.10.2011, Available from: http://www.epsos.eu/

EuroRec: European Institute for Health Records. (2010). 02.11.2010, Available from: http://www.eurorec.org

Kern, J. & Polašek, O. (2007). Information and Communication Technology in Familiy Practice in Croatia. *European Journal for Biomedical Informatics,* No.1, (2007), pp. 7-14

Khoja, S.; Scott, R.; Casbeer, A.; Mohsin, M.; Ishaq, A.F.M. & Gilani, S. (2007). e-Health readiness assessment tools for healthcare institutions in developing countries. *Telemedicine and e-Health,* Vol.4, No.13, (2007), pp. 425-431

Khoja, S.; Scott, R.; Ishaq, A.F.M. &; Mohsin, M. (2007). Validating eHealth Readiness Assessment Tools for Developing Countries, In: *e-Health International Journal,* 25.06.2010, Available from: http://www.ehealthinternational.net

Končar, M. & Gvozdanović, D. (2006). Primary healthcare information system – The Cornerstone for the next generation healthcare sector in Republic of Croatia. *Int J Med Inform,* No.75, (2006), pp. 306-314

Kralj, D. & Tonković, S. (2009). Implementation of e-Health Concept in Primary Health Care - Croatian Experiences, *Proceedings of 31st Int. Conf. on Information Technology Interfaces (ITI2009 Posters Abstracts),* pp. 5-6, ISBN 978-953-7138-15-8, Cavtat, Croatia, June 22-25, 2009

Kralj, D.; Tonković, S. & Končar, M. (2010). Use of Guidelines and Decision Support Systems within EHR Applications in Family Practice - Croatian Experience, *Proceedings of 12th Mediterranean Conference on Medical and Biological Engineering and Computing (MEDICON 2010),* pp. 928-931, ISBN 978-3-642-13038-0, Chalkidiki, Greece, May 27-30, 2010

Kralj, D.; Tonković, S. & Končar, M. (2011). A Survey on Patients' Privacy and Safety Protection with EMR Applications in Primary Care, *IFMBE Proceedings Volume 37: 5th European Conference of the International Federation for Medical and Biological Engineering,* pp. 1132-1135, ISBN 978-3-642-23507-8, Budapest, Hungary, September 14-18, 2011

Li, J. (2008). E-Health Readiness Framework from Electronic Health Records Perspective - Master Thesis. University of New South Wales, Sydney, Australia, November 2008. 25.06.2010, Available from: http://handle.unsw.edu.au/1959.4/42930

23

Psychomagnetobiology

José María De la Roca Chiapas[1,2]
[1]*Universidad de Guanajuato, División de Salud, Departamento de Psicología*
[2]*Organización Filosófica Nueva Acrópolis México*
México

1. Introduction

The magnetobiology is known in the scientific world as being the link between magnetic fields and the behavior of particular animal species (some migratory birds, dolphins, and ants)that navigate through the magnetic currents that are generated by the Earth, and have a special sense of orientation, which has been associated with genetic memory. This arises from an increased concentration of iron in the head, or from the presence of a chemical that is activated by the presence of magnetic fields, including those generated by human construction, allowing the assumption that such magnetic fields are observable by some birds (Hevers, 2010; Mouritsen, 2005; Wiltschko, 2007; Gegear, 2010; Oliveira, 2010).

In these species, the relationship between the animal and the strength of the magnetic field allows them to remember their previous travels, and this has a wide application, because the assumptions regarding changes in these magnetic fields suggest that magnetic fields can be linked to changes in migration flows (Lohmann, 2007), reproduction, or to the extinction of a species. This relationship between animals and the properties of the Earth is studied as a part of magnetobiology (Valentinuzzi, 2004; Temurvants & Shekhotkin, 2000).

On the other hand, psychobiology, or biological psychology, studies the physiological mechanisms and evolutionary relationship between the development of the body and brain with emotion, thought, and behavior. This has been amply demonstrated in studies of psychopathology and health psychology (Sánchez-Martín, 2011). For cases such as schizophrenia (Ritsner, 2006) or depression (Gartside, 2003), it was found that some hormones and neurotransmitters that can induce some personality traits (or variations of these neural substrates that may cause mood disorders) also influence those biological emotional states of being and pleasure (Zak & Fakhar, 2006) that are associated with an increase in particular neurotransmitters that also regulate or relieve stress (Heinrichs, 2003).

There are also known specific psychoneuroimmunological responses and reactions triggering autoimmune diseases, such as those caused by severe stress or a high-intensity emotional state. For example, some patients who are notified of a terminal illness have emotions that may trigger symptoms associated with these effects, which may activate the genes of some diseases such as lupus (Schattner, 2010), heart attacks, or cancer (Stürmer, 2006).

This chapter discusses the existence of a relationship between magnetism and the physiological responses of health and disease associated with emotional states, which is not a new concept, as many traditional medicines have assumed this relationship exists, in civilizations from different geographic locations, such as China (Rosch, 2009; Gulmen, 2004), Egypt, and many Mexican cultures (Bocanegra-García, 2009). Today it is known as magnetotherapy (Zyss, 2008).

This idea is strengthened by the somatic marker proposal, which poses that as there is a biological anticipatory response to the decisions we make, and that it is reinforced by stimuli from external perception, the consciousness and emotional states that can guide accompanying positive actions. For example, in the migratory birds discussed above, a strengthening of the biological response to the magnetic field intensity is expected, as the migration of the species depends on a successful response (Martínez-Selva, 2006).

We proposed to test the hypothesis of relationships among the body, mind, and consciousness as a way of showing what the above cultures, doctors, and healers have supposed for millennia: that a relationship between consciousness, mind, emotion, and the body exists, i.e., there is a two-way communication that can transform the emotions, perception, and biology from magnetic and electromagnetic fields that can influence biology.

An example of how changing a body's electromagnetic currents can alter the emotional state can be found in the electrical stimulator, which has proven effective for people with depression (Baeken & De Raedt, 2011), auditory hallucinations (Freitas, 2011), and chronic pain, and is a promising treatment in this area.

Another example is biological neurofeedback (Dias & van Deusen, 2011) which can change depressed or obese health patterns under transcranial magnetic stimulation or deep transcranial magnetic stimulation (Rosenberg, 2011).

This hypothesis raises the question concerning which current technology we have to measure magnetic fields in human beings and what the future options might be.

Knowing technological developments that can measure magnetic fields can help in biomedicine, as they could be used in early diagnostic techniques based on the measurement of magnetic changes that can anticipate changes in the biology, immunology and endocrinology of the body. Among the current applications available for this purpose, we note the Gas Discharge Visualization (Korotkov, 2010), Magnetic Scanner (Pacheco, 2010), and SQUIDS27 (Bryant, 2011) techniques.

Psychomagnetobiology is a new area of interdisciplinary research that includes psychology, medicine, biological engineering, and physics, and the following provides an overview of how one can use magnetism and electricity in diagnosis and treatment in both medicine and psychology(see figure 1).

2. Technologies that use electricity and magnetism for diagnosis and therapy

2.1 Microcurrent stimulation and cranial electrotherapy

Cranial Electrotherapy Stimulation (CES) is an experimental psychiatric treatment that applies a small, pulsed electric current through a patient's head (Smith, 2008). It has been shown to have beneficial effects forsome conditions, such as anxiety, depression, insomnia, and stress (Klawansky, 1995).

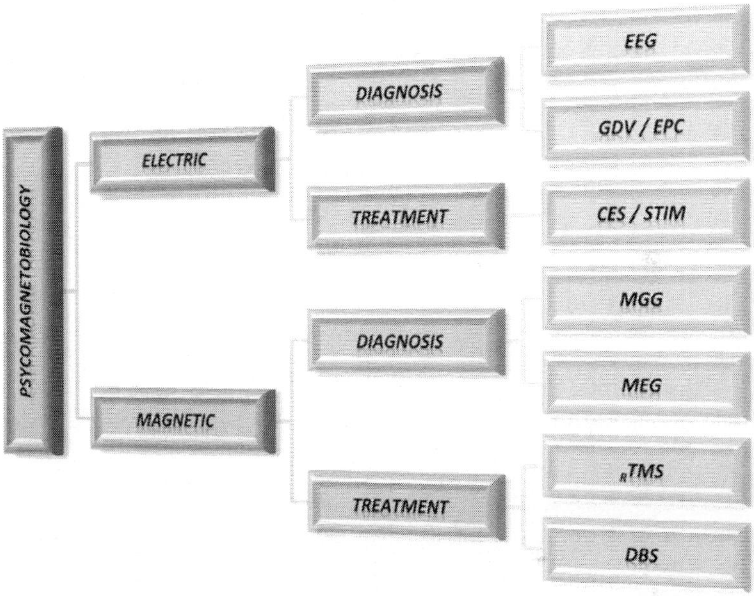

Fig. 1. Psychomagnetobiology

2.1.1 Early treatments

Electricity has been used in medicine since the ancient Greeks, who used eels for conditions such as rheumatism, gout, and pain. Unfortunately, because of a lack of legal controls, many charlatans took advantage of this situation, and captured the market. This led the Carnegie Foundation to carry out studies, and in 1910,it rejected electrotherapy as an acceptable medical method. The impact of this study has influenced physicians to this day (Fariña, 2010).

In the 1960s, Leduc and Rouxeau in France, initiated studies on the use of electricity in medicine using very low currents in the brain to induce sleep, and thus, introduced the term "electro-sleep". Note that sleep is induced after 4 to 5 hours using CES, and it is still unknown if it can induce rapid and consistent sleep (Fariña, 2010).

Electricity received another boost in its application to the brain when, in 1965,Melzack in Canada and Wall in Britain discovered a relationship between pain and the central nervous system, and tested the role of electricity in controlling pain (Melzack& Wall, 1965).

In 1967, when electrical stimulation was used to determine who really needed surgery to relieve pain, it was found that patients improved and responded therapeutically to a procedure that involved a distraction. This procedure was Transcutaneal Electrical Neuro Stimulation (TENS), a precursor of Microcurrent Electrical Therapy (MET). This method is different from MET, because TENS initially reduces pain by producing an alternative pain, and, therefore, is known as a "counter-irritant" (Debock, 2000). As the body adapts, the current is increased, even reaching levels not recommended as tolerable, or not required to stop the use of therapy. Using this method, the results are short term and recurrences are common. On the other hand, MET does not reach intolerable levels and the results are usually long lasting and positive (Fariña, 2010).

There are currently many research studies into CES in humans (Gunther & Phillips, 2010) and so far, 29 experimental animal studies have shown mostly positive results, with several using double-blind and placebo studies. No lasting adverse effects have been reported (Fariña, 2010).

CES has been approved by the US Food and Drug Administration (FDA) for use since 1979, and was reevaluated in 1986. Examples where the utility of CES/MET has been investigated are (Schmitt et al., 1986): discrete brain damage (reduction in pain and anxiety and increase in IQ); substance withdrawal syndrome (decrease in anxiety and increase in IQ), paraplegia and quadriplegia (decreased spasticity); cerebral paralysis (decrease in primitive reflexes); prisoners (reduced aggression); hypnotherapy (increases the speed and depth of the induction and reduces resistance to hypnotism); anesthesia (increases the effect of anesthesia by 37% and reduces postoperative pain); fibromyalgia (reduces pain and improves the quality of life) (Kirsch, 2006); and headaches (reduces many types of headache, such as migraine, tension, and headaches resistant to treatment where the patient has fibromyalgia and cancer) (Cork et al., 2004).

2.1.2 Mechanism of action

Studies have shown that, despite very low currents in the microampere range, 42% to 46% of the current passes through the cranial bone and enters the brain, focusing on the limbic system. It has been shown that this leads to an increase in the neurotransmitters dopamine, serotonin, and norepinephrine in the brain. The waveform used is as important as the current intensity, placement of electrodes, and exposure time (Kirsch, 2006).

2.1.3 Waveform

What really goes through the brain are unique waves that move the electrons and influence their frequency. The term used for this group of frequencies is "harmonic resonance", and using the above technology, it has been determined that the EEG changes to a more coherent resonance form, as observed in non-stressful conditions. This is comparable with results observed in deep meditation (Kirsch, 2006).

2.1.4 Microcurrent effects

Normalization of the electrical impulses reinforces the activity of the heart and blood circulation, andmicrovascular vessels are promoted; thus, cells are activated. The immune system's capacity increases, the rate of recovery doubles, healing ofwounds is promoted, and the sterilization effect suppresses bacterial growth. This technique is good for the treatment of patients with diseases associated with the feet, such as chronic pain, and reduces muscle fatigue (Kulkarni& Smith, 2000).(see figure)

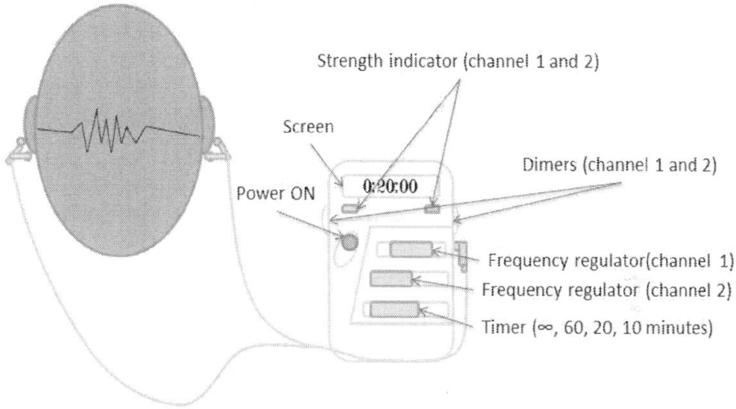

Stim diagram. The kit contains two channels, both with separate indicators and regulators. Dimmers are responsible for leveling the strength of the shock, while another regulator level the frequency. A timer is responsible for limiting the discharge time, shown on the screen. The voltage is transmitted to the patient who experiences the shock with the chosen parameters.

2.2 Gas discharge visualization and electrophotonic camera

Gas Discharge Visualization (GDV) is a technique based on the collection of signals from the body after electrical stimulation. The method is fully noninvasive, as it does not alter the physical and mental integrity of the patient.(see figure)

The functional basis of the GDV technique is the "crown effect" that occurs after passing a voltage through a conductor susceptible to discharge with the surrounding environment, creating a colorful halo around a material, based on the conducting components and the amount of volatile compounds in the environment. Using GDV, the medium is maintained at a constant voltage by a dielectric plate, and in the case of the body, the conductor is the crown of the system.

The variation of the intensity and wavelength of each signal generated can be measured according to the processes occurring within the body, and mainly the physiological state of the patient.

While it is not known exactly how this method amplifies the body's natural electromagnetic field, or how the patient's information is collected, the "entropy" is already established as a diagnostic method in the fields of medicine and psychology, with outstanding results.

GDV cameras are certified in Russia as medical instrumentation, and are freely used in hospitals and medical centers, while Europe is working on certification, and the United States is still developing the necessary research.

2.2.1 History

In 1939, Kirlian observed the formation of a halo of light after an electric shock on an X-ray machine. Researchers discovered that the phenomenon that bears his name (the Kirlian effect) was also observed in more than 30 patients, and his invention was supported in the USSR, where it was classified as "secret". In 1996, the Russian physicist Konstantin Korotkov at the University of St. Petersburg improved the Kirlian camera by adding a PC to allow processing and quantification of the data signals from the halo of light generated.

From the research of Mandel in Germany, Korotkov developed a methodology for medical diagnosis using fingers that generated a signal that could be used to diagnose the entire body's physiology.

The images obtained are known as beograms, GDVgrams or bioelectrograms.

2.2.2 Operation

The object to be scanned (e.g., a finger or plant) is placed on the surface of a glass cover that has an electroconductive layer underneath that generates luminescence by passing a discharge from the object to the conductive material. A CCD camera captures the halo of light around the object, and the signal is sent to a PC for processing and analysis (Korotkov & Popechitelev, 2002).

The computer-controlled parameters of the equipment are: pulse width (5.0ms), frequency (11.0 to 3.0kHz), amplitude voltage (1000.0 to 4000.0V), peak pulse power consumption (80watts), pulse current (1 mA), stability (0.1%), and the resolution of the CCDcamera (800 ×600pixels).

2.2.3 Applications

This technique has been used to monitor and diagnose disease. In the case of asthma, it can detect the developmentof the disease even before symptoms occur, allowing for early treatment. It can also monitor body functions during treatment and rehabilitation, providing a direct observation of drug efficacy and side effects (Alexandrova et al., 2003).

In cancer studies, statistical analysis shows differences in the beograms between healthy people and those with breast or lung cancer (Gagua et al., 2005), and during follow-up to radiation therapy, beograms show the effect on the physiological state of patients, depending on the entropic energy, which is correlated to the functional state of the organ (Gedevanishvili et al., 2004).

A study of subjects at risk of foot amputation from diabetes shows that an increase in the functional reserve of energy is a favorable sign for the recovery of the patient, a constant factor in chronic diseases (Olalde et al., 2004).

After operation, GDV can also detect and monitor the status of preoperative anxiety in patients, correlating low functional energy reserves with the Spielberger-Khaninscale (Polushin et al., 2004).

In cellular metabolism, GDV studies are correlated with metabolic processes and humoral regulatory processes at the level of the reflex nervous system. The photoelectric emission increases with the parameters of stress tolerance and decreases with a low energy index (Bundzenetal., 2003).

In the examination of blood using GDV, specifically for the electrophoretic mobility of erythrocytes, it has been used to characterize the membrane surface charge, an important factor in a wide variety of diseases that are mainly genetic in nature (Gertsenhtein & Panin, 2008).

Within psychology, there is a significant relationship between GDV beograms and the state of anxiety ,and to a lesser extent, a relationship to neuroticism. There was also a strong relationship observed with the degree of openness and empathy of a patient towards healthy subjects and athletes (Dobson & O'Keeffe, 2007; Polushinetal., 2003; Polushinetal., 2004).

Low levels of entropy in a beogram are correlated with acute stress (O'Keeffe, 2006). The GDV method can detect the influence of odorants in humans, which could be used to record the influence of environment on the psycho-emotional state (Priyatkinetal., 2006). GDV methodology can evaluate the overall improvement of an emotional state and eliminate nervous excitement during short-term rehabilitation (Sergeev & Pisareva, 2004).

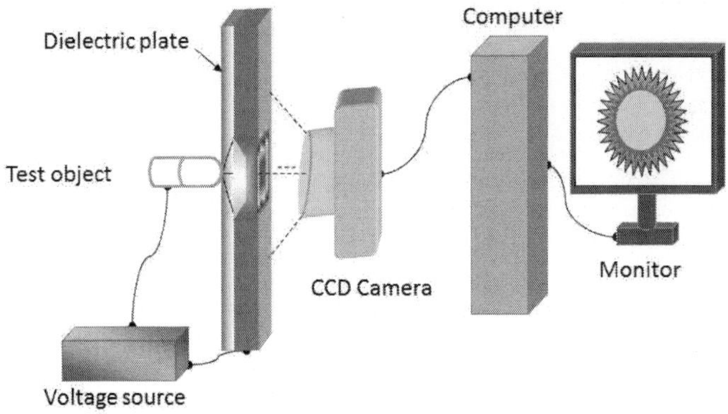

EPC Diagram. The "testing object" is placed on the "dielectric plate." Under the influence of a "voltage source", the object generates a luminous halo, which is captured by the "CCD camera" and sent to a "computer" for processing the signal.

2.3 Transcranial magnetic stimulation

Transcranial Magnetic Stimulation (TMS) is a noninvasive method that can depolarize or hyperpolarize neurons in the brain. TMS uses electromagnetic induction to induce weak electric currents in either specific or general parts of the brain.

It has been described as selective depolarization of the neurons in the neocortex or cerebral cortex, located between 1.5 and 2 cm below the cranial bone using magnetic pulses with specific intensity, either single or repetitive. This latter method is known as repetitive Transcranial Magnetic Stimulation or rTMS (Rothetal., 1994).

It is one of the latest tools in neuroscience that have been incorporated in both studies and research as therapeutic methods for the treatment of various diseases and neuropsychiatric disorders, among which are: depression, anxiety, attention deficit, hyperactivity, autism, tinnitus or unusual noise in the ear(s), post traumatic stress, phantom pain in people who have suffered limb amputation or central nervous system injuries, migraine headaches, decreased libido, some cases of schizophrenia and epilepsy, sleep disorders, obsessive-compulsive disorder, and bipolar disorder (Fitzgerald et al., 2006).

It is known to have neuro protective effects that help, at least temporarily, people affected by degenerative neurological diseases, such as multiple sclerosis, Parkinson's disease, and Alzheimer's disease, and impacts very favorably in the modulation of brain plasticity, which refers to the brain's ability to renew or reconnect neural circuits, and thus, acquire new skills and abilities and preserve memory (McDonald et al., 2011).

TMS uses a magnetic field oriented orthogonally to the plane of the coil. The magnetic field passes unimpeded through the skin and cranium, inducing a current in opposite directions in the brain to activate nearby nerve cells in the same way as currents applied directly to the cortical surface (Cacioppo et al., 2007).

The course of the field is difficult to predict, because the brain has an irregular shape and magnetic field lines are not distributed uniformly throughout the tissues or brain surface. Usually, the pulse only penetrates no more than 5 cm into the brain (Riehl, 2008). Depolarization from electromagnetic induction was originally discovered by Faraday (NIMH, 2009).

2.3.1 Clinical applications

From a therapeutic perspective, there are already a large number of studies that have shown that there are two sides to transcranial magnetic stimulation. Both TMS and rTMS have the great virtues of being harmless, but not innocuous, i.e., they are effective and can be classified as being safe. However, various measures need to be taken to ensure this (Rossini & Rossi, 2007). These techniques have been tested as a tool for treating depression and auditory hallucinations (Pascual-Leone et al., 2002) and for increasing attention (Fregni & Pascual-Leone, 2007).

2.3.2 Risks

The main contraindications for treatment are pregnant women, children under 6 years, patients with pacemakers, electrodes, or drug infusion pumps (Rossi, 2009), or patients with metallic implants in the head (Roth et al., 1992).

On the other hand, some patients subjected to cortical stimulation experience some side effects after application, which can be regarded as being minor and transient, including headaches, which can be mitigated by common analgesics (Wasserman, 1998). There have also been reports concerning patients with epilepsy or who take epileptogenic antidepressants who are unable to reach convulsive crises during treatment with transcranial magnetic stimulation (Duckworth, 2008). We have observed that at magnetic field intensities above 1Tesla and frequencies above 60 Hz can cause convulsions (Zelaya et al. 2010), and, therefore, we have suggested setting international standards for medical use.

2.4 Deep brain stimulation

Deep Brain Stimulation (DBS) was first developed as a treatment for Parkinson's disease, to reduce tremors, stiffness, difficulty in walking, and uncontrollable movements. In DBS, a pair of electrodes are implanted in the brain and controlled by a generator that is implanted in the chest. The stimulation is continuous at a frequency and level to suit the patient (Perlmutter & Mink, 2006). It has only recently been studied as a treatment for depression or OCD (obsessive-compulsive disorder).

It is currently available on an experimental basis. So far, very little research has been conducted on testing DBS for the treatment of depression (Mohr, 2011), but a few studies have been conducted showing that this treatment may be promising. In a trial using patients with severe depression that were treatment resistant, we observed that four of the six patients showed a marked improvement in their symptoms immediately after the procedure (Maybergetal., 2005). In another study on 10 patients with this disorder, we found that the improvement was consistent among the majority of patients 3 years after surgery (Greenbergetal., 2006).

2.4.1 How does it work?

DBS requires brain surgery. The head is shaved and then a screw is fixed to a frame that prevents the head from moving during surgery. Scans are taken of the head and brain using magnetic resonance. The surgeon uses these images as a guide during surgery. The patient is awake during the procedure to provide feedback to the surgeon. During this procedure,the patient feels no pain because the head is numbed using a local anesthetic.

Once ready for surgery, two well sare drilled in the head. From there, the surgeon inserts a thin tube into the brain to place the electrodes on either side of a specific part of the brain. In the case of depression, brain target area 25 is considered. This area has been found to be related to depression, hyperactivity, and mood disorders (Maybergetal., 2005). In the case of OCD, the electrodes are placed in a different part of the brain that is believed to be associated with the disorder.

After the electrodes have been implanted and the patient has provided feedback on the placement of the electrodes, the patient is placed under general anesthesia. The electrodes are connected to wires that run inside the body from the head to the chest, which are connected to two battery-powered generators. From here, electrical impulses are continuously delivered through the wires to the electrodes in the brain. Although it is unclear exactly how the device reduces depression or OCD, scientists believe that the pulses help to "restore" the area of the brain that is not working properly to function normally again (Perlmutter & Mink, 2006).

2.4.2 What are the side effects?

DBS has risks that are associated with any brain surgery. For example, the procedure can lead tobleeding in the brain or stroke, infection, disorientation or confusion, unwanted changes in mood, movement disorders, dizziness, and difficulty sleeping.

Because the procedure is still experimental, there may be other side effects that have not been identified. The long-term benefits are also unknown.

3. Diagnostic techniques for magnetism

3.1 Magnetogastrography

The use of sensors to measure magnetic activity generated by the body has been known since 1950 (Wenger et al., 1961; Wengeretal., 1957), although it has been "known" since ancient times for healing applications and diagnosis. It was in the 1970s that biomagnetic techniques began to expand their application and to become more common, with publications on ferromagnetic contamination in the lungs and other organs, as well as the detection and analysis of magnetic fields produced by bioelectric currents in human beings (Cohen, 1973; Cohen, 1969; Cohen et al., 1970; Benmair, et al., 1977; Frei et al., 1970).

Mechano-Magnetogastrography (M-MGG) is a biomagnetic technique used to determine the gastrointestinal activity of the stomach by determining the frequency of peristaltic contractions and gastric emptying half-time (Córdova et al., 2004; Córdova-Fraga et al., 2005).

Biomagnetic applications in the gastrointestinal system have resulted in the study of the transit time in different phases of the menstrual cycle in women or spatiotemporal assessment of the colon motility (Córdova-Fraga et al., 2005).

MGG is a technique that has advantages over current diagnostic techniques because it is noninvasive, lacks ionizing radiation, does not interfere with a patient's privacy, and provides reproducible results (De la Roca et al., 2007).

The reproducibility of measurements was analyzed in a study that measured the same patient over a period of several weeks evaluating the gastric emptying half-time, which showed a reproducibility coefficient above 85%. The remaining variation can be attributed to changes in motility of the same patients, depending on social and environmental conditions such as diet and health (De la Roca et al., 2007).

Several studies (De la Roca et al., 2007; Benmair & Dreyfus, 1977) have evaluated gastric emptying using magnetic tracers and the results have been presented in terms of half-time of emptying and peristaltic contractions in healthy male volunteers employing magnetic tracers in a yogurt vehicle test meal (Carneiro, 1977; Forsman, 2000), with similar results.

Gastric emptying has been evaluated in patients with functional dyspepsia, and a solid food test has been developed to compare results against benchmarks that primarily use the above type of food.

The esophageal transit time has also been evaluated. Techniques and instrumentation for biomagnetic studies permit the noninvasive functional evaluation of the gastrointestinal tract (Daghastanlietal., 1998; Córdova-Fraga et al., 2008).

We believe that the use of fluxgate sensors using magnetic markers can be used as a complement to manometric studies and are equivalent to centigraphy for clinical use.

Various studies have been performed using different test assemblies, and designs that we consider most relevant showing common patterns are presented below.

3.1.1 Magnetic stimulator

A magnetic stimulator has been used in experiments involving susceptometry (Carneiro et al., 2000) and magnetogastrography (Córdova et al., 2004). The magnetogastrograph (De la

Roca et al., 2007) was built by the Medical Physics Laboratory at the University of Guanajuato in Mexico.

The magnetic stimulator is composed of two identical coils, assembled as a Helmholtz coil array. This setting means that the coils are placed parallel to each other and share the same axis of symmetry, with the separation distance being equal to the radius of the coils.

The coils contain 60 turns composed of magnet gauge 4 copper wire (average radius =6 mm). The wire was wrapped around two aluminum supports that contain five layers of 12 turns of wire. The magnitude of the pulse field produced by this arrangement is of the order of a few millitesla.

This arrangement of coils connected in parallel has a resistance of 260 milliohms and an inductance of 0.928mH. The magnetic pulse is generated by a bank of six capacitors connected in parallel with an equivalent capacitance of 46mF. The capacitor bank is connected to the mains voltage (220V), and this voltage is rectified before reaching the capacitor bank. Once the capacitors are charged, the discharge produces a magnetic pulse of 32mT for a period of 17μs.

For field measurements, we used the above system with a Model 53 triaxial fluxgate (Physics Applet Systems),which is a solid state device used to measure the direction and magnitude of direct current magnetic fields, or variations thereof, with a frequency less than 100Hz and a magnetic field of 18mT. This device has an output in three axes that can transmit data from the measurements performed through a serial port at a frequency of 250 samples per second with a noise level of 3nT. This system is automated and operated from a PC via the LabVIEW software package both for stimulation and data acquisition.

(see figures)

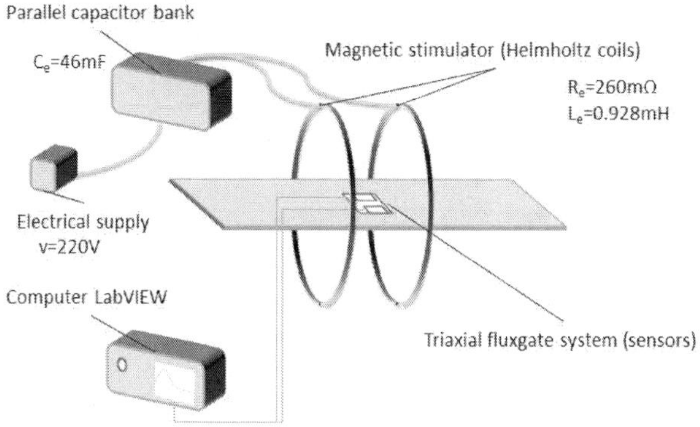

Magnet-gastrographer diagram. Helmholtz coils are responsible for generating the magnetic field, and receive the voltage from a bank of six capacitors in parallel. A triaxial fluxgate system detects the alignment of the magnetic markers, and information is recorded on a computer.

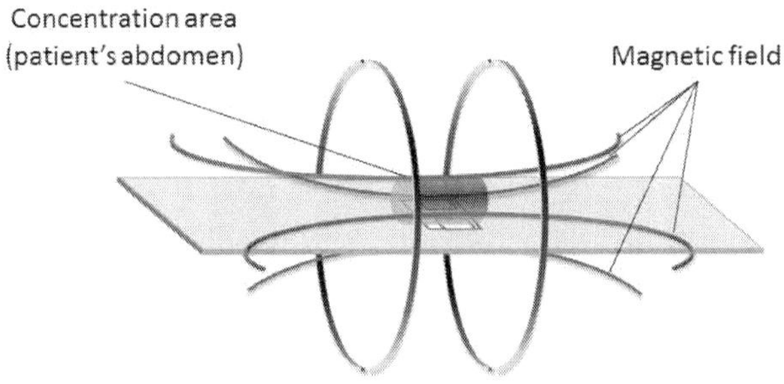

The stimulator generates a magnetic field is concentrated in the abdomen

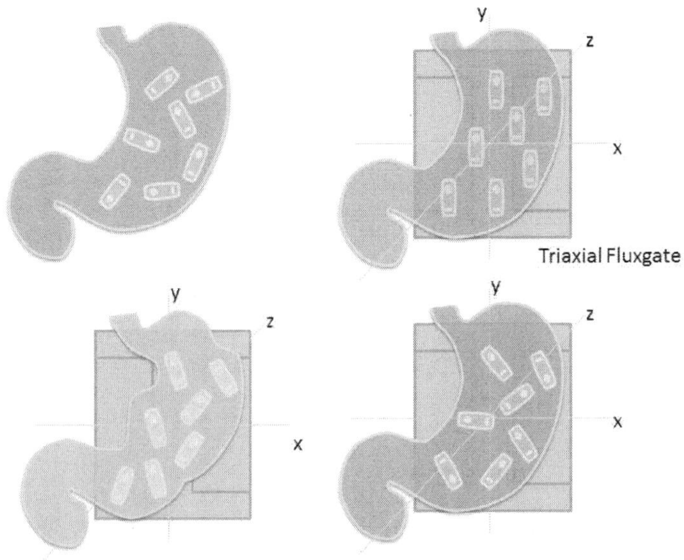

1. Stomach after eating markers, 2. Markers aligned by the magnetic field, located in triaxial plane, 3. Markers for gastric movement, 4. Misaligned markers after gastric movement.

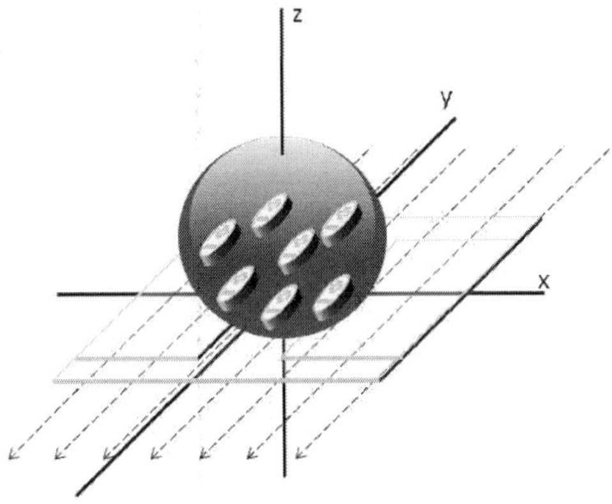

Diagram of the orientation of the markers on the triaxial sensor.

3.1.2 Magnetic contrast

Volunteers were asked to fast the previous evening and not to take any medication that would affect the gastric emptying time. The patients were asked to ingest a harmless dye and were placed in a prone position. Ten minutes after ingestion, the measurements began and were conducted every 10 minutes for a period of 1-2 hours.

In the case of semisolid food, the patients were given 250g of yogurt mixed with 4g of magnetite (Fe_3O_4). In the case of solid food in healthy volunteers (controls), this comprised a scrambled egg, a piece of bread and 250ml of peach juice. The bread contained 4g of magnetite for the MMGG and was made from milk, flour, eggs, and butter where the bread was in the form of a "hot cake"with a mass of approx. 30g (Reynaga, 2008).

3.2 Magnetic scanner

We have developed a device that is capable of creating a map of the magnetic fields obtained using magnetically marked phantoms, produced in the laboratory. This is a mobile automatic two-way device, developed to detect changes in magnetic flux, and is composed of on an array of magneto resistive sensors designed to detect magnetic fields of 100mT to 10nT (Pacheco, 2010).

4. Conclusions

Psychomagnetobiology is an interdisciplinary field that will help scientists propose strategies for the diagnosis and treatment of biological and psychological diseases, knowing that there is technology for electric or magnetic stimulation that has proven experimentally to be effective for the treatment of depression, anxiety, and in some cases, even hallucinations and addictions. It shows promise in this challenging landscape.

Both biological engineering and developments in technology are needed to implement new products in the service of human beings, but more research is required in joint efforts in psychology, medicine, and medical physics. Commitment is needed to continue working on this to help create the links needed to reach people in need.

We are currently developing new equipment and applications for research into missing areas, and the development of portable, magnetic and low-frequency equipment and software for the treatment of depression in Latin America.

Technology advances more each time to provide tools for the diagnosis and treatment of physical and mental illnesses, we have developed with several collaborators, technology to measure gastric emptying time, peristaltic contractions andtransit time in the gastrointestinal system (De la Roca-Chiapas JM et al, 2011), the influence of emotions on the symptoms of Dyspepsia (De la Roca-Chiapas et al, 2010), we have developed technology to measure magnetic fields on surfaces (Pacheco et al, 2008) , and we tried to measure tumor sizes (De la Roca-Chiapas, 2009) and now we are developing technology in electrical and magnetic microstimulation as tools that serve to treatment in people with anxiety, stress and depression.

There needs to be increasingly greater openness in science, allowing us to learn more about the man, and serve it better, this means leaving the arrogance to believe that science is "truth" and need to learn interrelated studies to do with people who think differently and in turn need projects to enter these sciences with integrators projects.

5. Future directions

Areas in which I think will developing the technology and where future research can focus are displayed in spaces that need to be covered in Figure 1. It's needed a portable and powerful magnetic technology for the treatment of depression. Lack the technological development of a scanner capable of measuring magnetic fields in the human body, and perhaps they are needed armored cameras, but I think the SQUID application for this is part of the answer, but today only deals to equip magnetoencephalography with the EEG, providing information on what brain areas are running the electric field lines. Similarly we believe that knowing how it behaves electric and magnetic fields in the human body can be used for the treatment and diagnosis.

I think in the future we will learn more about how magnetic fields of the human body and the planet affect us in the biological and psychological. We have technology that measures the order of femtoteslas, human magnetic fields, allowing us to understand how there is this mind-body-health interaction.

As for the GDV/EPC, in the future we will find a basic application that achieves characterize the behavior of fluids and tissues in humans, and their interaction with the environment.

In this sense, it is working at the University of Guanajuato to create models that seek to both basic research and the development of patents and technology with human sense.

I conclude by recalling that understanding the human being as an integral whole is an essential part of this work, since linking the mind, body and health consciousness, it is a model that seeks to achieve interdisciplinary in the service of man, speaking of the psycomagnetobiology, search of integrating different areas of expertise: medicine, psychology, physics and engineering. And this effort is retrieved from the traditional medicine of many cultures, including Mexico, China and Egypt, without being new, and that by proposing a new term is intended to entrench in a modern language, an expression that is natural multidimensional human.

As time passes, more and more will be heard: engineering biological and engineering psychological; science and technology for physical and mental health.

6. Acknowledgments

For their invaluable assistance in gathering information and format, to: BS. Jose Eduardo Lepez, and BS. Jorge Fernando Ortiz Paz for the collection of information and image design, this chapter has been possible thanks to support and UGTO/CA-37 UGTO/PTC-183 Promep, and PIFI funds from the University of Guanajuato.

7. References

Alexandrova, RA., Fedoseev, BG. & Korotkov KG. (2003). Analysis of the bioelectrograms of bronchial asthma patients, *In: Proceedings of conference "Measuring the human energy field: State of the science"*. Baltimore: National Institute of Health, pp.70–81.

Alexandrova, RA., Nemtsov, VI., Koshechkin, DV. & Ermolev SU. (2003). Analysis of holeodoron treatment effect on cholestasis syndrome patients. *In: Proceedings of VII International Scientific Congress on Bioelectrography.* St. Petersburg, Russia, pp. 4–6.

Baeken, C. & De Raedt, R. (2011). Neurobiological mechanisms of repetitive transcranial magnetic stimulation on the underlying neurocircuitry in unipolar depression. *Dialogues ClinNeurosci.* 13(1):139–45.

Benmair, Y., Dreyfuss, F., Fischel, B., Frei, EH. & Gilat T. (1977). Study of Gastric Emptying Using a Ferromagnetic Tracer, *Gastroenterology* 73:1041–1045.

Benmair, Y., Fischel, B., Frei, EH. & Gilat T. (1977). Evaluation of a Magnetic Method for the Measurement of Small Intestine Transit Time, *American Journal of Gastroenterology* 68:470–475.

Bocanegra-García, V., Del Rayo Camacho-Corona, M., Ramírez-Cabrera, M., Rivera, G. & Garza-González, E. (2009). The bioactivity of plant extracts against representative bacterial pathogens of the lower respiratory tract. *BMC Res Notes.* 1(2):95.

Bryant, HC., Adolphi, NL., Huber, DL., Fegan, DL., Monson, TC., Tessier, TE. & Flynn, ER. (2011). Magnetic Properties of Nanoparticles Useful for SQUID Relaxometry in Biomedical Applications, *J Magn Magn Mater*, 323(6):767–774.

Bundzen, PV., Korotkov, KG. & Belobaba, O. (2003). Correlation between the parameters of induced opto-electron emission (Kirlian effect) and the processes of corticovisceral regulation. *In: Proceedings of VII International Scientific Congress onBioelectrography*, St. Petersburg, Russia, pp.89–91.

Cacioppo, JT., Tassinary, LG. & Berntson, GG. (2007). *Handbook of psychophysiology* (3rd ed.). New York, NY: Cambridge Univ. Press. pp. 121.

Carneiro, A. (1999). Study of stomach Motility using the relaxation of magnetic tracers. *Phys Med Biol*, 44:1691–1697.

Carneiro, AA., Ferreira, ER., Moraes, DB., Sosa, M. & Baffa, O. Biomagnetismo: Aspectos Intrumentais e Aplicacoes, *Revista Brasileira de Física*, 22(3):324–338.

Cohen, D. (1969). Detection And Analysis of Magnetic Fields Produced By Bioelectric Currents In Humans, *Journal Of Applied Physics* 40(3):1046–1048.

Cohen, D. (1973). Ferromagnetic Contamination in the Lungs and Other Organs of the Human Body, *Science*, 180:743–748.

Cohen, D., Edelsack, EA. & Zimmerman, JE. (1970). Magnetocardiogram taken inside a shielded room with a superconducting point-contact magnetometer, *Appl Phys Lett*, 16:278–280.

Córdova-Fraga, T., Carneiro, AA., de Araujo, DB., Oliveira, RB., Sosa, M. & Baffa, O. (2005). Spatiotemporal evaluation of human colon motility using three-axis fluxgates and magnetic markers.Med, *Biol Eng Comput*, 43(6):712–715.

Córdova-Fraga, T., Gutierrez, JG., Sosa, AM., Vargas, LF. & Bernal, AJ. (2004). Gastric activity studies using a magnetic tracer, *Institute of Physics Publishing*, 25:1261–1270.

Córdova-Fraga, T., Sosa, M., Wiechers, C., De la Roca-Chiapas, JM., Maldonado Moreles, A., Bernal-Alvarado, J. & Huerta-Ranco, R. (2008). Effects of anatomical position on esophageal transit time: A biomagnetic diagnostic technique. *World J Gastroenterol*, 14(37):5707–5711.

Cork, RC., Wood, P., Ming, N., Shepher, C., Eddy, J. & Price, L. (2004) The effect of CES on pain associated with fibromyalgia. *The Internet Journal of Anesthesiology*; 8:2.

Daghastanli, NA., Braga, FJ., Oliveira, RB. & Baffa, O. (1998). Esophageal transit timeevaluated by a biomagnetic method, *PhysiolMeas* 19(3):413–20.

De la Roca Chiapas JM, Cordova Fraga T, Barbosa Sabanero G, Macias de la Cruz JH, Cano ME, Pacheco AH, Rivera Cisneros AR, Solis S, Sosa M. Aplicaciones interdisciplinarias entre Física, Medicina y Psicología.(2009) *Acta Universitaria*; 19(2) 5:9.

De la Roca-Chiapas JM, Cordova-Fraga T.(2011). Biomagnetic techniques for evaluating gastric emptying, peristaltic contraction and transit time. *World J Gastrointest* Pathophysiol 2(5): 65-71

De la Roca-Chiapas José Ma., Solís-Ortiz Silvia, Fajardo-Araujo Martha, Sosa Modesto, Córdova-Fraga Teodoro, Zarate Alma Rosa.(2010). Stress profile, coping style, anxiety, depression, and gastric emptying as predictors of functional dyspepsia: A case-control study. *Journal of Psychosomatic Research* 68: 73–81.

De la Roca-Chipas, JM., Hernández, SE., Solis, MS., Sosa, AM. & Córdova, FT. (2007). Magnetogastrography (MGG) reproducibility assessments of gastric emptying on healthy subjects, *Physiol Meas*, 28(2):175–183.

De Oliveira, JF., Wajnberg, E., Esquivel, DM., Weinkauf, S., Winklhofer, M. & Hanzlik, M. (2010). Ant antennae: are they sites for magnetoreception, *R Soc Interface*. 7(42):143–152.

Debock, P. (2000). European perspective: a comparison between TENS and MET, *Physical Therapy Pro*, pp:28–33.

Días, AM. & van Deusen, A. (2011). A new neurofeedback protocol for depression, *Span J Psychol*, 14(1):374–384.

Dobson, P. & O'Keeffe, E. (2007). Investigation into the GDV technique and personality. *In: Proceedings of the International Scientific Conference: Measuring energy fields*, Kamnik-Tunjice, Slovenia, pp:111–113.

Duckworth, K. (2008). "Transcranial Magnetic Stimulation (TMS)" (Review). *National Alliance on Mental Illness*, pp:12-15.

Fitzgerald, PB., Fountain, S. & Daskalakis, J. (2006). A comprehensive review of the effects of rTMS on motor cortical excitability and inhibition, *Clinical Neurophysiology*, 117(12):2584-2596.

Forsman, M. (2000). Intragastric movement assessment by measurement magnetic field decay of magnetised tracer particles in a solid meal, *Med Biol Eng Comput*, 38 169-174.

Fregni, F., & Pascual-Leone, A. (2007). Technology insight: noninvasive brain stimulation in neurology-perspectives on the therapeutic potential of rTMS and tDCS, *Nature Clinical Practice Neurology*, 3(7):383-393.

Frei, EH., Benmayr, Y., Yerashlmi, S. & Dreyfuss, F. (1970). Measurements of the emptying of the stomach with a magnetic tracer, *IEEE Trans Mag*, 6:348-9.

Freitas, C., Pearlman, C. & Pascual-Leone, A. (2011). Treatment of auditory verbal hallucinations with transcranial magnetic stimulation in a patient with psychotic major depression: One-year follow-up, *Neurocase*, 25:1-9.

Gagua, PO., Gedevanishvili, EG. & Korotkov, KG. Experimental study of the GDV technique application in oncology [in Russian], *J IzvestiaVuzovPriborostroenie*, 49(2):47-50.

Gartside, SE., Leitch, MM. & Young, AH. (2003). Altered glucocorticoid rhythm attenuates the ability of a chronic SSRI to elevate forebrain 5-HT: implications for the treatment of depression, *Neuropsychopharmacology*, 28(9):1572-1578.

Gedevanishvili, EG., Giorgobiani, LG. & Kapanidze, A. (2004). Estimation of radiotherapy effectiveness with gas discharge visualization (GDV). *In: Proceedings of VIII International Scientific Congress on Bioelectrography*. St. Petersburg, Russia, pp:98-99.

Gegear, RJ., Foley, LE., Casselman, A. & Reppert, SM. (2010). Animal cryptochromes mediate magnetoreception by an unconventional photochemical mechanism, *Nature*, 463(7282):804-807.

Gertsenhtein, SY., Panin, DN. (2008). Study of Blood Electric Properties by the Method of Gas-Discharge Visualization, *Dokl Phys*. 53:107-110.

Gilula, MF. & Barach, P. (2004) CES: a safe neuromedical treatment for anxiety, depression or insomnia. *South MJ* 97(12):1269-1270.

Greenberg, BD., Malone, DA., Friehs, GM., Rezai, AR., Kubu, CS., Malloy, PF., Salloway, SP., Okun, MS., Goodman, WK. & Rasmussen, SA. (2006). Three-year outcomes in deep brain stimulation for highly resistant obsessive compulsive disorder, *Neuropsychopharmacology*, 31(11):2384-2393.

Gulmen, FM. (2004). Energy medicine, *Am J Chin Med*, 32(5):651-658.

Gunther, M. & Phillips, KD. (2010). Cranial Electrotherapy Stimulation for the Treatment of Depression. *Journal of Psychosocial Nursing*, 48(11):37-42.

Heinrichs, M., Baumgartner, T., Kirschbaum, C. & Ehlert, U. (2003). Social support and oxytocin interact to suppress cortisol and subjective responses to psychosocial stress, *Biol Psychiatry*, 54(12):1389-1398.

Heyers, D., Zapka, M., Hoffmeister, M., Wild, JM. & Mouritsen, H. (2010). Magnetic field changes activate the trigeminal brainstem complex in a migratory bird. *Proc Natl Acad Sci U S A*. 107(20):9394-9399.

Kirsch, DL. (2006). CES in the treatment of fibromyalgia. PPM, 6(6):60-64.

Kirsch, DL. (2006). Microcurrent electrical therapy (MET): A tutorial, *PPM*, 6(7):59-64.

Korotkov, KG. & Popechitelev, EP. A Method for Gas-Discharge Visualization and an Automated System for Its Implementation, *Biomed Eng*, 36(1), 23-27.

Korotkov, KG., Matravers, P., Orlov, DV. & Williams, BO. (2010). Application of electrophoton capture (EPC) analysis based on gas discharge visualization (GDV) technique in medicine: a systematic review, *J Altern Complement Med*, 16(1):13–25.

Korotkova, AK. (2006). Gas discharge visualization bioelectrography method in studies of master-sportsmen's psychophysiology, *Abstract of a Ph.D. thesis in psychology [in Russian]*, St Petersburg, Russia.

Kostyuk, N., Rajnarayanan, V., Isokpehi, RD. & Cohly, HH. (2010). Autism from a Biometric Perspective, *Int J Environ Res Public Health*, 7:1984–1995.

Kulkarni, AD. & Smith, RB. (2000).The use of MET and CES in pain control, *Cl Pr Alt Med*, 2(2):99–102.

Lohmann, KJ., Lohmann, CM. & Putman, NF. (2007). Magnetic maps in animals: nature's GPS, *J Exp Biol*, 210(21):3697–705.

Martínez-Selva, JM., Sánchez-Navarro, JP., Bechara, A. & Román, F. (2006). Mecanismos cerebrales de la toma de decisiones. *Rev Neurol*, 42(7):411–418.

Mayberg, HS., Lozano, AM., Voon, V., McNeely, HE., Seminowicz, D., Hamani, C., Schwalb, JM. & Kennedy, SH. (2005). Deep brain stimulation for treatment-resistant depression. *Neuron*. 45(5):651–660.

McDonald, WM., Durkalski, V., Ball, ER., Holtzheimer, PE., Pavlicova, M., Lisanby, SH., Avery, D., Anderson, BS., Nahas, Z., Zarkowski, P., Sackeim, HA. & George, MS. (2011). Improving the antidepressant efficacy of transcranial magnetic stimulation: maximizing the number of stimulations and treatment location in treatment-resistant depression. *US National Library of Medicine National Institutes of Health Search*.

Melzack, R. & Wall, P. (1965). Pain mechanisms: A new theory, *Science, New Series*, 150(3699):971–979.

Mercola, JM. & Kirsch, DL. (1995). The basis for MET in conventional medical practice. *J of Adv in Med*, 8(2):107–120.

Mohr, P., Rodriguez, M., Slavíčková, A. & Hanka, J. (2011). The application of vagus nerve stimulation and deep brain stimulation in depression, *Neuropsychobiology*, 64(3):170–81.

Mouritsen, H. & Ritz, T. (2005). Magnetoreception and its use in bird navigation, *Curr Opin Neurobiol*, 15(4):406–414.

Narayanamurthy, G. & Veezhinathan, M. (2011). Design of Cranial Electrotherapy Stimulator and Analyzing It with EEG. *In: Power Electronics and Instrumentation Engineering Communications in Computer and Information Science*, 102(2):42–45.

NIMH (2009) Brain Stimulation Therapies.National Institute of Mental Health.2009-11-17.Retrieved 2010-07-14.

O'Keeffe, E. (2006). The GDV technique as an aid to stress assessment and its potential application in recruitment and selection of individuals suited to positions associated with high level of stress. *In: Proceedings of X International Scientific Congress on Bioelectrography*, St. Petersburg, Russia, pp:202–204.

Olalde, JA., Magarici, M., Amendola, F. & del-Castillo, O. (2004). Correlation between electrophoton values and diabetic foot amputation risk. *In: Proceedings of Conference: Neurobiotelekom*. St. Petersburg, Russia, pp:54–58.

Pacheco, AH., Cano, ME., Palomar-Lever, E., Córdova-Fraga, T., De la Roca, JM., Hernández-Sámano, A. & Felix-Medina, R. (2010). An XY Magnetic Scanning

Device for Magnetic Tracers: Preliminary Results, *International Journal of Bioelectromagnetism,* 12(2):81–84.

Pascual-Leone, A., Davey, N., Rothwell, J., Wassermann, EM. & Puri, BK. (2002). Handbook of Transcranial Magnetic Stimulation. Hodder Arnold.

Perlmutter, JS. & Mink, JW. (2006). Deep brain stimulation. *Annual Review of Neuroscience.* 29:229–257

Polushin, US., Korotkov, KG. & Korotkina, SA. (2004). Perspectives of the application of gas discharge visualization for the estimation of organism condition at critical states. *In: Proceedings of IX International Scientific Congress on Bioelectrography.* St. Petersburg, Russia, pp:115–116.

Polushin, US., Korotkov, KG., Strukov, EU. & Shirokov, DM. (2003). First experience of using GDV method in anesthetization and resuscitation. *In: Proceedings of VII International Scientific Congress on Bioelectrography.* St. Petersburg, Russia, pp:13–14.

Priyatkin, NS., Korotkov, KG. & Kuzemkin, VA. (2006). GDV bioelectrography in research of influence of odorous substances on psycho-physiological state of man [in Russian]. *J IzvestiaVuzovPriborostroenie,* 49(2):37–43.

Reynaga-Ornelas, MG., De la Roca-Chiapas, JM., Córdova-Fraga, T., Bernal, JJ. & Sosa, M. Solid Test Meal to Measure the Gastric Emptying with Magnetogastrography, *AIP Conference Proceedings - American Institute of Physics,* 1032(1):246.

Riehl, M. (2008). TMS Stimulator Design, In Wassermann, EM., Epstein, CM., Ziemann, U., Walsh, V., Paus, T., Lisanby, SH, *Oxford Handbook of Transcranial Stimulation,* Oxford University Press, pp.13–23,25–32.

Ritsner, M., Gibel, A., Ram, E., Maayan, R. & Weizman, A. (2006). Alterations in DHEA metabolism in schizophrenia: two-month case-control study, *Eur Neuropsychopharmacol,* 16(2):137–146.

Rosch, PJ. (2009). Bioelectromagnetic and subtle energy medicine: the interface between mind and matter, *Ann N Y Acad Sci,* 1172:297–311.

Rosenberg, O., Isserles, M., Levkovitz, Y., Kotler, M., Zangen, A. & Dannon, PN. (2011). Effectiveness of a second deep TMS in depression: A brief report, *Prog Neuropsychopharmacol Biol Psychiatry,* 35(4):1041–1044.

Rossi, S. (2009). The Safety of TMS Consensus Group, Safety, ethical considerations, and application guidelines for the use of transcranial magnetic stimulation in clinical practice and research, *Clinical Neurophysiology,* 120(12):2008–2039.

Rossini, P. & Rossi, S. (2007). Transcranial magnetic stimulation: diagnostic, therapeutic, and research potential, *Neurology,* 68(7):484–488.

Roth, BJ., Maccabee, PJ., Eberle, L., Amassian, VE., Hallett, M., Cadwell, J., Anselmi, GD. & Tatarian, GT. (1994). In-vitro evaluation of a four-leaf coil design for magnetic stimulation of peripheral nerve, *Electroenceph Clin Neurophysiol,* 93(1):68–74.

Roth, BJ., Pascual-Leone, A., Cohen, LG. & Hallett, M. (1992). The heating of metal electrodes during rapid-rate magnetic stimulation: A possible safety hazard, *Electroenceph.Clin.Neurophysiol,* 85(2):116–123.

Sánchez-Martín, JR., Azurmendi, A., Pascual-Sagastizabal, E., Cardas, J., Braza, F., Braza, P., Carreras, MR. & Muñoz, JM. Androgen levels and anger and impulsivity measures as predictors of physical, verbal and indirect aggression in boys and girls, *Psychoneuroendocrinology,* 36(5):750–760.

Schattner, E., Shahar, G., Lerman, S. & Shakra, MA. Depression in systemic lupus erythematosus: the key role of illness intrusiveness and concealment of symptoms, *Psychiatry*, 73(4):329–340.

Schmitt, R., Capo, T. & Boyd, E. (1986). Cranial Electrotherapy Stimulation as a Treatment for anxiety in chemically dependent persons, *Alcoholism: Clinical and Experimental Research*, 10(2)158–160.

Sergeev, SS. & Pisareva, SA. The use of gas-discharging visualization method (GDV) for monitoring a condition of the personnel at short-term rehabilitation. *In: Proceedings of VIII International Scientific Congress on Bioelectrography*, St. Petersburg, Russia, pp:128–129.

Sidney, K. (1995). Meta-Analysis of Randomized Controlled Trials of Cranial Electrostimulation: Efficacy in Treating Selected Psychological and Physiological Conditions, *Journal of Nervous & Mental Disease* 183(7):478–484.

Smith, RB. (2002). Microcurrent therapies: emerging theories of physiological information processing, *Neuro Rehab*, 17(1):3–7.

Smith, RB. (2008). Cranial Electrotherapy Stimulation: Its First Fifty Years

Strukov, EU. Facilities of gas discharge visualization method for assessment of functional state of organism in preoperational period [in Russian]. *Abstract of a medical doctoral candidate's thesis*. St Petersburg, Russia: Military Medical Academy.

Stürmer, T., Hasselbach, P. & Amelang, M. (2006). Personality, lifestyle, and risk of cardiovascular disease and cancer: follow-up of population based cohort, *BMJ*, 332(7554):1359.

Temuryants, NA., Shekhotkin, AV. (2000). The role of the pineal gland in magnetobiological effects, *Crit Rev Biomed Eng*, 28(1–2):307–321.

Valentinuzzi, ME. (2004). Magnetobiology: a historical view, *IEEEEng Med Biol Mag*, 23(3):85–94.

Wassermann, EM. (1998). Risk and safety of repetitive transcranial magnetic stimulation: report and suggested guidelines from the International Workshop on the Safety of Repetitive Transcranial Magnetic Stimulation, *Electroencephalography and clinical Neurophysiology*, 108(1):1–16.

Wenger, MA., Engel, BT., Clemens, TL. & Cullen, TD. (1961). Stomach Motility in Man as Recorder by the Magnetometer Method, *Gastroenterology*, 41:479–85.

Wenger, MA., Henderson, EB. & Dinnin, JS. (1957). Magnetometer method for recording gastric motility, *Science*, 125:192–195.

Wiltschko, W., Ford, H., Munro, U., Winklhofer, M. & Wiltschko, R. (2007). Magnetite-based magnetoreception: the effect of repeated pulsing on the orientation of migratory birds, *J Comp Physiol A Neuroethol Sens Neural Behav Physiol*, 193(5):515–22.

Woodbury, FM. (2010). Efecto de la microcorriente sobre síntomas de ansiedad, depresión, insomnio y dolor. *Revista Galenus*, 5.

Zak, PJ. & Fakhar, A. (2006). Neuroactive hormones and interpersonal trust: international evidence. *Econ Hum Biol*. 4(3):412–429.

Zelaya, RM., Saracco-Álvarez, RA. & González J. (2010). The transcraneal magnetic stimulation for the negative symptoms in schizofrenia: a review, Salud Ment, 33(2):169-178.

Zyss, T. (2008). Magnetotherapy, *Neuro Endocrinol Lett*, 29(1):161–201.

24

Study on the Mechanism of Traumatic Brain Injury

Yuelin Zhang[1], Shigeru Aomura[2],
Hiromichi Nakadate[2] and Satoshi Fujiwara[3]
[1]*Tokyo University of Agriculture and Technology,*
[2]*Tokyo Metropolitan University,*
[3]*Yokohama City University,*
Japan

1. Introduction

Skull fracture, intracranial hemorrhage, or cerebral injury can be caused in humans due to a strong impact to the head. The following 2 types of cerebral injuries are often observed: one type is cerebral contusion which is a local brain damage to the brain, and the other is diffuse axonal injury (DAI) which is a diffuse brain damage to the brain. In various head injuries caused by external impact, cerebral contusion and DAI mainly result in direct failure of the cerebral parenchyma.

Cerebral contusions can be either coup or contrecoup contusions that occur on either the same or the opposite side of impact, respectively (Yanagida et al., 1989). Cerebral contusions are caused by rapid pressure fluctuations transmitted to the brain surface via the cerebrospinal fluid (CSF) (Fujiwara et al., 1989, Zhang et al., 2001). The hypothesis that the brain surface is destroyed when the cerebral parenchyma collides with the skull, although intuitive, has never been observed (Gurdjian et al., 1966). The cavitation theory states that the pressure gradient generated in the CSF by impact causes contrecoup negative pressure on the opposite side of impact and forms cavitation bubbles; the subsequent collapse of the bubbles causes brain tissue damage. Although this theory can be trusted, no collapse of bubbles in the head has yet been observed (Gross, 1958). Although various theories report the generation mechanism of cerebral contusion, none can sufficiently explain the entire mechanism. For predicting the dynamic response of the human head, numerous cadaver and animal experiments have been performed (Nahum & Smith, 1977; Gennarelli, 1983); however, these experiments are difficult to conduct because of cost and/or ethical concerns. Furthermore, the finite element method is widely used to predict the dynamic responses of the human head (Aomura et al., 2002). Some researchers report the reconstruction of real-world brain injury cases using multibody dynamics and finite element method (Raul et al., 2006; Riordain et al., 2003; Doorly & Gilchrist, 2006). These studies demonstrate the effectiveness of these methods but do not explain the mechanism of the brain injuries themselves.

DAI is considered to be caused by strain to the brainstem due to the rotational movement of the head. When a human head receives a external impact, the cranium moves first and then the brain follows its movement; this delay becomes more remarkable inside the brain, and a large strain is generated in the deep brain. This large strain causes damage to the axons of nerve cells and results in DAI (Fujiwara et al., 1998; Ommaya & Gennarelli, 1974).

As described above, in the past few decades, in order to clarify the mechanism of cerebral contusion and DAI, the impact experiments using physical models and animals, numerical analysis by finite element method are performed as engineering approach. In recent years, in order to clarify the tolerance of impact at the cellular level, the impact experiments are performed using cultured neuronal cells and tissues as biological approach. However, these researches often focus on the mechanism of only one type of injury; can not to evaluate all types of traumatic brain injury comprehensively. Thus, future research should be performed concurrently engineering and biological approaches. Therefore, in this study, the reconstruction analyses of real-world brain injury accident cases are performed to understand the mechanism of cerebral contusion and the impact experiments of cultured cells are performed to understand the mechanism of DAI.

2. Finite-element human head model

A computer model was constructed using cross-sectional T1 weighted MRI data of a woman's head because it was recently decided that CT should not be used for research to avoid radiation exposure. The slice thickness of the data is 3.3mm, and the slice interval is 0.0mm. Both the internal and external boundary curves of the scalp, skull, CSF, brain, and brain stem were extracted by binary image processing of the MRI data to make the internal and external surfaces of each part of the model. Three-dimensional human head models with hexahedral elements were made between the internal and external surfaces of each part (Fig. 1). The three-layered structure of the skull, which consists of an outer table, diploe, and inner table, was also reproduced. Finally, the finite element model consisted of 147,723 nodes and 114,012 elements. The material properties of each part of the model are shown in Table 1 (Willinger & Baumgartner, 2003; Nishimoto et al., 1998; Viano et al., 1998). Elastic properties were assigned to the scalp (Willinger & Baumgartner, 2003) and skull (Nishimoto et al., 1998), and viscoelastic properties were assigned to the CSF, brain, and brain stem (Viano et al., 1998).

For verifying the finite element model, the numerical results were compared with those results of the cadaver experiment by Nahum (Nahum & Smith, 1977). The impact direction was along the specimen's mid-sagittal plane, and the head was rotated forward such that the Frankfort anatomical plane was inclined 45° from the horizontal plane. The outline of the experiment is shown in Fig. 2(a). In the experiment, a 5 kg iron impactor was impacted to the head at 6 m/s (used by Nahum). However, Nahum does not definitively show what types of padding materials were interposed between the skull and impactor; therefore, in numerical calculations of this study only the time-force history(Fig.2(b)) was used as described in the literature (Nahum & Smith, 1977). The restraint condition of the head was free because the cadaver subject was seated and not restrained around the neck. The slide-type contact condition was used between the skull and CSF, CSF and brain, and brain and brain stem.

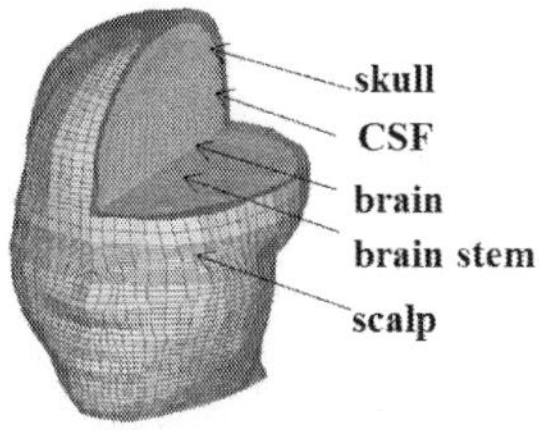

Fig. 1. Finite element human head model. The model consists of the scalp, skull (outer table, diploe, and inner table), CSF, brain, and brain stem.

	Scalp	Outer/inner table	Diploe	CSF	Brain	Brain stem
Density ρ (kg/m³)	1000	1456	850	1040	1040	1040
Young's Modulus E (MPa)	16.7	8750	4660	-	-	-
Bulk Modulus K (MPa)	-	7120	3470	2190	2190	2190
Short Time Shear Modulus G0 (MPa)	-	-	-	-	0.0125	0.0225
Long Time Modulus G∞ (MPa)	-	-	-	0.0005	0.0025	0.0045
Tangent Modulus (MPa)	-	4620	2170	-	-	-
Yield(MPa)	-	41.8	13.6	-	-	-
Poisson's Ratio ν (-)	0.42	0.25	0.25	-	-	-
Time Constant (1/s)	-	-	-	500000	80	80

Table 1. Material properties of the finite element human head model. Elastic properties were assigned to the scalp (Willinger & Baumgartner, 2003) and skull (Nishimoto et al., 1998), and viscoelastic properties were assigned to the CSF, brain, and brain stem (Viano et al., 1998).

The experimental pressure response given by Nahum and pressure response calculated using finite element model in this study are shown in Fig. 3. Although slight difference was observed between the experimental and numerical results, this model was corroborated by the experimental cadaver test and sufficiently predicted intracranial pressure.

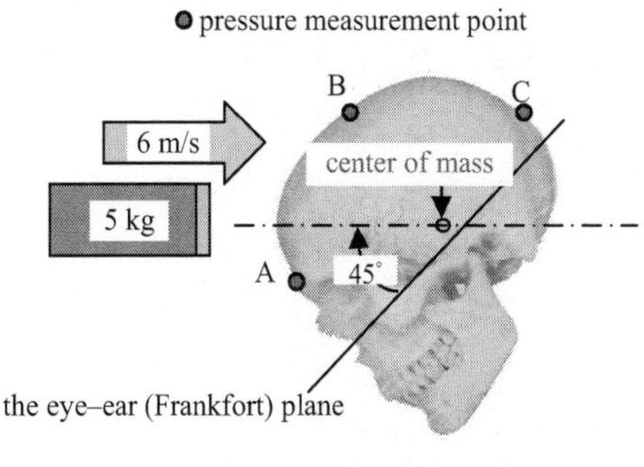

(a) The outline of the experiment of Nahum.

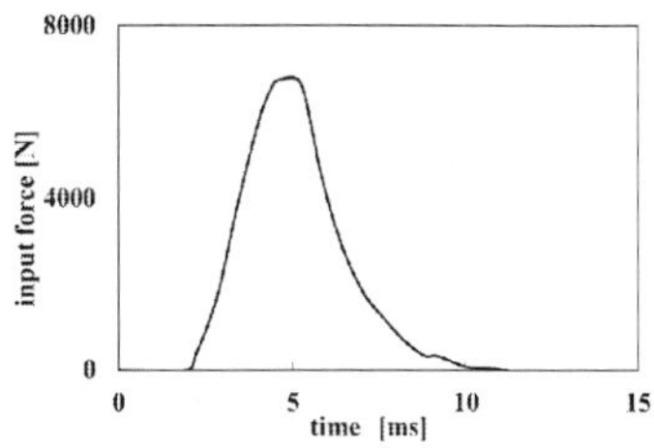

(b) The input force curve.

Fig. 2. Experiment by Nahum (Nahum & Smith, 1977). (a)The 5 kg iron impactor impacted the frontal region of the head at 6 m/s, and intracranial pressures were measured in the frontal (point A), parietal (point B) and occipital (point C) region of the head. (b) The input force curve obtained from the experiment.

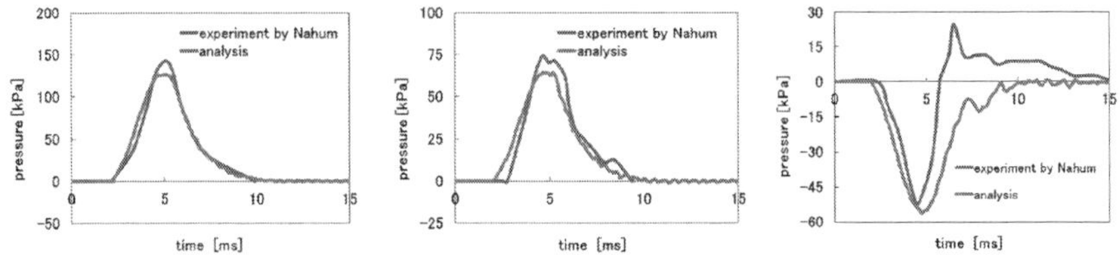

(a) Frontal region(point A) (b) Parietal region(point B) (c) Occipital region(point C)

Fig. 3. Comparison to the cadaver experiment by Nahum (Nahum & Smith, 1977) and numerical calculation. The validation demonstrates that this model is corroborated by an experimental cadaver test and sufficiently predicts intracranial pressure.

3. The mechanism of cerebral contusion

Fujiwara et al. analyzed 105 real-world fatal brain injury cases (Fujiwara et al., 1986). Coup contusions are caused more easily by direct blows to the head than contrecoup contusions, and contrecoup contusions are caused more easily by falls and fall-downs than coup contusions (Fujiwara et al., 1986). In this study, input force duration which is strongly related to the impact region on the human head, impact velocity, stiffness, mass or shape of the impact object, was focused. Previous studies (Aomura et al., 2008; Zhang et al., 2010) using impact experiments and finite element analysis of a water-filled acrylic container have showed that negative pressure inside the container is caused by deformation of the acrylic wall; this negative pressure tends to occur on the impact side when the force duration is short and on the opposite side of impact when the force duration is long.

In this chapter, for understanding the relationship between input force duration and dynamic response inside the skull, 9 real-world brain injury accident cases, including 3 coup contusion cases and 6 contrecoup contusion cases, were simulated using a finite element human head model. Numerical calculations were performed using LS-DYNA version 971.

3.1 Real-world brain injury accident cases

The autopsy results (performed by S. Fujiwara), in which the cause of death was cerebral contusion, are shown in Table 2. In these cases, the type of impact was classified as a blow, fall, or fall-down. In each type of impact, the contusion was classified as a coup or contrecoup contusion. Coup contusions are predominant in blows, and contrecoup contusions are predominant in falls and fall-downs. According to the postmortem data in Table 2, coup contusions tend to occur due to impacts by sharp-cornered objects (cases 1–3), and contrecoup contusions, due to impacts by objects with flat surfaces (cases 4 and 5). Contrecoup contusions are predominant in all the cases of falls and fall-downs (cases 6–9). In the simulations, the pressure threshold for causing cerebral contusion was -100 kPa. Skull fracturing was also simulated, because it was observed in all cases. The tensile stress thresholds for causing skull fracture were 70.5 MPa for the outer and inner tables and 21.4 MPa for the diploe (Nishimoto et al., 1998).

Case	Impact object	Impact region	Fracture region	Contusion region	
				Coup	Contrecoup
1	Beer bottle	Frontal region	Frontal region	Lower side of frontal lobe	
2	Wooden box (1.5 t)	Right temporal region	Right temporal region ~ right cranial fossa (semi) crushing	Right parietal lobe	
3	Sake bottle (empty: 700g)	Right parietal region	Right parietal region	Right parietal lobe	
4	Tank lorry	Parieto-occipital region	Occipital region (crushing)		Lower side of left and right frontal lobes Lower side of left temporal lobe
5	Steel Box (600 kg)	Occipital region	Occipital region		Lower side of frontal lobe Right and left temporal lobe poles

(a) Blows. The data include 3 coup and 2 contrecoup contusions.

Case	Impact object (height/weight)	Impact region	Fracture region	Contusion region	
				Coup	Contrecoup
6	Concrete (5.5 m)	Upper side of occipital region	Occipital region		Lower side of frontal lobe
7	Wooden deck (10 m)	Occipital region	Occipital region		Lower side of frontal lobe Frontal pole

(b) Falls. The data include 2 contrecoup contusions.

Case	Impact object (height/weight)	Impact region	Fracture region	Contusion region	
				Coup	Contrecoup
8	Asphalt (160 cm/58 kg)	Occipital region	Occipital region		Frontal pole
9	Asphalt (156 cm/59 kg)	Right occipital region	Right temporal region		Lower side of right frontal lobe Lower side of right temporal lobe Lateral surface of left temporal lobe

(c) Fall-downs. The data include 2 contrecoup contusions.

Table 2. Postmortem data (cause of death was cerebral contusion, 1968~1984). In these cases, the type of impact was classified as a blow, fall, or fall-down. In each type of the impact, the contusion was classified as a coup or contrecoup contusion.

3.2 Simulations of real-world brain injury accident cases

In order to begin the simulation, the relative velocity between the head and impact object, and the impact position of each case must be estimated. In this study, the impact positions are described in the postmortem data (Table 2, Impact Region). The relative velocities between the head and impact objects were estimated in order to generate negative pressure in the lesion area of the brain and fracture the skull in the fracture region described in the postmortem data. The simulations of the 9 cases are shown below.

[Case 1]

The frontal region of the head was impacted by a beer bottle (467 g), causing a skull fracture at the frontal region and a coup contusion at the lower side of the frontal lobe. In the simulation, the impact velocity (1-15 m/s) was applied to the node that constituted the beer bottle model (Fig. 4(a)). In order to determine the impact velocity of this case, the following 2 conditions had to be satisfied:

1. The negative pressure must be generated on the impact side only, because a coup contusion was observed.
2. The frontal skull must be fractured.

The impact velocity that satisfies these conditions was around 10 m/s. The intracranial pressure fluctuations of the impact side and its opposite side are shown in Fig. 4(b). The input force duration (i.e. the length of time that the impact object contacted the head) of this case was counted from the animation of the analysis result, was 1.4 ms.

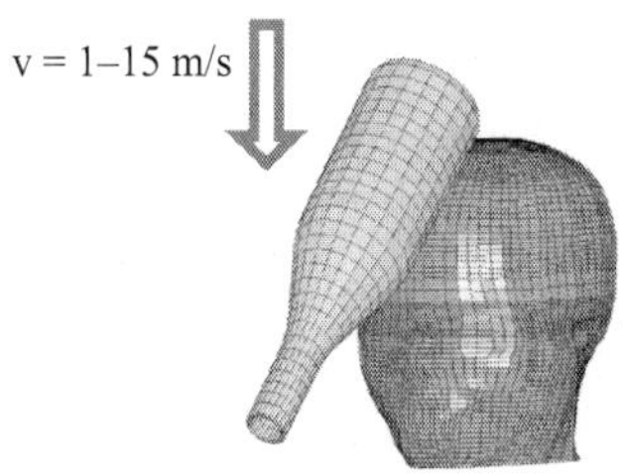

(a) Simulation outline

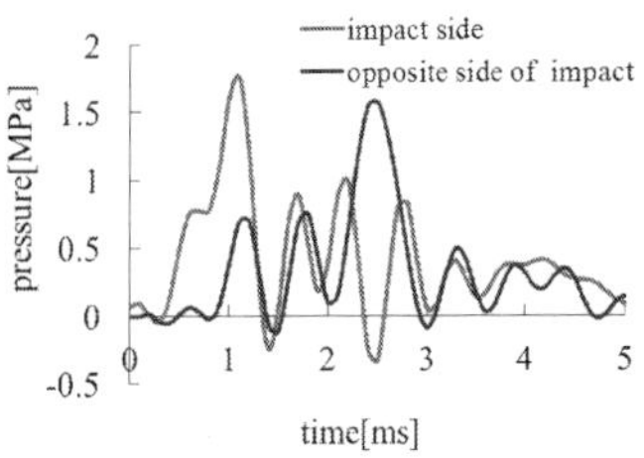

(b) Intracranial pressure fluctuations (v = 10 m/s)

Fig. 4. Simulation outline and results of case 1. (a) Simulation outline. The impact velocity (1–15 m/s) was applied to the node that constituted the beer bottle model. (b) The intracranial pressure fluctuations of the impact side and its opposite side. The results show that negative pressure occurred only on the impact side.

[Case 2]

The right temporal region of the head was impacted by a wooden box (1.5 t), causing a skull fracture from the right temporal region to the right cranial fossa and a coup contusion at the right parietal lobe. In the simulation, the impact velocity (1-15 m/s) was applied to the node that constituted the wooden box model (Fig. 5(a)). The impact velocity that satisfied this case was around 15 m/s, which caused negative pressure on the impact side (Fig. 5(b)) and skull fracture in the right temporal region of the head. The input force duration (i.e. the length of time that the impact object contacted the head) of this case was counted from the animation of the analysis result, was 2.7 ms.

[Case 3]

The right parietal region of the head was impacted by a sake bottle (700 g), causing a skull fracture at the right parietal region and a coup contusion at the right parietal lobe. In the simulation, the impact velocity (1-15 m/s) was applied to the node that constituted the sake bottle model (Fig. 6(a)). The impact velocity that satisfied this case was around 15m/s, which caused the negative pressure at the impact side (Fig.6(b)) and the skull fracture at the right parietal of the head. The input force duration (i.e. the length of time that the impact object contacted the head) of this case was counted from the animation of the analysis result, was 2.2 ms.

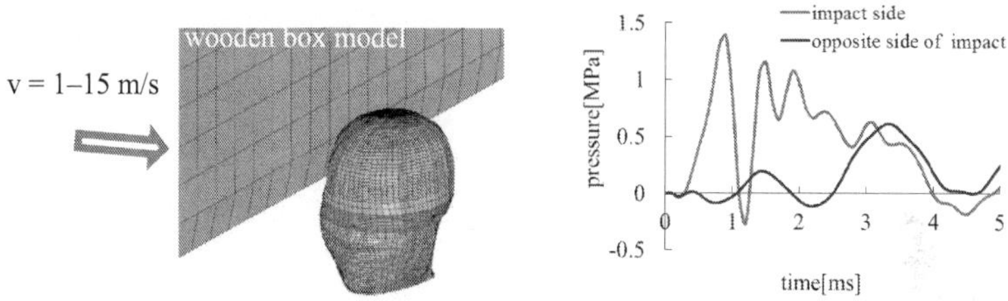

(a) Simulation outline (b) Intracranial pressure fluctuations (v = 15 m/s)

Fig. 5. Simulation outline and results of case 2. (a) Simulation outline. The impact velocity (1–15 m/s) was applied to the node that constituted the wooden box model. For better view, only part of the wooden box is displayed. (b) The intracranial pressure fluctuations of the impact side and its opposite side. The results show that negative pressure occurred only on the impact side.

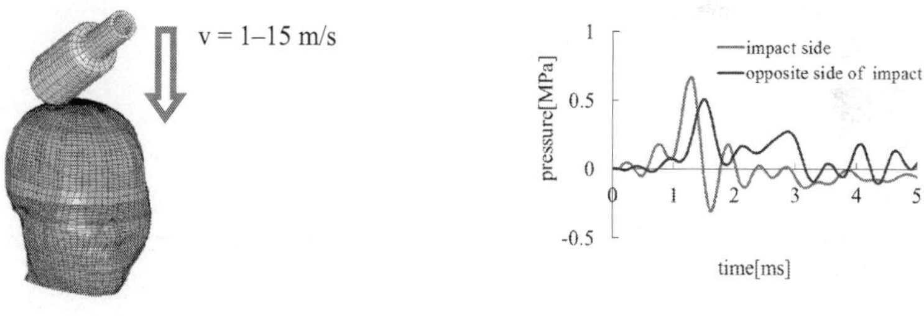

(a) Simulation outline (b) Intracranial pressure fluctuations (v = 15 m/s)

Fig. 6. Simulation outline and results of case 3. (a) Simulation outline. The impact velocity (1–15 m/s) was applied to the node that constituted the sake bottle model. (b) The intracranial pressure fluctuations of the impact side and its opposite side. The results show that negative pressure occurred only on the impact side.

[Case 4]

A man who was walking along the street was impacted by a tank lorry (6 t) at the parieto-occipital region of the head, causing a skull fracture at the occiput region and contrecoup contusions at the lower side of the left and right frontal lobes and in the lower side of left temporal lobe. In the simulation, the impact velocity (1–15 m/s) was applied to the node which constituted the tank lorry model (Fig.7(a)). The impact velocity which satisfied this case was around 10m/s, which caused the negative pressure at the opposite side of impact (Fig.7(b)) and the skull fracture at the occiput region of the head. The input force duration (i.e. the length of time that the impact object contacted the head) of this case was counted from the animation of the analysis result, was 3.7 ms.

[Case 5]

A man who was working at a construction yard was impacted by a steel trash box (600 kg) at the occipital region of the head, causing a skull fracture at the occipital region and contrecoup contusions in the lower side of the frontal lobe and the right and left temporal lobe poles. In the simulation, the impact velocity (1–15 m/s) was applied to the node which constituted the steel box model (Fig.8(a)). The impact velocity which satisfied this case was around 9.5m/s, which caused the negative pressure at the opposite side of impact (Fig.8(b)) and the skull fracture at the occipital region of the head. The input force duration (i.e. the length of time that the impact object contacted the head) of this case was counted from the animation of the analysis result, was 3.6 ms.

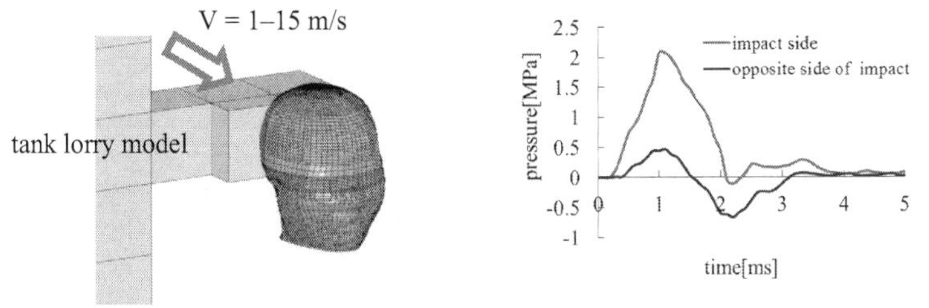

(a)Simulation outline (b) Intracranial pressure fluctuations (v = 10 m/s)

Fig. 7. Simulation outline and results of case 4. (a) Simulation outline. The impact velocity (1–15 m/s) was applied to the node that constituted the tank lorry model. For better view, only part of the tank lorry is displayed. (b) The intracranial pressure fluctuations of the impact side and its opposite side. The results show that negative pressure occurred only on the opposite side of impact.

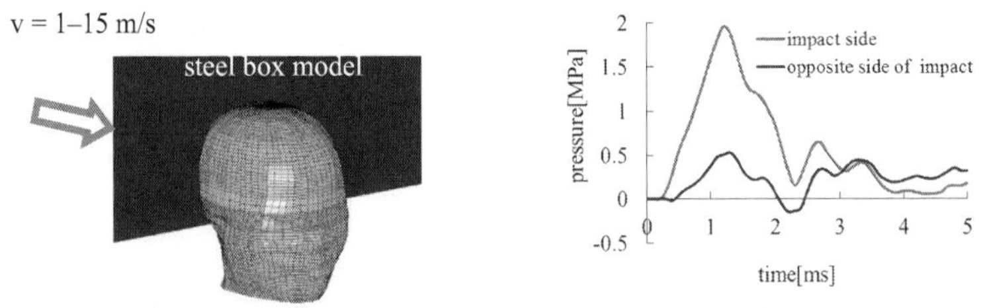

(a) Simulation outline (b) Intracranial pressure fluctuations (v = 9.5m/s)

Fig. 8. Simulation outline and results of case 5. (a) Simulation outline. The impact velocity (1–15 m/s) was applied to the node that constituted the steel box model. For better view, only part of the steel box is displayed. (b) The intracranial pressure fluctuations of the impact side and its opposite side. The results show that negative pressure occurred only on the opposite side of impact.

[Case 6]

A man fell from 5.5 m high onto a concrete road, and the upper side of the occipital region of the head was impacted, causing a skull fracture at the occiput region and a contrecoup contusion at the lower side of the frontal lobe. In the simulation, the impact velocity (1-10.4 m/s, from the law of conservation of mechanical energy, the maximum velocity was calculated to be 10.4 m/s) was applied to the node that constituted the head model (Fig.9(a)). The impact velocity that satisfied this case was 10.4 m/s, which caused negative pressure on the opposite side of impact (Fig.9(b)) and a skull fracture in the occiput region of the head. The input force duration (i.e. the length of time that the impact object contacted the head) of this case was counted from the animation of the analysis result, was 3.7 ms.

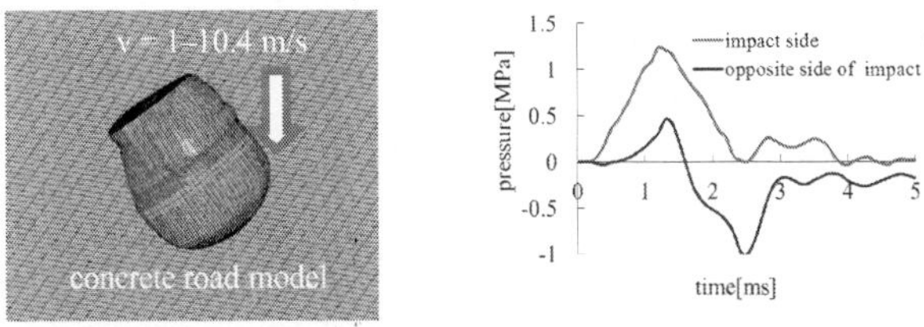

(a) Simulation outline (b) Intracranial pressure fluctuations (v = 10.4 m/s)

Fig. 9. Simulation outline and results of case 6. (a) Simulation outline. The impact velocity (1-10.4 m/s) was applied to the node that constituted the head model. For better view, only part of the concrete road model is displayed. (b) The intracranial pressure fluctuations of the impact side and its opposite side. The results show that negative pressure occurred only on the opposite side of impact.

[Case 7]

A sailor fell from 10 m high onto a deck, and the occipital region of head was impacted, causing a skull fracture in the occiput region and contrecoup contusions in the lower side of the frontal lobe and frontal pole. In the simulation, the impact velocity (1-14m/s, from the law of conservation of mechanical energy, the maximum velocity was calculated to be 14 m/s) was applied to the node that constituted the head model (Fig.10(a)). The impact velocity that satisfied this case was around 10 m/s, which caused negative pressure on the opposite side of impact (Fig.10(b)) and skull fracture in the occiput region of the head. The input force duration (i.e. the length of time that the impact object contacted the head) of this case was counted from the animation of the analysis result, was 3.6 ms.

[Case 8]

A man fell down onto an asphalt road, and the occipital region of the head was impacted, causing a skull fracture in the occiput region and a contrecoup contusion in the frontal pole. In the simulation, the impact velocity (1-15 m/s) was applied to the node which constituted the head model (Fig.11(a)). The impact velocity which satisfied this case was around 11m/s, which caused the negative pressure at the opposite side of impact (Fig.11(b)) and the skull fracture at the occiput region of the head. The input force duration (i.e. the length of time that the impact object contacted the head) of this case was counted from the animation of the analysis result, was 2.9 ms.

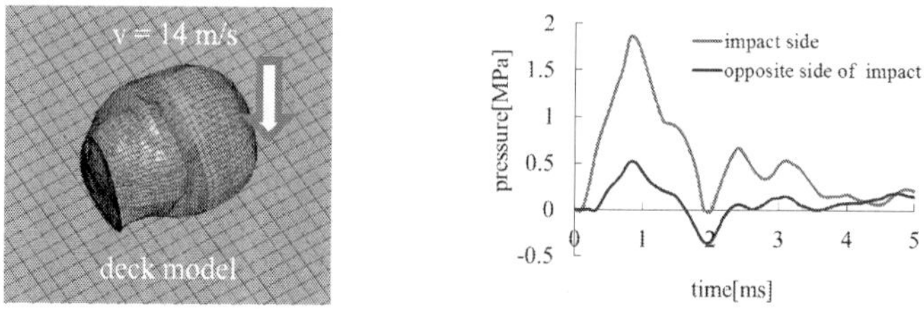

(a) Simulation outline (b) Intracranial pressure fluctuations (v = 10 m/s)

Fig. 10. Simulation outline and results of case 7. (a) Simulation outline. The impact velocity (1–14 m/s) was applied to thc nodc that constituted the head model. For better view, only part of the deck model is displayed. (b) The intracranial pressure fluctuations of the impact side and its opposite side. The results show that negative pressure occurred only on the opposite side of impact.

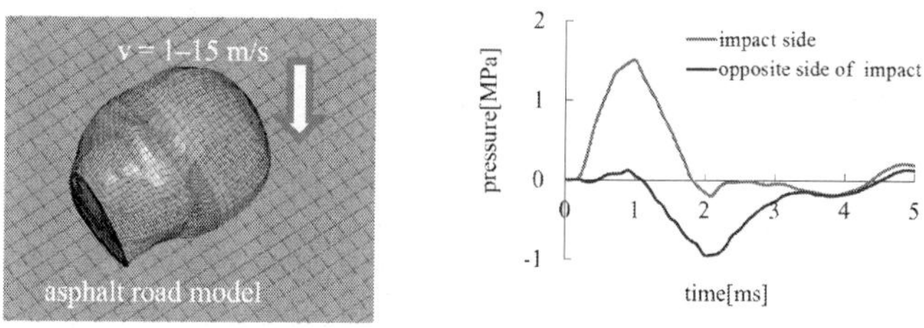

(a) Simulation outline (b) Intracranial pressure fluctuations (v = 11 m/s)

Fig. 11. Simulation outline and results of case 8. (a) Simulation outline. The impact velocity (1–15 m/s) was applied to the node that constituted the head model. For better view, only part of the asphalt road model is displayed. (b) The intracranial pressure fluctuations of the impact side and its opposite side. The results show that negative pressure occurred only on the opposite side of impact.

[Case 9]

A man fell down onto an asphalt road, and the right occipital region of the head was impacted, causing a skull fracture in the right temporal region and contrecoup contusions in the lower sides of the right frontal and right temporal lobe and on the lateral surface of the left temporal lobe. In the simulation, the impact velocity (1–15 m/s) was applied to the node which constituted the head model (Fig.12(a)). The impact velocity which satisfied this case was around 7m/s, which caused the negative pressure at the opposite side of impact (Fig.12(b)) and the skull fracture at the right occipital region of the head. The input force duration (i.e. the length of time that the impact object contacted the head) of this case was counted from the animation of the analysis result, was 3.4 ms.

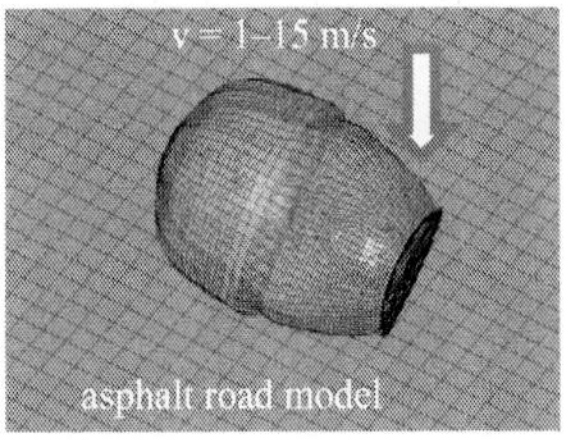

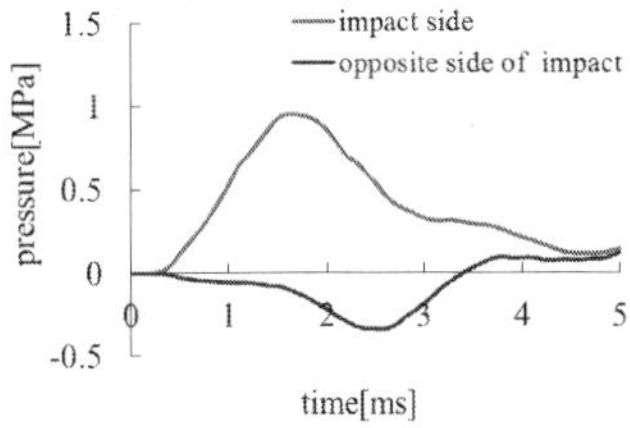

(a) Simulation outline (b) Intracranial pressure fluctuations (v = 7 m/s)

Fig. 12. Simulation outline and results of case 9. (a) Simulation outline. The impact velocity (1–15 m/s) was applied to the node that constituted the head model. For better view, only part of the asphalt road model is displayed. (b) The intracranial pressure fluctuations of the impact side and its opposite side. The results show that negative pressure occurred only on the opposite side of impact.

3.3 Relationship between force duration and contusion type

Coup and contrecoup contusions were classified according to the force duration which was obtained from the simulations (Table 3). In coup contusion cases, the input force durations were 1.4~2.7ms, and in contrecoup contusion cases, the input force durations were 2.9~3.7ms. Short (1.4~2.7ms) and long (2.9~3.7ms) force durations were obtained from coup and contrecoup contusion cases, respectively. These results show that when the head is impacted by sharp-cornered objects, coup contusions due to the short force durations are caused more easily; meanwhile, when the head is impacted by objects with flat surfaces, contrecoup contusions due to the long force durations are caused more easily.

	Case	Impact object	Impact region	Force duration
Coup contusion	1	Beer bottle	Frontal region	1.4 ms
	2	Wooden box (1.5 t)	Right temporal region	2.7 ms
	3	Sake bottle (empty: 700 g)	Right parietal region	2.2 ms
Contrecoup contusion	4	Tank lorry	Parietal occipital region	3.7 ms
	5	Steel Box (600 kg)	Occipital region	3.6 ms
	6	Concrete (5.5 m)	Upper side of occipital region	3.7 ms
	7	Wooden deck (10 m)	Occipital region	3.6 ms
	8	Asphalt (160 cm/58 kg)	Occipital region	2.9 ms
	9	Asphalt (156 cm/59 kg)	Right occipital region	3.4 ms

Table 3. Force durations obtained from the simulations. Short (1.4~2.7ms) and long (2.9~3.7ms) force durations were obtained from the coup and contrecoup contusion cases, respectively.

3.4 Summary of chapter 3

In this chapter, the relationship between the input force duration and the dynamic response of the human head were focused by reconstructing the real-world brain injury accident cases using the finite element human head model based on the contusions were caused by the negative pressure inside the skull. The results were shown, in the coup contusion cases, the impact objects were sharp so the short force durations were obtained and the negative pressure occurred at the impact side. In contrast, in the contrecoup contusion cases, the impact objects had flat surfaces so the long force durations were obtained and the negative pressure occurred at the opposite side of impact. In the other words, coup contusion tends to occur when the force duration is shorten, and contrecoup contusion tends to occur when the force duration is lengthen, so the force duration is shown to be the parameter for separating coup or contrecoup contusions.

4. The mechanism of DAI

Gennarelli et al. characterized the strain caused by a rotational acceleration load to the head, and proposed the strain threshold of DAI by using finite element models for the crania of human and baboon (Meaney et al., 1995; Susan et al., 1990). They observed the shear deformation generated in each part of the brain with a high speed camera when the head was rotated, and assumed that the strain that caused DAI was larger than 9.4%. Pfister et al. developed a device which could generate shear deformation of cells cultured on a plane by pulling the ground substance and made it possible to produce a strain up to 70% and a strain rate up to 90/s (Pfister et al., 2003). Laplaca et al. cultured cells in a gel and generated 3D deformation of the cells by producing a shear deformation of the gel (strain < 50%, strain rate < 30/s). Neuronal cells showed a lower tolerance to this strain than the glial cells (LaPlaca et al., 2005; Cullen et al., 2007).Tamura et al. analyzed the difference in strain caused by a tensile test between porcine brain tissue and nerve fiber in the white matter, and reported that the maximum neural fiber strain was ~25% of the level in the surrounding tissue (Tamura et al., 2006). Nakayama et al. showed morphological changes of axons and the progress of this damage over time caused by one-dimensional, horizontal oscillations of nerve cells (Nakayama et al., 2001). These data suggested that an axon would receive damage with a strain of larger than 10% and a strain rate of larger than 10/s.

In this chapter, in order to clarily the influence of the axonal damage on the damage of cells, the cytotoxicity and mortality of PC12 cell (rat adrenal pheochromocytoma cell) line were evaluated by applying huge acceleration to cells. Huge acceleration was generated by an impact machine and was given to 2 kinds of cells, i.e. with and without axons.

4.1 Cell culture

In this study, PC12 cell line (obtained from Riken Cell Bank, Tsukuba, Japan) was used. Cells were cultured in DMEM (Dulbecco's Modified Eagle's Medium; Gibco, Gland Island, NY, USA) supplemented with 10% FBS (fetal bovine serum), 10% HS (horse serum), and Pennicillin-Streptmycin (10U/ml, 100ng/ml, Sigma-Aldrich, St. Louis, MO, USA) in 95%Air, 5% CO2 at 37℃.

In the impact experiment, the PC12 cells with and without axons were used. Axons were developed by adding 50ng/ml NGF (nerve growth factor, 2.5S; Invitrogen, Carlsbad, CA, USA). The cells were seeded in PLL (poly-l-lysine)-coated dishes (Φ35mm) at a density of 1×104/cm2, and incubated for 5 days. Phase-contrast images of cells are shown in Fig. 13.

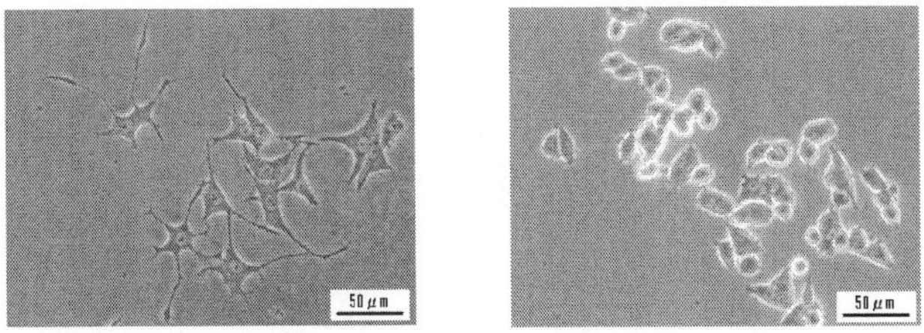

(a) PC12 cells with axons (b) PC12 cells without axons

Fig. 13. Phase-contrast images of PC12 cells cultured for 5days. (a) PC12 cells with axons. (b)PC12 cells without axons.

4.2 Impact experiment with huge acceleration

The outline of the impact experiment is shown in Fig. 14. The impact experiments were carried out with an SM-100-3P impact machine (AVEX Electronics Inc., PA, USA). The impact machine can accelerate the specimen, with a range of acceleration of 3~20000 G and for duration of 0.1~60ms.

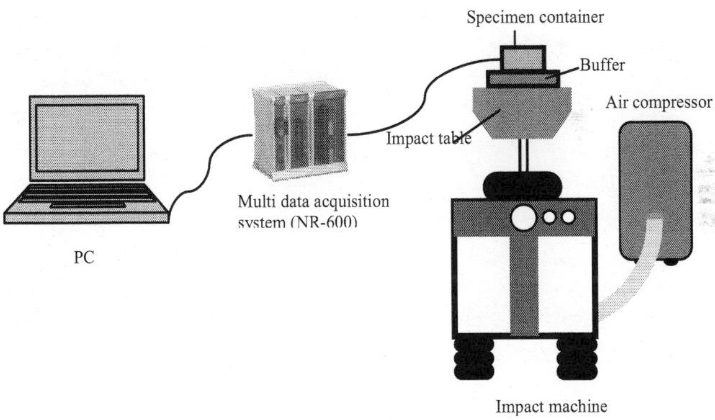

(a) Devices used for the impact experiments

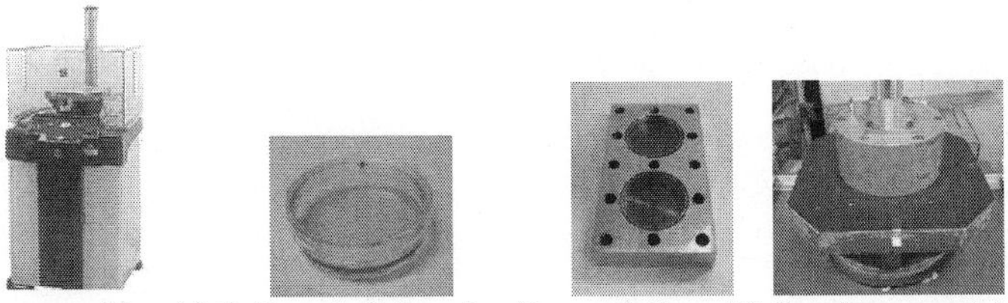

(b) Impact machine (c) Cultured dish and culture solution (d) Specimen container (e) Impact table

Fig. 14. Major components of the impact experiment. A dish seeded with PC12 cells was filled with culture solution (c), and fixed in position in a stainless plate (d). The plate was then fixed on the impact table (e).The impact table was elevated and dropped by the compressor.

A dish seeded with PC12 cells was filled with culture solution (Fig. 14(c)), and fixed in position in a stainless plate (Fig. 14(d)). The plate was then fixed on the impact table (Fig. 14(e)).The impact table was elevated and dropped by the compressor. The impact table collided against the buffer generating an impact with huge velocity to the dish.

The strain applied to the cultured dish was measured with a strain gauge (KFG-2N-120-C1; Kyowa Electronic Instruments Co.), which was attached to the bottom of the dish and connected to a multi-data acquisition system (NR-600; Keyence Co.). A total of 72 impact experiments were carried out, i.e. 6 experiments per condition. The input acceleration ranged from 3000 G to 10000 G, and the duration of all accelerations was 0.1ms.

4.3 Evaluation of Injury

4.3.1 Cytotoxicity of PC12 Cells

Cytotoxicity of cells was measured by the LDH (lactate dehydrogenase) assay. LDH is a soluble cytosolic enzyme that is released into the culture medium following loss of membrane integrity resulting from either apoptosis or necrosis.

After the impact, the culture solution in the dish was centrifuged for 10 minutes at 250 G, 100 μl of the reaction solution (cytotoxicity detection kit (LDH), Roche Diagnostics) was added to 100 μl of the supernatant. The reactions were incubated at room temperature for 30 min using 96-well plates (96-well Micro Test III assay Plate, BD Falcon), and 1N-HCl was added as a stop solution. The absorbance of each specimen was measured at 490 nm by a Microplate Reader (Model 680; Bio-Rad Laboratories). Similarly, the absorbance of the low control specimens (no load cells) and high control specimens (cells dissolved by 1% TritonX-100 in PBS) were measured. The cytotoxicity of PC12 cells was calculated by the following equation.

$$\text{Cytotoxicity}\ (\%) = (C - LC) / HC \times 100\% \tag{1}$$

where C is the LDH quantity (IU/l) obtained from the impact experiment specimen, LC is the LDH quantity (IU/l) obtained from the low control specimen, and HC is the LDH quantity (IU/l) obtained from the high control specimen.

4.3.2 Mortality of PC12 cells

Mortality of cells was measured by the dye exclusion method with trypan blue dye. This method determines cell viability by mixing a suspension of live cells with a dilute solution of trypan blue; cells that exclude dye are considered to be alive, while stained cells are considered to be dead.

After the impact, cells were separated from the dish with 0.25% Trypsin-EDTA (Gibco), collected in a microcentrifuge tube (1.5 ml), and centrifuged for 30 seconds at 2000 G.

$$\text{Mortality}\ (\%) = N/M \times 100\% \tag{2}$$

where N is the number of the dead cells and M is the total number of cells.

4.3.3 Morphological change of axon

When an axon is damaged, terminal swellings coincide with the detachment of the growth cones from the substrate. The detachment of the growth cones from the substrate destroys the cytoskeletal network, which determines and maintains cell shape, resulting in a spherical deformation of the axon. Terminal swellings form in the early stages of the injury. When the cytoskeletal destruction occurs at non-terminal sites along the axon, spherical deformations develop slowly, and these appear as beads. Beadings grow in the later stages of injury (Nakayama et al., 2001; Fujiwara et al., 2004).

After the impact, the morphological changes of the axons were observed with a phase-contrast microscope.

4.3.4 Statistical analysis

Statistical analysis of the cytotoxicity and mortality of cells with axons and without axons for each experimental condition were assessed with the t-test; $p < 0.05$ was considered to be statistically significant. Data were expressed as the mean ± standard error of the mean (SEM).

4.4 Results of damage evaluation

4.4.1 Strain and strain rate obtained from the impact experiments

The average strain and strain rate at the bottom of dish are shown in Table 4. As an example, the strain fluctuation when the peak of acceleration was 7000G is shown in Fig.15.

A strain from 0.035% to 0.201% and a strain rate from 6.67/s to19.02/s were measurable on the bottom of dish with the input accelerations from 3000 G to 10000 G. The strain measured at the bottom of dish had increased linearly as the input acceleration increased.

The strain rate tended to increase linearly as the input acceleration increased. However, when the input acceleration was 5000, 6000 and 8000 G, the strain rate was 13.02/s, 13.11/s, and 13.36/s, respectively. There was no significant difference between these strain rates. The strain rate obtained at 7000 G was 14.62/s, which was larger than the strain rate obtained at 8000G. It was difficult to control the duration of the acceleration accurately in the impact experiment when the input acceleration was very powerful. Although the strain obtained at 8000 G was larger than the strain obtained at 7000G, the duration of 8000 G became longer than the duration of 7000 G, resulting in the smaller strain rate at 8000 G.

Condition number	Peak acceleration [G]	Duration [ms]	Average strain [%]	Average strain rate (1/s)
1	3000	0.1	0.035	6.67
2	5000	0.1	0.065	13.02
3	6000	0.1	0.148	13.11
4	7000	0.1	0.164	14.62
5	8000	0.1	0.187	13.36
6	10000	0.1	0.201	19.02

Table 4. Strain and strain rates obtained from the impact experiments. The strain rate tended to increase linearly as the input acceleration increased.

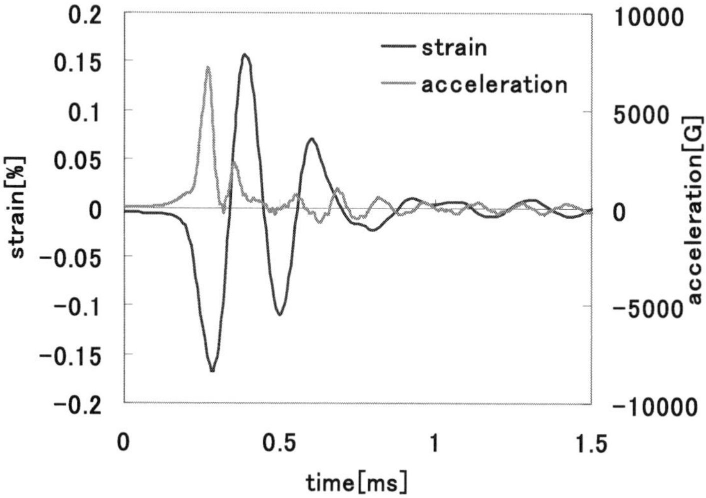

Fig. 15. Strain fluctuation when the peak of the acceleration was 7000 G. The strain of this input was 0.164%.

4.4.2 Cytotoxicity of PC12 cells

Cytotoxicity of cells with and without axons immediately after the impact experiment is shown in Fig.16. The relationship between the input acceleration and cytotoxicity of cells is shown in Fig.16 (a), the relationship between the strain and cytotoxicity of cells is shown in Fig.16 (b), and the relationship between the strain rate and cytotoxicity of cells is shown in Fig.16(c). Since the input of the impact experiment was acceleration, the strain rate could not be controlled in detail; the data obtained from 5000-8000G were concentrated on around 14/s as shown in Table 4.

Cytotoxicity of cells seemed to increase as the input acceleration and strain increased, but these relationships did not show strong correlations (Figs. 16(a), and 16(b)). Although the tendency that cytotoxicity of cells increased as the strain rate increased was shown, the correlation could not be quantitatively evaluated, because in the small strain rate range around 14/s cytotoxicity of cells did not increase monotonically.

For the two results obtained from 3000 and 5000 G (correspond to 0.035% and 0.065% in the strain, and to 6.67/s and 13.02/s in the strain rate), cytotoxicity of cells with axons was not significantly higher than in cells without axons. When the input acceleration was larger than 6000G, the strain was larger than 0.15%, and the strain rate was larger than 13.11/s, cytotoxicity of cells with axons was significantly higher than in cells without axons (Figs. 16(a), 16(b), and 16(c); $*p<0.05$).

Therefore, it appeared that cytotoxicity of cells increased as the strain rate increased, and cells with axons were more easily damaged than cells without axons when the strain rate was larger than 13.11/s.

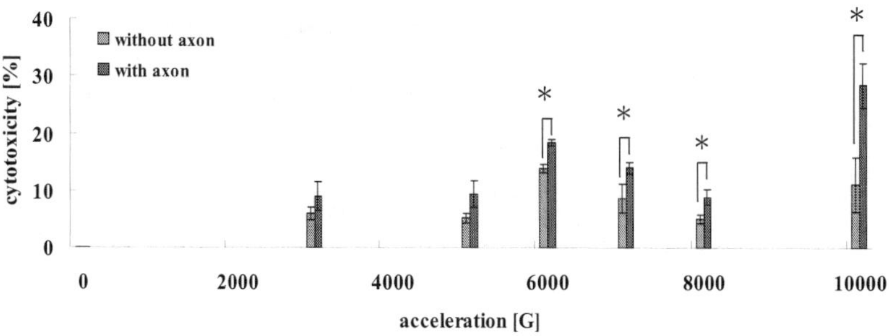

(a) Relationship between the input acceleration and cytotoxicity of PC12 cells

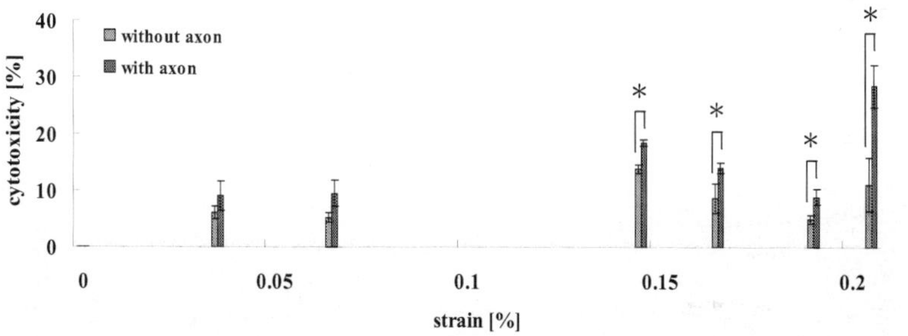

(b) Relationship between the strain and cytotoxicity of PC12 cells

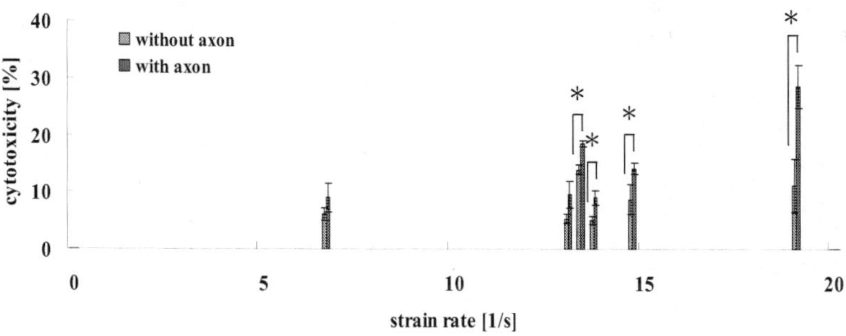

(c) Relationship between the strain rate and cytotoxicity of PC12 cells

Fig. 16. Experimental results of cytotoxicity of PC12 cells. Error bars represent SEM. (* $p < 0.05$)

4.4.3 Mortality of PC12 cells

Mortality of cells with and without axons immedieately after the impact experiment is shown in Fig. 17. The relationship between the input acceleration and mortality of cells is shown in Fig. 17(a), the relationship between the strain and mortality of cells is shown in Fig. 17(b), and the relationship between the strain rate and mortality of cells is shown in Fig. 17(c).

Mortality of cells seemed to increase as the input acceleration and strain increased, but these relationships did not show strong correlations (Fig. 17(a), and 17(b)). Although the tendency that mortality of cells increased as the strain rate increased was shown, the correlation could not be quantitatively evaluated, because in the small strain rate range around 14/s mortality of cells did not increase monotonically.

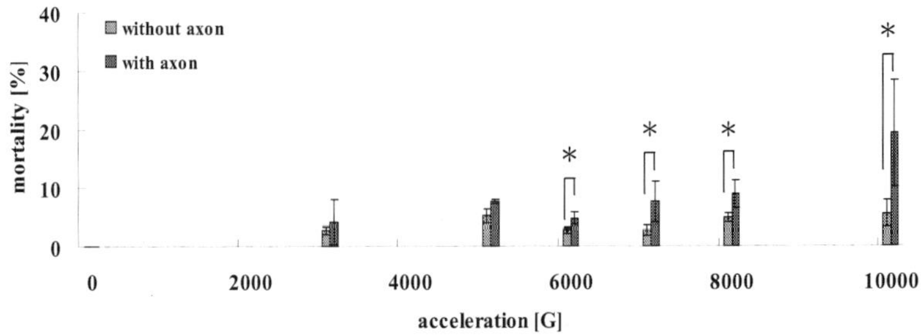

(a) Relationship between the input acceleration and mortality of PC12 cells

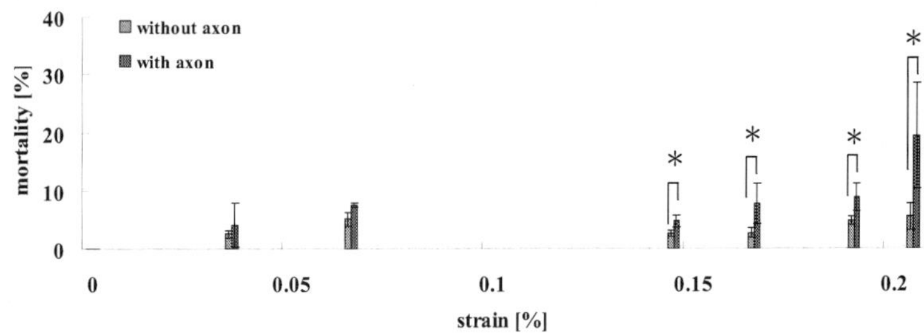

(b) Relationship between the strain and mortality of PC12 cells

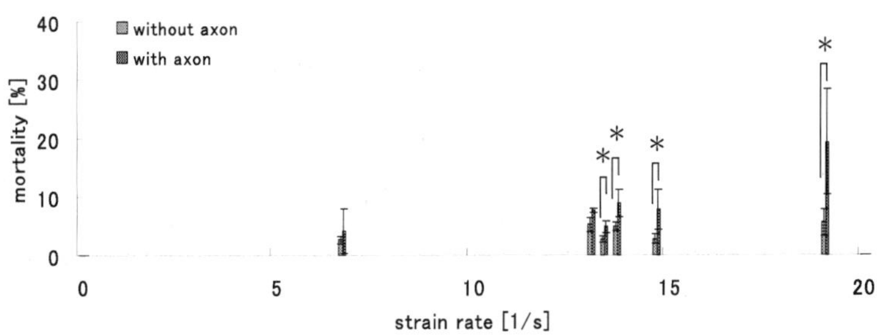

(c) Relationship between the strain rate and mortality of PC12 cells

Fig. 17. Experimental result of mortality of PC12 cells · Error bars represent SEM. (* $p < 0.05$)

For the two results obtained from 3000 and 5000 G (correspond to 0.035% and 0.065% in the strain, and to 6.67/s and 13.02/s in the strain rate), mortality of cells with axons was not significantly higher than in cells without axons. When the input acceleration was larger than 6000 G, the strain was larger than 0.15%, and the strain rate was larger than 13.11/s, mortality of cells with axons was significantly higher than in cells without axons (Figs. 17(a), 17(b), and 17(c); $^{*}p<0.05$).

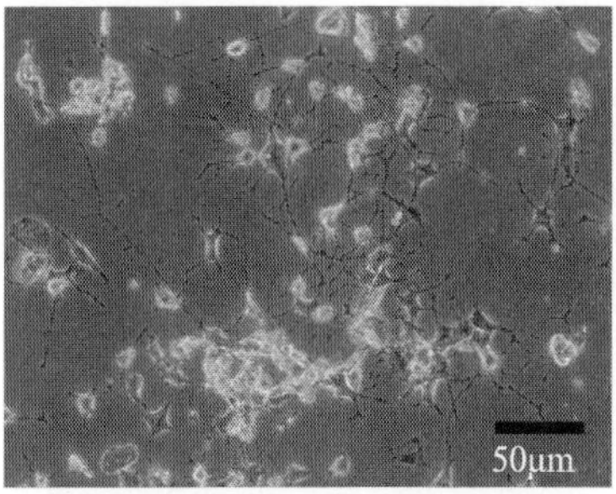

(a-1) Cells with axons, control

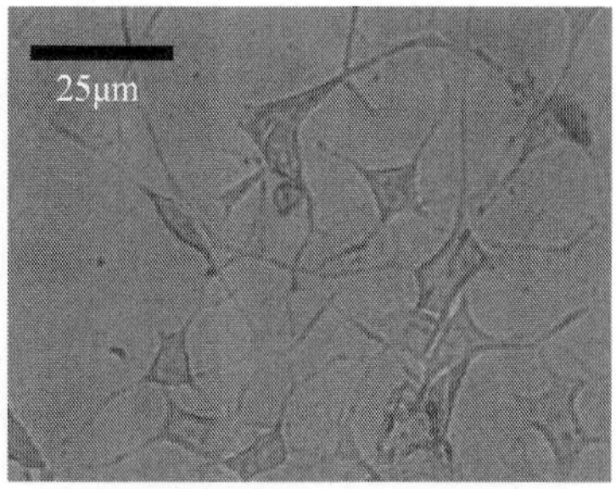

(a-2) Cells with axons, control

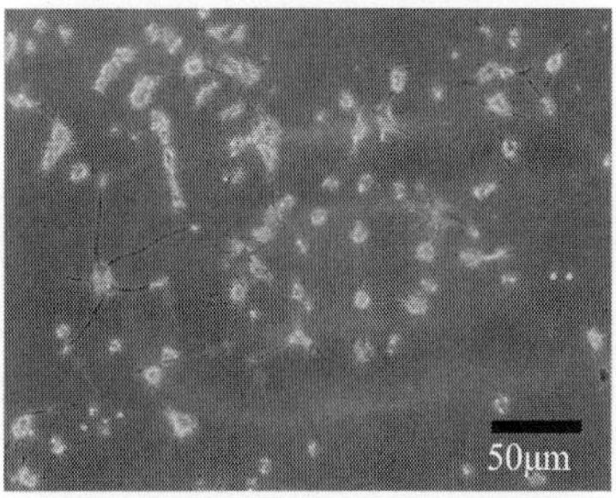

(b-1) Cells with axons, strain rate=19.02/s, immediately after the impact

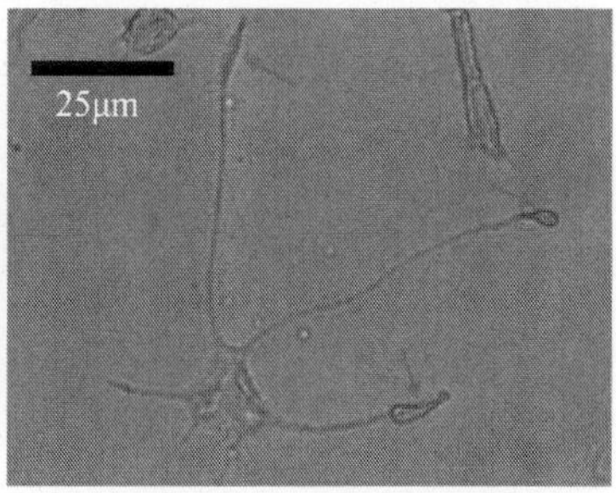

(b-2) Cells with axons, strain rate=19.02/s, immediately after the impact

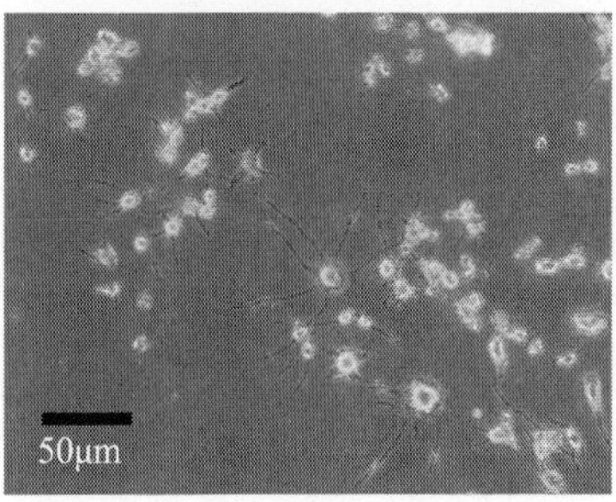

(c-1) Cells with axons, strain rate=19.02/s, 4 h after the impact

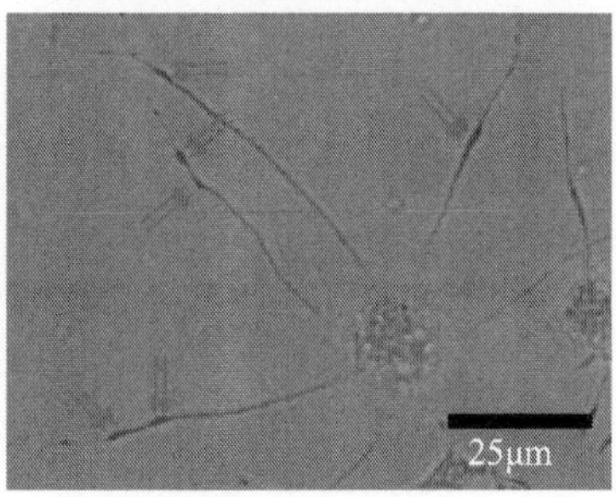

(c-2) Cells with axons, strain rate=19.02/s, 4 h after the impact

Fig. 18. Phase-contrast images of PC12 cells, control (a-1, a-2), immediately after the impact (b-1, b-2) and 4 h after the impact(c-1,c-2). For a clearer view, (a-1), (b-1), and (c-1) are enlarged in (a-2), (b-2), and (c-2), respectively. Terminal swellings are indicated with single arrows and beadings are indicated with double arrows.

Therefore, it appeared that mortality of cells increased as the strain rate increased, and cells with axons had an increased mortality than cells without axons when the strain rate was larger than 13.11/s.

4.4.4 Morphological change

In order to observe damage to axons, cells with axons were observed with a phase-contrast microscope. Phase-contrast images of cells with axons on the dish are shown in Fig.18.

Phase-contrast images of cells with axons before the experiments (control) are shown in Figs. 18(a-1) and 18(a-2). Cells extending their axons and a network creates with these axons can be observed. Cells and their axons attached to the substrate. Terminal swellings or the beadings of axons are not observed at this stage. Phase-contrast images of cells immediately after the impact with the strain rate of 19.02/s are shown in Figs. 18(b-1) and 18(b-2); terminal swellings of axons are indicated with single arrows in the figures. Terminal swellings can be observed when the terminals of axons detach from the substrate. Since beading occurs in the later stages of damage, beading can not be observed yet at this stage. Phase-contrast images of cells 4 h after the impact with the strain rate of 19.02/s are shown in Figs. 18(c-1) and 18(c-2); beadings in the damaged regions are indicated with double arrows in the figures. Although beadings can not be observed in the images immediately after the impact as shown in Figs. 18(b-1) and 18(b-2), beadings can be clearly observed in the images taken after 4 h as shown in Figs. 18(c-1) and 18(c-2).

4.5 Summary of chapter 4

In this chapter, in order to study the influence of the axonal damage on cell damage, an impact experiment with huge acceleration was performed on PC12 cell line. In order to evaluate damage to axon, the impact experiments were performed on cells with and without axons. The strain at the bottom of cultured dish was measured, and the strain rate was calculated. The cytotoxicity and mortality of PC12 cells were evaluated by the input acceleration, strain and strain rate. As a result, the strain rate seemed to be the most appropriate to evaluate the cytotoxicity and mortality of cells. The cytotoxicity and mortality of cells increased as the strain rate increased, and cells with axons were more easily damaged and had an increased mortality than cells without axons when the strain rate was larger than 13.11/s. These data suggest that the presence of axons increased the cytotoxicity and mortality of cells.

5. Conclusion

In this study, to elucidate the mechanics of head injuries, the engineering approach using finite element analysis and the biological approach using cultured cells are performed. In the engineering approach, the results of the reconstruction of the real-world brain injury accident cases are shown, in the coup contusion cases, the negative pressure occurred at the impact side and it had direct correlation with the short force durations. In contrast, in the contrecoup contusion cases, the negative pressure occurred at the opposite side of impact and it had direct correlation with the long force durations. As the result, the force duration is shown to be the parameter for separating coup or contrecoup contusions. In the biological approach, the results of the impact experiments using the cultured cells are shown, the strain rate seemed to be the most appropriate to evaluate the cytotoxicity and mortality of cells. Damage to axons was confirmed by terminal swellings and beadings of the axons. These data indicated that the presence of axons increased the cytotoxicity and mortality of cells.

6. Future directions

In the future works, in order to evaluate all types of traumatic brain injury comprehensively, the tolerance of nerve damage which is obtained from the impact experiment of cultured cells is applied to numerical analysis. Therefore, to construct a human head finite element model containing the nerve fibers, a method to accurately measure the material properties of nerve fibers have to be developed and the structure of the neural network inside the skull have to be clarified by the image processing.

7. Acknowledgement

We thank Associate Prof. Atsushi Senoo (Tokyo Metropolitan University, Faculty of Health Sciences, Division of Radiological Sciences) for his assistance in photographing MRI data to construct the finite element human head model.

8. References

Aomura, S.; Fujiwara, S & Ikoma, T. (2002). The Study on the Influence of Different Interface Conditions on the Response of Finite Element Human Head Models under Occipital Impact Loading, *JSME International Journal, Series C*, Vol.46, No.2, pp.583-593.

Aomura, S.; Zhang, Y.; Fujiwara, S. & Nishimura, A. (2008). Dynamic Analysis of Cerebral Contusion under Impact Loading, *Journal of Biomechanical Science and Engineering*, Vol. 3, No. 4, pp.499-509.

Cullen D.K.; Simon C.M. & LaPlaca M.C. (2007). Strain rate-dependent induction of reactive astrogliosis and cell death in three-dimensional neuronal-astrocytic co-cultures, *Brain Research*, Vol.1158, pp.103-115.

Doorly, M.C. & Gilchrist, M.D. (2006). The Use of Accident Reconstruction for the Analysis of Traumatic Brain Injury Due to Head Impacts Arising from Falls, *Computer Methods in Biomechanics and Biomedical Engineering*, Vol.9, No.6, pp.371-377.

Fujiwara S.; Ogawa Y.; Hirabayashi M.; Inamura K. & Aihara H. (1998). Biomechanics of Cerebral Contusion and Diffuse Axonal Injury, *Proceedings of the 6th Indo Pacific Congress on Legal Medicine and Forensic Sciences*, pp.1003-1006.

Fujiwara S.; Yanagisawa A.; Sato H.; Shindo Y.; Koide K. & Nishimura A. (2004). DAI Diagnosis Using β-APP mRNA Expression Analysis and its Application to Forensic Medicine, *Research and Practice in Forensic Medicine*, Vol.47, pp.85-90.

Fujiwara, S.; Yanagida, Y. & Mizoi, Y. (1989). Impact Induced Intra-cranial Pressure Caused by an Accelerated Motion of the Head or by Skull Deformation: An Experimental Study Using Physical Models of the Head and Neck, and Ones of the Skull, *Forensic Science International*, Vol.43, pp.159-169.

Fujiwara, S.; Yanagida, Y.; Fukunaga, T.; Mizoi, Y. & Tatsuno, Y. (1986). Studies on Cerebral Contusion in the Fatal Cases by Blow, Fall and Fall Down, *The Japanese Journal of Legal Medicine*, Vol.40, No.4, pp.377-383.

Gennarelli, T.A. (1983). Head Injury in Man and Experimental Animals: Clinical Aspects, *Acta Neurochirurgica*, Suppl.32, pp.1-32.

Gross, A.G. (1958). A New Theory on the Dynamics of Brain Concussion and Brain Injury, *Journal of Neurosurgery*, Vol.15, pp.548-561.

Gurdjian, E.S.; Lissner, H.R.; & Hodson, V.R. (1966). Mechanism of Head Injury, *Clinical Neurosurgery*, Vol.12, pp.112-128.

LaPlaca M.C.; Cullen D.K.; McLoughlin J.J. & Cargill R.S. (2005). High rate shear strain of three-dimensional neural cell cultures: a new in vitro traumatic brain injury model, *Journal of Biomechanics*, Vol.38, No.5, pp.1093-1105.

Meaney D.F.; Smith D.H.; Shreiber D.I.; Bain A.C.; Miller R.T.; Ross D.T. & Gennarelli T.A. (1995). Biomechanical Analysis of Experimental Diffuse Axonal Injury, *Journal of Neurotrauma*, Vol.12, No.4, pp.689-694.

Nahum, A.M. & Smith, R. (1977), Intracranial Pressure Dynamics during Head Impact, *Proceeding of 21st Stapp car Crash Conference*, pp.339-366.

Nakayama Y.; Aoki Y. & Niitsu H. (2001). Studies on the mechanisms responsible for the formation of focal swellings on neuronal processes using a novel in vitro model of axonal injury, *Journal of Neurotrauma*, Vol.18, No.5, pp.545-554.

Nishimoto, T.; Murakami, S.; Abe, T. & Ono, K. (1998). Mechanical Properties of Human Cranium and Effect of Cranial on Extradural Hematoma, *Transactions of the Japan Society of Mechanical Engineers, Part A*, Vol.61, No.591, pp. 2386-2392.

Ommaya A.K. & Gennarelli T.A. (1974). Cerebral concussion and traumatic unconsciousness, correlation of experimental and clinical observations on blunt head injuries, *Brain*, Vol.97, pp.633-654.

Pfister B.J.; Weihs T.P.; Betenbaugh M. & Bao G. (2003). An in vitro Uniaxial Stretch Model for Axonal Injury, *Annals of Biomedical Engin_eering*, Vol.31, No.5, pp.589-598.

Raul, J.S.; Baumgartner, D.; Willinger, R. & Ludes, B. (2006). Finite Element Modelling of Human Head Injuries Caused by a Fall, *International Journal of Legal Medicine*, Vol.120, No.4, pp.212-218.

Riordain, K.O.; Thomas, P.M.; Phillips, J.P. & Gilchrist, M.D. (2003). Reconstruction of Real Word Head Injury Accidents Resulting from Falls using Multibody Dynamics, *Clinical Biomechanics*, Vol.18, pp.590-600.

Susan S.M.; Lawrence E.T. & Thomas G. (1990). Physical Model Simulation of Brain Injury in the Primate, *Journal of Biomechanics*, Vol.23, No.8, pp.823-836.

Tamura A.; Nagayama K. & Matsumoto T. (2006). Measurement of Nerve Fiber Strain in Brain Tissue Subjected to Uniaxial Stretch (Comparison Between Local Strain of Nerve Fiber and Global Strain of Brain Tissue), *Journal of Biomechanical Science and Engineering*, Vol.1, No.2, pp.304-315.

Viano, D.C.; Casson, I.R.; Pellman, E.J.; Zhang, L.; King, A.I. & Yang, K.H. (1998). Concussion in Professional Football Brain Responses by Finite Element Analysis: Part 9, *Neurosurgery*, Vol.57, No.5, pp.891-916.

Willinger, R. & Baumgartner, D. (2003). Human Head Tolerance Limits to Specific Injury Mechanisms, *International Journal of Crashworthiness*, Vol.6, No.8, pp.605-617.

Yanagida, Y.; Fujiwara, S. & Mizoi, Y. (1989). Differences in the Intra-cranial Pressure Caused by a 'Blow' and/or a'Fall' – An Experimental Study Using Physical Models of the Head and Neck, *Forensic Science International*, Vol.41, pp.135-145.

Zhang, L.; Hardy, W.N.; Omori, K.; Yang, K.H.; & King, A.I. (2001). Recent Advances in Cerebral Injury Research: A New Model and New Experimental Data, *Proceedings of the ASME Bioengineering Conference*, pp.831-832.

Zhang, Y.; Aomura, S.; Nakadate, H. & Fujiwara, S. (2010). Study on the Mechanism of Cerebral Contusion Based on Judicial Autopsy Report, *Proceedings of the 6th World Congress on Biomechanics*, Vol.31, pp.505-508.

25

Residual Stresses and Cracking in Dental Restorations due to Resin Contraction Considering In-Depth Young's Modulus Variation

Estevam Barbosa de Las Casas, João Batista Novaes Jr., Elissa Talma, Willian Henrique Vasconcelos, Tulimar P. Machado Cornacchia, Iracema Maria Utsch Braga, Carlos Alberto Cimini Jr. and Rodrigo Guerra Peixoto

Universidade Federal de Minas Gerais
Universidade de Campinas
Brazil

1. Introduction

Composite resins have been increasingly used as restorative material, both in anterior and posterior teeth, where they replace metal restorations. Its aesthetic characteristics, coupled with improved physical properties have made their use extend from just anterior teeth to also include posterior teeth. The use of such material in oral regions subjected to higher loading makes it important to account for the effect of residual stresses arising during polymerization, induced by resin contraction (Ausiello, Apicilla and Davidson 2002). Different reports can be found in the literature focused in this aspect and using different approaches, such as X-ray micro-computed tomography (Sun, Eidelman and Gibson 2009), 3D evaluation of the marginal adaptation (Kakaboura et al 2007) and 3 D deformation analysis from MCT images (Chiang et al 2010). These authors agree in the critical role played by resin contraction in restoration success. The Finite Element Method can therefore be a useful tool to investigate the cracking of interfaces, stress concentrations in the internal angles and effects of variations in the mechanical properties in the overall behavior of the resin-based dental restorations.

Some composite resins for dentistry use are the result of the interaction of an organic matrix, a coupling agent and an inorganic material, since it was first devised by Bowen et al. (1983). In the last decades, industry has altered significantly the inorganic part of this composition. As a result, composite hybrid resins, with the inclusion of nanoparticles have not only improved strength and abrasion resistance but also presented greater polishing characteristics. Nevertheless, their physicochemical properties are still dependent of the polymerization of the resin matrix, induced by light penetration with 400 to 500 nm wave lengths, the peak absorption of camphorquinone (Braga et al., 2005).

The beginning of the polymerization process of the resinous matrix happens when it is irradiated with an external source, and stops when the maximum conversion of the monomers is reached, which varies with time of exposure to light, quality of the polymerizing agent and depth of light penetration (Jandt et al., 2000; Felix et al., 2006; Jong et al., 2007; Ceballos et al., 2009; Ferracane, 2005). The degree of conversion of the resin matrix can then be associated directly to the physical properties of the restoration, as well as its strength under dental loading (Peutzfeldt et al., 2000; Sakaguchiet al., 1991).

When a composed resin is applied directly to dental tissues, after the hybridization by the adhesive agent of the cavity walls, the requirement is to rigidly connect enamel and dentine to the restoring material, in the attempt to generate a solid and continuous body as a mechanically ideal restoration. The ideal restoration would be totally impermeable to the infiltration of fluids and resistant to the opening of gaps in the tooth-restoration interface.

The use of the composed resin as restorative material implies in the polymerization of the resinous matrix and in its fixation to the cavity walls. However, during the polymerization the resinous matrix suffers contraction, which can surpass the adhesive rupture resistance, leading to imperfections in the restoration as marginal gaps, cracking, hypersensitivity and infiltration. The reduction of the generated residual stresses can be obtained in different ways during polymerization: (i) when a controlled fluid flow is allowed during the process (Braga et al.,2005); (ii) by the use of devices with the *soft-start* technique (Yoshikawa et al., 2001); (iii) reducing the associated factor C in the layers deposition (Ceballos et al., 2009; Petrovic et al., 2010); (iv) through the application of resinous material with low modulus of elasticity that can deform without producing high residual stresses (Dietschi et al., 2002); and (v) using a method of improving marginal adaptation by eliminating stress concentration points during resin photo-polymerization (Petrovic et al., 2010).

After polymerization, the composite resin exposition to the humid oral environment leads to water penetration to the inner regions of the restored cavity, causing volumetric hygroscopic expansion. Due to the penetration of water inside the hydrophilic organic matrix, a gradual expansion occurs, until a balanced value is eventually reached.

The aim of this study is to quantify the effect of the use of two different irradiation sources (halogen and second-generation LED) on the elastic modulus and the degree cure during the polymerization process of a nanofilled composite restorative material. The effect of the variation of the elastic modulus on the polymerization residual stresses is then accessed by means of3-D finite element simulations, in order to understand the mechanical response of a cylindrical Class I restoration under polymerization contraction.

2. Material and methods

2.1 Evaluation of composite resin mechanical properties

A composite resin (Filtek Z250, 3M Co., St Paul., MN, USA) and two different irradiation sources, XL3000 (halogen - 3M) and Elipar Freeligth 2 (LED - 3M ESPE), were used to evaluate, *in vitro*, the degree of conversion and the Young's modulus (also modulus of elasticity or elastic modulus) distribution along sample height. This last parameter was then used to examine, through a computer simulation, the effect of through-height stiffness variation in expected polymerization residual stresses.

2.1.1 Evaluation of the Degree of Conversion

To measure the Degree of Conversion (DC), test samples were prepared in standardized plastic molds with diameter of 4 mm and height of 2 mm and 4 mm. Four groups of samples were prepared, each one with three samples (n=3). Three measurements were performed for each sample. The groups were classified as: Group 1 (G1) - XL 3000, 2 mm height; Group 2 (G2) - Elipar, 2 mm height; Group 3 (G3)- XL3000, 4 mm height; Group 4 (G4) - Elipar, 4 mm height. The moulds were filled to the top in one step, and irradiated during a period of 40 seconds. After that, they were stored in a dark environment. The Degree of Conversion (DC) was measured at the base of the samples. Raman spectra were obtained on a JobinYvon/Horiba LABRAM-HR 800 spectrograph equipped with a He-Ne laser (632.8nm). The power in each sample was around 7mW. The Raman signal was collected by an Olympus BHX microscope provided with objectives (10x, 50x and 100x). The detector used was a N_2 liquid cooled CCD (Charge-Couple Device) of the Spectrum One, back illuminated. Depending on the sample background fluorescence, the acquisition time ranged from 10 to 30 seconds. To reduce signal/noise ratio, spectra were acquired 5 times after a 5 minutes photobleaching. Collected Raman spectra were analyzed and optimized with Labspec 1.1 and PeakFit v4. Spectra collected were averaged. The background was corrected and if necessary, normalized and peak deconvoluted.

The samples were excited by laser in the region between 2000 to 1000 cm^{-1} after five 60 second accumulations in order to evaluate the conversion proportion of the vinylic function in aliphatic function, comparing the residual non-polymerized methacrylate band C=C (1640cm^{-1}) to the aromatic 1610cm^{-1} C=C stretching band used as reference. The DC value was defined as given in Eq. (1),

$$DC(\%) - 100x\ [1 - Rp/\ Rnp] \tag{1}$$

where Rp and Rnp are the signals for the polymerized resin and non-polymerized resin. The degree of conversion was determined at three locations and the mean value calculated for each of the three specimens. From these three averages a new mean value was calculated.

2.1.2 Young's modulus measurement

Three specimens were prepared for each condition in order to measure the modulus of elasticity (Young's modulus) and were stored dry at room temperature for at least 24 hours before testing. All these specimens were prepared with 4 mm height, and the radiation source was kept at a distance between 1 and 2 mm. Therefore, there were also four groups of specimens for Young's modulus measurement: Group 1 (G1) - XL 3000, light source at 1 mm distance; Group 2 (G2) - XL3000, light source at 2 mm distance; Group 3 (G3)-Elipar, light source at 1 mm distance; Group 4 (G4) - Elipar, light source at 2 mm distance. For each group, three specimens were made (n=3) and, for each specimen, three indentations were done at four different depths (0.5, 1.5, 2.5 and 3.5 mm). The indentations were performed using a micro-durometer Shimadzu, at a speed of 2.6 mN/sand kept for 5 seconds. The values of Young's modulus and hardness were obtained for each depth in order to detect through-depth changes in the mechanical properties.

2.2 Finite element simulation

To simulate the restoration, a cylindrical model with a cavity was created to represent the dentine. On the cavity's inner walls an adhesive layer was applied, followed by the resin addition and then polymerization is performed. Despite being an axisymmetric problem, a three dimensional model was necessary due to software limitations to represent the adhesive material. Previous works in the literature describe numerical analysis of resin expansion, but disregarded the stiffness variation due to the light activation of the resin (Rüttermann et al., 2007; Carvalho Filho, 2005; Ausiello et al., 2002).

To simulate both the dentine and the resin regions, ten-nodded tetrahedral elements were used, with three degrees of freedom at each node. Program Ansys, release 10, was used in the analyses. Figure 1 represents the geometry of the model. A special element with a constitutive model developed for brittle materials was used for the adhesive layer in order to simulate cracking. This material constitutive model has a cutoff that imposes a limit to normal and tangential stresses, after which fracture occurs.

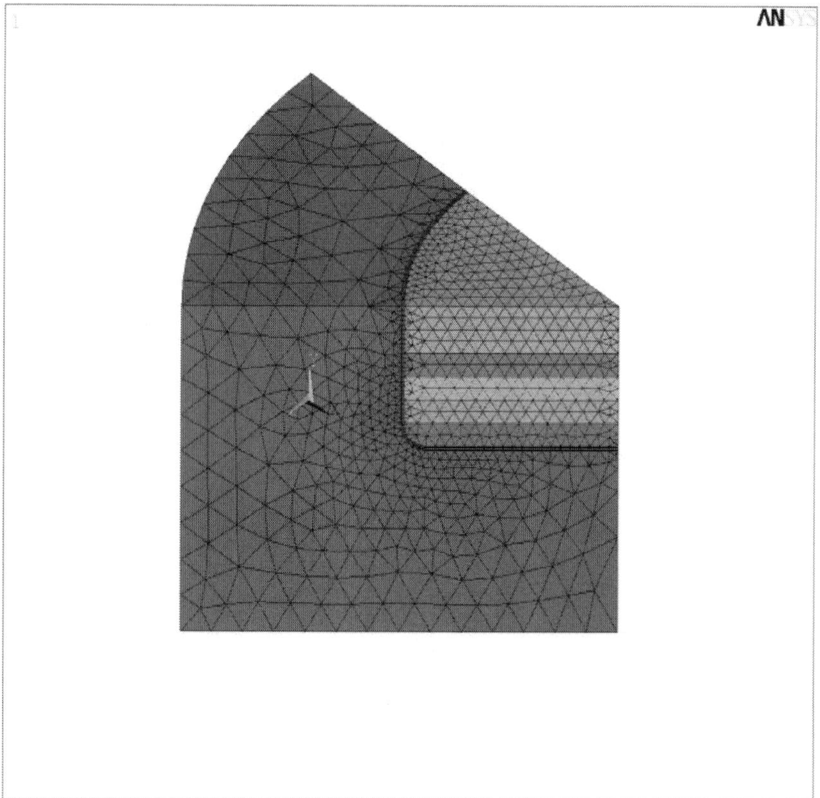

Fig. 1. Geometric model

Boundary conditions were imposed so as to restrict displacements at the base and non-vertical displacements in the faces, consistent with the restoration axisymmetry. Figure 2 shows dentine with the cavity, and Table 1 its material properties according to Ausiello et al. (2002). It is assumed that the dentine is under small displacements, with elastic behavior, and there is no stiffness variation. It is also considered homogeneous and isotropic. The analysis is then linear for this component.

The adhesive is represented by a thin layer with low traction strength. This material model introduces a nonlinear effect to the model, besides demanding a three dimensional geometric model. The traction at the interface was limited to 45 MPa, as indicated in the literature (Ausielo et al, 2002). In the process of solving the equations, the program verifies if this limit is exceeded at each iteration. If so, a crack is generated. Later, if compression at a normal direction to the crack's plane occurs, the crack is closed.

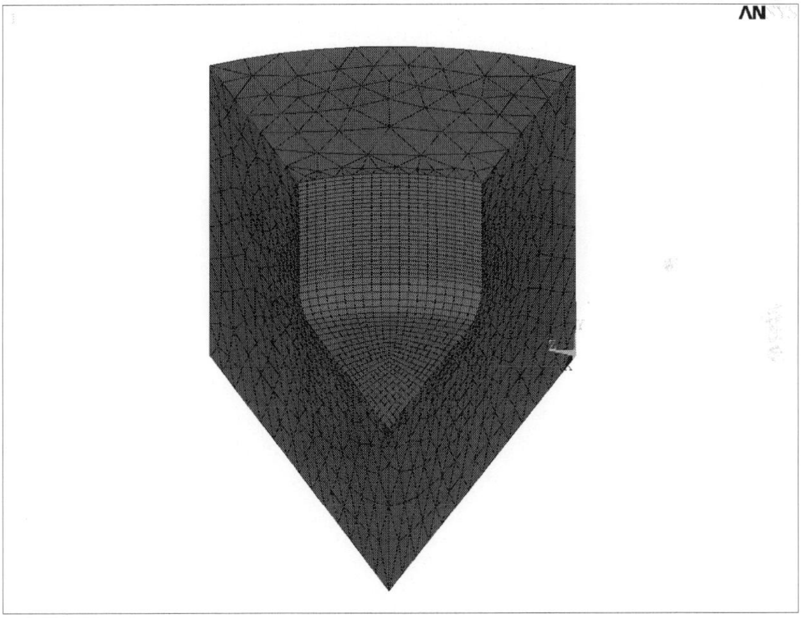

Fig. 2. Discrete model

Material	Young's Modulus	Poisson ratio
Dentine	18000 MPa	0.31
Adhesive	1000 MPa	0.30

Table 1. Material properties for dentine and adhesive (Ausielo et al, 2002)

Figure 3 shows the adhesive layer, and Table 1 presents its material mechanical properties (Ausielo et al, 2002).

The geometry of the resin was divided in six layers, each one with a half millimeter height. To these layers different values for the Young's modulus were assigned, which were measured from the laboratory experiments, as described in item 2.1.2.

In order to impose a volumetric contraction, a thermal expansion coefficient was introduced, and set to 0.01 $^{o}C^{-1}$. Then, a temperature variation was applied to the resin in the model, being negative to contraction and positive to expansion, calculated so as to produce the desired resin contraction.

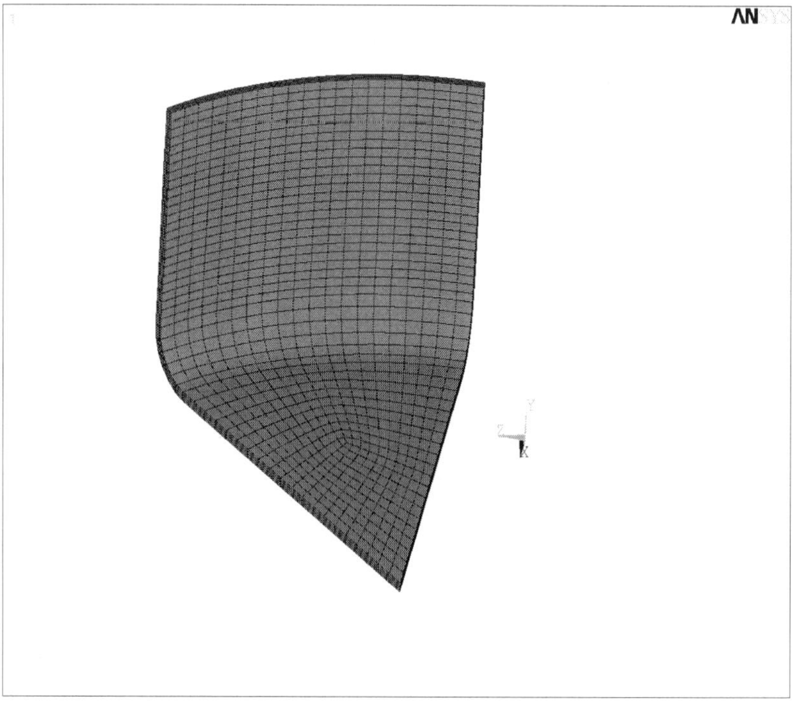

Fig. 3. Interface layer model

Two different clinical situations were studied. First, the cavity complete filling in a single step (here called *"one increment technique"*), consisting in filling the whole cavity with resin and then polymerizing it in one step. Then, the cavity filling in steps (here called *"horizontal incremental technique"*) consisting in filling the cavity with resin one layer at a time, polymerizing it and moving to the next, outer layer. A new layer of resin is added, and the process is repeated until the resin reaches the top of the cavity. This way, the layers will be thin, causing less stiffness variation, as indicated by the experimental results. For this study, the cavity was considered filled with three increments of equal thickness.

In the first method (one increment technique) the Young's modulus variation is significant, and its value will be smaller on the top of the restoration. The polymerization is simulated using the *Birth and Death* resource available in the software, which reduces the "dead" element's stiffness to a very low value, practically eliminating the contribution of that region's stiffness from the analysis. This resource allows the user to activate only part of the domain in one step, and then consider previously "dead" regions for further load steps.

To simulate the horizontal incremental technique, three layers were created. The two lowest were initially "killed" and a temperature variation applied at the top layer. The numerical system was solved. Then, the middle layer was "born" or activated, the temperature variation was applied, and the new system was solved. The same process was followed by the third layer.

This technique of simulation was similar to the one increment technique, but now the layers were polymerized from the bottom to the top, with the layer activation sequence following a downward sequence. An incremental iterative Newton-Raphson algorithm with a force based convergence criteria was used. The stopping criterion is given in Eq. (2), with $\beta = 0.001$ (F_{int} is the internal force and F_{ext} is the external force):

$$\left\| F_{int} - F_{ext} \right\| < \beta \cdot \left\| F_{ext} \right\| \tag{2}$$

3. Results

3.1 Degree of Conversion (DC)

The Raman test results for XL3000 (G1 and G3) and Elipar (G2 and G4) groups are respectively presented in Figures 4 and 5.

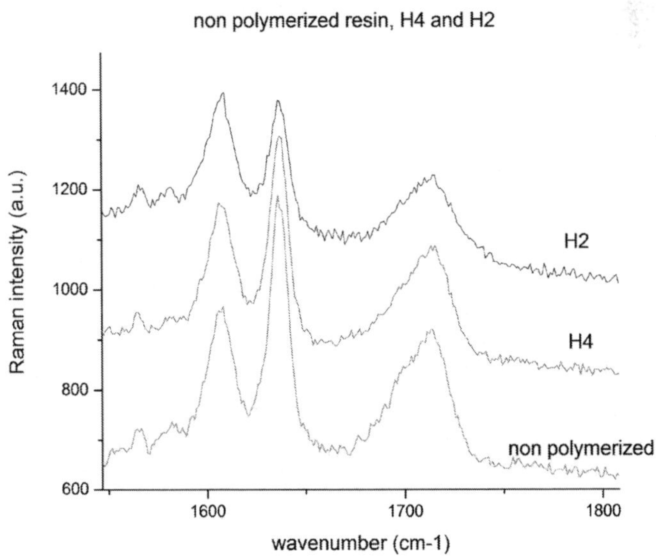

Fig. 4. Raman test results for XL3000 polymerization device and thicknesses of 2 mm (H2-G1) and 4mm (H4-G3)

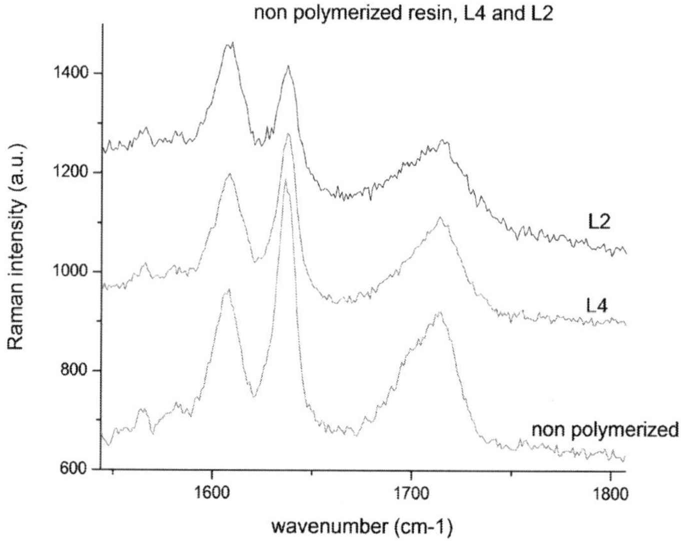

Fig. 5. Raman test results for Elipar polymerization device and thicknesses of 2 mm (L2-G2) and 4mm (L4-G4)

The measured average degrees of conversion values are listed in Table 2 for the four groups.

Sample height	XL3000 - QTH		Elipar Freeligth 2 - LED	
2mm	55 %	±3 %	59%	± 3 %
4mm	26%	± 1 %	32%	± 2 %

Table 2. Degree of conversion (in %) for Z350 resin measured using the Raman technique

The results for DC fit into a normal distribution, and three-way ANOVA model was used to analyze the influence of mode of cure sample height. Comparisons of the QTH (XL3000) and LED (Elipar Freeligth 2) curing methods showed significant influence of initial height in the degree of conversion ($p < 0.05$). For higher initial height, it was observed a sharp reduction in DC values. As for different irradiation techniques, it did not produce significant difference between the groups with the same initial height (2 or 4mm).

3.2 Young's modulus

The Young's modulus (E) showed a decrease for points located farther away from the light sources, as it is shown in Table 3, for both curing methods, regardless of the distance between the sample and the light source.

Group-depth	E (GPa)		W	p
	Average	Std Dev		
G1-0.5 mm	20.094	1.4360	0.678	0.0089
G1-1.5 mm	19.375	0.6461	0.9526	0.6901
G1-2.5 mm	17.720	0.8739	0.9351	0.9351
G1-3.5 mm	12.288	1.7453	0.9194	0.4180
G2-0.5 mm	19.004	1.4362	0.8287	0.0497
G2-1.5 mm	18.071	1.1987	0.838	0.0649
G2-2.5 mm	15.947	0.7665	0.9426	0.5816
G2-3.5 mm	10.755	0.6570	0.9247	0.4457
G3-0.5 mm	19.288	2.0709	0.9658	0.8331
G3-1.5 mm	18.221	1.4476	0.9018	0.3252
G3-2.5 mm	17.146	1.3244	0.9489	0.6501
G3-3.5 mm	15.226	1.2777	0.8505	0.0858
G4-0.5 mm	19.876	1.5748	0.7793	0.0157
G4-1.5 mm	19.056	1.5425	0.9095	0.3659
G4-2.5 mm	18.147	1.2606	0.9711	0.8905
G4-3.5 mm	16.016	1.3564	0.9736	0.9132

Table 3. Young's modulus (in GPa) variations with depth for different curing devices

Comparisons (Dunn method)	Differences	z calculed	z critical	p
G1-0.5mm x G1-1.5mm	2.3333	0.4698	2.638	ns
G1-0.5mm x G1-2.5mm	13.3333	2.6846	2.638	< 0.05
G1-0.5mm x G1-3.5mm	23.2222	4.6757	2.638	< 0.05
G1-1.5mm x G1-2.5mm	11	2.2148	2.638	ns
G1-1.5mm x G1-3.5mm	20.8889	4.2059	2.638	< 0.05
G1-2.5mm x G1-3.5mm	9.8889	1.9911	2.638	ns

Table 4. Young's modulus (in GPa). Variations with depth for group G1, for different depth values, XL3000at distance of 1 mm

Comparisons (Dunn method)	Differences	z calculed	z critical	p
G2-0.5mm x G2-1.5mm	4.5556	0.9172	2.638	ns
G2-0.5mm x G2-2.5mm	15.4444	3.1097	2.638	< 0.05
G2-0.5mm x G2-3.5mm	24.6667	4.9666	2.638	< 0.05
G2-1.5mm x G2-2.5mm	10.8889	2.1924	2.638	ns
G2-1.5mm x G2-3.5mm	20.1111	4.0493	2.638	< 0.05
G2-2.5mm x G2-3.5mm	9.2222	1.8569	2.638	ns

Table 5. Young's modulus (in GPa). Variations with depth for group G2, for different depth values, XL3000 for distance of 2 mm

After verifying that the results do not follow a normal distribution, Kruskal-Wallis analysis was used to statistically determine the significance of the variation in the obtained data. The test did not indicate significant differences in elastic modulus between the depths of 0.5 and 1.5 mm for the QTH device, not even by increasing the position of the polymerization tip by 1 mm. At each 2 mm in depth a statistically significant variation was observed for the elastic modulus.

Comparisons (Dunn method)	Differences	z calculed	z critical	p
G3-0.5mm x G3-1.5mm	3.7222	0.7495	2.638	ns
G3-0.5mm x G3-2.5mm	10.5556	2.1253	2.638	ns
G3-0.5mm x G3-3.5mm	20.1667	4.0605	2.638	< 0.05
G3-1.5mm x G3-2.5mm	6.8333	1.3759	2.638	ns
G3-1.5mm x G3-3.5mm	16.4444	3.311	2.638	< 0.05
G3-2.5mm x G3-3.5mm	9.6111	1.9352	2.638	ns

Table 6. Young's modulus (in GPa). Variations with depth for group G3, for different depth values, Elipar distance of 1mm

Comparisons (Dunn method)	Differences	z calculed	z critical	p
G4-0.5mm x G4-1.5mm	5.3889	1.085	2.638	ns
G4-0.5mm x G4-2.5mm	10	2.0135	2.638	ns
G4-0.5mm x G4-3.5mm	21.5	4.329	2.638	< 0.05
G4-1.5mm x G4 -2.5mm	4.6111	0.9284	2.638	ns
G4-1.5mm x G4-3.5mm	16.1111	3.2439	2.638	< 0.05
G4-2.5mm x G4-3.5mm	11.5	2.3155	2.638	ns

Table 7. Young's modulus (in GPa). Variations with depth for group G4, for different depth values, Elipar distance of 2 mm

For LED polymerization, the results also failed the normality assumption. Kruskal-Wallis analysis did not indicate statistically significant differences in elastic modulus between the depths of 0.5, 1.5 and 2.5 mm for the LED device, not even by increasing the position of the polymerization tip by 1 mm. As for the comparison between 0.5 mm depth and 3.5, $p<0.05$ was obtained, as well as with the distances of 1.5 and 3.5 mm. The LED device showed an improved polymerization performance at 2.5 mm depth, but results showed that at each 2 mm in depth a statistically significant variation has occurred for the elastic modulus.

The variation in the polymerization device`s tip from the sample did not affect the obtained stiffness results, as shown by a comparison between tables 4 and 5 and 6 and 7.

3.3 Numerical results

The mechanical properties for the resin used in the finite element model were the Young's modulus measured at the four different depths presented on Table 8 and the Poisson's ratio equal to 0.3 throughout the resin model. For the finite element simulation it was used the lowest values measured for the Young's modulus (Group 2 - XL3000, light source at 2 mm distance). In this group it was also verified the highest variations on the Young's modulus with respect to the depth (Tables 3 to 7).

Depth (mm)	Young's Modulus (GPa) for the resin	
	Test results for Group 2 (G2) - XL3000, light source at 2 mm distance	Properties used in the Finite Element simulations
0.5	19.004	19.0
1.5	18.071	18.1
2.5	15.947	15.9
3.5	10.755	10.8

Table 8. Young's modulus used in the finite element model (E) for the resin according to depth

The following figures show the first principal stress (σ_1), in MPa, after the polymerization contraction. Figures 6 to 8 show the simulation results for resin contraction in the three-layers horizontal incremental technique. The first principal stresses (σ_1) representing maximum tension are shown, as all the materials have a reduced strength for traction.

Figure 9 depicts the stress values after filling the restoration in a single step (one layer technique). Then, in Fig. 10, the simulation was repeated keeping the Young's modulus for the resin constant, that is, neglecting the variation due to incomplete polymerization. The results are given for both filling techniques.

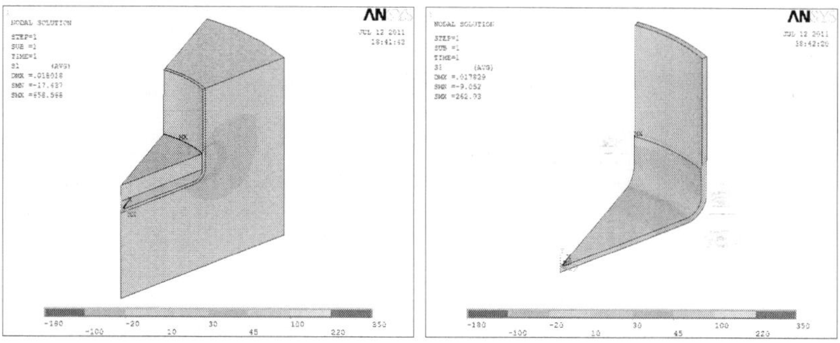

Fig. 6. First principal stresses (σ_1- MPa) for first layer in three-layers horizontal increment technique - restoration on the left and interface on the right

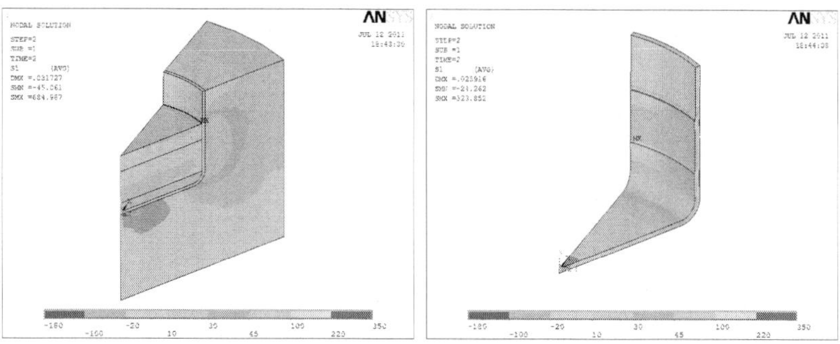

Fig. 7. First principal stresses (σ_1- MPa) for second layer in three-layers horizontal incremental technique - restoration on the left and interface on the right

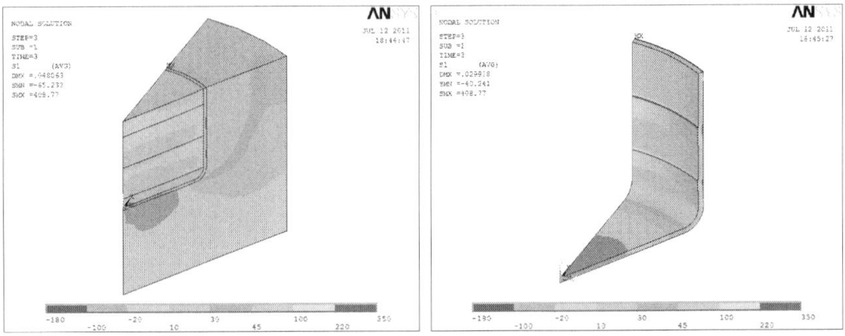

Fig. 8. Final first principal stresses (σ_1- MPa) in three-layers horizontal incremental technique - restoration on the left and interface on the right

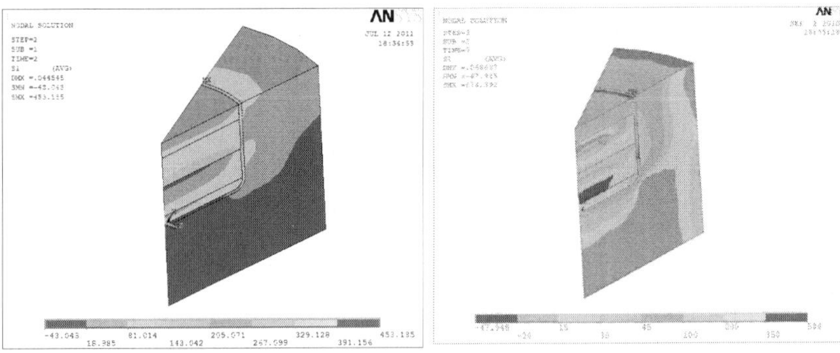

Fig. 9. Final first principal stresses (σ_1- MPa) horizontal incremental technique (2 layers) and one increment (or bulk) filling

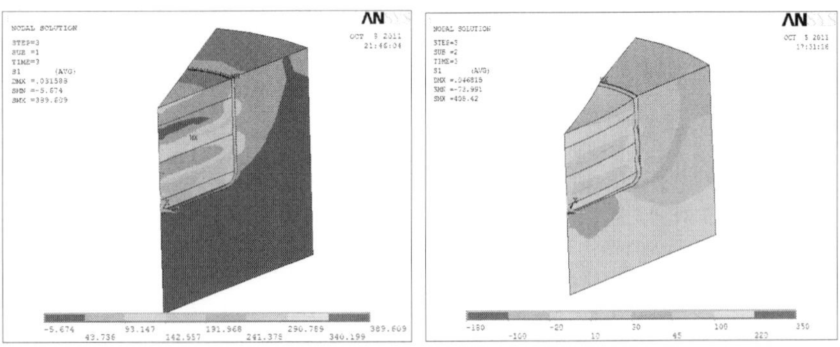

Fig. 10. Final first principal stresses (σ_1- MPa) three and one increment technique with constant E - restoration and dentine

4. Discussion

The study of residual stresses in dental restorations using a finite element simulation tries to reproduce *in silico* a phenomenon frequently observed in dental clinic. By including in the simulation the sequence of cavity filling, the variation in modulus of elasticity resulting from light penetration and the stress relief due to cracking the computational model can represent the process with the inclusion of key aspects of the restoration.

In order to consider the change in properties along the depth of the layers, experimental evaluation of this mechanical property was made, for different light sources and tip positions, as well as for hardness and degree of conversion based on micro-hardness.

Many authors use the degree of conversion associated to harness to verify the effectiveness of the polymerization of composite resins (Kawaguchi et al., 1989; Chung & Greener, 1990). The evaluation of micro-hardness is influenced not only by its degree of conversion, but also by the percentage of filler and presence or absence of oxygen (Peutzfeld, 1997; Yap et al., 2002; Halvorson et al., 2002). As the composite's viscous deformation is a time-dependent event, slower curing rates may provide extended periods where the material is able to yield to contraction forces before acquiring higher elastic modulus (Feilzer et al., 1993). In fact, reducing polymerization rates in composites has been shown to lower stress levels significantly (Bouschlicher & Rueggeberg, 2000; Lim et al., 2002).

There is a direct relationship between the degree of conversion of a resin and its modulus of elasticity. The maximum polymerization of a given resin implies in higher modulus of elasticity and higher contractive stresses in the tooth-resin restoration interface (Davdison-Kaban, 1997). As a consequence, higher mechanical properties for the composite resin results in a corresponding higher value for residual stresses at the adhesive interface (Braem et al., 1987; Silikas et al., 2000).

The degree of conversion was obtained by the Raman method. As for the Young's modulus associated to micro-hardness, the measurements were performed changing the distance from the resin to the tip of the device from 1 to 2 mm. Results showed DC results ranging from 55 and 60% for 2 mm depth, unchanged regardless of the polymerization technique or distance to the tip. For 4 mm depth, DC felt to between 26 and 32% for the two devices, showing a reduction with depth, which can lead to deterioration in its mechanical properties and a reduction in polymerization contraction (Ceballos et al., 2009).

The measurement of the modulus of elasticity showed, for all tested groups, a statistically relevant reduction at each 2 mm depth increase, regardless of the polymerization technology used.

The results obtained for Young's modulus presented a statistically significant reduction for each 2 mm variation in depth, regardless of the curing method. These results reinforce the idea of avoiding to apply layers thicker than 2 mm, which will assure a minimum of non-homogeneity in the material's stiffness, for any restoration volume or configuration factor (Chiang et al., 2010).

According to Dewaele et al. (2009), who investigated different polymerization protocols, the reduction in contraction is directly related to the reduction in the degree of cure. Cho et al. (2011), in an analysis of the particles movement in resin restorations, observed that it depends on the degree of conversion and the contraction value, and that a mathematical equation can be derived for the particles' displacements, especially for those below a 3.5 mm depth.

The computer simulations show a clear stress concentration between the cavity walls and the restoration material, especially in the regions with more abrupt geometry changes corresponding to restoration internal angles, as well as interface rupture at different points of the wall. Stresses are higher at the interface due to the change in stiffness at that point.. These results agree with the conclusions of Chiang et al. (2010), which also verified gap formation in cylindrical restorations with and without the use of an adhesive layer, both numerically and experimentally, through the use of micro-CT images. Their results pointed to higher stresses for adhesives with smaller modulus of elasticity, sometimes higher than the adhesive limit strength.

Most other regions of the restoration stay under stresses lower than 200 MPa. Stress concentration patterns, that is, final stresses after the polymerization process, are dependent of the curing technique. Stress levels indicate that, without subsequent relief, restoration can be easily damaged by additional loading such as temperature variation or biting. During the polymerization process, as the sequence in Figures 6, 7 and 8 shows, stresses redistribute and vary in the different parts of the restoration, reaching intermediate values that can lead to fracture in the interface and damage at the resin. The limit in stresses at the cement provide a buffer for dentine, as very high stresses are not transmitted through the interface layer, that cracks and avoid compromising the tissue.

As for a comparison between the three polymerization techniques, one, two and three increments, it is evident that higher stresses occur for the last option. Figures 8, 9 and 10 show higher peak stresses at dentine and resin for less incremental filling techniques (two and one layer, respectively).

In Figure 9 different filling techniques are explored. First, on the left, instead of three layers, only two 1.5 mm layers were considered. In the right side, bulk or one increment technique was used. In this case, the effect of the variation of Young's modulus with depth is expected to be more important.

In order to examine the influence of the variation in stiffness on the final results, two models were developed with constant resin modulus of elasticity. The results are shown in Fig. 10, both for the complete restoration and for dentine, and show a reduction in stress levels. The real, variable distribution of Young's modulus through depth leads to an increase in stresses in the restoration. This effect is more pronounced for the one increment technique, as expected, as the stiffness variation is larger, and are in agreement with the work of Chiang et al., 2010.

When the influence of the cavity size and incremental restoration technique were analyzed in Class I restorations, it was verified that the adhesive was damaged in several locations, and cracks were occurring in the interface.

He et al. (2007) observed that the size of the restoration and the restoration technique affected its overall behavior. Incremental filling of the cavity reduced the stress levels in large cavities, but did not affect the resulting tractions for small restorations. The authors suggested that incremental technique be used in large restorations with a high C factor.

Sun et al. (2009) noted the occurrence of contraction at the top and base of the restorations, fact also observed in the present finite element simulation. Gaps formation is directly connected to the C factor and volume of composite resin, eventually leading to micro-leakages. The authors concluded that neither C-factor nor sample volume affects polymerization shrinkage at a constant Degree Conversion. They observed in an analysis with a micro-CT that resin contraction occurred independently of the geometry. Using either μCt or infiltration with dyes, if was possible to verify the occurrence of infiltration and its dependence on the C factor and resin volume.

As for Young's modulus and DC values for composite resin, it was expected that a stiffness reduction along the axial direction would lead to a reduction in residual stress levels. This was verified by Oliveira et al. (2010), using resins with low modulus of elasticity. The resulting gaps, even though reduced after hygroscopic expansion, were permanent, being observed even 4 years after treatment (Krämer et al., 2009). The complex behavior of light activated resins and the several parameters involved in its use, as discussed, reinforce the need and importance of further study in the area and the need to consider different aspects in the definition of the clinical restoration procedure (Kakaboura et al., 2007).

5. Concluding remarks

The results described in the previous sections point to the following conclusions:

- The polymerization device, when comparing Elipar and laser-driven devices, used to cure the resin, did not affect significantly the degree of cure (DC) of the examined samples.
- As for the thickness of the sample, for both polymerization devices, the results proved a high correlation between depth and DC value.
- The stiffness of the composite resin was affected by the thickness of the sample. This effect was more pronounced for depths larger than 2 mm
- The numerical analysis showed that layered techniques lead to improved stress distribution and reduced residual stresses in cylindrical restorations.
- The variation in elastic modulus in layers with thickness smaller than 2 mm is not pronounced. As for 3 mm layers, the resulting stress distribution is significantly different when compared with the results for a homogeneous stiffness through restoration thickness.
- The deterioration of the modulus of elasticity in thick layers led to a reduction in stress concentration in the model. Other relevant information, such as reduction in strength, change in contraction and quality of adhesion of the interface should be also investigated for a more complete picture of this case.
- Current recommendations for restricting layer thickness to 2 mm are in accordance with the obtained results.

6. Future directions

The reported results show that a refinement in finite element analysis can deepen the knowledge in the mechanical behavior of resin restorations, providing a tool to improve clinical success. Future work directions should include, among other aspects:

- examine the effect of hygroscopic expansion on the residual stress distribution;
- include inclined layers as an alternative to horizontal layers in the models;
- simulate drop-shaped cavities and restorations;
- study the consequences of the residual stresses and cracks in the performance of the restoration.

7. Acknowledgments

The authors kindly acknowledge the support of the Brazilian funding agencies FAPEMIG and CNPq in the development of this work.

8. References

Ansys Release 10.0.

Ausiello, P.; Apicella, A. & Davidson, C.L. (2002). Effect of adhesive layer properties on stress distribution in composite restorations - a 3D finite element analysis. *Dental Materials,* Vol.18, No.4, pp. 295-303, ISSN 0109-5641

Bouschlicher, M.R. & Rueggeberg, F.A. (2000). Effect of ramped light intensity on polymerization force and conversion in a photoactivated composite. *Journal of Esthetic Dentistry,* Vol.12, No.6, pp. 328-339, ISSN 1040-1466

Bowen R.L.; Nemoto, K. & Rapson, J.E. (1983). Adhesive bonding of various materials to hard tooth tissues: forces developing in composite materials during hardening. *Journal of the American Dental Association,* Vol.106, No.4, pp.475–477, ISSN 0002-8177

Braem, M.; Lambrechts, P.; Vanherle, G. & Davidson, C.L. (1987). Stiffness increase during the setting of dental composite resins. *Journal of Dental Research,* Vol.66, No.12, pp. 1713–1716, ISSN 0022-0345

Braga, R.R.; Ballestera, R.Y. & Ferracane, J.L. (2005). Factors involved in the development of polymerization shrinkage stress in resin-composites: A systematic Review. *Dental Materials,* Vol. 21, pp. 962–970, ISSN 0109-5641

Carvalho Filho, F. (2005). Modelagem via método dos elementos finitos da contração de resinas odontológicas fotopolimerizáveis, M. Sc. thesis, Structural Engineering, Engineering School, Federal University of Minas Gerais, UFMG (in Portuguese)

Ceballos, L.; Fuentes, M.V.; Tafalla, H.; Martínez, A.; Flores, J. & Rodríguez, J. (2009). Curing effectiveness of resin composites at different exposure times using LED and halogen units. *Journal of Clinical and Experimental Dentistry,* Vol.1, No.1, pp. 8-13, ISSN 1989-5488

Chiang, Y.C.; Rösch, P.; Dabanoglu, A.; Linc, C.P.; Hickel, R. & Kunzelmann, K.H. (2010). Polymerization composite shrinkage evaluation with 3D deformation analysis from μCT images. *Dental Materials,* Vol.26, No.3, pp. 223–231, ISSN 0109-5641

Cho, E.; Sadr, A.; Inai, N. & Tagami, J. (2011). Evaluation of resin composite polymerization by three dimensional micro-CT imaging and nanoindentation. *Dental Materials,* Vol.27, No.11, pp. 1070-1078, ISSN 0109-5641

Chung, K.H. & Greener, E.H. (1990). Correlation between degree of conversion filler concentration and mechanical properties of posterior composite resins. *Journal of Oral Rehabilitation,* Vol.17, No.5, pp. 487–494, ISSN 0305-182X

Dewaele, M.; Asmussen, E.; Peutzfeldt, A.; Munksgaard, E.C.; Benetti, A.R.; Finné, G.; Leloup, G. & Devaux, J. (2009). Influence of curing protocol on selected properties of light-curing polymers: degree of conversion, volume contraction, elastic modulus, and glass transition temperature. *Dental Materials*, Vol.25, No.12, pp. 1576-1584, ISSN 0109-5641

Dietschi, D.; Monasevic, M.; Krejci, I. & Davidson, C. (2002). Marginal and internal adaptation of class II restorations after immediate or delayed composite placement. *Journal of Dentistry*, Vol.30, Nos.5-6, pp. 259–269, ISSN 0300-5712

Feilzer, A.J.; De Gee, A.J. & Davidson C.L. (1993). Setting stresses in composites for two different curing modes. *Dental Materials*, Vol.9, No.1, pp. 2–5, ISSN 0109-5641

Felix, C.A.; Price, R.B.T. & Andreou, P. (2006). Effect of reduced exposure times on the microhardness of 10 composites cured by high power LED and QTH curing lights. *Journal of the Canadian Dental Association*, Vol.72, No.2, pp. 147a–147g, ISSN 0008-3372

Ferracane, J.L. (2005). Developing a more complete understanding of stresses produced in dental composites during polymerization. *Dental Materials*, Vol.21, No.1, pp. 36–42, ISSN 0109-5641

Halvorson, R.H.; Erickson, R.L. & Davidson, C. L. (2002). Energy dependent polymerization of resin-based composite. *Dental Materials*, Vol.18, No.6, pp. 463–469, ISSN 0109-5641

He, Z.; Shimada, Y. & Tagami, J. (2007). The effects of cavity size and incremental technique on micro-tensile bond strength of resin composite in Class I cavities. *Dental Materials*, Vol.23, No.5, pp. 533–538, ISSN 0109-5641

Jandt, K.D.; Mills, R.W.; Blackwell, G.B. & Ashworth, S.H. (2000). Depth of cure and compressive strength of dental composites cured with blue light emitting diodes (LEDs). *Dental Materials*, Vol.16, No.1, pp. 41–47, ISSN 0109-5641

Jong, L.C.G.; Opdam, N.J.M.; Bronkhorst, E. M.; Roeters, J.J.M.; Wolke, J.G.C. & Geitenbeek, B. (2007). The effectiveness of different polymerization protocols for class II composite resin restorations. *Journal of Dentistry*, Vol.35, No.6, pp. 513-520, ISSN 0300-5712

Kakaboura, A.; Rahiotis, C.; Watts, D.; Silikas, N. & Eliades, G. (2007). 3D-marginal adaptation versus setting shrinkage in light-cured microhybrid resin composites. *Dental Materials*, Vol.23, No.3, pp. 272–278, ISSN 0109-5641

Kawaguchi, M.; Fukushima, T. & Horibe, T. (1989). Effect of monomer structure on the mechanical properties of light cured composite resins. *Dental Materials Journal*, Vol.8, No.1, pp. 40–45, ISSN 0287-4547

Krämer, N.; Reinelt, C.; Richter, G.; Petschelt, A. & Frankenberger, R. (2009). Nanohybrid vs. fine hybrid composite in Class II cavities: Clinical results and margin analysis after four years. *Dental Materials*, Vol.25, No.6, pp. 750–759, ISSN 0109-5641

Lim, B.-S.; Ferracane, J.L.; Sakaguchi, R.L. & Condon, J.R. (2002). Reduction of polymerization contraction stress for dental composites by two-step light-activation. *Dental Materials*, Vol.18, No.6, pp. 436–444, ISSN 0109-5641

Oliveira, L.C.A.; Duarte Jr., S.; Araujo, C.A. & Abrahão, A. (2010). Effect of low-elastic modulus liner and base as stress-absorbing layer in composite resin restorations. *Dental Materials*, Vol.26, No.3, pp. e159–e169, ISSN 0109-5641

Petrovic, L.M.; Drobac, M.R.; Stojanac, I.L. & Atanackovic, T.M. (2010). A method of improving marginal adaptation by elimination of singular stress point in composite restorations during resin photo-polymerization. *Dental Materials;* Vol.26, No.5, pp. 449–455, ISSN 0109-5641

Peutzfeld, A. (1997). Resin composites in dentistry: The monomer systems. *European Journal of Oral Sciences,* Vol.105, No.2, pp. 97–116, ISSN 1600-0722

Peutzfeldt, A.; Sahafi, A. & Asmussen, E. (2000). Characterization of resin composites polymerized with plasma arc curing units. *Dental Materials,* Vol.16, No.5, pp. 330–336, ISSN 0109-5641

Rüttermann, S.; Krüger, S.; Raab, W. & Janda, R. (2007). Polymerization shrinkage and hygroscopic expansion of contemporary posterior resin-based filling materials—A comparative study. *Journal of Dentistry,* Vol. 35, No.10, pp. 806-813, ISSN 0300-5712

Sakaguchi, R. L.; Sasik, C. T.; Bunczak, M.A. & Douglas, W.H. (1991). Strain gauge method for measuring polymerization contraction of resin composite restoratives. *Journal of Dentistry,* Vol.19, No.5, pp. 312–316, ISSN 0300-5712

Silikas, N.; Eliades, G. & Watts, D.C. (2000). Light intensity effects on resin-composite degree of conversion and shrinkage strain. *Dental Materials,* Vol.16, No.4, pp. 292–296, ISSN 0109-5641

Sun, J.; Eidelman, N. & Gibson, S.L. (2009). 3D mapping of polymerization shrinkage using X-ray micro-computed tomography to predict microleakage. *Dental Materials,* Vol.25, No.3, pp. 314–320, ISSN 0109-5641

Yap, A.U.; Soh M.S. & Siow, K. S (2002). Effectiveness of composite cure with pulse activation and soft-start polymerization. *Operative Dentistry,* Vol.27, No.1, pp. 44–49, ISSN 0361-7734

Yoshikawa, T.; Burrow, M.F. & Tagami, J. (2001). A light curing method for improving marginal sealing and cavity wall adaptation of resin composite restorations. *Dental Materials,* Vol.17, No,4, pp. 359-366, ISSN 0109-5641

26

Genetic Engineering in a Computer Science Curriculum

Nevena Ackovska[1], Liljana Bozinovska[2] and Stevo Bozinovski[2]
[1]*University Sts Cyril and Methodius, Institute of Informatics,*
[2]*South Carolina State University,*
[1]*Macedonia*
[2]*USA*

1. Introduction

Traditionally genetic engineering is understood as a molecular biology discipline. The tools used in molecular biology are specific, mostly used by people who come from biological or medical background, which made the discipline distant from classical Computer Science. In this paper we would like to address computer science auditorium and point out the importance of understanding genetic engineering.

Although the term "genetic engineering" was coined 1951 in a science fiction novel by Williamson (reprinted in (Williamson, 2002)), it was not until 1970s when the first achievements in DNA modification showed that genetic engineering is actually happening. As in all of the sciences, genetic engineering has its own milestones. In this introductory part we will describe the earliest genetic engineering achievements, using computer science terminology.

Through the prism of computer science terms, the best way to look at DNA is that it represents a string of letters, written in four letter alphabet. The string might be interpreted as a text subject to processes such as transcription and translation (Watson & Crick, 1953), or as database and software for processes in a cell (Bozinovski and Bozinovska, 1987; Bozinovski et al., 2000). The first genetic engineering achievement was the *cut-and-paste* operation of a DNA segment. Using two types of enzymes, restriction enzymes for cut operation, and DNA ligase for join operation, a segment from one DNA was cut and pasted in another DNA. Actually, the achievement was greater, since the DNA of two living forms, the bacterial phage lambda and monkey virus SV40, were (re)combined into a new DNA (Jackson et al., 1972). The second achievement, in 1973, was *prepare-and-copy* operation. A DNA fragment was inserted in a plasmid (pSC101) and put into a bacterium (Escherichia coli) and was replicated inside the bacterium. This experiment has another important point: a fragment was prepared outside a cell (in vitro) and was replicated inside a cell (in vivo). The cell machinery processed (replicated) the foreign piece of software as its own. That was the first step or cell (re)programming. In 1974 the first transgenic animal was created, by inserting a foreign DNA into a mouse embryo. In 1977 and 1978 the first human proteins (somatostatin and insulin) were produced inside a bacterium. Bacteria produced human insulin become commercially available in 1982 opening market for various types of genetically engineered products, making genetic engineering a new industry. Important achievement happened in 2010 by which a complete synthesized genome was introduced into a bacterial cell which had no DNA (Gibson et al., 2010). Therefore, a new life form was created with complete software prepared outside the cell. The bacterium was named Synthia and is the first synthetic life form. All of these examples and many more, represent the milestones that the science and technology of genetic engineering have already made possible for humans to use.

As computer engineers, it is our view that genetic engineering is a type of (software) engineering, and the way of doing genetic engineering is a way of programming and reprogramming a DNA. As today many computer science curricula contain a bioinformatics course, we argue that Computer Science curriculum should contain courses in genetic engineering as well. Since Computer science in part is about programming, genetic reprogramming can be viewed as important part of the Computer Science education. We will also present our experience in teaching genetic engineering to computer science students.

In this paper we will first describe natural way of doing genetic engineering. That is the way the Nature was doing genetic engineering long before it became known to humans. Then, we will describe a metaphor that can be used in education of Computer Science students. Afterwards we will describe our approach to introducing genetic engineering into Computer Science curriculum, including also lab exercises.

This paper addresses mainly the computer science auditorium. We present some elementary knowledge in molecular biology, but the concepts are presented through (computer) engineering terms. However, the notion presented here might be of interest for other scientists coming from biological sciences background.

2. Genetic engineering before Genetic Engineering

Genetic engineering, by human definition, is a process of human produced genotypic effect in order to obtain some phenotypic effects. Phenotypic effects can be at molecular level, such as production of a new protein, or at higher level, producing visible effect either in the structure or in the behavior of an organism. Usually, it is achieved by planned DNA alternation, in order to (re)program behavior of a cell or a multicellular organism.

The nature has been doing genetic engineering for a very long time. Some of the life forms on the Earth survive using sort of "genetic engineering". The question we will start our presentation here is how we can help Computer Science students to understand the concept of Genetic Engineering? We believe that the following story of phage lambda is an inspirational approach toward understanding genetic engineering for computer science students and professionals alike, if we can level the terminology used in classical Genetic engineering to Computer Science. As we have stated before, the way the story is been transferred to Computer Science students enables them to understand the life cycle of phage lambda. The simplicity and the clarity of the terminology seem to be of high importance in order for these students to understand complex biological processes. Even more, the story explains one way of genetic engineering done by the Nature itself.

"Consider a life form, a bacterium named Escherichia coli. It is a prokaryote, it does not have a nucleus inside the cell. It is a life form that is capable of self reproduction. We call it a single cell organism. Its chromosome is a circular one. Every twenty minutes it replicates itself, provided there are favorable conditions in the environment. The new bacterium is pretty much the copy of the previous one.

Now consider another life form, namely phage λ (lambda). It is a life form which cannot reproduce itself. So, the phage lambda needs a host organism to reproduce and E. coli is such a host. A phage (or bacteriophage) is a virus to a bacterium: it can replicate inside a bacterium and eventually destroy it. It is interesting that a phage is harmless to human cells and to all other eukaryotic cells (cell that do have a nucleus).

The phage lambda is a life form with head-and-tail appearance. The head contains the DNA as a single chromosome. The phage DNA is double stranded. It contains the phage genome, i.e. the set of all phage genes. The tail is used to insert the DNA into a bacterial cell. Once inside a bacterium, the phage chromosome exhibits two possible behaviors: lysogenic and lytic. Lysogenic behavior occurs if the phage chromosome remains its linear form. It then integrates into the bacterial chromosome and becomes segment of that chromosome. When bacterium replicates its chromosome, the phage segment is also replicated. However, under some condition, such as environment stress, linear phage chromosome leaves the bacterium chromosome, and exhibits lytic behavior. It is not necessary that a phage has a lysogenic behavior; it might start its lytic behavior immediately after entering a bacterial cell. The lytic behavior starts with transforming the linear phage chromosome into a circular one. That is preprogrammed into the sticky ends of both side of the linear chromosome. The site of sticking the both strands together is named a cos site. Once into its circular form phage chromosome replicates inside bacterium and creates new phage life forms. Eventually bacterium explodes releasing phages into the environment outside the bacterium.

Since the replication inside a bacterium is lethal for the bacterium, a simple immune system was designed in bacterial evolution: restriction enzymes. Restriction enzymes (or endonucleases) are enzymes able to recognize a foreign DNA and cut it, rendering it non reproducible. Restriction enzymes are probably the first form of immune system in organisms."

The story of phage lambda seems to be very simple. However, it explains one of the Nature's life cycles in a simplified manner, understandable for engineering students. From the above example the students can learn about three mechanisms how a bacterial genome can be modified:

1. by incorporating a linear DNA segment into the bacterial chromosome,
2. by adding a separate circular chromosome into the bacterium and creating a two-chromosome system inside the bacterium,
3. by producing environment stress that would activate some genetic response of inserted DNA segments.

In the following section we elaborate on other terminology modification in order to explain processes and actors in genetic engineering to (computer) engineers.

3. Leveling the terminology: Metaphors for understanding genetics

For computer science, genetic engineering and cell (re)programming can be viewed as kind of software engineering. A software sequence is written, and then inserted into genetic machinery for compilation and execution. Now, if we "translate" the biological processes into terminology that computer science students understand, we obtain greater results and better understanding of these rather complicated processes. In the sequel we will consider some metaphors that can be used in teaching computer science students concepts of genetic engineering.

A metaphor is understood as a paradigm transformation; using knowledge from a familiar system in order to understand the phenomena in another system. The first metaphor explaining genetic processes was the biochemistry metaphor, which basically relied on the fact that DNA is an acid. Obviously the acid metaphor was not good enough to explain the life processes; the fact that the DNA is an acid cannot explain information that is stored into a DNA. Another metaphor proposed in 1953 (Watson & Crick, 1953) stated that the DNA is a sequence of letters, actually a text where information is stored. Today it is a dominant metaphor. The principal processes named transcription and translation (Crick, 1958) are linguistic, text processing terms. In 1985 the relation between genetic engineering and robotics was pointed out (Bozinovski, 1985). An observation that DNA is actually a database was first made in 1987 (Bozinovski, 1987; Bozinovski & Bozinovska, 1987; Demeester et al. 2004; Pirim, 2005). Afterwards, new metaphor for genetic engineering was proposed, the robotics and flexible manufacturing metaphor, which proposed a viewpoint that the cell is a flexible manufacturing system. According to that metaphor, some molecular structures should be viewed as cell robots, an example being the tRNA, which is a transporting robot. Related to the flexible manufacturing metaphor is the systems software metaphor (Bozinovski et al. 2000; Bozinovski et al 2001; Danchin & Noria 2004, Ackovska & Bozinovski, 2008; Ackovska et al. 2008).

The latest metaphor is very comprehendible for computer science and computer engineering students. It uses the concept of a genetic file as a logical segment on DNA. In the cell processes related to manufacturing (e.g. protein biosynthesis) the genetic files are considered existing and read-only. In this paper we are focused on files that can be altered, such as updated, created, written, inserted into another files, and otherwise manipulated. This also happens in nature, but more importantly, it is a basis of genetic engineering. In the following section we address the issue of writing in genetic files, and creating genetic file systems and genetic disks.

4. Genetic files, disks, and genetic file systems

When studying genetics engineering and genetics in general, the crucial concept is the concept of gene. Thus, a very natural question is "What is a gene?" A usual answer is that a gene is a segment of a DNA that encodes for either protein or RNA. Also, one could encounter slightly different definitions (Brown, 2002).

In computer science and engineering a usual reasoning on an information processing system considers the files of that system. So, for genetic information processing we might ask the question "what are the files of the genetic information processing system?" Is the concept of a gene corresponding to the concept of a file? Having that as a starting point, in this section we will present our understanding of DNA organization and DNA computing in terms of files and related concepts.

Looking for a concept of a file in DNA, we found that the transcription units (or scriptons (Ratner, 1975)) are analogous to cell files. A transcription unit is a segment of DNA that eventually becomes transcribed to RNA. In prokaryotes, a transcription unit often produces a transcript with several genes (so-called polycistronic RNA). In eukaryotes it produces a precursor RNA (pre-RNA), which contains the information about a single gene, but in order to obtain it, additional processing needs to be performed.

The eukaryotic files are rather complex and contain segments of a gene, interleaved with segments that do not belong to the gene. Those segments are known as introns, as opposite to exons (gene expressing segments). To the people involved with genetics, there is a standard question considering this phenomenon: how did it happen that eukaryotic genes became segmented? However, for computer engineers introduced to the concept of a file, the answer is straightforward - busy files are fragmented. Defragmentation is sometimes needed in computer file systems. Moreover, it is expected that between two fragments of a file an entire different file could be expected. This fact points to the concept of distributed file systems (Nutt, 1992; Tanenbaum, 1994; Tanenbaum & Van Steen, 2007). And indeed, this is the case in molecular genetics: After the first evidence that Tetrahymena ribozyme is actually an intron (Kruger et al., 1982), more evidence has been found that genetic files could be found within a complete different file (Been, 2006).

The cell files contain genes and other important sequences. Some files are executable ones, they will produce cell robots. Cell robots are either enzymes (protein based) or ribozymes (RNA based enzymes). Besides genes, which contain program files, the file system contains files that are not genes; they are data structures, some of which can be used as template for pattern recognition.

We believe that while the genes are the proper concept when talking about heredity, the concept of a file is very useful in describing the DNA transcription process. This makes the first step in the analogy between the computer systems and genetic systems. The cell, especially the eukaryotic cell, undergoes extensive file processing: from copying the pre-RNA file until obtaining the RNA message. This process includes operations like: cut (introns), join (exons), right append (trailer string), left append (header string), letter replacement and so on, which are standard file processing operations in every modern computer operating system (Bozinovski et al., 2001).

Under genetic disk (or cell disk) we understand a cell chromosome. For example, human genome is a distributed file system that resides on 46 (or 23 pairs) disks in each cell. There are exceptions, for example gonad cells have only 23 cell disks. In some organisms besides main genomic system there is a satellite chromosome system. An example is the bacterium E. coli which contains its chromosome, but it can also contain satellite chromosomes from life forms such as phages and plasmids. So, under the concept of genetic disk we include both main, cell-replicating chromosomes, as well as the satellite, independently replicating chromosomes, such as plasmid chromosomes or phage chromosomes. Examples of satellite chromosomes in eukaryotic cells are mitochondria DNA.

We define disk segment as a set of files that will be written on a genetic disk. Under the genetic file system we understand ordered set of genetic files. Usually, genetic disks contain files in strict order. Our approach understands genome (set of all genes in a life form) as part of the cell file system.

Therefore, this approach toward genetic engineering starts with understanding that the DNA is cell operating system which resides on cell disks (chromosomes). Set of chromosomes can be viewed as an array of genetic disks.

In the sequel we will often use the terminology of genetic disks and disk segments to refer to a chromosome or DNA sequence. Here we will first describe the phage lambda and its genetic disk. The DNA of phage lambda is double stranded and circular one. A double stranded DNA allows storing gens on both strands, so that gens can be copied and processed by reading them on both sides, in opposite directions. Figure 1 describes behaviour of a phage DNA in a cell of bacterium E. coli.

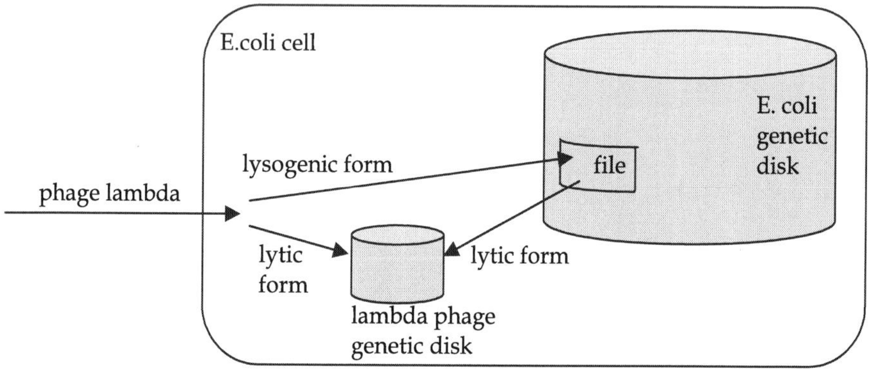

Fig. 1. Phage lambda DNA enters into an E. coli bacterium. The lambda DNA either becomes a file into the bacterium system disk or becomes own system disk.

Figure 1 shows two forms of existence of phage lambda DNA in a bacterium E. coli. It may integrate, as a disk segment (its linear form) into the E.coli DNA disk (lysogenic existence). However, it may encircle (its circular form) and form its own system disk (lytic existence). Once becoming a system disk, it replicates and forms new phages.

The phage lambda genetic disk is a file system that contains set of genes (genome) that can be divided into functional groups. According to the systems software metaphor the genes are viewed as source program files that are compiled into proteins. The phage genetic disk also contains two data files and they are not compiled.

5. Education of computer science students in genetic engineering

Contemporary education of computer science students is often related through molecular genetic through various forms of Bioinformatics courses. Bioinformatics is about genetic sequences that are stored on databases, usually available on the World Wide Web. Many institutions offer digital encyclopedias related to molecular biology. Many applications are built for using the knowledge stored in databases, such as searching various forms of similarities among genetic sequences and predicting genes in a genetic sequence (Xiong, 2006). The goal of post genome informatics (Kanehisa, 2000) is to understand the information in genetic sequences, including function of all the genes and other functional sentences. At this point, Genetic Engineering is usually not part of bioinformatics courses.

We propose that genetic engineering should be included in Computer Science curriculum. One way of doing that is through the existing bioinformatics related courses. Example is the elective undergraduate course CS495 Biocomputing and Bioinformatics which is part of the Computer Science curriculum of the South Carolina State University, or the courses Intelligent Systems (Madevska-Bogdanova & Ackovska, 2009), DNA Programming and Bioinformatics at the Institute of Informatics, University Sts Cyril and Methodius. The other approach is introducing a separate course.

In genetic engineering related course students will be able to learn programming life forms. So far, they are capable of programming robots through various type of robotics courses contemporary found in Computer Science curricula. However, Genetic engineering is a way of designing, writing, and executing programs for living beings: it is about designing new genes and genomes and consequently, their phenotypes. Therefore it is interesting for the students to learn how to program DNA in order to design life form robots.

The core of genetic engineering is creation of a file or set of files that will be written on a genetic disk. There are several ways how to obtain a genetic file. Examples are: 1) cut a file or segment from existing disk (using restriction enzymes), 2) copy a file from existing disk (copy on mRNA and then synthesize complementary DNA, cDNA), and 3) synthesize a human made (artificial) file or segment.

In this section we will be focused on genetic disk segments, and genetic tools as ways of creating genetic source programs that would be executed by the cell. We shall explain the way we represent the theoretical knowledge, including restriction enzymes, engineered genetics disks, artificial chromosomes and the process of transferring the source genes into host systems and creating genomic libraries.

5.1 Theoretical knowledge

When creating a curriculum it is always a question which topics should be primarily covered. When designing an interdisciplinary course, such as Genetics Engineering for Computer science students, it is even more difficult to make such a decision. It would depend on how much time or space the instructor has available for the course. The course can be separate, usually graduate course, for example on Physiology Engineering (Bozinovski and Bozinovska, 2011), or it can a part of an undergraduate course, for example on Bioinformatics. In any case, organization of genetic files, genetic disks, and related operating systems and robotics metaphors for understanding genetics is a good introduction to the subject. Other topics might include: sequencing, amplification, modifying enzymes, cloning, screening, applications, and state of the art. A good textbook might be Nichol's book (Nicholl, 2008).

5.1.1 A tool for genetic engineering: restriction enzymes

One of most used DNA modifying enzymes are restriction enzymes. They are tools for cutting a DNA string. Restriction enzymes, also known as endonucleases, are DNA cutting bionanorobots.

Restriction enzymes are naturally used by bacteria which use them as a natural defense mechanism to cut an invading phage DNA. Many bacterial restriction enzymes have been found and they are named according to the bacteria they are isolated from and the order (first, second, third etc.) in which they are isolated. For example EcoRI means first isolated restriction enzyme from *Esherichia coli*, HindIII means the third isolated restriction enzyme from bacteria *Haemophilus influenzae*, and PstI means the first restriction enzyme extracted from *Providencia stuartii.*

Genetic engineering relies upon ability to cleave (cut, splice) and ligate (paste) a functional piece of DNA predictably and precisely. Example is cutting a gene from a DNA. One should look for restriction sites on both sides of the gene and then use specific restriction enzymes that will cut at the observed restriction sites. As a result a DNA fragment (genetic disk segment) is obtained, which contains the gene of interest. That fragment should be inserted into another, recipient DNA. The same restriction enzymes are also used to cut the recipient DNA into which the fragment will be inserted. This cut-and-paste operation is one of the ways of engineering a genetic disk.

Each restriction enzyme recognizes a specific nucleotide sequence in the DNA, called a restriction site, and cuts the DNA molecule at only that specific sequence. Many restriction enzymes leave a short length of unpaired bases, called a "sticky" end, at the DNA site where they cut. Other restriction enzymes make a cut across both strands creating double-stranded DNA fragments with "blunt" ends. In general, restriction sites are palindromic, meaning the sequence of bases reads the same forwards as it does backwards on the opposite DNA strand. Example of a palindromic restriction site recognized by restriction enzyme HindIII is given in Figure 2. As Figure 2 shows, HindIII cuts the DNA at last letters of the palindrome and leaves two one-stranded ends of DNA, named sticky ends.

```
5'-N-N-N-A-A-G-C-T-T-N-N-N-N-
3'-N-N-N-T-T-C-G-A A-N-N-N-N-
```

Fig. 2. A two strand palindromic string in a DNA. This particular one is recognized by a HindIII restriction enzyme. Arrows show the cut sites, leaving sticky ends at the cut.

A DNA in presence of particular restriction enzymes will be cut at all the corresponding restriction sites. For example, HindIII restriction enzymes will cut the lambda phage chromosome into 8 segments (or fragments).

5.1.2 Engineered source disks

A genetic program is a file written on a genetic disk that contains a code for specific function in a cell. The program can be created and written by a human, which is essence of cell (re) programming. The written program is called source program, and the disk the program is written on is named source disk. A source disk is usually prepared outside a target organism. There are basically two types of source disks: engineered genetic compact disks and artificial chromosome disks.

A) Engineered Genetic Compact Disk. Engineered compact disk is based either on a plasmid or a phage. Usually a natural plasmid (or phage) is loaded with an engineered DNA sequence.

For computer engineers, it can be viewed as a rather small capacity disk media such as compact disk (CD). A cell can be viewed as a computer system that also contains a separate disk replicator, so that a particular CD can be replicated by the cell information processing system. A plasmid and phage can be inserted in a cell using natural way: just put a cell and plasmids into a favorable environment, and a plasmid (or phage) will enter the cell.

A typical example is the engineered plasmid pBR322, which is used for transferring a particular disk segment into bacterium E. coli. Plasmid pBR322 was engineered out of three natural E. coli plasmids: R1 plasmid, containing amp^R gene, which provides resistance to ampicillin, R6-5 plasmid, containing tet^R gene which provides resistance to tetracycline, and pMB1 plasmid, containing replication origin (ori) segment. There is an ori part in a genetic disk which makes the disk replicable. There are specific spots on the pBR322 where restriction enzymes such as EcoRI, SalI, PstI, Pvuil, and HindIII can make the disk open for inserting a file. After insertion of the disk segment, the plasmid disk has extended its used disk space. Plasmid pBR322 has capacity of accepting disk segments of about 10 Kbp (Brown, 2001).

B) Artificial chromosome. Artificial chromosome is an engineered genetic disk which has organization of a natural chromosome, but is much shorter. An example of artificial chromosome is the Yeast artificial chromosome (YAC). Figure 3 shows a procedure of insertion of a DNA fragment into a Yeast artificial chromosome.

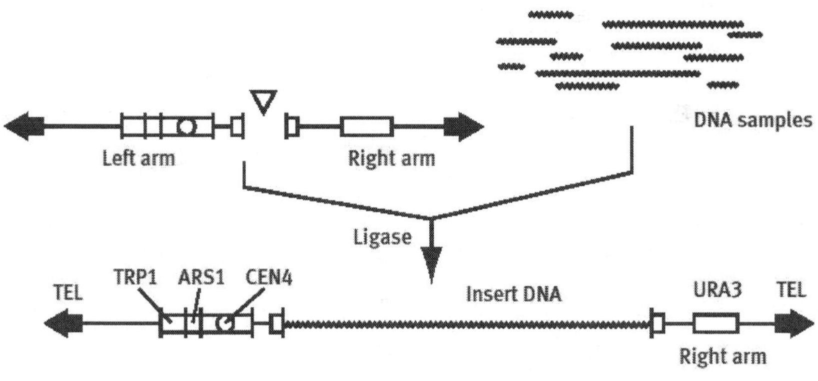

Fig. 3. File insertion into a Yeast artificial chromosome

Figure 3 shows how a DNA fragment is inserted into an artificial chromosome in order to be transferred into a cell. A chromosome of a eukaryote (yeast is a one-cell eukaryote) contains specific DNA part such as telomeric DNA (TEL1), replication origin (ori), replication sequences (ARS1), and centromeric DNA (CEN4). Centromeric DNA enables segregation of the DNA at the time of cell division. Selectable markers are genes that allow distinguishing cells that have this artificial chromosome. For example, for the pYAC2 chromosome, the genes are: amp^R, ura3, and trpI. Artificial chromosomes possess important property, they do not transfer files into the main, cell replicating disk(s) of the cell. Instead they remain as a separate disk, in addition to the cell chromosome disks. The inserted DNA is possibly an engineered one, which acts as part of the chromosome system of the cell where the artificial chromosome is inserted.

There are several types of artificial chromosomes. One is the Bacterial Artificial Chromosome (BAC), which is based on plasmid F and can accept segments between 80-300Kbp. The Yeast Artificial Chromosome (YAC) is often used for transferring files into yeast (Burke et al, 1987). A YAC is able to accept disk segments of Mbp size. Mammalian artificial chromosomes (MAC) (Grimes & Cooke, 1998) as well as Human Artificial Chromosomes (HAC) (Larin & Mejia , 2002) were also engineered. Recently a plant artificial chromosome with length of 30 Mbp was reported (Ananiev et al, 2009).

5.1.3 Transferring source disks into cell file systems

Engineered genetic compact disks are plasmids (or phages). They are transferred into a cell by simply mixing cells and plasmids under favorable conditions; the plasmids will enter the cells. In genetic engineering those source disks are named vectors, pointing out their inherent transferring ability.

There is no natural way of inserting a rather large artificial chromosome into a cell. Usual procedure is electroporation (Rebersek & Miklavcic, 2011), by which the artificial chromosome is forced into a cell as a high energy particle. Once inside a cell, an artificial chromosome behaves in principle like other cell chromosomes; it just has much less files than the natural chromosomes.

5.1.4 Arrays of genetic disks: Genomic libraries

Genetic engineering can create new life forms or modify existing life forms. Example of modified life forms are so called transgenic organisms, which in their genome contain genes from another organism. For example, it is possible to include a gene of a human in a bacterium.

There are other applications that are more oriented toward file systems rather than the primary intention of modifying an existing mechanism. One such application is creating an array of genetic disks to store a particular genome. Figure 4 (Ackovska et al., 2010) shows creation of a human genomic library. The human genome (all human genes) are kept into array of transgenic disks, each disk is a bacterial genome in which a human gene is inserted.

In humans there are 23 pairs of disks on which the cell operating system resides. They are marked F1-F22 and M1-M22 on Figure 4, pointing out that F23 disk represents the X chromosome and M23 disk represents the Y chromosome. The capacity of those disks is between 50 and 230 Mbp. The density of files on disks is low, only about 5% of the entire DNA contains genes. The other parts are control sequences, data structures, and also areas which, by today's knowledge, contain no meaningful information. Some of human cell files are longer than 100 Kbp, so BAC disks are used (Osoegawa et al., 2001). In such a case, about 30,000 disks, which means 30,000 bacteria are needed to store the human genome.

The obtained set of files contains the whole genome, but is not the true representative of the cell file system and cell operating system, as it is in the original 23 pairs of disks. However, a transgenic disk array allows access to a particular segment and set of files faster and in a way more convenient for study. So called arrayed genomic libraries, arranged as a matrix, are built for easier access of a particular segment.

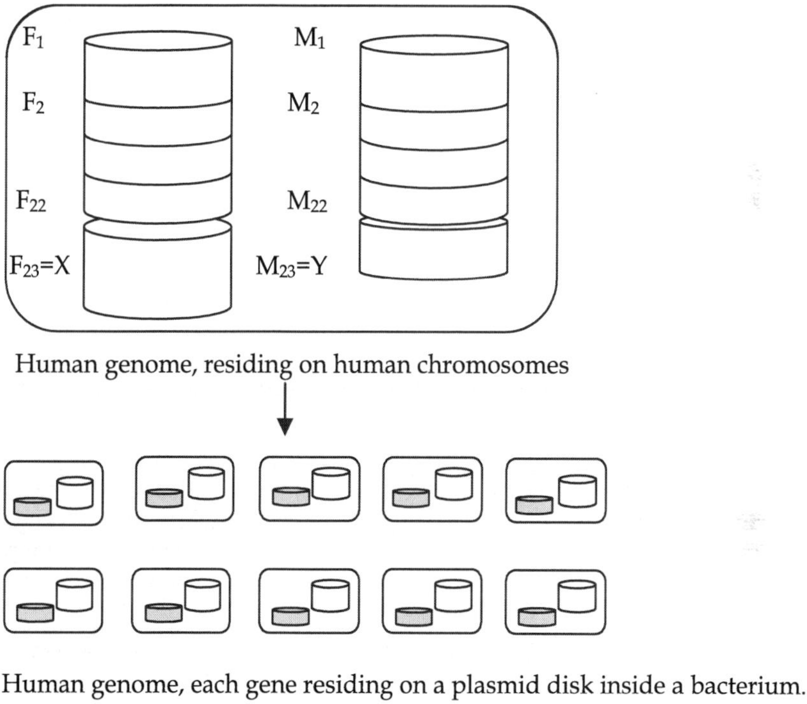

Fig. 4. Creating genomic library on a transgenic disks array

5.2 A lab experience in genetic engineering for computer science students

In addition to knowledge to be conveyed to students as lectures, lab experience is important part of every course. Working in labs with tools for genetic engineering is very different from the everyday practice for computer science students. If one is going to expose computer science students to work in a genetic lab, there are basically two ways of doing that: 1) lab work is carried out in a computer science lab, or similar, in which limited number of equipment and tools for genetic engineering can be installed; 2) lab work is carried out in a specialized lab, for example a molecular biology lab, which already has all the genetic engineering equipment and tools. The tools for genetic engineering include instruments such as water baths, dry baths, centrifuges, incubation ovens, spectrophotometers, electrophoresis chambers, polymerase chain reactors, and electroporators, among others. The lab activities can be carried out as regular lab activities inside a Computer Science course, such as Bioinformatics course. Another way of carrying out genetic engineering labs is an extracurricular activity, for example activity funded by a research project. In short, here we describe two lab exercises and the way to organize this specific lab practice so it can become closer to Computer science students.

5.2.1 Lab example 1: Extracting DNA from human saliva cells

First, we will describe a lab activity that does not require many specialized devices, and as such this activity can be carried out inside a computer lab. As introduction to this lab activity one should mention that, DNA is most important molecule for life. It carries hereditary information and also manages production of proteins and manages processes in a cell. Human genome is organized in linear chromosomes, and somatic cells such a saliva cells have 46 chromosomes. The total length of all chromosomes is about 2 m. However, DNA is invisible, it is a nanostructure, and its total width is 2 nm.

Understanding and working with DNA is one crucial educational task in hands-on lab experience for a Computer Science student. A DNA sample can be obtained from human blood, such as in medicine or in forensics. In lab practices for Computer Science obtaining DNA sample from human saliva is preferable approach. Therefore, in this lab task a computer science student will be able to extract her/his own DNA from her/his saliva.

The important part of "hardware" needed for this exercise, not usually used by CS students, is an incubator, for example an incubation oven, which can keep a temperature of 50°C for some time. There are devices such as water bath, that keeps water on that temperature, and students insert their lab tubs into that water for some time. The simplest approach is to take any heating source, take a thermometer, heat the water until thermometer shows around the desired temperature, and put the lab tubes in such water for needed time. If conditions allow, a water bath might be purchased. However, a lab kit that contains necessary tools, such as enzymes, tubes etc, should be purchased. There are many vendors of these types of kits, one example is BioRad.

The detailed explanation of the lab activity for extraction a human DNA from human saliva cells is given in Figure 5. It shows detailed flow of the processing of the tube in which the saliva is placed up until the DNA is visible in the same tube. It is not necessary to give the students task in detailed terms. As the reader may notice, the explanation written for CS students differs significantly than the explanation found in lab manuals for biology or medical students. Computer science students are accustomed to process thinking. Given below is a description of the task.

Step 1. **Collect cells.** You can collect thousand of cells from the inside of your mouth just by gently chewing your cheeks and rinsing your mouth with water.

Step 2. **Break open (lyse) the cells.** Use provided *lysis buffer*. It will break open the cell membrane and nucleus membrane and release DNA.

Step 3. **Remove proteins.** Use provided enzymes named *proteases*. They will remove all the proteins in your solution along with proteins that keep DNA as a thread. Proteases work best at 50°C. So you incubate (in a water bath previously warmed up to 50°C) your solution together with enzymes to that temperature.

Step 4. **Condense DNA, make it visible.** Use salt and cold alcohol. It will precipate DNA out of the solution, and you can see it as a mass of white threads.

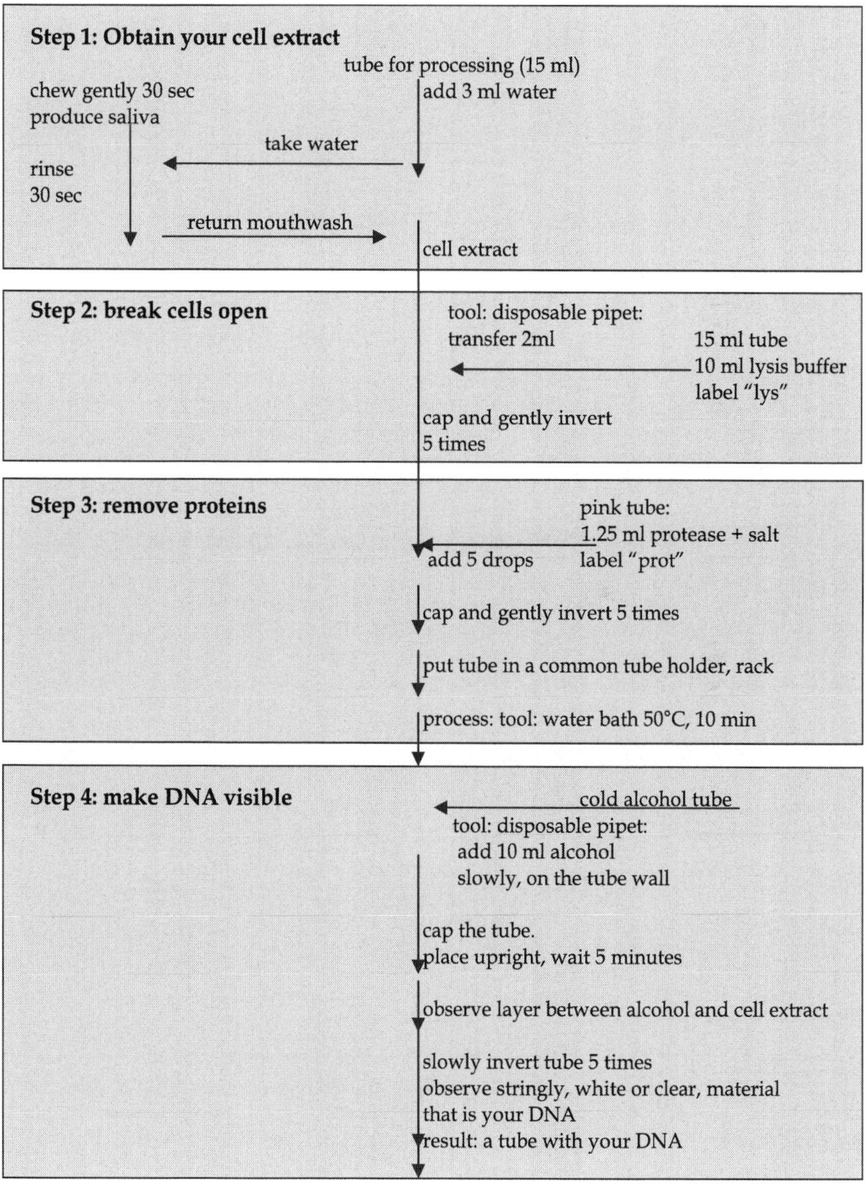

Fig. 5. Lab procedure for extracting DNA from human saliva cells

5.2.2 Organization of a lab for computer science students

Organization of the laboratory is important for any lab activity. It is especially important for computer science students working with tools such as lab tubes and pipets, which are not part of their regular computer science lab activity.

A workstation should be prepared, which can be for one student or shared by more than one student. Each student has her/his processing tube, in which she/he puts the saliva and then processes it using the provided tools such as lysis buffer and protease enzymes. The equipment, such as Water Bath, is shared by all the students. All the processing tubes are put in a rack and then placed in the Water Bath for incubation. Some tools needed for processing are kept in the refrigerator, such as alcohol. This part is very different form everything the Computer Science students are accustomed to.

5.2.3 Lab example 2: Finding shortest file segment obtained by a restriction enzyme

Here we describe a lab that introduces hands-on experience with restriction enzymes to computer science students. For Computer Science students the easiest way to understand restriction enzymes is that they are type of cell robots that are able to cut DNA at a particular point. In this lab exercise the fragments are obtained from a DNA and their length is estimated. This exercise uses a classical lab technique named agarose gel electrophoresis to estimate length of a particular DNA fragment. Since specialized equipment, electrophoresis chamber, is used, this activity might be easier if carried out in a biology lab.

The task description is as follows: DNA of a phage lambda is given. Also, given are three restriction enzymes: EcoRI, PsfI, and HindIII. Cut the lambda DNA with each enzyme. Determine which restriction enzyme will obtain DNA fragments with minimum length.

The lab procedure is performed in parallel on four processing tubes. One tube is lambda DNA, the second is lambda+EcoRI, the third is lambda+HindIII, the forth is lambda+PstI. They are centrifuged and then put into an incubator with temperature that is best for enzymes. The enzymes cut the DNA into number of fragments.

The following is more elaborated description of the lab procedure for obtaining fragments of the phage lambda genome processed by various restriction enzymes:

Step 1. Obtain DNA fragments

Put restriction enzymes into three tubes with DNA, the fourth is just DNA. Mix the tubes, possibly in a centrifuge, heat the tubes at 37°C for 30 min, possibly in a water bath. Result: each tube contains fragmented DNA.

Step 2. Distinguish fragments by their lengths

Put marker dye into tubes, mix, possibly with centrifuge, prepare agarose gel wells, put the tube content into the gel wells, and perform electrophoresis at 100V for 30 min. Result: The resulting gel contains information how far in the electrical field the fragments travelled. However, the result is not visible for human eyes.

Step 3. Visualize DNA fragments

Put colouring marker on the gel, wait, then wash the gel. Result: Visible lanes of DNA fragments with different travelling paths.

If the exercise is done correctly there is a visible result of the procedure, which can be analyzed and/or photographed. On a solid rectangle piece of gel, there are 4 visible vertical lanes. Each lane has horizontal bars, each bar representing DNA fragments with various lengths. The first lane contains uncut DNA (single fragment), the second lane contains fragments cut by PstI, the third and the fourth lanes contain fragments cut by EcoRI and HindIII respectively. It can be observed that the horizontal bar at longest distance is in the lane where fragments cut by PstI are positioned. Therefore, the answer to this lab task is: If a lambda DNA is processed with three restriction enzymes, EcoRI, PstI, and HindIII, the shortest DNA fragment will be obtained by PstI restriction enzyme.

The lab exercise is carried out in groups, each group having own lab workstation with all the tubes and materials necessary. The devices like electrophoresis chamber and water bath might be common for the groups.

6. Implementation

This approach has been successfully implemented to at least two Universities: South Carolina State University in Orangeburg, SC, USA and St. Cyril and Methodius University in Skopje, Macedonia. It is applied in the courses CS495 Biocomputing and Bioinformatics (South Carolina state University), and partly in the course DNA Programming, Intelligent Systems and Bioinformatics (Sts Cyril and Methodius University). During lab activities part of which are described here, computer science students are given opportunity to obtain hands on experience with bionanorobots and other nano structures used in genetic engineering. Each lab has a lab quiz that asks students to relate the observed knowledge with their background knowledge in robotics, flexible manufacturing, and operating systems. Students show enthusiastic interest in learning steps toward genetic engineering.

7. Conclusion

The paper describes an innovative approach toward education of Computer Science students and specialists in genetic engineering. We argue that genetic engineering is good way of evolution for classical engineering and that it should be part of computer science education. Computer science is about programming and reprogramming, and cell (re)programming is essence of genetic engineering and of creating new organisms.

For a long time computer science is involved in creating artificial creatures such as robots. However, biological robots, such as bionanorobots, were not part of computer science education. We argue that the students should be familiarized with possibility of programming DNA that will compile into a bionanorobot.

Appropriate language should be used in explaining molecular genetics to computer science students. This paper proposes use of the computer science related metaphors, such as robotics and flexible manufacturing metaphor as well as operating systems and systems software metaphor.

This approach has been successfully implemented to at least two Universities: South Carolina State University (SCSU) in Orangeburg, SC, USA and Sts. Cyril and Methodius University in Skopje, Macedonia. It is applied in the course CS495 Biocomputing and bioinformatics in SCSU, and the course Bioinformatics, Intelligent Systems, and DNA

Programming at the Faculty of Natural Sciences and Mathematics at Sts. Cyril and Methodius University. The terminology used in these courses is adapted toward computer engineering way of thinking. The addressed issues are strongly connected to the terms of files, disks, operating systems, file processing, robots etc. This enables the computer science students better understanding of some of the most complicated processes known to man, the processes of life. Students are given opportunity to obtain hands on experience with bionanorobots, such as restriction enzymes. Computer Science student have shown interest toward understanding and reprogramming DNA. In addition to theoretical lectures, the students participate in extracurricular activities which give them hands on-experience with DNA manipulation. It seems that this way of reasoning makes students curious for additional knowledge in Genetic Engineering. Many of these students have expressed interest for the upcoming master's degree program related to biorobotics at SCSU. Some of the students, who graduated at the University St. Cyril and Methodius, and have taken classes that support Genetic Engineering education, are already students in some of the Europe's Genetics Engineering masters programmes.

We believe that we should continue towards further research for appropriate metaphors in relation between computer science and genetic engineering. We also believe that we should enrich the student work with more practical implementation of the concepts presented in this paper.

8. Acknowledgment

This work was supported in part by the NSF grant EPS-0903795-2010-702 awarded to South Carolina State University in 2009.

9. References

Ackovska N., Bozinovska L. & Bozinovski S (2010) Artificial chromosomes as genetic disks: A systems software metaphor for genetic engineering, *Proceedings of IEEE SouthestCon 2010*, pp. 324-327, 978-1-4244-5853-0, Charlotte, NC, March 18-21, 2010

Ackovska N. & Bozinovski S. (2008), Next Generation Operating Systems: A Biologically Inspired Future, *Proceedings of 2nd Annual IEEE Systems Conference*, pp. 1-7,978-1-4244-2150-3, Montreal, Canada, April 7-10, 2008

Ackovska N., Bozinovski S. & Jovancevski G. (2008a). Real-Time Systems - Biologically Inspired Future, *Journal of Computers*, Vol. 3, No.3, (March 2008), pp. 56-63, 1796-203X, 2008.

Ackovska N., Bozinovski S. & Jovancevski G. (2008b). File system organization in minimal biological system, *Proceedings of the 6th International Conference on Informatics and Information Technology*, pp. 44-47, 978-9989-668-78-4, Bitola, Macedonia, February 10-14, 2008

Ackovska N., Bozinovski S. & Jovancevski G. (2007). A New Frontier for Real - Time systems - Lessons from Molecular Biology, Proceedings of IEEE SoutheastCon 2007, pp.224-228, 1-4244-1029-0, Richmond, VA, March 22-25, (2007)

Ananiev E., Wu C., Chamberlin M., Switashev S., Schwartz C., Gordon-Kamm W. & Tingey S. (1985). Artificial chromosome formation in maize, *Chromosoma,* Vol. 118, No. 2, pp. 157-177, ISSN : 0009-9515, 1985

Been M. (2006). Versatility of Self-Cleaving Ribozymes, *Science*, Vol. 313, pp. 1745-1747, ISSN: 0036-8075, 2006

Bozinovski S. (1985) Guest Editor's Introduction, *Automatika, Vol. 26 (3-4), Special Issue on Biocybernetics*, pp. 128, Zagreb, ISSN: 0005-1144, 1985

Bozinovski S. (1987) Flexible manufacturing systems: Biocybernetics approach (In Russian), *Problems in Manufacturing and Control*, Vol. 16, pp. 31-34, ISSN: 0234- 6206, 1987

Bozinovski S. & Bozinovska L. (1987), Flexible production lines in genetics: a model of protein biosynthesis process, *Proceedings of International Conference on Robotics*, pp.1-4, Dubrovnik, Yugoslavia, 1987

Bozinovski S., Mueller B. & diPrimio F. (2000). Biomimetic autonomous factories: Autonomous manufacturing systems and systems software, *GMD Report*, No. 115, German National Research Center for Information Technology, Bonn, ISSN: 1435-2702, 2000

Bozinovski S. & Bozinovska L. (2001), Manufacturing science and protein biosynthesis, In N. Calaos, W. Badawy, S. Bozinovski (eds.) *Proceedings of SCI Conference 2001, Vol. XV*, pp. 59-64, ISBN : 980-07-7555-2, Orlando, FL, 2001

Bozinovski S., Jovancevski G. & Bozinovska N. (2001). DNA as a real time, database operating system, In N. Calaos, W. Badawy, S. Bozinovski (eds.) *Proceedings of SCI Conference 2001*, VOL XV : pp. 65-70, ISBN: 980-07-7555-2, Orlando, FL, 2001

Bozinovski S. & Bozinovska L. (2011). Human Body Parts Making: Educational Challenges for Engineered Physiology, Biorobotics, and Biofabrication, *Proceedings of IEEE SoutheastCon 2011*, pp. 307-308, ISBN: 978-1-61284-737-5 , Nashville, TN, 2011

Brown T. A. (2001). *Genetics, A Molecular Approach*, Nelson Thomas, ISBN 0-7487-4370-7, 2001

Brown T.A. (2002), *Genomes*, 2-nd Ed., Willey-Liss, ISBN: 0-471-31681-0, 2002

Burke D., Carle M. & Olson M. (1987). Cloning of large segments of exogenous DNA into yeast by means of artificial chromosome vectors, *Science*, No. 236, pp. 806-812, ISSN : 0036-8075, 1987

Crick F. (1958). On protein synthesis, *Proceedings of Symposium on Society for Experimental Biology*, No.12, pp. 138-163, ISSN: 0081-1386, 1958

Demeester L. ; Eichler K & Loch C. H. (2004). Organic Production Systems: What the Biological Cell Can Teach Us About Manufacturing, *Manufacturing and Service Operation Management*, Vol. 6, No. 2, INFORMS, pp. 115-132, ISSN: 1523-4814, 2004

Danchin A. & Noria S. (2004). Genome structure, operating systems and the image of the machine in *Molecules in Time and Scpace: Bacterial Shape, Division, and Phylogeny*, Vicente M., Tamames J., Valencia A., Mingorance J. (eds.), pp. 195-208, Kluwer, ISBN: 0-306-4857-8, 2004

Gibson D., Glass J., Lartigue C., Noskov V., Chuang R., Algire M., Benders G., Montague M., Ma L., Moodie M., Merryman C., Vashee S., Krishnakumar R., Assad-Garcia N., Andrews-Pfannkoch C., Denisova E., Young L., Oi Z-O., Segall-Shapiro T., Calvey C., Parmar P., Hutchison C., Smith H. & Venter C. (2010). Creation of a bacterial cell controlled by a chemically synthesized genome, *Science*, Vol. 329 (5987): 52–56. 2010

Grimes B. & Cooke H. (1998) Engineering mammalian chromosomes, *Human Molecular Genetics*, Vol. 7, No.10, pp. 1635-1640, ISSN: 0964-6906, 1998

Jackson D., Symons R. & Berg P. (1972) Biochemical method for inserting new genetic information into DNA of Simian Virus 40: Circular SV40 DNA molecules containing lambda phage genes and the galactose operon of Escherichia coli. *Proceedings of National Academy of Sciences*, 69 (10): 2904–2909, 1972.

Kruger K., Grabowski P. J., Zaug A. J., Sands J., Gottschling D. E. & Cech T. R. (1982). Self-splicing RNA: Autoexcision and autocyclization of the ribosomal RNA intervening sequence of tetrahymena, *Cell*, Vol.31, pp. 147-157 , ISSN: 0092-8674, 1982

Kanehisa M. (2000). *Post-genome Informatics*, Oxford University Press, ISBN: 0-19-850326-1, 2000

Larin Z. & Mejia . (2002). Advances in human artificial chromosome technology, *Trends in Genetics*, Vol. 18, No.6, pp. 313-319, ISSN: 0168-9525, 2002

Madevska-Bogdanova A. & Ackovska N. (2009), Different Approach to Information Technology - Teaching the Intelligent Systems Course in Technology, Education and Development, Lazinica A. & Calafate C. (eds), pp. 357-366, 978-953-307-007-0, In-Teh, Vukovar, Croatia, 2009

Nicholl D. (2008). *An Introduction to Genetic Engineering*, Cambridge University Press, ISBN: 051-80867-7, 2008

Nutt G. (1992). *Centralized and Distributed Operating Systems*, Prentice Hall, ISBN 0-13-122326-7, 1992

Osoegawa K., Mammoser A., Wu C., Frengen E., Zeng C., Catanese J., & de Jong P. (2001). A Bacterial Artificial Chromosome Library for Sequencing the Complete Human Genome, *Genome Research*, No. 11, pp.483–96, ISSN: 1088-9051, 2001

Pirim H. (2005). Biological Cell's production system, *Proceedings of 35th International Conference on Computers and Industrial Engineering*, pp. 1571-1575, Istabul, Turkey, 2005

Ratner V. (1975). Control Systems in Molecular Genetics, (In Russian) *Nauka*, Novosibirsk, 1975

Rebersek M. & Miklavcic D. (2011) Advantages and disadvantages of different concepts of electroporation pulse generation. *Automatika 42(1):, Special Issue on Recent Advances in Biomedical Engineering*, pp. 12-19, ISSN 0005-1114, 2011

Ren X., Tihimic C., Katoh M., Kurimasa A., Inoue T. & Oshimura M. (2006). Human artificial chromosome vectors meet stem cells, *Stem Cells Reviews and Reports*, Vol. 2, No.1, pp. 43-50, ISSN: 1558-6804, 2006

Tanenbaum A. (1995). *Distributed Operating Systems*, Prentice Hall, ISBN 10: 0321-99084, 1994

Tanenbaum A. & Van Steen M. (2007). *Distributed Systems; Principles and Paradigms.* ISBN 0-13-239227-5, Prentice Hall, 2007

Watson J. & Crick F. (1953). Molecular structure of nucleic acids: a structure of deoxyribose nucleic acid, *Nature*, No. 171, pp. 737-738, ISSN: 0028-0836, 1953

Williamson J. (2002) Dragon's island and other stories. Five Star, ISBN-10: 0786243147

Xiong J.(2006). *Essential Bioinformatics*, Cambridge University Press, ISBN-10 0-521-60082-0, 2006

Zaibak F., Kozlovski J., Vadolas J., Sarsero J., Williamson R. & Howden S. (2009). Integration of functional bacterial artificial chromosomes into human cord blood-derived multipotent stem cells, *Gene Therapy*, Vol. 16, No.3, pp. 404-414, ISSN: 0969-7128, 2009

27

Design of a PC-Based Electrocardiogram (ECG) Recorder as - Internet Appliance

Mahmud Hasan
Computer Science Program, Faculty of Science, University Brunei Darussalam
Brunei

1. Introduction

The advancement of medical science contributes towards lengthening the human life expectancy. Therefore the proportion of the elder people in the society is increasing. And taking proper care of these people should, most certainly, be one of the prime responsibilities of the society. ECG is the only way to check the heart condition, and if ECG can be done frequently, then it is easier for the physician to identify a problem from the ECG's history of a person (it has long been preferred by physicians).

The importance of ECG as a medical tool has led to the development of various types of ECG recording system. The developed systems vary from a simple ECG recorder that can only monitor the ECG signal to a sophisticated system with computer analysis and database. With the use of the computer, patients can record and save their reliable ECG data by themselves at home. Moreover, the Internet services like e-mail and File Transfer Protocol (FTP) can be used as a communication tool to send the recorded ECG data to the medical center. What they need is an ECG data acquisition system at home, which is easy for recording, viewing and sending the ECG data to the medical center with reliable accuracy. To send the ECG data over Internet, the recorded ECG data should be made into a form suitable for transmission; for example, the size and the fidelity of the ECG data should be taken into consideration.

This chapter will explain step by step development work to produce an ECG data acquisition system that is suitable for use at home and for transmitting ECG data over Internet. The system consists of an ECG recorder hardware that is used as a computer peripheral connected to the computer via USB port and software written to display the ECG data. The recorder hardware performs amplification, proper filtering and analog-to-digital conversion to the ECG signal. An 8-bit microcontroller is used to control the hardware and to communicate with the computer. The hardware is portable, battery-powered and its design emphasizes on low power consumption. The device should be isolated from the 240V power line; thus, working independently in a robust and reliable mode. The ECG signal was over sampled at 500 samples per second to improve its fidelity. The software can be written in Visual C++ or Java programming language. It will communicate with the hardware to control its recording process, monitor its battery status and display the ECG signal in real-time while recording is in process with the indication of bad or good ECG data. The software should provide a graphical user interface (GUI), which help general user to work with this system. Besides that, it detects the presence of the heartbeat, calculates the current heartbeat rate and beat-to-beat interval while recording the ECG data in memory. To make a reasonable file size for easy transmission over the Internet, a lossless compression can be performed to the ECG data before it is saved into a file.

Leveraging the growing impact of the Internet on healthcare, this device can be used for cardiac research, cardiac rehabilitation, cardiac activities follow-up (like Arrhythmia and Pacemaker), sports, emergency unit (wireless ECG transfer by wireless Internet) as well as regular cardiac care for improving health. This system can be expand according to the organizational need. A hospital database can be developed where the individual patient will upload their ECG information regularly from home for diagnostic purposes.

1.1 Objective

The objectives of this chapter are:

- To demonstrate a development process of a portable and reliable system that enables the recording of patient's ECG at home.
- To show how to recondition the recorded data that will be suitable for transmission over the Internet and suitable for use in the analysis and measurement of PQRST waves of the patient's ECG.
- To show how to develop software that must have the basic functions to get data from the hardware and send through the network.

2. Background study

2.1 The heart wiring

When the heart is working properly, it is a masterpiece of timed precision, with heart valves opening and closing on cue to prevent backward blood flow. Heart valves, chambers, electrical impulses, coronary arteries and veins all of these must be in perfect working order for the heart to function at its best.

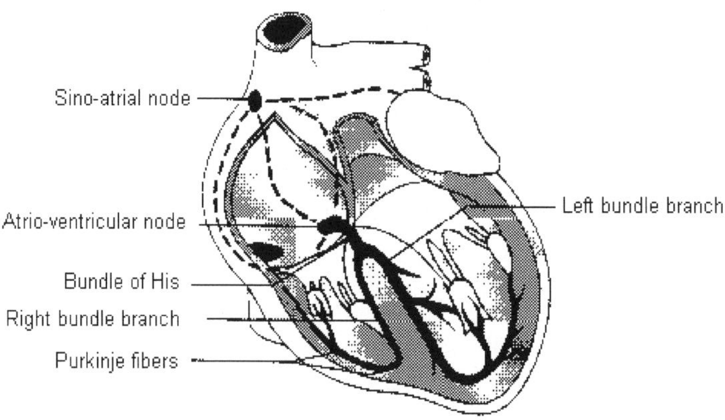

Fig. 1. Anatomy of the heart

2.2 The surface electrodes

The electrodes for surface recording of biopotential are generally made of silver-silver chloride (Ag-AgCl). This disposable foam-pad consists of an Ag-AgCl metal contact button at the top of a hollow column that is filled with a conductive gel. Most bioelectric measurements an interference level of 1 to 10μV peak-to-peak (pp) or less than 1% of the pp value of an ECG, is acceptable.

2.3 Interference

The capacitances between the patient, the power lines and ground cause a small interference current to flow through the body. These capacitances cause an interference current of 0.5μA_{pp} to flow from the power supply lines (220V, 50Hz) through the body to ground [9]. A typical situation with a mean current of 10nA_{pp} in the wires, mean electrode impedance of 20KΩ and a relative difference electrode impedance of 50%, leads to an unacceptable high interference level of 200μV_{pp}. There are two ways by which a high common mode voltage may cause interference. The first, obvious way is when the common mode rejection ratio of the amplifier is limited. Second, and much more important way a high common mode voltage may cause interference is when there are differences in electrode impedance and input impedance whish convert common mode voltage into a differential input voltage. There are three situations.

- The amplifier common is connected to ground. The amount of interference current Z_{rl} is determined mainly by the capacitance between patient's body and the main power supply (C_{pow}). In a typical situation (C_{pow} = 3pF, Z_{rl} = 20KΩ) the common mode voltage is an acceptable 10mV_{pp}.
- The amplifier common is not connected to ground. The resulting current through the impedance of the electrode-skin interface of the right leg electrode depends on the values C_{pow}, capacitance between body and ground (C_{body}), capacitance between amplifier common and main power supply (C_{sup}) and between amplifier common and ground (C_{iso}). It can be calculated that under typical conditions (Cbody = 300pF, Cpow = 3pF, Zrl = 20KΩ), the common mode voltage will be small, 1mVpp.
- In all cases, the common mode voltage can be largely reduced if a driven right leg circuit is added. An extra amplifier drives the patient to the same voltages, as the voltage of the amplifier common mode voltage can be made much smaller this way than the voltage across Z_{rl}.

2.4 Data acquisition system

With the analog low-pass filter, high frequency noise and interference can be removed from the signal path prior to the analog-to-digital conversion. Using a sampling frequency (f_s), typically called the Nyquist rate. If there is a portion of the input signal that resides in the frequency domain above $f_s/2$, that portion will fold back into the bandwidth of interest with the amplitude preserved [15]. This frequency folding phenomena can be eliminated or significantly reduced by using analog low-pass filter prior to the ADC input. Consequently, this signal will not be aliased into the final sampled output. There are two regions of the analog low-pass filter illustrated in Figure 2. The region to the left is within the bandwidth of DC to $f_s/2$. The second region, which is shaded, illustrates the transition band of the filter. Since this region is greater than $f_s/2$, signals within this frequency band will be aliased into the output of the sampling system. The effects of this error can be minimized by moving the corner frequency of the filter lower than $f_s/2$ or increasing the order of the filter. In both cases, the minimum gain of the filter at $f_s/2$ should be less than the signal-to-noise ratio (SNR) of the sampling system.

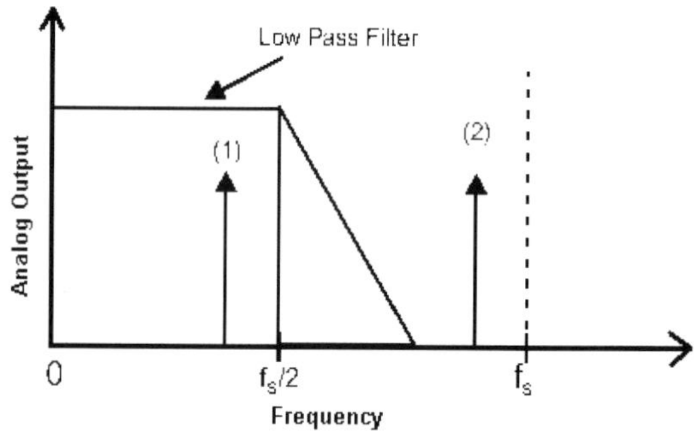

Fig. 2. Frequency Response of Low Pass Filter

2.5 Passive filters

Passive, low pass filters are realized with resistors and capacitors. The realization of single and double pole low-pass filters are shown in Figure 3. This value of resistor could create an undesirable voltage drop or make impedance matching difficult. Consequently, passive filters are typically used to implement a single pole.

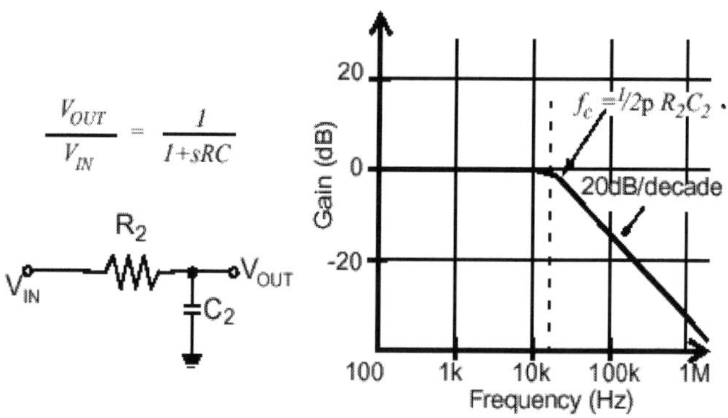

Fig. 3. Passive, Low-pass Filter

2.6 Active filters

The active filter offers the advantage of providing isolation between stages [11]. This is possible by taking advantage of the high input impedance and low output impedance of the operational amplifier. In all cases, the order of the filter is determined by the number of capacitors at the input and in the feedback loop of the amplifier. The Double Pole, Voltage Controlled Voltage Source is better known as the Sallen-Key filter realization. This filter is configured so the DC gain is positive. In the Sallen-Key Filter realization shown in Figure 4, the DC gain is greater than one. In the realization shown in Figure 5, the DC gain is equal to one. In both cases, the order of the filters is equal to two. The poles of these filters are determined by the resistors and capacitors values of R1, R2, C1 and C2.

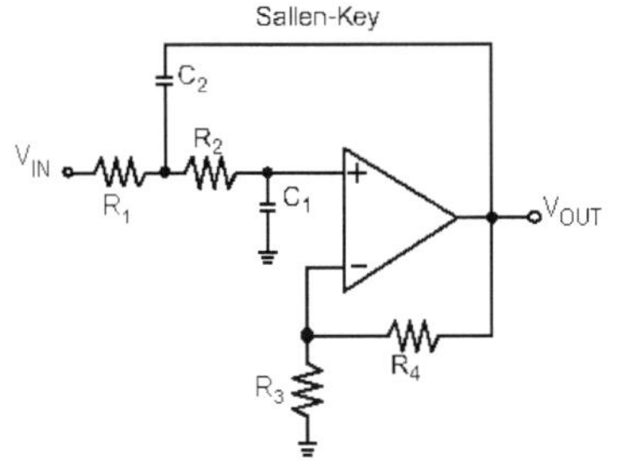

$$\frac{V_{OUT}}{V_{IN}} = \frac{K/(R_1R_2C_1C_2)}{s^2+s(1/R_1C_2+1/R_2C_2+1/R_2C_1-K/R_2C_1+1/R_1R_2C_1C_2)}$$

$$K = 1 + R_4/R_3$$

Fig. 4. Sallen-Key filter with DC gain greater than one

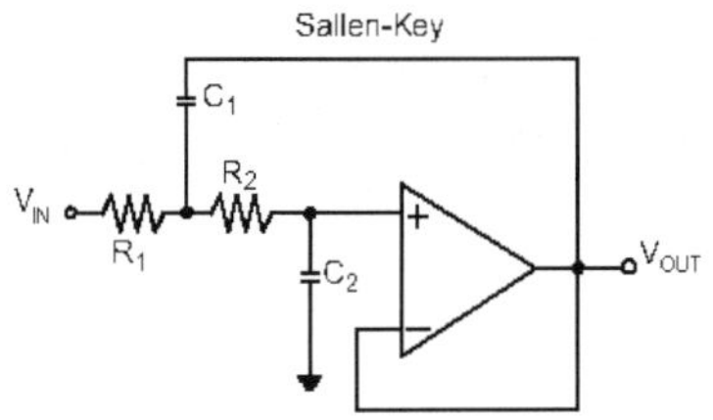

Fig. 5. Sallen-Key filter with DC gain equal to one.

2.7 Low power design

It is possible to have the system to manage its own power consumption by software control utilizing a microcontroller. Some microcontroller like the PICmicro™ family from Microchip can source up to 20mA of current and provides power to other components. In this case, one can simply connect the Vdd pin of an external component to an input-output (IO) pin of the microcontroller. Currently, most of the op-amps, analog-to-digital converter (ADC), and other devices manufactured today are low powered and therefore can be powered by this technique. Many techniques are used to reduce power consumption in the microcontroller. The most commonly used methods are SLEEP mode and external events. The microcontroller can periodically wake-up from sleep using the Watchdog Timer or external interrupt, execute code and then go back into SLEEP Mode.

2.8 Data compression

In these applications, the loss of even a single bit could be catastrophic. In the case of ECG file, it is important to preserve the actual recorded ECG data when transmitting to the physician for later analysis. Thus, the lossless compression technique is more suitable to be used for the compression of ECG data. Huffman codes have the unique prefix attribute, which means they can be correctly decoded despite being variable length.

2.9 Heartbeat detection techniques

The recognition of almost all ECG parameters is based on a fixed point identifiable at each cycle. R-peak is suitable for use as the datum point, because it has the largest amplitude and sharpest waveform that can be extracted from ECG. For the detection of R-peak, the amplitude level triggering method is based on the square of the derivative. The high frequency components of an original signal are indicated by differentiating the filtered ECG signal. The reliability of the identification is increased by squaring this differentiated value, which will highlight the high frequency components. After this processing, the R-peak can be detected by determining the known amplitude level as a triggering level. The triggering level can also be adaptively determined. Thus, the value of the triggering level is dependent on the upper values of the ECG signal. The R-wave triggering threshold value can be determined by try and error to find out the most suitable value [19]. The value of the triggering threshold can adaptively change with the base line value of the ECG signal. The R-peak can be recognized by determining the squared value that is greater than the R-wave triggering value. The current RR-interval can be calculated by differentiating the previous R-wave time with the current R-wave time and the heartbeat can be calculated by the following formula.

$$
\begin{aligned}
&RR\,\mathrm{int}\,erval = Xms \\
&Beat\,/\,Second = \frac{1}{X}\times 1000 \\
&\therefore\ Beat\,/\,Minute = \frac{1}{X}\times 1000\times 60 = \frac{60000}{X}
\end{aligned}
\tag{1}
$$

3. Hardware design

3.1 Block diagram of the hardware design

The proposed block diagram of the ECG recorder is shown in Figure 6. Three electrodes were used in the ECG recorder; two electrodes are used to sense the ECG signal and the other one is for noise reduction. The weak ECG signal acquired from electrodes is first amplified by the preamplifier with a gain of about 500 before it is filtered by a 96Hz low-pass filter to eliminate most of the electromagnetic noise. The offset null circuit is to eliminate the DC voltage between the two electrodes. The filtered signal is further amplified to about 1V and the offset of the signal is shifted to 1.25V by another stage of amplifier. It is necessary to shift the signal offset to 1.25V so that all the negative voltage is shifted to positive because the ADC accepts pseudo-differential inputs ranging from 0V to reference voltage of 2.50V. The amplified signal is digitized by a 12-bit ADC sampled at 500 samples per second before it is sent to the microcontroller via 3-wire serial interface. In the block diagram, there is a power supply unit that produces +5V and -5V needed by the analog circuits. The power supply for analog circuit can be shutoff by a control line connected to the microcontroller. Besides that, this unit can detect the battery level and signal the microcontroller in case of battery low. The recorder has an 8-bit microcontroller to control its operations like initializing the ECG recording circle, stop recording, shutdown the circuits when there is no activity and monitor the battery status. It also implements the communication protocol between recorder and the computer. The ECG recorder is physically isolated from the 240V power line using opto-isolator for the safety of the patient.

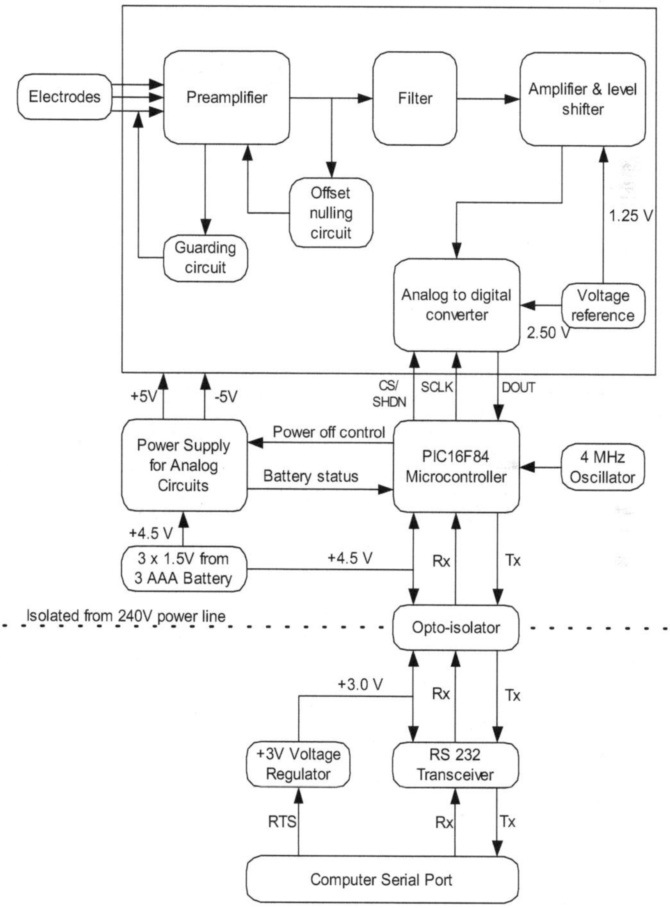

Fig. 6. Block Diagram of the ECG Recorder

3.2 Amplifier design

The amplification of ECG signal can be divided into two stages, the preamplification stage has a gain of about 500 to improve Common Mode Rejection Ratio (CMRR) and the second stage of amplification has a gain of two to make the overall gain of 1000 that will amplify the signal voltage to about 1.0V so that it is high enough to input to the ADC. The 50 Hz line interference can be sufficiently reduced by having a third electrode connected to the amplifier's common ground, which put the patient's body voltage potential to the amplifier's common voltage. The ECG recorder is optically isolated from the main power line and the amplifier is powered by battery, which delivers very clear voltage supply. DC input voltage of up to 200mV should not result in saturation of the amplifier. The INA118 uses a single external resistor to set gain from 1 to 10000. It is laser trimmed for very low offset voltage (50μV) and high CMRR (110dB at 1000 gain). It operates with power supplies as low as ±1.35V and quiescent current is only 350μA, which is very suitable for battery operation. The INA118 has eight pins which are the positive input pin (V_{in}^+), negative input pin (V_{in}^-), positive voltage supply pin (V^+), negative voltage supply pin (V^-), output reference pin (Ref), two pins for gain setting (R_G) and output pin (V_o). To set G to 500, In the recorder design, two 51Ω resistors are connected in series between the two R_G pins to set the amplifier gain to 491.

$$500 = 1 + \frac{50K\Omega}{R_G} \tag{2}$$

$$R_G = \frac{50K\Omega}{500-1} = 100.2\Omega$$

The LMC6464 quad Operational Amplifier (OA) from National Semiconductor is used in the second stage of signal amplification. The filtered ECG signal is input to the inverting input of the OA through a 10KΩ resistor and the output is feedback to the inverting input pin by a 20KΩ resistor to set the inverting amplifier gain to two. The offset of the ECG signal is shifted to +1.25V by connecting the non-inverting input of the OA to a +1.25V voltage reference through a 10KΩ resistor. A 20KΩ resistor is then connected between the ground and the non-inverting input to make the amplifier balance.

3.3 Filter design

The filtering system for the ECG recorder can be divided into two parts, the low-pass filter and the high-pass filter. The low-pass filter is a second order Butterworth Filter designed to give a cutoff frequency of 96Hz. At this cutoff frequency, most of the electromagnetic noise will be filtered out. The LMC6464 OA is used to build the filter with two resistors and two capacitors connected to form a Sallen-Key configuration as shown in Figure 9. The values of the two resistors were 8.2KΩ and 15KΩ and the values of the two capacitors are 0.1μF and 0.22μF. The calculation of cutoff frequency (f_c) is as follows:

$$\begin{aligned} f_c &= \frac{1}{2\pi\sqrt{R_1R_2C_1C_2}} \\ &= \frac{1}{2\pi\sqrt{(8.2K)(15K)(0.22\mu)(0.1\mu)}} \\ &= 96.8Hz \end{aligned} \tag{3}$$

The high-pass filter has a cutoff frequency of 0.3Hz to eliminate the DC signal. It was built by using a LMC6464 OA, a 1MΩ resistor and a 0.47μF capacitor to form an integrator circuit. The output of the preamplifier was integrated and connected back to the Ref pin of the INA118. Cutoff frequency calculation for the high-pass filter is given by equation 4.

$$f_c = \frac{1}{2\pi(1M)(0.47\mu)} \tag{4}$$
$$= 0.3Hz$$

3.4 Electrodes, wires and guarding circuit

The electrode that has been selected for the ECG recorder is the disposable foam electrode. Two electrodes are used to form a single lead pair where one will be placed on the left arm and the other will be placed on the right arm. Another electrode, which is used for noise reduction will be placed on the right leg or hand. The lead wires have to be made short, preferably less than one meter to reduce the electromagnetic interference. The length of the lead wires must be equal so that the difference of impedance in the two lead wires can be minimized. The difference of impedance in the lead wires can cause the potential divider effect, which converts the common mode voltage to differential voltage. The wires used in the ECG recorder were shielded with a single guarding circuit to drive the shield back to common mode voltage. The guarding circuit consists of the LMC6464 OA connected as a uni-gain amplifier. The common mode voltage from the INA118 was input to the non-inverting input of the OA and the output was feedback to the inverting input. The high input impedance from the non-inverting input of the OA will isolate the guarding circuit from the IA so that the operation of the IA will not be interrupted.

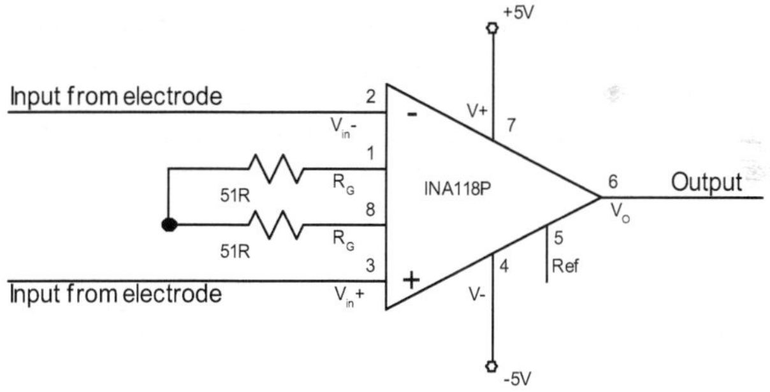

Fig. 7. Circuit Diagram for the Instrumentation Amplifier

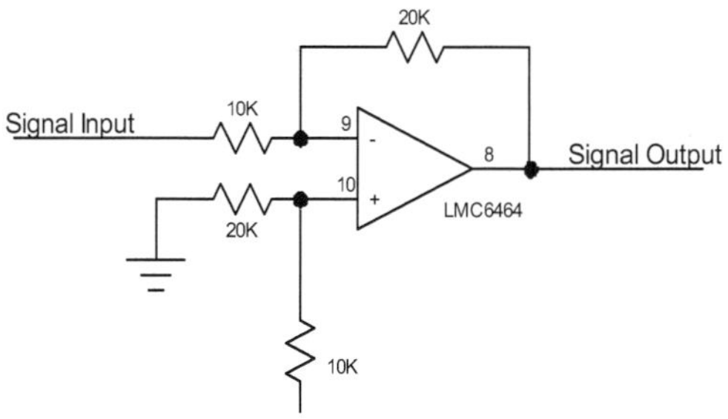

Fig. 8. Circuit Diagram for the SecondStage Amplifier

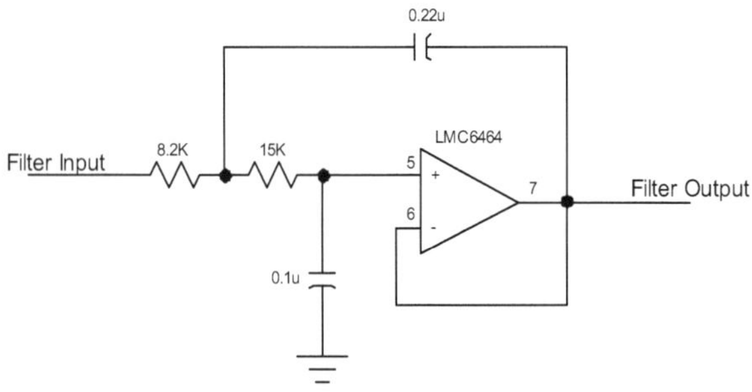

Fig. 9. Circuit Diagram for the Low Pass Filter

3.5 Analog to digital converter

The MAX145 ADC from MAXIM Integrated Product was selected in the development of the ECG recorder. It is a serial 12-bit ADC with low power consumption, automatic shutdown and fast wake-up time. It has an internal track-and-hold circuitry eliminating the need for external sample-and-hold amplifier. The reference voltage of 2.5V was used in the ECG recorder to limit the Quantization Noise to $1mV_{PP}$. A serial ADC has more complicated data transfer process compared to parallel ADC. However, a serial ADC has been chosen to minimize number of pin used for data transfer because the PIC16F84 microcontroller that is used to control the ADC has limited number of IO pin. In addition, a serial ADC will use up less space to make the recorder compact. The MAX145 pin 2 and pin 3 are pseudo-differential inputs which only accept input signal ranging from zero to a reference voltage set at pin 5, which is 2.5V in the ECG recorder design. The pin 2 of MAX145 is connected to the ground and the analog ECG signal is input to the pin 3 of MAX145. Because MAX145 only accept positive input voltage, the offset of the ECG signal is shifted to 1.25V before it is input to the pin 3 of MAX145.

Only three pins need to be connected to the microcontroller from MAX145, via the pin 7 (DOUT), pin 8 (SCLK) and pin 6 (active low chip select/active high shutdown). Pin 7 and 8 is used for reading out the digitized ECG sample serially and pin 6 is a control pin to activate the analog-to-digital conversion process. The serial data output format for MAX145 is a stream of 16-bit data stream. The first bit must be logic high to indicate the end of conversion. The next three bits must clock out high followed by the 12 bits of data in MSB-first format. After the last bit has been read out, additional serial clock pulses will clock out trailing zeros. DOUT changes on the falling edge of SCLK. That means the DOUT pin should be sampled when SCLK is high.

3.6 Power supply unit

The basic function of the power supply unit is to produce +5V and -5V from a single +4.5V supply from the battery. The MAX681 voltage converter is used to convert +4.5V to both +9V and -9V. It is a monolithic, dual charge-pump converter that provides positive and negative outputs of two times a positive input voltage. The +9V is regulated to +5V by using the MAX666 voltage regulator and the -9V is regulated to -5V by using the MAX664 voltage regulator. With this configuration, the input voltage from the battery can drop to +3V without affecting the output voltage of the power supply unit. This is because MAX681 voltage converter can convert the +3V to +6V for the MAX666 voltage regulator and -6V for the MAX664 voltage regulator.

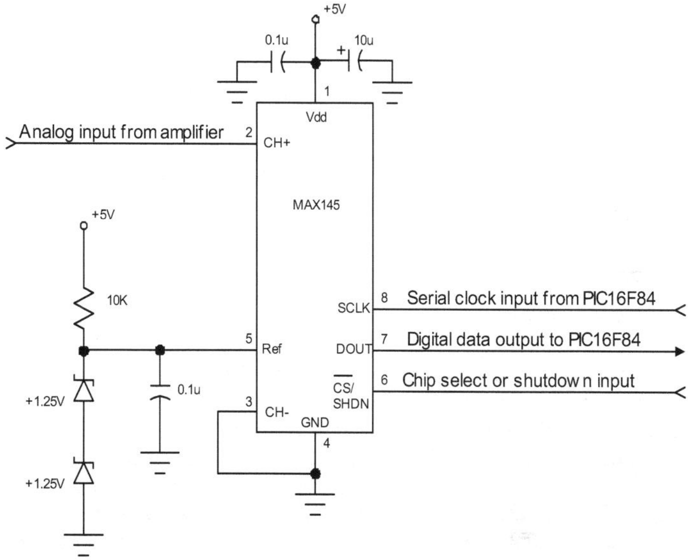

Fig. 10. Circuit Diagram for the ADC

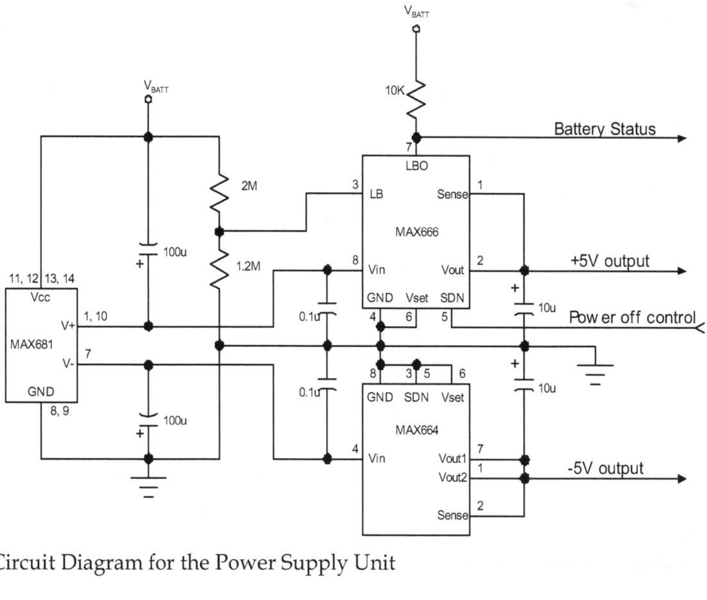

Fig. 11. Circuit Diagram for the Power Supply Unit

The MAX666 contains on-chip circuitry for low power detection. If the voltage at pin 3 of MAX666 falls below the regulator's internal reference of 1.3V, then pin 7 or the Low Battery Output pin goes low. The threshold for low battery indication can be set by using two external resistors with the values of 2MΩ and 1.2MΩ to form a voltage divider to the supply voltage. The divided voltage is then input to pin 3 of MAX666. The MAX666 can be shutdown by logic input at pin 5. When in Shutdown State, the maximum drain current is limited to 12μA, which is desired for low power design.

3.7 Microcontroller

The microcontroller acts as an intelligent unit to perform all the operation of the ECG recorder such as power management, ECG samples data acquisition and implementation of the computer interfacing protocol. Microcontroller selected for the ECG recorder is the PIC16F84 from Microchip Technology Inc. It is a low cost 8-bit microcontroller operating at the speed of 4MHz. The microcontroller has pins connected to the ADC, power supply unit and the opto-isolator. Pin 18 (RA1), pin 1 (RA2) and pin 2 (RA3) of the PIC16F84 microcontroller are connected to the MAX145 ADC. RA1 is the clock output to clock out serial data from the ADC. It is connected to the SCLK pin of the ADC. RA2 is the serial data input pin to receive the serial data from the ADC. It is connected to the DOUT pin of the ADC. RA3 is the chip-select output pin, which will power up the ADC when RA3 is high and shutdown the ADC when RA3 is low. It is connected to the pin 6 of the MAX145 ADC. Pin 3 (RA4) and pin 17 (RA0) are connected to the power supply unit. RA4 is an output pin to power off the analog circuitry and RA0 is the input pin for battery status. Pin 6 (RB0) and pin 7 (RB1) are used for serial data transfer with the computer. RB0 is for receiving data and RB1 is for transmitting data.

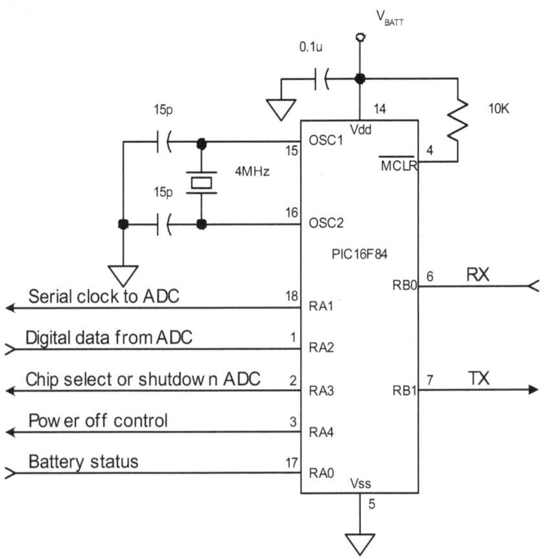

Fig. 12. Circuit Diagram for the Microcontroller

The flowchart for the microcontroller firmware is shown in Figure 17. Once the microcontroller power is up or being reset, it sets its IO pins direction by setting the internal registers, TRIS A and TRIS B [20]. RB0, RA0 and RA2 are set as input pins whereas RB1, RA1, RA3 and RA4 are set as output pins. The microcontroller then set all the output pins' initial state to logic high.

After initialization, it enters the Ready State. The Ready State puts the microcontroller in SLEEP mode and puts the ECG recorder to the lowest power consumption while waiting for the present of data from the computer serial port. Before entering the SLEEP mode, the microcontroller will enable RB0 pin interrupt.

When in SLEEP mode, the microcontroller will eventually wake up by the watchdog timer and go back to SLEEP mode. When a start-bit is detected at RB0 pin, the microcontroller will wake up, send back an "OK" string to the computer and wait for the command string from the computer. It then parses the command to determine whether the computer wants to start recording ECG or wants to check battery status. If the command is not valid, the microcontroller will reset.

In the check battery routine, the microcontroller will check the status of RA0 pin and send back the battery status to the computer. The routine then goes back to Ready State. In the record ECG routine, the microcontroller initializes its internal timer to start the analog-to-digital conversion of the ECG signal every two milliseconds. It sends one ECG sample together with the battery status to the computer every two milliseconds. The record ECG routine is designed such that the computer has to send back an acknowledgement byte to the microcontroller before 255 samples of ECG data have been sent to the computer. This is to prevent the recording process to run continuously without knowing whether the computer is receiving the ECG data. The recording process will stop and go back to SLEEP mode if there is no acknowledgement received from the computer after 255 samples have been sent to the computer.

3.8 Opto-isolator

The H11L1 opto-isolator is used to isolate the ECG recorder from the 240V power line. It has an infrared emitting diode optically coupled to a high-speed integrated detector with Schmitt trigger output. The H11L1 can isolate maximum peak voltage of 7500V before the isolation breaks down. For the ECG recorder, two H11L1 opto-isolators are used to isolate the transmit data and receive data lines for the serial port. With the use of opto-isolator, there will be no electrical path connecting the patient and the computer, which is then connected to the 240V power line.

3.9 RS-232 transceiver to USB

The RS-232 transceiver is used to convert the TTL level logic at the ECG recorder to RS-232 level logic at the serial comport and vice versa. The MAX3232 low-power RS-232 transceiver is used in the ECG recorder. It requires four 0.1μF external capacitors to operate and typical supply current of only 300μA. The low power consumption of this component makes it possible to be powered by the RTS line of the computer serial port. This part cannot be powered by the battery because it is not isolated from the 240V power line by the opto-isolator.

3.10 Communication protocol between computer and ECG recorder

The ECG recorder is interfaced to the computer via RS-232 port with the setting of 19200 baud, 8 bit data, no parity bit and one stop bit. To activate the ECG recorder, the computer has to send a set of commands to the ECG recorder. The communication starts with a function call from the computer software either to get the battery status of the ECG recorder or to start a recording process.

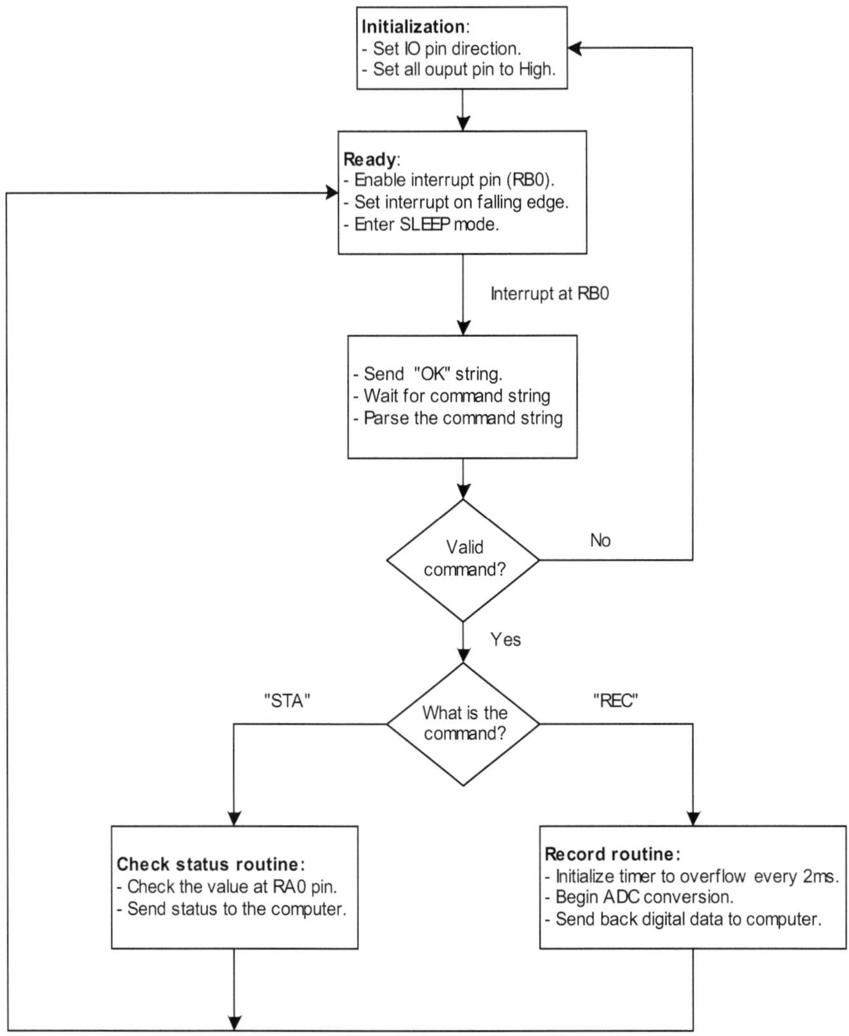

Fig. 13. Flow Chart for Microcontroller Firmware

To get the battery status of the ECG recorder, the computer will first send a one-byte data with hexadecimal value of '0xAA' to wakeup the ECG recorder. Upon receiving the one byte data, the ECG recorder will wakeup from sleep, power up the analog circuit and send back an "OK" string to indicate that it is now ready to receive a command from the computer. The command format begins with one byte of 'SOH' ASCII character and then followed by three letters string. To get the battery status, the letter string is "STA". When the ECG recorder receives a 'SOH' followed by a "STA" string, it will check the battery status and send back the battery status to the computer. It first sends a "SOH" byte followed by the status byte, which is an ASCII letter 'L' if battery level is low and an ASCII letter 'H' if battery level is normal. After sending the status byte to the computer, the ECG recorder goes back to sleep mode.

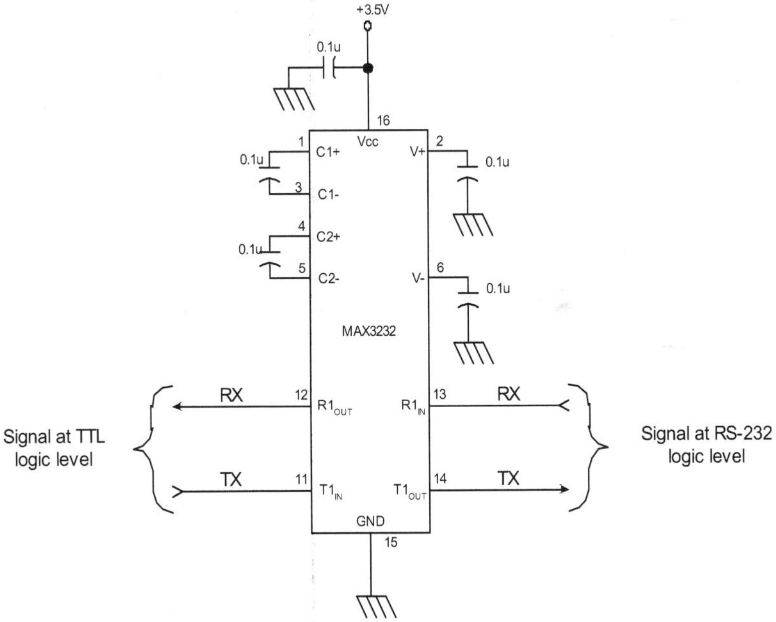

Fig. 14. Circuit Diagram for the RS-232 Transceiver

To start the ECG recording process, the computer sends a byte with value '0xAA' to the recorder. Then the ECG recorder wakes up from sleep, power up the analog circuit and sends back an "OK" string to the computer. The computer then sends a 'SOH' byte followed by a "REC" string command to the ECG recorder. When the ECG recorder receive the "REC" string command, it will initiate the ECG recording process and send back a 'SOH' byte to the computer to signal that the ECG samples are coming. Then it sends a sequence of ECG sample to the computer, two bytes of data per sample. Before the ECG recorder has sent 255 samples, the computer must send a byte with hexadecimal value '0xff' to the ECG recorder to continue the recording process. Otherwise, the ECG recorder will stop recording and go back to sleep mode. The communication protocol is illustrated by Figure 15.

4. Software design

The software design part involves the design of multiple functioning objects and the design of data flow between them [21, 22]. The functions and data structures of several main objects in the ECG software are described in the following sections. The algorithms used in the compression of ECG data and heartbeat detection are described in the Data Compression Unit and the Heartbeat Detection Unit.

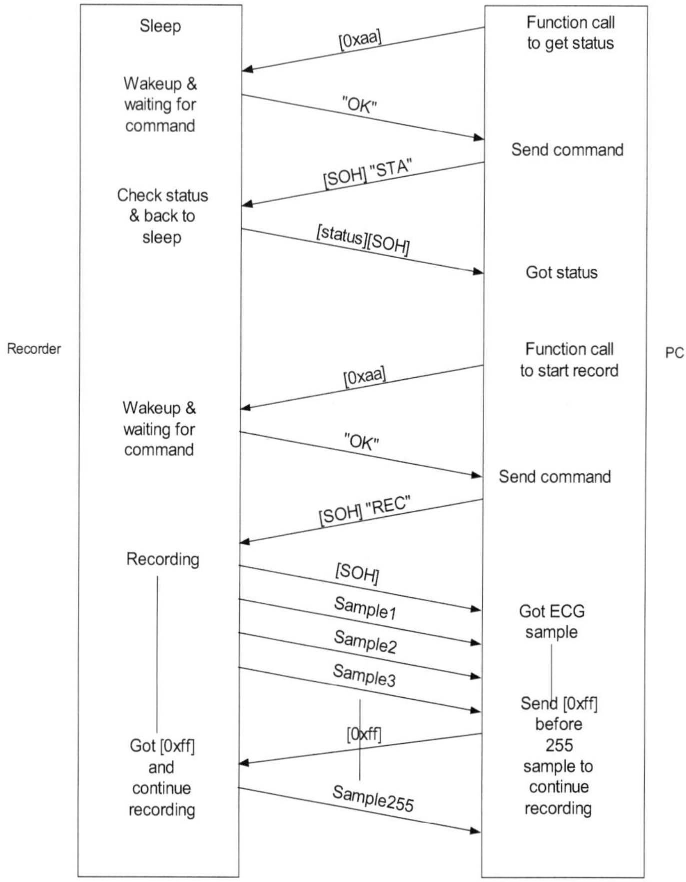

Fig. 15. Communication Protocol Between the Recorder and Computer

4.1 Data flow diagram

The data flow diagram in Figure 20 shows the flow of information between different objects and variables for the ECG recorder software. The object can be hardware, Graphic User Interface (GUI), file on disk, variable in the program memory or running thread. The information can be in the form of command or variable passed from one object to another.

The GUI objects are objects that interact with the user. They are the objects that the user can see in the main window or as a dialog box. The GUI objects in the data flow diagram together with their description are listed in the Table 1.

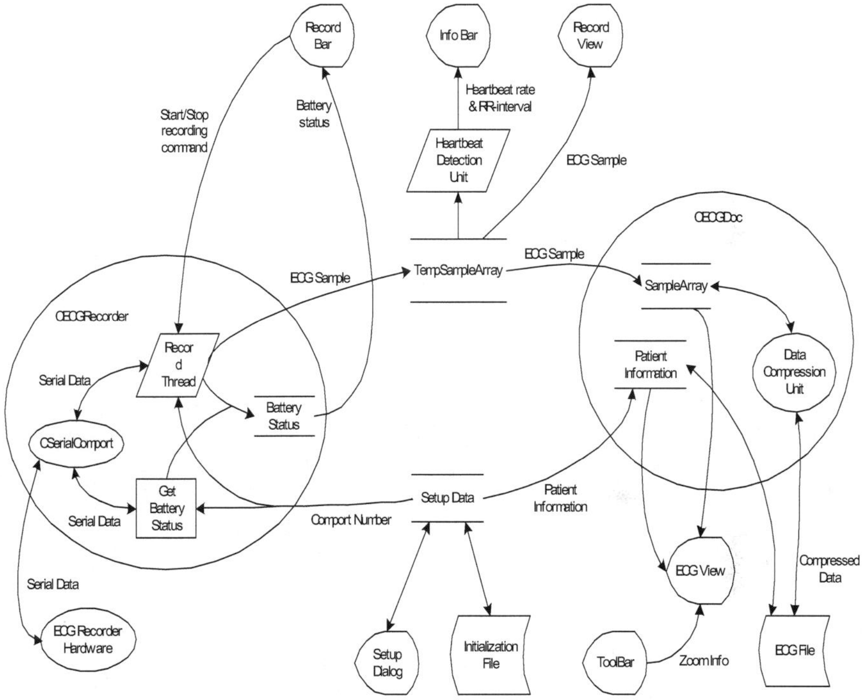

Fig. 16. Data Flow Diagram for the ECG Software

The recording process is initiated by the user from the Record Bar. When a Start Recording command is received by the CECGRecorder object, it will start the Record Thread. The Record Thread then activates the appropriate serial port and start sending and receiving serial data from the ECG recorder hardware. The Record Thread will decode the serial data into digital samples of ECG signal and the battery status. The ECG samples are then appended to the TempSampleArray, an instance of CWordArr that represents ECG signal in the memory. The battery status will be stored in a variable that later will be used to update the battery status display at the Record Bar. While the TempSampleArray represents the recording ECG signal in the memory, Record View displays it in graphical form. The Record View constantly reads the TempSampleArray and updates its display so that the user will see the real-time signal. Meanwhile, another thread, the Heartbeat Detection Unit will examine the recording signal to check whether a heartbeat is present in the signal. If a heartbeat is detected, the thread then calculates the current heartbeat rate and updates the Info Bar.

GUI object	Description
Record Bar	This is the control panel for the ECG recorder to start or stop the ECG recording process. It displays the battery status of the ECG recorder, the start time and the time elapsed.
Info Bar	Displays the heartbeat rate and the RR-interval. It also displays animation when a heartbeat is detected by the program.
Record View	Displays the real-time graph of the ECG signal when the recording process is running.
ECG View	Displays the recorded ECG signal or the ECG document in a graph. This object enables the user to scroll through the whole ECG document by a Scroll Bar. It also enables the ECG signal to be zoomed to 5 different sizes.
Setup Dialog	This dialog box is for the user to set the name of serial port where the ECG recorder hardware has been connected. Besides that, the user can also set the patient's information here.

Table 1. Description for the GUI Objects

When the recording process is stopped by the user, a new CECGDoc object will be created. The TempSampleArray will be copied to another instance of CWordArr class, which is the SampleArray and the patient information from the setup data will be copied to the member variable of the CECGDoc. The CECGDoc object represents the recorded ECG signal in the memory. It includes every detail of the recorded ECG such as the record time, the length of the recorded ECG and information of the patient, to whom the ECG belongs. The CECGDoc is graphically displayed by the CECGView. In the CECGView, one can see everything in the CECGDoc. It includes five types of zoom view to view the recorded ECG signal in different sizes. The zoom size of the CECGView can be controlled by the user in Tool Bar or in program menu. The CECGDoc can be saved on a disk as an ECG file. Actually, the patient information and the SampleArray are saved to the file when a CECGDoc is saved. The patient information is saved directly to the ECG file while the SampleArray will be compressed first before it is saved to the ECG file. The Data Compression Unit is responsible to compress and decompress the SampleArray.

4.2 Main frame window

The main frame window is the main display for the ECG software that is showed when the program starts. Like other standard window program, it has a main menu, toolbar, status bar, minimize box, maximize box and close box. It is a Multiple Document Interface (MDI) frame, which may contain several child frames so that two or more ECG files can be viewed at the same time. If the main frame window is closed, the program will also be terminated.

4.3 CECGRecorder class and the recording thread

CECGRecorder is a class that abstractly represents the ECG recorder in the ECG software. This class provides all the functions to control the ECG recorder hardware. All the low-level protocols to communicate with the hardware are automatically handled here. To use the CECGRecorder class, one must call the Activate function first and pass two arguments with it. One argument is strings to specify the name of serial port that connects to the recorder hardware, and the other argument is a pointer to the data structure to store the ECG samples when recording ECG. The member functions of this class are listed in the Table 2.

Member Function	Description
BatteryStatus	Method to return the battery status of the ECG recorder hardware.
StartRecord	Method to start the record thread.
StopRecord	Method to stop the record thread.
IsRecording	Method to check whether the record thread is running.
Activate	Method to activate the CECGRecorder.
DeActivate	Method to deactivate the CECGRecorder.
IsActivated	Method to check whether the CECGRecorder is activated.
HardwareAvailable	Method to check whether the recorder hardware is still connecting to the activated comport.

Table 2. Member Function for CECGRecorder Class

4.4 Data structure of the ECG signal

CWordArr Class represents the ECG signal in the program memory. It is a thread-safe array, which enables multiple threads to add data to it and get data from it at the same time without blocking each other. Each element of the CWordArr consists of 16-bit word, which manages to hold a 12-bit ECG sample. An ECG sample can only be added to the top of the CWordArr so that the position of ECG samples in the CWordArr will follow exactly like the ECG signal. When reading from the CWordArr, ECG sample in the CWordArr can be read out at any position and will not be deleted from the CWordArr. It is designed to be like this so that multiple threads can read out ECG sample in the CWordArr at different position simultaneously. Beside adding and reading ECG sample, the CWordArr class includes method to get the length of the ECG sample.

4.5 Data compression unit

The Data Compression Unit compresses the SampleArray into a compressed data stream before it is saved to a file. The compression process is divided into two steps. First, the ECG samples stored in the 16-bit array are converted to a stream of 12-bit ECG samples stored in CByteArray. In this step, no compression is actually done except to eliminate the redundant bits in the SampleArray. Then the CByteArray data stream is compressed by using Huffman algorithm. To implement the Huffman algorithm, the frequency of occurrence of each byte in the CByteArray is counted and the result is stored in the Counts array. The Counts array is then scaled down so that they fit in a byte and then stored as initial weights in the NODE array. From the NODE array, a Huffman tree is built. The Huffman tree is then converted to Huffman codes by a function that recursively walks through the tree, adding the child bits to each code until it gets to a leaf. When it gets to a leaf, it stores the code value in the CODE element and return. The Counts array, which has been scaled down, is saved in the ECG file so that the Huffman tree can be rebuilt in the data expansion process. When the Huffman codes are available, the CByteArray can be compressed by saving the Huffman code correspondence to each byte in the CByteArray into the ECG file. The Data Compression Unit is also responsible to expand the compressed data to SampleArray. The expansion process is also divided to two steps. First, it converts the Huffman codes to CByteArray and then converts the CByteArray to SampleArray.

4.6 Heartbeat detection unit

The Heartbeat Detection Unit is a thread that detects the present of heartbeat in the ECG signal. The algorithm used to detect the heartbeat is to find the presence of R-wave in the signal by amplitude triggering method. In this method, the average value of the signal is calculated by taking the latest 1000 samples into calculation. The triggering threshold is set to 600 units higher than the calculated average value. This value is determined by trial and error to find the most suitable value. Then, the ECG sample is read in one by one. An R-wave is considered detected when it can fulfill the follows conditions.

- The ECG sample value is higher than the triggering threshold.
- The differential value between the current ECG sample and the previous one is greater than three units.
- Four consecutive decrease of sample value followed by four consecutive increase of sample value is detected.

5. Discussion

The ECG recorder has been constructed prototype on a board and tested for its electrical characteristics. The microcontroller firmware is tested by software simulation before it is transferred to the PIC16F84 microcontroller. The microcontroller can successfully get the ECG samples from the ADC and send it to the computer. To test for the stability of the recorder, it is put in record mode for long duration and it is able to continuously sending data to the computer for more than 3 hours. When the recorder is in recording mode, it automatically goes back to power saving mode if the ECG recorder is disconnected from the computer. At battery low condition, the recorder can still work until the battery voltage drops to less than +3V. The battery low indicator will turn on when the battery level drop below +3.5V and left some time for the user to stop the recorder before it stop working by itself.

5.1 Testing for the amplifier gain

The voltage gain for every stage of the amplifier was measured. By using a sinusoidal signal with frequency of 20Hz, the peak-to-peak voltage at the input and output is measured by an oscilloscope. The measurement result for the preamplifier and second stage amplifier are shown in the Figure 17 and Figure 18. From the Figure 17 and Figure 18, the voltage gain for the preamplifier is 497.2 and the voltage gain for the second stage amplifier is 2.0. Thus, the total voltage gain for the two amplifiers is 994.4.

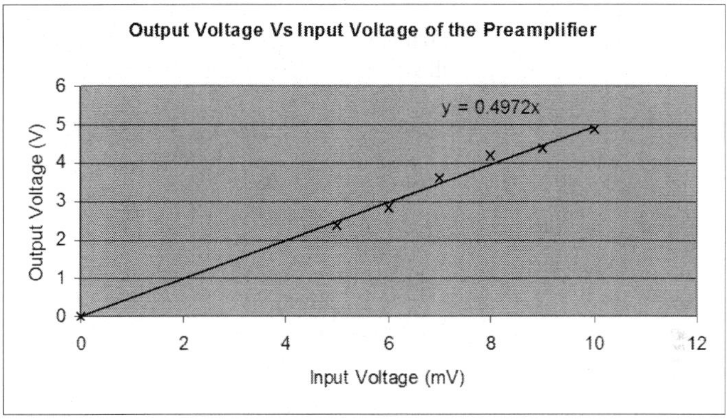

Fig. 17. Gain Measurement for the Preamplifier

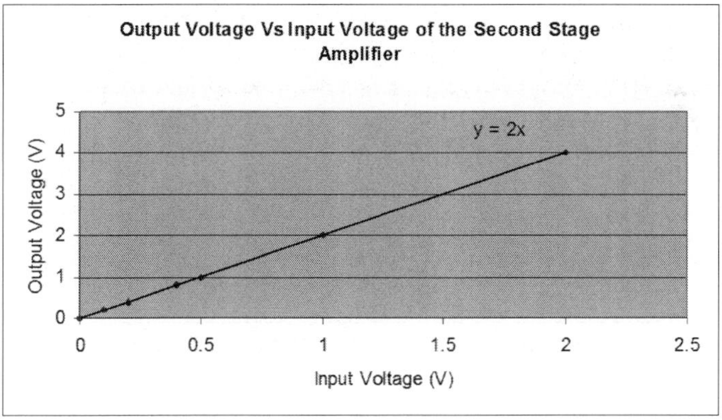

Fig. 18. Gain Measurement for the Second Stage Amplifier

5.2 Testing for the filter

To measure the frequency response for the analog circuit, a sinusoidal signal with different frequency was applied to the differential input of the preamplifier. The input signal is set to voltage of 25mV and then the output voltage for every frequency at the final stage amplifier was measured by an oscilloscope. From the measured result, a graph was plotted to find the cutoff frequency for the high pass filter and the low pass filter. Figure 19 shows the measurement result for frequency response. From the Figure 19, the cutoff frequency for high pass filter was 0.23Hz and the cutoff frequency for low pass filter was 79Hz.

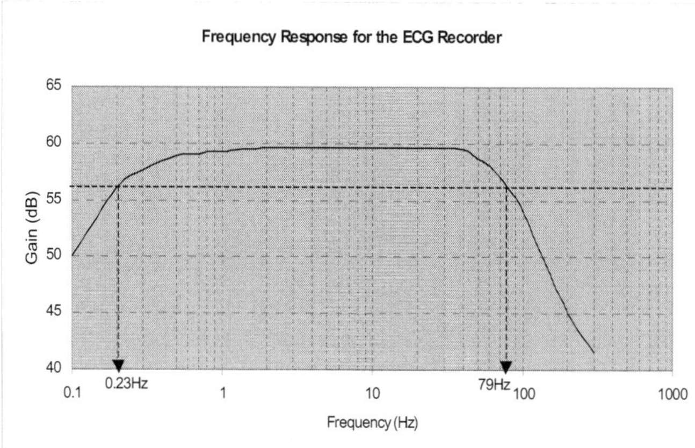

Fig. 19. Frequency Response for the Analog Circuit

5.3 Total current consumption

The total current consumption for the ECG recorder was measured with ammeter. Measurements have been made when the recorder was in power saving mode and active mode. The measurement results are shown in Table 3. As we can see in Table 6, the ECG recorder consumes very little power with only 1.85mA in power saving mode and 6.50mA in active mode.

Recorder Operation State	Total Current Consumption (mA)
Power Saving Mode	1.85
Active Mode (Recording ECG)	6.50

Table 3. Measurement for the Total Current Consumption

5.4 The ECG software

The ECG software can communicate with the recorder hardware and get data from the recorder. The recorded ECG signal can be displayed at five different scales, via 5mm/mV, 10mm/mV, 20mm/mV, 40mm/mV, and 80mm/mV. The P, Q, R, S and T waves of the ECG signal can be clearly displayed at the scale of 10mm/mV, 20mm/mV, 40mm/mV, and 80mm/m. The recorded ECG signal has noise level of about 0.12mV and can be noticed when displayed at the scale of 40mm/mv and 80mm/mV. The heartbeat detection unit can detect the heartbeat quite well when there is no movement artifact present. Therefore, the patient should prevent large movement when the recording is in progress to reduce the movement artifact noise

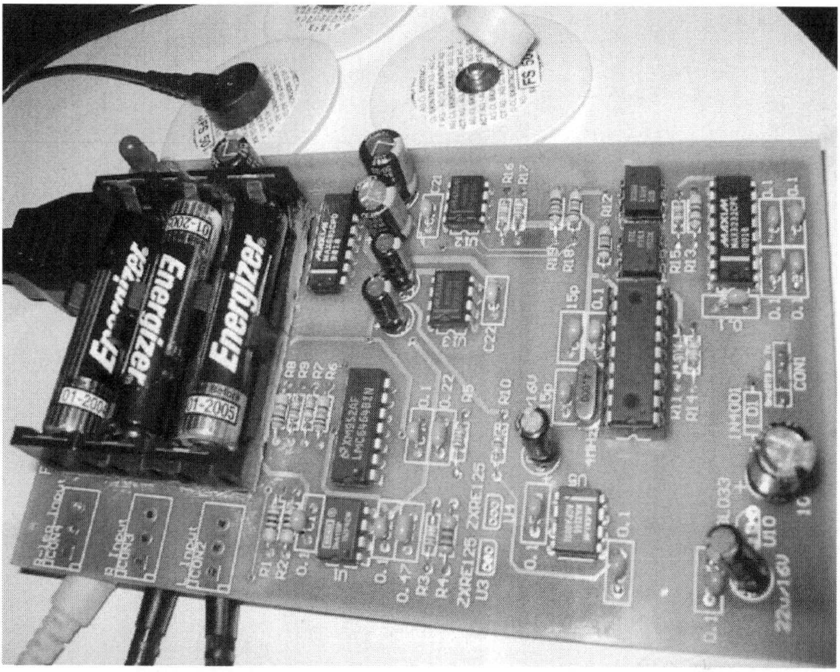

Fig. 20. The actual PC-based Electrocardiogram (ECG) recorder as - Internet appliance

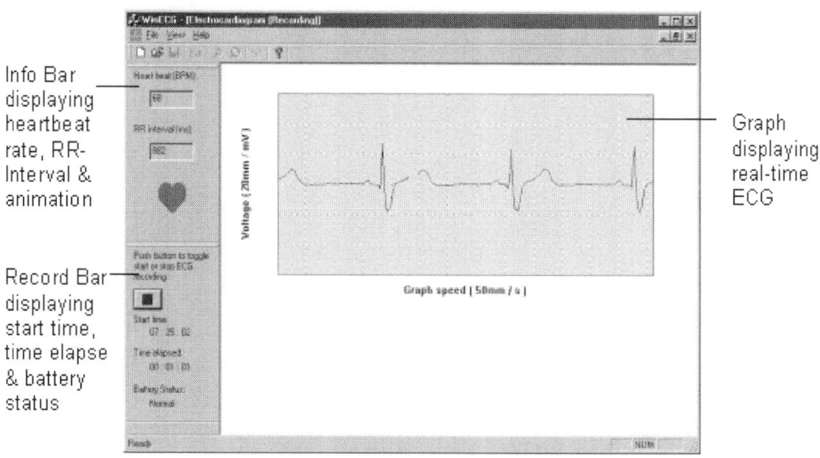

Fig. 21. Recording View for the ECG Software

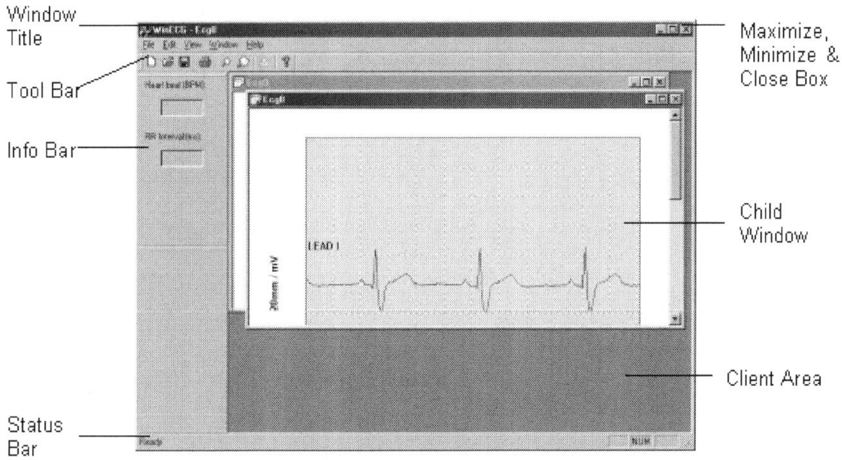

Fig. 22. Main Window for the ECG Software

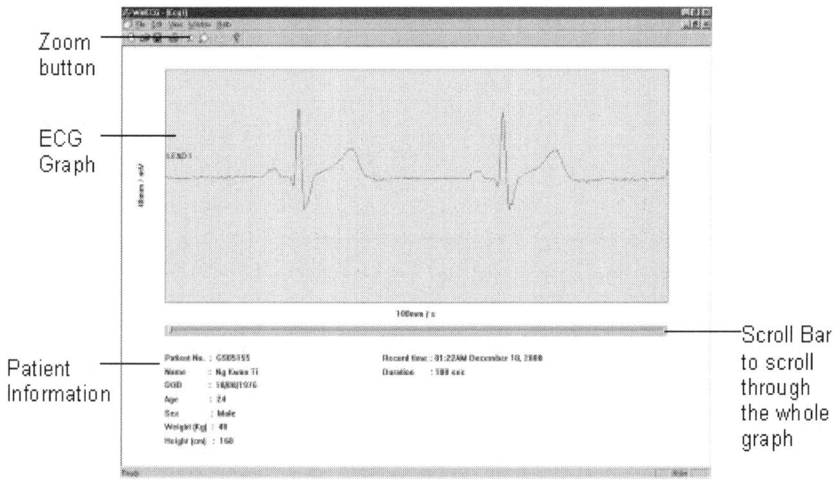

Fig. 23. Document View for the ECG Software

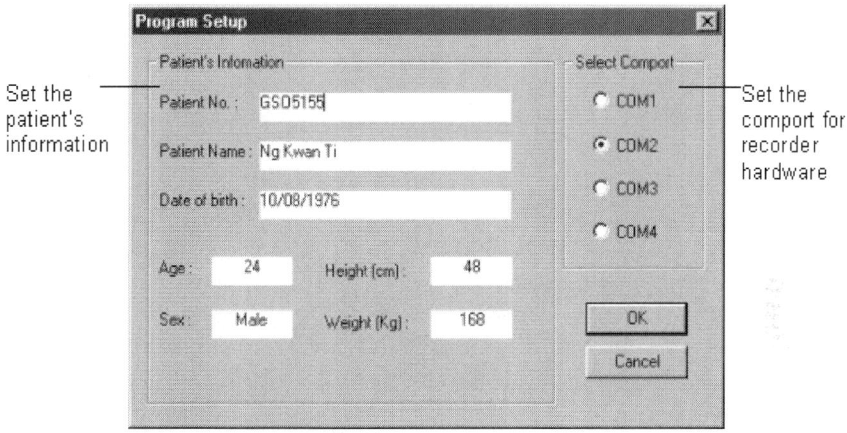

Fig. 24. Setup Dialog for the ECG Software

5.5 ECG file size

The graph in Figure 25 shows the size of the ECG files and its record duration. The increasing rate for the ECG file is approximately 0.5236 kilobyte per second. If the result is compared with the increasing rate without compression, which is 0.7324 kilobyte per second, the compression ratio achieved is 39.9%.

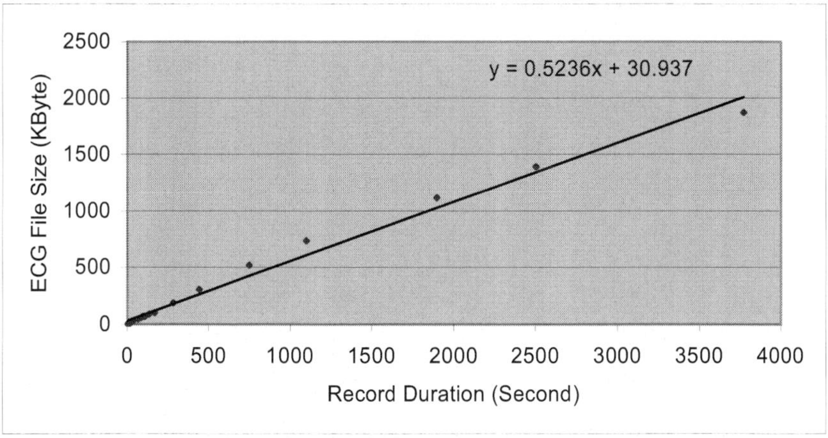

Fig. 25. ECG File Size versus Record Duration Graph

6. Conclusion

Electrocardiogram (ECG) has long been used as an important medical tool in monitoring patient's heart activities. In some cases, the patient has to go to the medical center very often to record their ECG for the diagnostic of the physician. This chapter describes the design and development of an electrocardiogram (ECG) recorder for single-lead recording that enables the recording of ECG at home and development of software to receive the ECG data from the recorder. The ECG data is saved in a compressed format for easy transmission over the Internet. The ECG recorder is a battery-powered device and its design emphasises on low power consumption. The ECG recorder is used as a peripheral connected to the computer via RS-232 port as well as USB simulator. The software was can be developed using Visual C++ or Java programming language. This design has been tested with the real patient and the ECG output has been verified by the medical doctors. The software can display the ECG data and clearly show the P, Q, R, S and T waves for diagnosis. The system consists of ECG recorder hardware and a software program. The recorder hardware has the following characteristics:

- It is battery powered and small in size. Therefore, it is very portable and easy to use.
- It provides amplification, noise filtering, analog-to-digital conversion and data acquisition of ECG signal. In addition, it has the ability to monitor its battery status and manage its power usage.
- It samples the ECG signal at high resolution of 12-bit and with the sampling rate of 500 samples per second. Therefore, the digitized ECG signal is suitable for use in the analysis and measurement of PQRST waves of the patient's ECG.
- This battery operated portable device has safety medical standards that comply with IEC601-1, AAMI EC11 (protective class).

The ECG software has the following characteristics:

- It can control the recorder hardware and get the digitized ECG data from the hardware via serial port.
- It provides the display of the real time ECG signal, patient's heartbeat rate and the battery status when recording ECG. When viewing the recorded ECG signal, the user can scroll through the signal by a scroll bar. Besides that, the ECG signal can be zoomed to five different sizes.
- It compresses the ECG data before saving the data to a file and expands it when the file is loaded. This makes the ECG file small and easy to send through the Internet.

6.1 Suggestion for future expansion

The following improvements can be made to make the system more powerful and useful.

- The program can be expanded to be a client-server program so that the patient's ECG file can update directly to the medical center's database and thus providing a more secure transmission.
- The security part of the program can be further improved by providing some data encryption to the ECG file so that only the intended person can view the patient's ECG data.
- Besides that, the program can be developed so that it includes digital filter to further reduce the noise level.

- The prototype can be expanded to make it work with handheld devices such as palm top to make the recorder mobile. The ECG recorded at the handheld device can then be downloaded on the computer.
- To make the recorder a wireless device by adding the radio communication circuitry to the recorder hardware and computer.
- To view of more flexibility, this device can be modified further to work with direct telephone line interface whereby the communication and ECG data will be transferred to the server automatically. A modem and a communication protocol need to be embedded with this device.

7. References

Application of Embedded Technology on a Portable ECG Recorder, Posted on April 8, 2010 by China Papers, http://mt.china-papers.com/2/?p=116829

Bonnie C. Baker, Anti-aliasing, analog filters for data acquisition systems, Microchip Technology Inc., 1999.

Claydokjun S and Chitsakul K, "Real Time Electrocardiogram Compression Technique Using Wavelet transform On MCS-51," 16th Biennial International Eurasip Conference Biosignal 2002.

Claydokjun S and Chitsakul K, "Real Time Electrocardiogram Compression Technique Using Wavelet transform On MCS-51," 16th Biennial International Eurasip Conference Biosignal 2002.

Daskalov, I. K., I. I. Christov, Electrocardiogram Signal Preprocessing for Automatic Detectioin of QRS boundaries, *Medical Engineering & Physics* 21, 1999, pp 37–44.

Edmond Zahedi, Wong Meng Meng, Chye Jun Lee, Development of a Portable Electrocardiogram Event Recorder with Digital Memory, Department of Electrical, Electronic and System Engineering, Universiti Kebangsaan Malaysia, 1999.

Farah Magrabi, Nigel H. Lovell, Branko G. Celler, (1999) A web-based approach for electrocardiogram monitoring in the home, *International Journal of Medical Informatics* 54, 1999, pp 145–153.

Ho, C.S.; Chiang, T.K.; Lin, C.H.; Lin, P.Y.; Cheng, J.L.; Ho, S.H.; , "Design of portable ECG recorder with USB storage. Electron Devices and Solid-State Circuits, 2007. EDSSC 2007. IEEE Conference.

ITU SG-2 Q14/2 Document 2/195 (Rev.1)-E "Telemedicine Directory". by Rapporteur for Question 14/2; 6 July 2001.

James W.Grier.Comparison of three handheld 1-lead ECG / EKG recorders. NDSUEDU.2008.

John D. Halamka, Carsten Osterland, Charles Safran, CareWeb™, a Web-based Medical Record for an Integrated Health Care Delivery System, *International Journal of Medical Informatics* 54, 1999, pp 1–8.

K. Janda, K. Chitsakul, Portable ECG monitor/record with wireless data transmission, The 3rd International Symposium on Biomedical Engineering (ISBME 2008).

Kohki Shinozaki Risk management of QT-prolonging Drugs by community pharmacists by using a mobile electrocardiography.The Pharmaceutical Society of Japan.2010.

Metting , A. C. Van Rijn, A. Peper, C. A. Grimbergen, High Quality Recording of Bioelectric Events: Interference Reduction, Theory and Practice, Academic Medical Center, Netherlands, 1998.

Metting, A. C. Van Rijn, A. Peper, C. A. Grimbergen, Amplifiers for Bioelectric Events: a Design with a Minimal Number of Parts, Academic Medical Center, 1998.

Metting, A. C. Van Rijn, A. Peper, C. A. Grimbergen, High Quality Recording of Bioelectric Events II: A Low-noise, Low-power Multichannel Amplifier Design, Academic Medical Center, Netherlands, 1998.

Tamas Hornos, Wireless ECG/EEG with the MSP430 Microcontroller,Dept. Of Electronics and Electrical Engineering, University of Glasgow, Thesis for Master of Science, 2009

Tikkanen, P. E., L. C. Sellin, H. O. Kinnunen, H. V. Huikuri, Using simulated noise to define optimal QT intervals for computer analysis of ambulatory ECG, *Medical Engineering & Physic* 21, 1998, pp 15–25.

28

Implications of Corporate Yoga: A Review

Rudra B. Bhandari[1], Churna B. Bhandari[2], Balkrishna Acharya[3], Pranav Pandya[4], Kartar Singh[5], Vinod K. Katiyar[6] and Ganesh D. Sharma[7]

[1]*University of Patanjali, Haridwar, Uttarakhand,*
[2]*Department of Physics, Case Western University, Ohio,*
[3]*University of Patanjali, Haridwar, Uttarakhand,*
[4]*Dev Sanskriti Vishwavidyalaya, Uttarakhand,*
[5]*University of Patanjali, Haridwar, Uttarakhand,*
[6]*Department of Mathematics, Indian Institute of Technology, Roorkee, Uttarakhand,*
[7]*Department of Yogic Sciences, University of Patanjali, Haridwar, Uttarakhand,*
[1,3,4,5,6,7]*India*
[2]*USA*

1. Introduction

Yoga is an art of life management and a universal means for self realization. Health benefits and improvement of human intelligence are inseparable byproducts of yoga practices that can be achieved by every practitioner. Aurobindo (1999) defines yoga as "a practical discipline incorporating a wide variety of practices whose goal is the development of a state of mental and physical health, well-being, inner harmony and ultimately a union of the human individual with the universal and transcendent existence". Yoga is an ancient discipline designed to bring balance and health to the physical, mental, emotional, and spiritual dimensions of the individual (Iyengar, 1976). In contemporary scenario, a part of oriental wisdom, yoga has been widely known even in western countries and a substantial number of people have been practicing it for different purposes such as physical fitness, flexibility, stress management, psychological well being, emotional rectification, good habits cultivation and disease management as adjunct therapy. Only USA invests 5.7 billion US dollars annually for yoga classes and yoga products (Macy, 2008). A substantial number of women have been found practicing yoga in UK and other countries. The emergence of many more yoga studios in Europe and South Asia and research studies made pertaining diverse efficacies of yoga portray its ascending popularity and scientific validation and standardization by scientific community.

At present, there are number of scientific researches that substantiate preventive, rehabilitative, therapeutic and excelling powers of yoga at individual and corporate levels (Becker, 2000; Jacobs, 2001; Khalsa, 2004; Ornish, 2009). One of the most exciting developments in the last few decades is the cross fertilization of western science with ideas from Eastern wisdom system such as yoga. With increasing precision, scientists are able to look at the body, mind and spirit and detect the sometime subtle changes than practitioners of yoga and meditation undergo. A scientific interpretation of yogic effects has been made on the basis of bio-psycho-socio-spiritual research model (Evans et al., 2009).

On the other hand, a flood of chronic diseases (cardiac problems, diabetes, cancer, lower back pain, obesity, depression etc.) (World Economic Forum [WEF], 2010, p. 9), organizational misbehaviors (work place incivility, insidious and insulting behaviors, social undermining, theft of company assets, acts of destructiveness, vandalism and sabotage, substance abuse and misconduct perpetrated against fellow employees) (Fox & Spector, 2005), interpersonal conflict/work-life conflict and dearth of spiritual leadership have been met as the precursors for global recessions and workplace disharmony. Therefore, most of the today's successful companies of the world have prioritized workplace yoga/spirituality as an emerging avenue for corporate- wellness (CW) and excellence (CE).

"The business of business and business of life are one. The reason for living and working is to act and the reason to act is to seek excellence in everything that you do" (Sinclair, n.d, as cited in Pruzen & Pruzan, 2001). This quotation from a CEO and chairman of a leading company (Tan Range Exploration, Ltd., USA/Tanzania) portrays the relevance of spiritual insight for business management and performance excellence. Persistent practice of yoga and allied disciplines as a part of corporate culture improves somatic, psychic, social and spiritual health and intelligence of an individual and organizational workforce.

Additionally, levels of four human intelligences- spiritual (SI), emotional (EI), creative (CI) and rational (RI), acquired by an individual govern his/her way of feeling, thinking and behavior and undoubtedly can be regarded as the determiners of human personality and human excellence too. Optimal health (physical, mental, social and spiritual) and the four elements of intelligence (SI, EI, CI and RI) that can be acquired and sustained by prolonged yoga practices underpin individual or CW and CE.

Health problems- stress or distress, obesity, low backache, respiratory disorders, cardiovascular problems, digestive disorders and genitourinary disorders are prevalent at corporate world and cause a huge decline in the corporate health and wealth. On the other hand, regular yoga practice is found more helpful for total health promotion, disease prevention and rehabilitation as well. Particularly, yoga has been found effective to manage work related stress, respiratory disorders (asthma, pulmonary tuberculosis, pleural effusion, obstructive pulmonary diseases, chronic bronchitis), cardiovascular disorders (ischemic heart disease, coronary artery disease, angina, chronic heart failure, hypertension), digestive disorders (irritable bowel syndrome, hyperacidity, colitis, indigestion, diabetes, gastroesophageal reflux disease, hepatitis, gall stones, celiac disease) and genitourinary problems (urinary stress incontinence, women sexuality, climacteric syndrome, premature ejaculation, pregnancy outcomes, labor pain and duration). Thus, this writing is contained with sub-headings that describe the efficacy of CY to manage aforesaid health problems.

Being a secular, global, holistic and cost effective tool for boosting holistic health and awakening four faculties of human intelligence, yoga needs to include as a part of corporate culture along with scientific researches to substantiate its multidimensional efficacies. So the prime theme of this chapter is to highlight contemporary significance of corporate yoga (CY) to enrich health, happiness and harmony at workplace by promoting CW and CE. More specifically, the chapter is intended to argue-

1. The concept and contemporary significance of CY
2. Link among yoga, health care and four human intelligences
3. Efficacy of yoga for CW and CE
4. Preventive and therapeutic value of yoga relating to work related stress, respiratory disorders, cardiovascular disorders, digestive disorders and genitourinary disorders.

2. Contemporary significance of CY

Sages of yore have argued eternal significance of yoga for the welfare of entire mankind and global harmony. Same has been reinstated by contemporary enlightened masters such as Shriram Sharma Acharya, Swami Vivekananda, Maharishi Aurovindo, Swami Shivanand and Swami Rama so forth on the basis of their experiential and experimental knowledge. The father of scientific spirituality, Shriram Sharma Acharya defines yoga as "an art of living". This contemporized definition of yoga implies that yoga is nearer to life business or management. Correspondingly, business of business and business of life are one and the reason for living and working is to seek excellence in everything that we do (Sinclair, n.d, as cited in Pruzen & Pruzan, 2001). Interestingly, this indicates art of self business (yoga) as a foundation of sustainable corporate business and success. This substantiates the contemporary significance of CY for CW and CE. The contemporary significance of CY for corporate success can be concisely discussed in three sub heads- concept, popularity and health impacts of yoga for the ease of readers' comprehension.

2.1 Concept of Yoga

Yoga is a Sanskrit word that means union, to yoke or to unify; the merging of the microcosm of our existence in our body with the macrocosm. In other words, this also implies the fusion of embodied consciousness with cosmic consciousness (Chaoul & Cohen, 2010). The famous yoga exponent, sage Patanjali defines the yoga as "the inhibition of psychic modifications (Patanjali Yoga Sutra, 1:2)" that ultimately results in the fission of *Prakriti* (the equilibrium condition of three strands- *sat, raj* and *tam* that is eternal but changeable) and *Purusha* (pure consciousness that is immortal, eternal, omnipresent, omniscience and omnipotent). The next famous ancient text of yoga, Shrimad Bhagvat Geeta (SBG) defines the yoga as "a state of mental equanimity at each moment of the life" (SBG, 2:47). Subsequently, SBG also defines yoga from the behavioral perspective as "the excellence in action" (SBG, 2:48). In the West, yoga is often referred to as a mind-body technique from Asia, usually categorized as meditation (for those seated practices) and yoga (practices that include movement and the active participation of the body) (Chaoul & Cohen, 2010). Thus, yoga is perceived as an overarching category that includes all Asian mind-body practices, whether from India (Hatha yoga, etc.), Tibet (Tsa lung Trul khor [rTsa rlung 'Phrul 'khor]), China (T'ai chi, qi gong) or other Asian origin. Nonetheless, in Indian context, yoga is more than mind-body practices that also incorporates spiritual practices.

Basically, four major streams of yoga: *Karma Yoga* (The yogic path of undertaking selfless deeds by using attained wisdom, power and prosperity), *Bhakti Yoga* (The yogic path of devotion), *Jnana Yoga* (The yogic path that prioritizes rational thinking over knowledge), and *Raj Yoga* (The eightfold yogic path synthesized by sage Patanjali 5000 years ago) can be met in Indian classical texts. However, Raj Yoga as conceptualized by sage Patanjali is supposed to have synthesized all yogic paths as a garland. It has metaphorically comprised of eight subsequent limbs (a tree of eight limbs): *Yama* (universal ethics/social codes), *Niyama* (individual ethics), *Asana* (physical postures), *Pranayama* (breath control), *Pratyahara* (control of the senses), *Dharana* (concentration), *Dhyan* (meditation), and *Samadhi* (bliss). Indeed, this path of *Raj Yoga* is an integral form of *Karma Yoga, Bhakti Yoga,* and *Jnana Yoga* that can be adopted by any individual for total health and ascetic elevation (spiritual advancement). Correspondingly, Satyanand (2000) argued that from the perspective of yoga psychology (*Raj Yoga*), human personality can be categorized into four types: dynamic, emotive, rational and volitional (p. 16).

Karma Yoga is preferred yogic path for an individual with active personality who can traverse inner journey of psychic refinement through selfless deeds. An individual with emotive personality may love *Ishwarparnidhan* (*Bhakti Yoga*) for psychic refinement and subsequently inhibition of psychic modifications. The path of *Jnana Yoga* is an optimal yogic way that prioritized by rational personalities. Eminent yoga scholar and seer, Patanjali put forth *Raj Yoga* (the royal path of yoga) that is equally applicable to each aspirant desired for perfect health, happiness, harmony, and ultimate bliss. Obviously, that is an integral and concise yogic way for all possible personalities.

2.2 Popularity of Yoga

Popularity of yoga practice in the West is in ascending order since 1960 and particularly in UK, where yoga classes are open to everyone although women tend to make up 70 to 90 per cent of the student base of most classes as well as the majority of yoga teachers (Newcombe, 2007). Moreover, perceived better physical health and emotional well-being by the yoga practice is an important reason for women's more participation in the classes. Additionally, yoga also served as an important support for women becoming more aware of feelings of alienation from traditional biomedical practitioners. "Only US invest $5.7 billion dollars per year in yoga classes by involving 15.8 million people. Among US yoga practitioners, 72.2 percent are women who practice yoga to be slim, flexible, de-stressed and attractive (Macy, 2008). In a national population-based telephone survey (n = 2055), 3.8% of respondents reported using yoga in the previous year and cited wellness (64%) and specific health conditions (48%) as the motivation for doing yoga (Saper et al., 2004). In South Asian countries, everyone has craze for yoga and yoga has greater space in corporate circles too. Turnover of yoga business in Asia is more than 50 crore per year and a large number of corporate personnel are being trained in yogic ways of stress management and mind management in Pure Yoga Studio of the Hong Kong (Singh, 2009). Moreover, the rise of yoga masters like Swami Ramdev has promoted mass media communication of yoga worldwide.

2.3 Yoga versus health

A famous yoga exponent of contemporary time, Aurobindo (1999) defines yoga as "a practical discipline incorporating a wide variety of practices whose goal is the development of a state of mental and physical health, well-being, inner harmony and ultimately a union of the human individual with the universal and transcendent existence". Iyengar (1976) defines yoga as an ancient discipline designed to bring balance and health to the physical, mental, emotional, and spiritual dimensions of the individual. These two definitions of the yoga given by Aurobindo and Iyengar clearly hint its bio-psycho-socio-spiritual efficacy for attainment and maintenance of total health (physical, mental, social and spiritual health) as an elementary benefit and a byproduct if practiced persistently.

The *Hatha Yoga* is widely known in the present scenario, especially in the west, is supposed to be an elementary practice for the practice of *Raj Yoga* which includes body cleansing techniques (*Shatkarmas*), postural exercises (*Asanas*), gestures (*Mudras*), psychic locks (*Bandhas*), breath control (*Pranayama*), concentration (*Dharana*) and meditation (*Dhyana*).

Yoga practice consists of the five-principles including proper relaxation, proper exercise, proper breathing, proper diet, positive thinking and meditation (Chanavirut, Khaidjapho, Jaree & Pongnaratorn, 2006). Impacts of yoga practices can be better explained via bio-psycho-socio-spiritual model- at physical level it improves musculoskeletal functioning, cardiopulmonary status, autonomic nervous system (ANS) response and endocrine functioning; at psychosocial level, it enhances self-esteem, social support and positive mood; and at spiritual level it elevates compassionate understanding and mindfulness (Evans et al., 2009). Same hypothesis is supported as "well-rounded yoga practice may have benefits on structural, physiological, psycho-emotional and spiritual levels" (Herrick & Ainsworth, 2000).

Mechanisms underlying the modulating effects of yogic cognitive-behavioral practices (e.g., meditation, *Asanas*, *Pranayama*, caloric restriction) on human physiology can be classified into four transduction pathways: humoral factors, nervous system activity, cell trafficking, and bio-electromagnetism that shed light how yogic practices might optimize health, delay aging, and ameliorate chronic illness and stress from disability (illness and stress from disability) (Kuntsevich, Bushell, &Theise, 2010). Moreover, they provided standpoints for in-depth study of underlying mechanisms by postulating three possible hypotheses regarding mechanisms of yogic effects. Correspondingly, yogic practices may: 1) promote restoration of physiologic setpoints to normal after derangements secondary to disease or injury, 2) promote homeostatic negative feedback loops over non-homeostatic positive feedback loops in molecular and cellular interactions, and 3) quench abnormal ''noise'' in cellular and molecular signaling networks arising from environmental or internal stress. The detailed elaboration of the proposed hypotheses is beyond the scope of this writing unless it is quite intriguing and comprehensive that includes all possible modes of varied yogic effects (effects of *Asanas*, *Pranayams*, varieties of meditations and caloric restriction) till now.

It is claimed that these techniques bring an individual to a state of perfect health, stillness and heightened awareness by increasing the body's store of *prana*, or flow of vital energy (Kulkarni & Bera, 2009; Nayak & Shankar, 2004).Other claimed benefits of regular yoga practice leads to suppleness, muscular strength, feelings of well-being, reduction of sympathetic drive, pain control and longevity (Brown & Gerbarg, 2009; Garfinkel & Schumacher, 2000; Lipton, 2008). Yogic breathing exercises allegedly reduce muscular spasms and expand available lung capacity (Brown & Gerbarg, 2005).Yoga is thus advocated as a symptomatic treatment for a wide range of conditions, including anxiety, arthritis, back pain, cardiovascular problems, gastrointestinal complaints, headaches, insomnia, premenstrual syndrome, respiratory problems and stress (Ernst & Soo, 2010). However, substantial evidences from clinical trials also should be undertaken to generalize the therapeutic efficacy of yoga.

3. Yogic prescription for CW and CE

Yogic prescription (YP) is a sort of yogic capsule that is comprised of yogic practices from all major yogic streams (*Jnana, Bhakti, Karma and Raj*) and designed as per workplace problems met at individual and organizational level. YP presumes nine hurdles (physical or mental illness, dullness, doubt, procastination, laziness, over indulgence, delusion, inability and instability) behind inidvidual and corporate failure and basically targets their dissolution (Pandya, 2006, p. 118) via its prolonged practice. The components of YP may vary as per nature of participants and workplace. Nonetheless, YP considers four possbile types of human personality (rational, emotive, dyanmic, and volitional) and incorporates yogic practices from aforesaid four yogic streams accordingly. Dissolution of these hurdles via sustained YP practice leads to complete harmony (homogenity among feeling, thinking and action), harmony leads to talent, talent results in creativity and innovations, creativity results in perfection that further results in excellence as depicted in Figure 1.

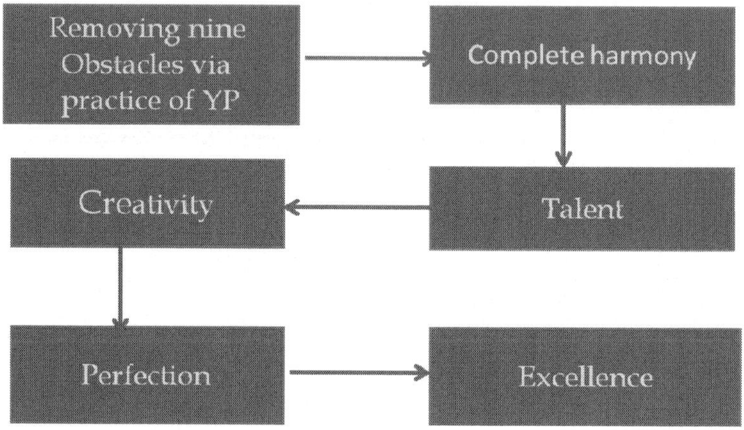

Fig. 1. Tentative model showing emergence of excellence via YP practice.

YPs have been found effective for health promotion and diseases management. Mind-body interventions derived from yoga (including breathing, meditation, postures, concentration and visualization) ameliorate stress-related mental and physical disorders—asthma, high blood pressure, cardiac illness, elevated cholesterol, IBS, cancer, insomnia, multiple sclerosis, and fibromyalgia (Becker 2000; Jacobs 2001). Curative effect of yoga has been seen in psychiatric problems, cardiovascular problems (CAD, hypertension), respiratory disorders (Bronchial asthma, OPD, pneumonia etc.), diabetes, neurological problems, musculoskeletal disorders, and others (Khalsa 2004). Ornish (2009) asserted that lifestyle changes (yogic way of living) could be considered not only as preventing chronic diseases but also reversing their progression—as an intensive non-surgical, non-pharmacological intervention. Moreover, the coronary heart disease, prostate and breast cancer, diabetes, and obesity account for 75% of health-care costs, yet the progression of these diseases can be stopped or even reversed with intensive lifestyle changes. Falus et al. (2010) highlighted the considerable connection between the length of telomeres and intensive changes in lifestyle and nutrition as well as behavioral and psychological factors. Epel et al. (2009) concluded that some forms of meditation might have salutary effects on telomere length by reducing cognitive stress and stress arousal and increasing positive states of mind and hormonal factors that might promote telomere maintenance. Between times one (before the Life Force Yoga program) and two (two weeks after learning it), participants reported 64% decrease in total mood disturbance, 53% decrease in average depression scores and overall mood disturbance continued to drop after two months (Bennett, Weintraub & Khalsa 2008).

Besides, the enhancement of SI, EI, CI and RI and their harmonious interplay by yogic practices is also substantiated by various scientific researches which are deemed essential for love and happiness at workplace: visionary leadership, sound management practices, creativity and innovations, and optimal work performance. Interestingly, levels of SI and EI are more about love and happiness at workplace. Moreover, happiness assists organization's members to be more productive, creative, fulfilled and with high morale that lead to outstanding performance and therefore, have a direct impact on organization's financial success (Claude & Zamor, 2003).

But the level of these four intelligences varies from person to person as per their personality types (dynamic, emotive, rational and mystic). Therefore, that holistic YP designed to promote CW and CE needs to include selected practices from *Ganan, Bhakti, Karma and Raj yoga.* Moreover, YP must include yogic practices of gross body, subtle body and causal body. As per author's self experience, pervious research findings and needs assessed in corporate companies, different tentative YPs can be designed that need to be tested to assess their effectiveness for promotion of four human intelligences and holistic health.

3.1 Yoga for CW

Yoga may be an integral part of worksite health promotion program (WHPP). "WHPP is an organized program in the worksite that is intended to assist employees and their family members (and/or retirees) in making voluntary behavior changes which reduce their health and injury risks, improve their health consumer skills and enhance their individual productivity and well-being whereas wellness is an intentional choice of a lifestyle characterized by personal responsibility, moderation, and maximum personal enhancement of physical, mental, emotional and spiritual health. Wellness programs typically begin by focusing on the reduction of health risks and then target issues that affect personal productivity, general well being, quality of work-life, personal growth, and other areas of interest" (Hunnicutt & Chapman, 2006, p. 4). On the other hand, CW is a good physical, mental, social and spiritual health of an individual and organizational workforce.

Royal path of yoga includes subsequent steps: *Yam, Niyam, Asana, Pranayama, Pratyahara, Dharana, Dhyan* and *Samadhi*. *Yama* (social codes) is the practice of improving social health and harmony that incorpates five vows: non-violence, truthfulness, non-stealing, non-possessiveness and celibacy. *Niyam* (moral codes) is the practice for creating homogeneity and harmony among feelings, thinking and action and comprised of five code of conducts- purity, contentment, austerity, self-study and complete surrender to God.

Asana (posture) is the practice for improving physical health, physical flexibility and fitness; overcoming conflicts, and maintaining steady posture for meditation. Yoga quietens the body and mind through vascular and muscular relaxation (Monro, 1995). Maintaining of posture was thought to lead strengthening and relaxation of voluntary muscles and eventually to control over the autonomic nervous system (ANS) (Vahia et al. 2004). In the same way, another study had reported that intensive practice of postural sequences as *Surya Namaskar* for longer than 10 minutes was associated with sufficiently elevated metabolic and heart response to improve cardio-respiratory fitness (Hagins et al., 2007). The continuous extension and flexion of muscles during yoga poses is associated with activation of antagonistic neuromuscular system as well as tendon-organ feedback resulting in increased range of motion and relaxation (Riley, 2004).

Pranayama is the fourth step in the *Ashtanga* yoga system of Patanjali. The control of the breath leads to the control of the life force or *prana* and mind. The ancient yogis have propounded many breathing techniques to maximize the benefits of *prana* at somatic and psychic level. The word "*Pranayama*" is made up of two words, *Prana* and *Ayama*. *Prana* stands for the capacity to keep body alive by air, i.e breath and *Ayama* means expansion, stretching or extension and control of breath. Thus, Pranayama means the art of controlling breath. *Pranayama* is basically undertaken for somatic and psychic purification, regulation of *prana* to each body organ and to optimize the cardio-pulmonary and autonomic functions. The ancient yogis of yore searched the intimate connection between breath and mind. Breath control has indirect influence over the mind thereby showing mind-body interplay. Breathing is an automatic process controlled by the autonomic nervous system. The science of bio-energy including the breathing movements is the practical yoga par excellence. One of the main texts of *Hatha Yoga, Hatha Yoga Pradeepika*(HP) advocates that unsteady flow of *prana* in body leads to unsteady mind and vice-versa (HP, 2:2). The ancient yoga texts state that *Pranayam* practiced properly can cure all diseases, but if practiced wrongly can onset diseases. Therefore, *Pranayama* needs to be learned under the supervision of an experienced teacher by taking needful precautions.

Breathing is the most important bodily function. Learning of breath control helps control body metabolism. There are generally 10 types of *Pranayama* (techniques of breath control) but five (*Bhastrika, Kapalbhati, Anulom-Vilom, Bharamari* and *Udgeeth Pranayama*) of them are found more in practice due to their prominent benefits. *Pranayam* (breathing mechanics for control and expansion of *prana*) is the practice for attaining a sound mental health by channeling *pranic* flow in subtle energy channels, expanding and controlling *pranic* energy. Its regular practice regulates secretions of endocrine hormones and neuro-hormones. The voluntary control of breath can modulate autonomic nervous system functions including cardiac vagal tone as measured by heart rate variability (Lehrer 1999; Sovik 2000), vigilance and attention (Fokkema 1999), chemoreceptor and baroreflex sensitivity (Bernardi 2001; Spicuzza 2000), as well as the level of central nervous excitation (Brown & Gerbarg 2005). *Pranayam* like *Ujjayi* breathing increases vagal tone, heart rate variability (HRV) (Telles and Desiraju 1992) and respiratory sinus arrhythmia (RSA) (Carney et al. 1995) by inducing parasympathetic activity through numerous mechanisms, including slow breath rate, contraction of the laryngeal musculature, inspiration against airway resistance and breath holds (Cappo & Holmes 1984). Furthermore, they emphasized that slow breathing with prolonged expiration was shown to reduce psychological and physiological arousal, anxiety, panic disorder, depression, IBS, early Alzheimer's disease and obesity (Friedman & Thayer 1998; Haug et al. 1994). Thus, *Pranayam* is the best practice of boosting morale, will power, self-confidence and mind-body health.

Deep yoga breathing exercises like *Bhastrika* reduce the work load on the heart in two ways. Firstly, deep breathing leads to more efficient lungs, which means more oxygen is brought into contact with blood sent to the lungs by the heart. So, the heart doesn't have to work hard to deliver oxygen to the tissues. Secondly, deep breathing leads to a greater pressure differential in the lungs, which leads to an increase in the circulation, thus resting the heart a little. Deep breathing improves the quality of the blood by promoting increased oxygenation in the lungs and thereby aiding the elimination of toxins and morbid matters; increases the digestion and assimilation of food by promoting enriched oxygen supply to stomach; and improves the health of the nervous system, including the brain, spinal cord, nerve centers and nerves by promoting supply of oxygenated blood accompanied by nutrients. This improves the health of the whole body, since the nervous system communicates to all parts of the body. Moreover, it rejuvenates glands, especially the pituitary and pineal glands. The brain has a special affinity for oxygen, requiring three times more oxygen than the rest of the body. This has far-reaching effects on well being. The movements of the diaphragm during the deep breathing exercise massage the abdominal organs - the stomach, small intestine, liver and pancreas. The upper movement of the diaphragm also massages the heart. This stimulates the blood circulation in these organs. The lungs become healthy and powerful, a good insurance against respiratory problems. Deep and slow yoga breathing reduces the work load for the heart. The result is more efficient and stronger heart that operates better and lasts longer. It also means controlled blood pressure and less chances of heart disease. Deep, slow breathing assists in weight control. If we are overweight, the extra oxygen burns up the excess fat more efficiently. If we are underweight, the extra oxygen feeds the starving tissues and glands. Slow, deep and rhythmic breathing causes a reflex stimulation of the parasympathetic nervous system which results in a reduction in the heart rate and relaxation of the muscles. These two factors cause a reflex relaxation of the mind, since the mind and body are very interdependent. In addition, oxygenation of the brain tends to normalize brain function and reduce excessive anxiety levels. The breathing exercises cause subsequent contractions of lung tissues thereby increasing elasticity of the lungs and rib cage. This creates an increased breathing capacity all day, not just during the actual exercise period.

Alternate Nostril Breathing (ANB) produces optimum functions to both sides of the brain-optimum creativity and optimum logical verbal activity. Regulated and harmonious rhythms of left and right nostrils calm the mind and the nervous system. Substantial studies have proven that the nasal cycle is associated with brain function. The electrical activity of the brain was found to be greater on the opposite side of decongested nostril. The right side of the brain controls creative activity while the left side controls logical verbal activity. The researches have shown that predominance of left nostril activates the right side of the brain thereby bettering creative performance. Similarly, the predominance of the right nostril activates the left side of the brain and betters verbal skills.

The concept of yoga therapy seems more advance and ancient compared to modern medical science. Yoga therapy advocates that manifestation of every disease accompanies with unrhythmic breathing and disturbed nasal cycles. Moreover, the onset of each disease can be perceived just by checking nasal cycle. Alternate nostril breathing technique is met efficacious to regulate alternate predominant flow of left and right nostril and hence activation of just two opposite sides of the brain. This clears blockage of the nasal passage and reestablishes the natural nasal cycle. For example, the yogis have known for a long time that prolonged breathing through the left nostril only (over a period of years) causes asthma. They also knew that this so-called incurable disease can be easily cured by teaching the patient to breathe through the right nostril and then to prevent its recurrence by practicing the alternate nostril breathing technique. The yogis also believed that diabetes is caused to a large extent by breathing mainly through the right nostril.

Pratyhara (senses withdrawal) is the practice of conserving energy or *prana* by diverting senses inward from their external objects to seal outward *pranic* flow. It is an introspective practice of increasing bio-immunity, psycho-immunity and spiritual immunity at large. The prevalent practice like *Yoga Nidra* comes under *Pratyahara* in which practitioner goes in relaxed meditative state and gets dissociated from wish to act. Kjaer et al. (2002) made a study to investigate whether endogenous dopamine release increased during loss of executive control in meditation (*Yoga Nidra*) and found a 65% increase in endogenous dopamine release, concomitant increase in theta activity, decreased desire for action and heightened sensory imagery.

Dharana (concentration) is the practice of hitting target by being pin pointed. i.e., hundred percent focused mental flow at a particular target. The practice like mindful awareness, mindful based stress reduction technique, guided imagery and advance stage of *Yoga Nidra* come under this. Siegel (2009) hypothesized that mindful awareness induced internal attunement thereby catalyzing the fundamental process of integration. Moreover, he asserted that integration—the linkage of differentiated elements of a system led to the flexible, adaptive, and coherent flow of energy and information in the brain, the mind and relationships. *Dharana* has shown remarkable effect on brain activity. The brain is an electrochemical organ that uses electromagnetic energy to function. Electrical activity emanating from the brain is displayed in the form of brainwaves. There are four categories of these brainwaves. They range from delta with high amplitude and low frequency to beta with the low amplitude and high frequency. Men, women and children of all ages experience the same characteristic brainwaves. They are consistent across cultures and country boundaries. During meditation brain waves alter. Emission of Beta waves (13-30 cycles per second) is an indication of awaking awareness, extroversion, concentration, logical thinking and active conversation. A debater would be in high beta. A person making a speech, or a teacher, or a talk show host would all be in beta when they are engaged in their work. Emission of Alpha (7-13 cycles per second) is associated with relaxation, non-arousal, meditation and hypnosis. Emission of Theta (4-7 cycles per second) is associated with the activities like dreaming, day-dreaming, creativity, meditation, paranormal phenomena, Extra Sensory Perception (ESP) and shamanic journeys. Emission of Delta (1.5-4 or less cycles per second) is an indicator of deep and dreamless sleep. Mindfulness meditation and related techniques are intended to train attention for the sake of provoking insight. It can be thought as the opposite of attention deficit disorder. A wider, more flexible attention span makes it easier to be aware of a situation, easier to be objective in emotionally or morally difficult situations and easier to achieve a state of responsive, creative awareness or 'flow'.

Dhyan (meditation) is the prolonged concentration on a particular target that culminates in self-realization and paranormal accomplishments. The subsequent practice of meditation is supportive for awakening ESP and reaching self-realization. Neuroimaging studies had shown that meditation resulted in activation of the prefrontal cortex, the thalamus and inhibitory thalamic reticular nucleus and a resultant functional deafferentation of the parietal lobe (Mohandas, 2008). He further asserted that neurochemicals' (GABA, endogenous dopamine, epinephrine, nor-epinephrine, encephalin, acetylcholine etc.) changes as a result of meditative practice involved all the major neurotransmitter systems that contributed to ameliorate anxiety, depressive symptomatology and psycotogenic property. Meditation works because of the relationship between the amygdala and the prefrontal cortex. Simply, the amygdala is the part of the brain that decides when to get angry or anxious (among other things) and the pre-frontal cortex is the part that makes us stop and think about things (it is also known as the inhibitory centre). Moreover, intuitive flashes and ESPs are very common when mind gets tranquilized and calm in deep meditative stage. In such condition there happens harmonious interplay among conscious, subconscious and unconscious minds thereby causing intuition and ESPs.

Samadhi (trance or super-consciousness) is fusion of embodied consciousness with cosmic consciousness; a steady feeling of holism and interconnectedness. As per yoga, *Samadhi* is supposed as the stage of total health where an aspirant gets freed from the effects of three strands—*Sat, Raj and Tam* and realizes one's real self. On other word, it is *Nirudha* stage of psyche that represents the total health.

3.2 Yoga for CE

Leadership is one of the most important components of CE and is more about putting first things first to translate vision into action. Prolonged yoga practice is deemed responsive to develop spiritual traits- self awareness, field independence, humility, tendency to ask fundamentals- why; ability to reframe, positive use of adversity and sense of vocation (Zohar, 2005) that are essential for effective leadership and translating holy organizational vision into action. Correspondingly, this sub head will advocate yogic efficacy for promoting organizational excellence thereby excelling leadership and four human intelligences (SI, EI, CI and RI).

CE is the function of four intelligences—SI (farsightedness, serenity, discriminative wisdom, personal meaning production, critical existential thinking, transcedental awareness and concious state expension), EI (affectionate and loving relationship with family and society; memorizing God's compassion is unbounded, transfer of privilege, career development, team building, empathy, sound leadership and civility), CI (creativity and innovations) and RI (good managerial capabilities, job placements and technical performances) born by an organization family. The optimal level of these intelligences among organization family members can be induced by inculcating yogic culture among them. On the basis of the ladder proposed by *Raj yoga,* an interesting model for achieving CE can be set to overcome the nine hurdles. Removing aforesaid hurdles by appropriate yogic practices induces inner harmony; inner harmony induces talent, talent leads to creativity and innovations; creativity and innovation lead to perfection; and perfection culminates in excellence. On the other hand, employee health and performance are closely linked to each other. Good workers' health leads to productivity at the work; productivity at the work leads to business competitiveness; business competitiveness leads to economic development and prosperity; economic prosperity leads to social well being and wealth; social well being and wealth again help maintain good employee health (Burton, 2010) as depicted in Figure 2.

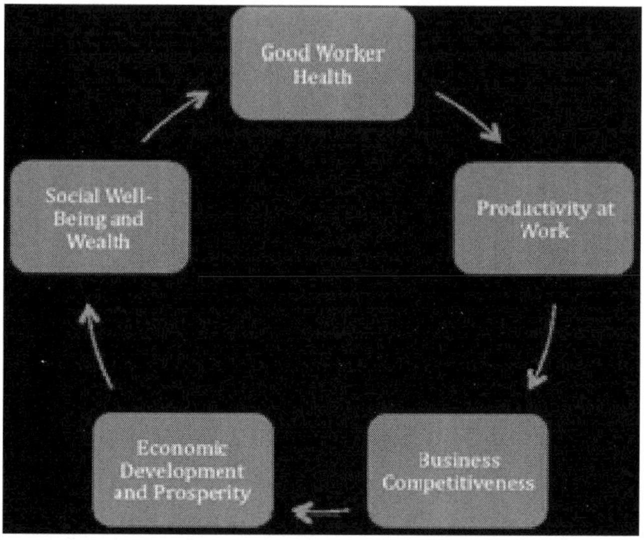

Fig. 2. Relationship between Health and Wealth.

This hierarchical relationship between health and wealth also displays the high possibility of achieving CW and CE via yoga practices. Therefore, total health and perfection need to be developed first at individual level for CW and CE by adopting persistent yoga practices. This may be plausiable by developing corporate yoga culture to provide equal chance of practicing yoga for each and every organizational family member.

4. Preventive and therapeutic value of Yoga

Preventive and therapeutic value of yoga has been argued as a side benefit of yogic practices especially associated with gross and subtle body and most of the yoga practitioners have been found to have the same concern. Substantial scientific studies undertaken have also attempted to substantiate the preventive and curative value of yoga practices like cleansing techniques (*Shatkriyas*), postures (*Asanas*), breathing techniques (*Pranayamas*), gestures (*Mudras*), psychic locks (*Bandhas*), concentration (*Dharana*) and meditation (*Dhyan*). As far as preventive and curative value of CY for CW is concerned, it is deemed contextual to discuss efficacy of CY in the connection of the most prevalent corporate health problems such as work related stress, respiratory problems, cardiovascular problems, digestive problems and genitourinary problems.

4.1 Yoga versus stress

Globalization, technological advancements, intermixing of work cultures, recessions and subsequent changes in the nature of work are in fast pace. Consequently, stress is found with everyone at workplace whether rich or poor, young or old, male or female; no one is immune from it. Stress may be the biggest single cause for illness or premature death. WHO has declared stress as worldwide epidemic and reported job stress as "the twentieth-century disease". The American Institute of Stress (AIS) states that stress related illness costs economy more than $ 100 billion per year. Additionally, AIS estimated in 2001 that stress costs organizations $ 300 billion in healthcare, workers compensation, absenteeism, and turnover. The productivity losses hover around $17 billion annually. Every health problem from simple headache to heart attack, from psychosomatic disorders to stroke can be linked to stress that is called the plague of the 21st century. Stress-related illness and injuries account for almost three-fourths of employee absenteeism.

A growing body of research evidence supports the belief that certain yoga techniques may improve physical and mental health through down-regulation of the hypothalamic-pituitary-adrenal (HPA) axis and the sympathetic nervous system (SNS) (Ross & Thomas, 2010). The HPA axis and SNS are triggered as a response to a physical or psychologic demand (stressor), leading to a cascade of physiologic, behavioral, and psychologic effects, primarily as a result of the release of cortisol and catecholamines (epinephrine and norepinephrine). This response leads to the mobilization of energy needed to combat the stressor through the classic "fight or flight"syndrome. Over time, the constant state of hypervigilence resulting from repeated firing of the HPA axis and SNS can lead to dysregulation of the system and ultimately diseases such as obesity, diabetes, autoimmune disorders, depression, substance abuse, and cardiovascular disease (Sterling, 2004; McEwen, 2000, as cited in Ross & Thomas, 2010). Conversely, substantial studies have shown yoga to have an immediate downregulating effect on both the SNS/HPA axis response to stress. Studies show that yoga decreases levels of salivary cortisol (Michalsen, 2005; West, 2004), blood glucose (Gokal & Shillito, 2007; Khatri et al. 2007) as well as plasma rennin levels, and 24-hour urine norepinephrine and epinephrine levels (Selvamurthy et al., 1998). Yoga significantly decreases heart rate and systolic and diastolic blood pressure (Damodaran et al., 2002; McCaffrey, Ruknui, Hatthakit & Kasetsomboon, 2005; Selvamurthy et al., 1998) (as cited in Ross & Thomas, 2010) . Studies suggest that yoga reverses the negative impact of stress on the immune system by increasing levels of immunoglobulin A (Stuck et al., 2003) as well as natural killer cells (Rao et al., 2008) (as cited in Ross & Thomas, 2010). Yoga has been found to decrease markers of inflammation such as high sensitivity C-reactive protein as well as inflammatory cytokines such as interleukin-6 (Pullen et al., 2008) and lymphocyte-1B (Schultz et al., 2007) (as cited in Ross & Thomas, 2010).

Aforementioned studies show that yoga has an immediate quieting effect on the SNS or HPA axis response to stress unless the precise mechanism of action has not been determined. The proposed hypotheses substantiate that yoga exercises cause a shift toward parasympathetic nervous system dominance, possibly via direct vagal stimulation (Innes, Bourguignon and Taylor, 2005); significant reductions in low-frequency heart rate variability (HRV)—a sign of sympathetic nervous system activation—in depressed patients following an 8-week yoga intervention (Shapiro et al., 2007); decrease in anxiety (Gupta et al., 2006; Michalsen, 2005; Telles et al., 2006; West, 2004) and increase in emotional, social, and spiritual well-being(Moadel et al., 2007) (as cited in Ross &Thomas, 2010).

4.2 Yoga versus respiratory problems

Yogic practices are always undertaken with synchronization of action, mental awareness and breathing pattern. Particularly, *Pranayam, Bandha, Mudra and Asana* incorporate systemic and subsequent inhalation, exhalation, inner breath retention and outer breath retentions; contraction and relaxation of lung tissues and chest wall thereby affecting the cardiopulmonary function (lung function, heart rate, breath rate, heart rate variability, oxygen consumption, and CO_2 expulsion), endocrine secretions and neural secretions and function of associated visceral organs. *Asanas* (postures) are basically somatic techniques for physical conditioning; *Pranayam* is a technique for breath control (inhalation, exhalation and retention) and expansion of *prana* (life energy) that strengthens respiratory muscles and better ventilation; a *Mudra* (gesture) is a sort of seal- a body movement to hold energy, or concentrate awareness; and a *Bandha* is an energy lock, using muscular constriction to focus awareness (Raub, 2002). Early studies (Joshi et al., 1992; Makwana et al., 1988) reported improvement in some, but not all, measures of ventilation after breath control exercises alone. For example, Joshi et al. (1992) followed lung function in 75 males and females with an average age of 18.5 years during yoga breath-control exercises. After 6 weeks of practice, they reported significant increases in forced vital capacity (FVC), forced expiratory volume in 1 second (FEV1), peak expiratory flow rate (PEFR), maximum voluntary ventilation (MVV), as well as a significant decrease in breathing frequency (fB), and prolongation of breath-holding time. Other studies reported similar improvement in lung function after practicing yoga postures alone or combined with other yoga techniques. Konar et al. (2000) reported that the practice of *Sarvangasana* (shoulder stand) twice daily for 2 weeks significantly reduced resting HR and left ventricular end-diastolic volume in 8 healthy male subjects. Birkel and Edgren (2000) reported that yoga postures, breath control, and relaxation techniques taught to 287 college students (89 men and 198 women) in two 50-minute class meetings for 15 weeks significantly improved FVC of the lungs measured by spirometry. In a similar study, 1 hour of yoga practice each day for 12 weeks significantly improved FVC, FEV1, and PEFR in 60 healthy young women having 17 to 28 years of age(Yadav & Das, 2001).

Moreover, yogic interventions are also found beneficial for improving ailments like asthma (Bhagwat, Soman, & Bhole, 1981; Bhole, 1967; Nagendra & Nagarathna, 1986; Nagendra & Nagarathna, 1985; Jain & Talukdar, 1993; Sabina et al., 2005; Singh, Wisniewski, Britton, & Tattersfield, 1990; Vedanthan et al., 1998), pulmonary tuberculosis (Milani, Valli & Bhole, 1992; Prakasamma & Bhaduri, 2004; Visweswaraiah & Telles, 2004), pleural effusion (Prakasamma & Bhaduri, 1984), rhinitis (Sim, 1981), sinusitis(Rabago et al., 2002), chronic obstructive pulmonary diseases (Behera, 1998; Donesky-Cuenco, Nguyen, Paul & Carrieri-Kohlman, 2009; Kamath & Chauhan, 1982; Pomidori, Camigotto, Amatya, Bernardi & Cogo, 2009; Tandon, 1978), chronic bronchitis (Behera, 1998) (as cited in McCall, 2009).

Controlled clinical studies have shown that an integrated approach of yoga therapy (consisted of yoga exercises and postures for 25 minutes; slow, deep breathing for 10 minutes; slow mental chanting for 15 minutes; and a devotional session as a daily practice) to be beneficial in the clinical management of asthma. A 65-minute daily practice of yoga for 2 weeks improved PEFR, medication use, and asthma attack frequency in 53 patients when compared to an age-, gender-, and clinically matched control group (Nagarathna & Nagendra, 1985). In a long-term, follow-up (3 to 54 months) prospective study (Nagendra & Nagarathna, 1986) made among 570 asthmatics showed overall significant improvement in PEFR after a similar yoga training program. The greatest improvement was found in patients who had practiced yoga most frequently and intensively thereby showing asthma medication reduction among approximately 70% of the practitioners. The effects of two

Pranayamas on lung function, airway reactivity, respiratory symptoms, and medication use were assessed in 18 patients with mild asthma in a randomized, double-blind, placebo-controlled, crossover trial (Singh et al., 1990). The subjects were taught *Pranayamas* by using a breathing device called the Pink City lung (PCL; Pulmotech, Jaipur, India) exerciser that could be used with a matched placebo breathing device.

After a baseline measurement, the subjects were undergone through the practice of slow deep breathing for 15 minutes, two times a day for consecutive 2-week periods, randomly alternating the breathing devices for each practice period. Measured lung function variables (FEV1, FVC, PEFR), symptom scores, and medication use improved with the PCL device with small and statistically insignificant changes. However, there was a statistically significant increase in the dose of histamine required to produce a 20% decrease in FEV1, a provocative airway test commonly used to assess lung responsiveness to nonspecific bronchoconstrictors. The findings indicate that *Pranyama* may lead to an overall clinical improvement in mild asthma. In a subsequent letter to the editor, Stanescu (1990) commented on possible autonomic mechanisms suggested by Singh et al. (1990) that might lead to reduced airway responsiveness. Studies previously conducted by Stanescu et al. (1981) on healthy subjects showed the efficacy of controlled yoga breathing techniques (i.e., slow, near VC maneuvers accompanied by apnea at end inspiration and end expiration) for significant lowering of ventilatory responsiveness to increased carbon dioxide. Two early studies (Behera & Jindal, 1990; Jain & Talukdar, 1993) reported on quality of life benefits provided by the effects of various yoga exercises among asthmatics. Behera & Jindal (1990) assessed the benefits of daily yoga exercises contained with breath control and postures, over a 6- to 8-week period in 41 asthmatics. Although the authors reported an overall subjective improvement in asthma symptoms, objective lung function measurements showed improvement in some, no change and reduced in some. Jain and Talukdar (1993) reported a similar overall effect of yoga therapy on exercise capacity in 46 asthmatics and reported improvement in a 12-minute walking test, a modified Harvard step test, and a more subjective index of exercise tolerance. However, it was unclear if the improvements were due, in part, to a placebo response. In the more recent literature (after 1995), breath-control and relaxation techniques in both children and adults with asthma have been reported to improve some, but not all, measures of lung function (e.g., PEFR, MVV, FEV1, and FVC), decrease usage of medication, and increase exercise tolerance (Blanc-Gras et al., 1996; Khanam et al., 1996; Manocha et al., 2002; Sathyaprabha et al., 2001; Vedanthan et al., 1998). Large variability in the subject population, questionable compliance in the yoga treatment groups, and potentially adverse outcomes in some subjects further complicates interpretation of the effects specific to a particular relaxation technique (Ritz, 2001). Further studies are warranted, therefore, to better understand the mechanisms of response to yogic intervention and to determine its clinical value for asthmatics.

Behera (1998) reported improvement in shortness of breath and some lung function parameters in patients (*n*= 15) with the history of chronic bronchitis and age range 48 to 75 years (58.9 6±11.1 years) who received yoga therapy that consisted of breath control and 8 types of *asanas* for a period of 4 weeks. The patients had baseline assessment of their history of chronic bronchitis, including spirometry, medication strategy, and exercise tolerance. They were instructed yogic postures (e.g., *Vajrasana, Simhasana, Sarvangasana, Chakrasana & Matsyasana*) and breathing techniques for 1 week and were encouraged to practice daily with follow-up yoga sessions each subsequent week along with medication. Reevaluated clinical status and pulmonary function revealed a significant improvement in FEV1 and PEFR after second week and significant improvements in VC and PEFR after fourth week excluding a patient's reporting of perceptual decrease in shortness of breath. No changes were noted in the amount of medication taken. This preliminary study (with poor research design) was made among few patients for short duration. Unfortunately, no other studies examining the possible benefits of yoga on chronic obstructive lung disease have been published yet and hence generalization of the outcomes needs further studies to eliminate its limitations.

4.3 Yoga versus cardiovascular problems

Cardiovascular disease continues to be a significant health issue, contributing to more deaths than any other disease in developed countries while becoming the leading cause of death in developing countries worldwide (Yach, Leeder, Bell, & Kistnasamy, 2005, as cited in deJong, 2009). Although the risk factors for cardiovascular disease are well known, they remain poorly controlled in the United States (Glover, Grerenlund, Ayala, & Croft, 2005) leading to increased costs for treatment (American Heart Association, 2005, as cited in deJong, 2009). Smoking, hypertension, diabetes mellitus, obesity, poor dietary patterns, physical inactivity, alcohol consumption, elevated blood apolipoprotein levels, and psychosocial factors are estimated nine risk factors that account for approximately 90% of population-attributed risk for cardiovascular disease (Yusuf et al., 2004, as cited in deJong, 2009). Besides, emotional stress is one more major cause in the pathogenesis of cardiac diseases like ischemic heart disease (IHD) (Eastwood &Trevelyan, 1971, as cited in Ornish et al., 1983). Some emotions and behaviors are associated with IHD include intense anxiety, depression, feelings of helplessness, and "type A behavior," characterized by ambitiousness, competitiveness, impatience, and a sense of time urgency (Hackett & Rosenbaum , 1980, as cited in Ornish et al, 1983). Significant lipid risk factors for CVD are increased levels of serum cholesterol and triglycerides, increased low-density lipoprotein (LDL) cholesterol, decreased high-density lipoprotein (HDL) cholesterol, and increased concentration of apoB-carrying lipoproteins (Raub, 2002). In fact, Chiuve, McCullough, Sacks and Rimm (2006) estimated that 62% of all coronary events could be avoided if all men adhered to a low-risk lifestyle that included smoking abstinence, regular exercise, healthy diet, moderate alcohol intake, and the maintenance of a healthy weight (as cited in deJong, 2009). Consistent citation was also made by Ornish et al. (1983) that concluded that bio-behavioral techniques such as yoga (meditation, pranayama, and progressive relaxation) may reduce some of the cardiovascular risk factors- BP (Bensen, 1977) and plasma cholesterol levels (Patel, 1976; Cooper & Aygen, 1979). Yoga's potential benefit to patients with CVD has been reported by limited literature (Raub, 2002). Adoption of a yoga lifestyle can significantly reduce many of the risk factors for CVD, including increased body weight, altered blood lipid profile, and elevated blood pressure (BP) (Mahajan et al., 1999; Manchanda et al., 2000; Schmidt et al., 1997, as cited in Raub, 2002). As cited in Field (2010), Yogendra et al. (2004) reported benefits of one year long yoga life style among the patients of advanced coronary artery disease. They found 23% reduction in cholesterol in the yoga group as compared to 4% in the standard treatment control group. Besides, serum low density lipids also seen reduced more in the yoga group (26% versus 3% in the control group). In a similar study on coronary artery disease, a dietary change plus yoga group was compared to a group who only made dietary changes (Manchanda et al., 2000, as cited in Field, 2010). After one year of weekly sessions, the yoga group had fewer anginal episodes per week, improved exercise capacity, decreased body weight and lower serum total cholesterol levels. Low-density lipoprotein, cholesterol and triglyceride levels also decreased in the yoga group. Revascularization procedures (coronary angioplasty or bypass surgery) were less frequently required in the yoga group, and coronary angiography showed that more lesions regressed (20% versus 2%) and fewer lesions progressed (5% versus 37%) in the dietary change plus yoga group. Pullen et al. (2009) also reported improved cardiovascular endurance and decreased inflammatory markers (Interleukin-6 and C- reactive protein) in heart failure patients thereby showing similar effects of yoga as massage therapy. Schmidt et al. (1997) reported that a 3-month residential training program of yoga, meditation, and vegetarian nutrition decreased body mass, total serum and LDL cholesterol, fibrinogen, and BP (as cited in Raub, 2002). Mahajan et al. (1999) reported a similar reduction in risk factors for patients with coronary artery disease (CAD) and documented angina (chest pain) where subjects with risk factors for CAD were randomly assigned to a yoga intervention group (*n*=5 52) or a control group (*n* =5 41) (as cited in Raub, 2002). Both groups received lifestyle advice and the intervention group received additional yoga training. Serial evaluations at 4, 10, and 14 weeks showed a regular decrease in all lipid parameters, except for HDL, only in the patients with angina receiving yoga intervention. The most impressive of these studies was a 1-year prospective, randomized controlled trial of 42 men with angiographically documented CAD (Manchanda et al., 2000, as cited in Raub, 2002). A subgroup (*n* =5 21) treated with an active program of risk factor and diet control along with yoga and moderate aerobic exercise showed significant reduction in angina, improved exercise capacity, and greater reductions in body weight, total cholesterol, LDL cholesterol, and triglyceride than the control group (*n* = 5 21) treated conventionally with risk factor control and the American Heart Association (AHA) Step I diet.

Revascularization procedures also were less frequent in the yoga group and coronary angiography repeated at 1 year showed a significant regression of atherosclerotic lesions. The Lifestyle Heart Trial (Ornish et al., 1998) demonstrated that intensive lifestyle changes could lead to regression of CAD after only 1 year of a 5-year program. Forty-eight (48) patients with moderate-to-severe CAD were randomized to an intensive lifestyle change group or to a usual-care group. The lifestyle changes consisted of a 10% fat whole-food vegetarian diet, aerobic exercise, stress management training (yoga and meditation), smoking cessation, and group psychologic support. Clinical status was followed by quantitative coronary angiography and frequency of cardiac events. Of the 35 patients completing the 5-year follow-up, 20 in the experimental group showed a 4.5% relative improvement in cardiovascular status after 1 year and a 7.9% relative improvement after 5 years. The control group had a relative worsening of cardiovascular status after 1 and 5 years (5.4% and 27.7%, respectively), and more than twice as many cardiac events. Intensive lifestyle changes/yogic life style, therefore, can cause a regression of CAD. Nonetheless, the sparse of randomized controlled studies for assessing the efficacy of yogic intervention on CVD, especially in comparison to the conventional practice of Western medicine, has made it difficult to assess the direct benefits of an integrated yoga practice on patients with CAD.

Another most prevalent risk factor for cardiac problems is hypertension. Early studies on yoga intervention for hypertension investigated the value of total body relaxation postures, primarily *Savasana* (Chaudhary et al., 1988; Mogra and Singh, 1986, as cited in Raub, 2002). The authors reported reductions in BP that were similar to control by drug therapy or biofeedback;

however, small numbers of subjects were utilized in the studies and there were no controls. I hour daily yoga practice of three month decreased blood pressure, blood glucose, cholesterol and triglycerides and improved subjective well-being and quality of life among mild to moderate hypertensive participants (Damodaran et al., 2002, as cited in Field, 2010).

Yoga exercises twice a day for 11 weeks were found to be as effective as standard medical treatment in controlling measured variables of hypertension (Murugesan et al., 2000). In a randomized study, 33 hypertensive patients with 35 to 65 years of age, were assigned into three groups receiving yoga therapy, physician-provided medication, and no treatment (control group). Preanalysis/postanalysis regarding systolic and diastolic blood pressure, pulse rate, and body weight revealed that both the treatment groups (i.e., yoga and drug) were effective in controlling hypertension. Twenty male patients with essential hypertension (EH) were treated for 3 weeks with postural tilt stimulus (tilt table) or with postural yoga *asanas* to restore normal baroreflex sensitivity (Selvamurthy et al., 1998). Progressive autonomic changes were assessed by cardiovascular responses to head-up tilt and cold pressor stimulus, electroencephalographic indices, blood catecholamines, and plasma rennin activity. There was a significant reduction in blood pressure after 3 weeks in both treatment groups, indicating a gradual improvement in baroreflex sensitivity. A similar improvement in baroreflex sensitivity, and significant reductions in systolic and diastolic blood pressure, were seen in 81 patients (58-61 years of age) with stable chronic heart failure (CHF) who practiced slow and deep breathing (Bernardi et al., 2002). The same authors (Bernardi et al., 1998) previously reported that a slow rate of breathing in patients with CHF increases resting oxygen saturation, improves ventilation/perfusion mismatching, and improves exercise tolerance. These changes were obtained by simply modifying the breathing pattern, from a resting, spontaneous ventilation of approximately 15 breaths per minute to 6 breaths per minute, which seems to cause a relative increase in vagal activity and a decrease in sympathetic activity. The effects on baroreflex sensitivity were similar to those obtained with captopril treatment in patients with CHF (Osterziel et al., 1988). Captopril belongs to a group of drugs called angiotensin-converting enzyme (ACE) inhibitors that help to lower blood pressure and make the heart beat stronger. This medication is used to treat hypertension (high blood pressure) and heart failure.

4.4 Yoga versus digestive problems

Hectic and unnatural corporate life style (fast food, materialistic relationship, hectic schedule, distanced natural environment, odd duty hours, smoking, alcoholism, poor intake of mental and emotional diet etc.) has been a sufficient condition to trigger and progress digestive problems like hyper acidity, irritable bowel syndrome, gastritis, pancreatitis, flatulence, ulcerative colitis, diabetes, inflammatory bowel disease, constipation, indigestion, hiccups, gastroesophageal reflux disease (GERD), hepatitis, gall stones, celiac disease among corporate workforces. Additionally, because of being a major system of nutrients absorption and morbid matter elimination, disordered digestive system is sufficient to disturb homeostasis and to trigger varieties of somatic and psychological problems. Sages of yore have rightly spoken that good digestion is a key to radiant health and is the function of psychological well being. Yoga views the digestive system as a very sensitive mirror of the mind and encourages examining overall lifestyle choices, emotions and other mental components in the diagnosis and healing of the digestive problems (Butera, 2010, p. 14).

Within a few seconds of "flight or fight" response happened in the central nervous system due to distress, most of the blood in the body gets shunted out from the digestive system and into the major muscle groups. This negatively impacts on the contractions of the digestive muscles that help move food through the body as well as the fluids and secretions that are needed for healthy digestion. Consequently, persistent mental distress results in esophagus spasms, indigestion, nausea, diarrhea, constipation, stomach ulcers, celiacs disease, irritable bowel syndrome as well as other more severe digestive ailments.

Yogic life style (regular practice of a complete yogic approach including selected- cleansing techniques, postures, gestures, psychic locks, concentration, meditation, natural diet as per body constitution and season, exercising charter of righteousness, and observance of social and moral codes) is found beneficial for the proper digestion and elimination, and healing of various digestive disorders like hyper acidity, irritable bowel syndrome, gastritis, pancreatitis, flatulence, ulcerative colitis, diabetes, inflammatory bowel disease, constipation, indigestion, hiccups, Gastroesophageal reflux disease (GERD), Hepatitis, Gall stones, Celiac disease etc.

Practice of yogic postures causes sponge like squeezing in the soft tissues of the digestive organs, and encourages stale and waste-bearing fluids to be out of the tissues thereby facilitating the elimination of the morbid matters and subsequently supply of essential nutrients to these areas. Subsequent opening and stretching of digestive organs during the practice of yogic postures regulates the Peristalsis movement that is a key involuntary process for the proper digestion and elimination. Besides, yogic breathing exercises send oxygen deep into the cells of the body and help it to absorb nutrients and excrete morbid matters thoroughly. On the other hand, efficacy of Yoga for stress management, rebalance of the autonomic nervous system to create deep relaxation and dominate parasympathetic system is well documented.

Langhorst et al. (2007) analyzed the effects of a comprehensive lifestyle modification program (a structured 60-hour training program over a period of 10 weeks which included stress management training, psycho-educational elements, and self-care strategies) on health-related quality-of-life, psychological distress, and clinical parameters in 60 patients with ulcerative colitis (UC). The 60 patients were randomly assigned to an intervention group or a usual-care control group. Comparison of the measurements taken at baseline, after 3 and 12 months showed significant improvement in the quality of life and emotional well-being of the participants as compared to controls.

4.5 Yoga versus genitourinary disorders

Most of the corporate workforces have been competing for material prosperity and focused on sensual indulgences. The most fashionable one is over and multi-partner romantic relationship. Prevalent dress codes, especially girls', unnatural food at cafeteria, pornographic literatures and audio-visual aids and western corporate culture are serving as the best catalysts to provoke more lust and engage in frequent sexual activities. The incestuous workplaces are in ascending order. Consequently, corporate workforces are extremely prone to the genitourinary problems and seriously loosing their health and wealth. Hence, it seems quite contextual to address significance of CY for managing the genitourinary problems. As yoga argued, over sexual activities result in suppressed immunity, low self-esteem, low morale and different health problems, especially genitourinary problems such as urinary stress incontinence, poor sexual orgasm, HIV AIDS, syphilis, infertility, miscarriage, premature ejaculation (PE), climacteric syndrome and pregnancy problems.

The efficacy of mind-body intervention like yoga was supposed effective means for bettering genitourinary health for long. Yoga has been found effective to promote genitourinary health and heal the concerned problems like urinary stress incontinence (Milani, Valli & Bhole, 1992), women sexuality (Brotto, Krychman & Jacobson, 2008; Dhikav et al., 2007), climacteric syndrome (Chattha et al., 2008), PE (Dhikav et al., 2007), pregnancy outcomes (birth weight, preterm labor, and IUGR either in isolation or associated with PIH) (Narendran et al., 2005), labor pain and duration (Chuntharapat, Petpichetchian & Hatthakit, 2008). Interestingly, Yoga appeared as a non-pharmacological measure for improving female sexual functions (Dhikav et al., 2007). Dhikav et al. (2010) also reported that after the completion of yoga sessions; the female sexual functions scores were significantly improved ($P< 0.0001$). The improvement occurred in all six domains of female sexual function index (FSFI) (i.e., desire, arousal, lubrication, orgasm, satisfaction, and pain) was more in older women (age > 45 years) compared with younger women (age < 45 years) thereby proving yoga as an effective method of improving all domains of sexual functions in women. Considering widespread acceptability of yoga, non-pharmacological nature, and apparent beneficial effects in the present study, this modality deserves further study. Chattha et al. (2008) studied the effect of 8 week-integrated yoga program consisted of breathing practices, sun salutation and cyclic meditation on cognitive functions in climacteric syndrome by sampling 120 premenopausal women between 40 and 55 years with follicle-stimulating hormone level equal to 15miu/ml. Sample was randomly assigned in two groups as participants and controls and participants were allowed to practice yoga module one hour per day, 5 day per week for 8 weeks. In yoga group they reported improvement on flushes and night sweats; and cognitive functions such as remote memory, mental balance, attention and concentration, delayed and immediate recall, verbal retention and recognition tests after 8 week. Dhikav et al. (2007) conducted another study to know if yoga could be tried as a treatment option in PE and to compare it with fluoxetine. For the same, they sampled 68 patients (38 yoga group; 30 fluoxetine group) attending the outpatient department of psychiatry of a tertiary care hospital and employed both subjective and objective assessment tools to evaluate the efficacy of the yoga and fluoxetine in PE and found that all 38 patients (25–65.7% = good, 13–34.2% = fair) belonging to yoga and 25 out of 30 of thefluoxetine group (82.3%) had statistically significant improvement in PE thereby showing yoga as a feasible, safe, effective and acceptable non-pharmacological option for PE. Nonetheless, more studies involving larger patients could be carried out to establish its utility in this condition. Vaze and Joshi (2010) also concluded that Yoga as a free-of-cost noninvasive method that is fairly effective and is strongly recommended to all women of menopausal age. Another study conducted by Brotto et al. (2008) reported that Eastern techniques like acupuncture, yoga, mindfulness and other forms of spiritual practice might offer a unique approach to enhance women's sexuality. However, it needs the development of sound theory and controlled studies; they might be the key for improving women's lack of sexual satisfaction. Narendran et al. (2005) conducted a study to assess the effect of yoga on pregnancy outcomes and recruited 335 women with 18-20 weeks of pregnancy. Yoga program including selected postures, breathing techniques and meditation was given to 169 women of yoga group one hour daily until delivery whereas 166 women of control group were suggested to go for 30 minutes walk twice a day during the study. Intervened integrated yoga approach during pregnancy was found safe thereby showing improvement in birth weight, preterm labor, and IUGR either in isolation or associated with PIH, with no increased complications in yoga group as compared to control group. Chuntharapat et al.'s (2008) findings suggested that 30 min of yoga practice at least three times per week for 10 weeks is an effective complementary means for facilitating maternal comfort, decreasing pain during labor and 2 hour post delivery, and shortening the length of labor that highlighted yoga as an alternative nursing intervention to improve the quality of maternal and child health care.

5. Summary

In 21st century the corporate world is associated with the most tension giving elements such as competition, deadlines, market conditions and above all the desire to reach high on the corporate ladder. These four elements are ultimately responsible to impair the harmonious interplay of body, mind and spirit thereby leading to various health problems among corporate workforces. On the other hand, yoga seems as an emerging avenue for the worldwide corporate health and wealth. The packaging of CY for corporate life style is the best preventive and therapeutic measure to optimize organizational health and culture as well. Persistent practice of CY by a corporate executive makes him/her healthy and wealthy. CY will prove to be an art and science of life for a corporate executive.

Yoga is an ultimate attempt for the fusion of embodied consciousness with supreme consciousness that subsequently proceeds from the practice of social adjustment (*Yam*), moral observance (*Niyam*), postures (*Asana*), breathing mechanics (*Pranayama*), senses withdrawal (*Prathyara*), concentration (*Dharana*), meditation (*Dhyan*) and super-consciousness (*Samadhi*). Regular practice of yoga is supposed to empower corporate health, happiness and harmony and hence wealth too.

The relevance and popularity of yoga is ascending in the entire West and Europe. Particularly, in UK and USA, yoga has become more popular where the women form 70-90% of the student population. Nonetheless, it is difficult to say in numerical figures exactly how many people are benefiting from yoga around the world. But one can easily notice that a huge number of people especially the women have been practicing yoga daily. The participation of a huge number of women itself signifies how important the yoga is for the health and the happiness. This trend also recommends that yoga must be taken seriously into the consideration as a part of workplace curriculum or culture to promote CW, CE and corporate social responsibility (CSR).

The CY will consists of normal subtle yogic warming up exercises, postures, yogic breathing exercises(*pranayama*), gestures, psychic locks, concentration, meditation, and spiritual counseling. CY can be taught collectively and practiced individually in order to gain its wholesome effects. Impacts of CY practices can be better explained via bio-psycho-socio-spiritual model- at physical level it improves musculoskeletal functioning, cardiopulmonary status, ANS response and endocrine functioning; at psychosocial level, it enhances self-esteem, social support and positive mood; and at spiritual level it elevates compassionate understanding and mindfulness.

The progress of CY practice will positively produce prolonged physical, mental, emotional, social and spiritual effects on executives. This will also help in producing effective leadership in corporate world. Nurturing effective leaders is one of the most important functions of the corporate excellence. This aspect also can be achieved by persistent practice of CY. There is no other method better than yoga that can make a corporate executive physically fit, mentally alert, emotionally rectified, socially adapted, rationally positive, completely self analytic and spiritually elevated.

Particularly, work related stress, respiratory problems, cardiac problems, digestive problems and genitourinary problems are seen improved by the specific and regular yoga practice. Mechanisms underlying the modulating effects of yogic cognitive-behavioral practices (eg, meditation, *Asanas, Pranayama,* caloric restriction) on human physiology can be classified into four transduction pathways: humoral factors, nervous system activity, cell trafficking, and bio-electromagnetism that shed light how yogic practices might optimize health, delay aging, and ameliorate chronic illness and stress from disability (illness and stress from disability). That implies that yoga is a cost effective and common avenue to minimize medical expenditure and maximize corporate performance and productivity.

Promotion of total health, happiness, harmony and four human intelligences- rational intelligence, creative intelligence, emotional intelligence and spiritual intelligence are side benefits of CY practice. Scientific validation and standardization of the effects of yoga practices at individual and corporate level follows bio-psycho-socio-spiritual research model and substantiate efficacy of CY for CW and CE. The general mechanism of yogic effects and efficacy of yoga for managing work stress, and improving health problems related to stress, respiratory, cardiopulmonary, digestive and genitourinary systems in organizational family is portrayed on the basis of concerned research findings. Regular practice of yoga or CY culture is directly linked to wellness and optimal intelligences of organizational family. Good employees' health leads to productivity at work, productivity at work leads to business competitiveness, business competitiveness leads to economic prosperity and well-being which is again associated with employees' good health.

Cognitive intelligence that can be slightly enhanced and maintained through yoga practice is helpful for sound managerial capabilities and technical skill empowerment. Creative intelligence and concentration promoted by yoga practice is supportive for the generation of creative and innovative ideas. Emotional intelligence that can be remarkably increased by yoga practice is the key for galvanizing leadership, team building, optimal interpersonal relationship and harmony. Spiritual intelligence that can be increased subsequently via yoga practices is near to the corporate social responsibility, holism, empathy, farsightedness, compassion and universal love. Thus, it can be concluded that CY is a cost-effective, eternal and universal means for workplace wellness and excellence that needs to be included as an indispensable part of corporate culture.

6. References

American Institute of Stress. (2011). *Effects of stress.* Retrieved May 31, 2011 from http://www.stress.org/topic-effects.htm

Aurobindo, S. (1999). *The Synthesis of Yoga* (5th ed.). Pondicherry, India: Sri Aurobindo Ashram Publication Department.

Becker, I. (2000). *Use of yoga in psychiatry and medicine.* In P. R. Muskin (Ed), *Complementary and alternative medicine and psychiatry* (pp. 107- 145). Washington, D.C.: American Psychiatric Press, Inc.

Behera, D. (1998). Yoga therapy in chronic bronchitis. *Journal of the Associations of Physicians of India, 46,* 207–208.

Behera, D. & Jindal, S. K. (1990). Effect of yogic exercises in bronchial asthma. *Lung India, 8*(4), 187-189.

Bennett, S. M., Weintraub, A. & Khalsa, S. B. (2008). Initial evaluation of the LifeForce Yoga® Program as a therapeutic intervention for depression. *International Journal of Yoga Therapy, 18,* 49-56. Retrieved from http://www.yogafordepression.com/IJYT-2008-Bennett.pdf

Bernadi, L., Gabutti, A., Porta, C. & Spicuzza, L. (2001). Slow breathing reduces chemoreflex response to hypoxia and hypercapnia, and increases baroreflex sensitivity. *Journal of hypertension, 19,* 2221- 2229.

Bernardi, L., Porta, C., Spicuzza, L., Bellwon, J., Spadacini, G., Frey, A. W., …Tramarin, R. (2002). Slow breathing increases arterial baroreflex sensitivity in patients with chronic heart failure. *Circulation, 105,* 143–145.

Bernardi, L., Spadacini, G., Bellwon, J., Hajric, R., Roskamm, H., & Frey, A. W. (1998). Effect of breathing rate on oxygen saturation and exercise performance in chronic heart failure.Lancet, 351, 1308–1311.*British Medical Journal (Clin Res Ed), 291,* 1077 . doi: 10.1136/bmj.291.6502.1077

Birkel, D. A. & Edgren, L. (2000). Hatha Yoga: Improved vital capacity of college students. *Alternative Therapy and Health Medicine,* 6(6), 55-63.

Blanc-Gras, N., Benchetrit, G. & Gellego, J. (1996). Voluntary control of breathing pattern in asthmatic children. *Perceptual Motor Skills, 83* (3 Pt 2), 1384-1386.

Brotto, L. A., Krychman, M., & Jacobson, P. (2008). Eastern approaches for enhancing women's sexuality: Mindfulness, acupuncture, and yoga. *Journal of Sex Medicine, 5,* 2741–2748.

Brown, R. P., & Gerbarg, P. L. (2009). Yoga breathing, meditation, and longevity. *Annals of the New York Academy of Sciences,* 1172, 54–62.

Brown, R. P. & Gerbarg, P. L. (2005). Sudarshan Kriya Yoga Breathing in the treatment of stress, anxiety, and depression: Part I - Neurophysiological model. *Journal of Alternative and Complementary Medicine, 11,* 189–201.

Brown, R. P. & Gerbarg, P. L. (2005). Sudarshan KriyaYoga breathing in the treatment of stress, anxiety, and depression: Part II: Clinical applications and guidelines. *Journal of Alternative and Complementary Medicine, 11,* 711–717.

Burton, J. (2010, February). *WHO Healthy Workplace Framework and Model, Background and Supporting Literature and Practices.* Submitted to Evelyn Kortum WHO Headquarters, Geneva, Switzerland. Retrieved at www.who.int/entity/occupational../healthy_workplace_framework.

Butera, K. (2010). Yoga therapy for the digestive health. *Yoga Living, xii*(ii), 14. Retrieved from http://yogalivingmagazine.com/wp-content/issues/2010/sept/YogaWebFall10%201_16.pdf.

Cappo, B. M. & Holmes, D. S. (1984). The utility of prolonged respiratory exhalation for reducing physiological and psychological arousal in non-threatening and threatening situations. *Journal of Psychosomatic Research, 28*, 265–273.

Carney, R. M., Saunders R. D., Freedland, K. E., Stein, P., Rich, M. W., & Jaffe, A. S. (1995). Association of depression with reduced heart rate variability in coronary artery disease. *American Journal of Cardiology, 76*, 562–564.

Chaoul, M. A. & Cohen, L. (2010). Rethinkging Yoga and the Application of Yoga in Modern Medicine. *Crosscurrents, 60*(2), 144-167. doi:10.1111/j.1939-3881.2010.00117.x

Chattha, R., Nagarathna, R., Padmalatha, V., & Nagendra, H. (2008). Effect of yoga on cognitive functions in climacteric syndrome: a randomized control study. *BJOG, 115*, 991-1000. doi: 10.1111/j.1471-0528.2008.01749.x

Chuntharapat, S., Petpichetchian, W., & Hatthakit, U. (2008). Yoga during pregnancy: Effects on maternal comfort, labor pain and birth outcomes. *Complementary Therapies in Clinical Practice, 14*, 105–115.

Claude, J., & Zamor, G. (2003). Workplace spirituality and organizational performance. *Public administration review, 63*(3): 355-362.

Damodaran, A., Malathi, A., Patil, N., Shah, N., Suryavansihi & Marathe, S. (2002). Therapeutic potential of yoga practices in modifying cardiovascular risk profile in middle aged men and women. *Journal of the Association of Physicians of India, 50*(5), 633-640.

deJong, A. (2009). Cardiovascular disease: Using a polypill, lifestyle modification, or a combined approach to reducing overall risk. *ACSM's Health & Fitness Journal, 13*(6), 38-40.

Dhikav, V., Karmarkar, G., Gupta, M., & Anand, K. S. (2007). Yoga in premature ejaculation: A comparative trial with fluoxetine. *Journal of Sex Medicine, 4*, 1726–1732.

Dhikav, V., Karmarkar, G., Gupta, R., Verma, M., Gupta, R., Gupta, S., & Anand, K. S. (2010). Yoga in female sexual functions. *Journal of Sex Medicine, 7*, 964–970.

Epel, E., Daubenmier, J., Moskowitz, J. T., Folkman, S., & Blackburn, E. (2009). Can meditation slow rate of cellular aging? Cognitive stress, mindfulness, and telomeres. Can meditation slow rate of cellular aging? Cognitive stress, mindfulness, and telomeres. *Annals of New York Academy of Science, 1172*, 34-53.

Ernst, E., & Soo, M. L. (2010). How effective is yoga? A concise overview of systematic reviews. *Complementary Therapies, 15*(4), 274–279. doi:10.1111/j.2042-7166.2010.01049.x

Evans, S., Tsao, J. C. I., Sternlieb, B., & Zeltzer, L. K. (2009). Using the biopsycosocial model to understand the health benefits of yoga. *Journal of complementary and integrative medicine, 6*(1): Article 15. doi: 10.2202/1553-3840.1183

Falus, A., Marton, I., Borbényi, E., Tahy, A., Karádi, P., Aradi, J., ...Kopp, M. (2010). The 2009 Nobel Prize in Medicine and its surprising message: style is associated with telomerase activity. *Orv Hetil., 13*, 151(24), 965-970.

Field, T. (2010). Yoga clinical research review. *Complementary Therapies in Clinical Practice xxx*, 1-8.

Fokkema, D. S. (1999). The psychobiology of strained breathing and its cardiovascular implications: A functional system review. *Psychophysiology, 36*(2), 164-175.

Fox, S., & Spector, P. E. (2005). *Counterproductive work behavior: Investigations of actors and targets.* Washington, DC: American Psychological Association.

Friedman, B. H. & Thayer, J. F. (1998). Autonomic balance revisited: panic anxiety and heart rate variability. *Journal of Psychosomatic Research, 44*, 133–151. from http://www.who.int/chp/chronic_disease_report/en/.

Garfinkel, M., & Schumacher, H. R. Jr. (2000).Yoga. *Rheumatic Disease Clinics of North America, 26*, 123- 32.

Glover, M. J., Grerenlund, K. J., Ayala, C. & Croft, J. B. (2005). Racial/ethnic disparities in prevalence, treatment, and control of hypertension V United States, 1999-2002. *Morbidity and Mortality Weekly Report, 54*, 7-9.

Gokal, R., & Shillito, L. (2007). Positive impact of yoga and pranayam on obesity, hypertension, blood sugar, and cholesterol: A pilot assessment. *Journal of Alternative and Complementary Medicine, 13*, 1056–1057.

Hagins, M., Moore, W. & Rundle, A. (2007). Does practicing hatha yoga satisfy recommendations for intensity of physical activity which improves and maintains health and cardiovascular fitness? *BMC Complementary and Alternative Medicine, 30*, 7-40

Haug, T. T., Svebak, S., Hausken, T., Wilhelmsen, I., Berstad, A. & Vrsin, H. (1994). Low vagal activity as mediating mechanism for the relationship between personality factors and gastric symptoms in functional dyspepsia. *Psychosomatic Medicine, 56*, 181–186.

Herrick, C. M., & Ainsworth, A. D. (2000). Yoga as a Self-Care Strategy. *Nursing Forum, 35* (2), 32-36.

Hunnicutt, D. & Chapman, L. S. (2006). Planning wellness getting off a good start. *Absolute Advantage, 5*(4), 4. Retrieved from http://www.welcoa.org/freeresources/pdf/financial_wellness.pdf

Iyengar, B. K. S. (1976). *Light on Yoga* (2nd ed.). New York: Schocken Books.

Jacobs, G. D. (2001). Clinical applications of the relaxation response and mind-body interventions. *Journal of Alternative and Complementary Medicine, 7* (Suppl 1), S93-S101.

Jain, S. C. & Talukdar, B. (1993). Evaluation of Yoga Training Programmae for Patients of bronchial asthma. *Singapore Medical Journal, 34*(4), 306-308.

Joshi, L. N., Joshi, V. D. & Gokhale, L. V. (1992). Effect of short term Pranayama practice on breathing rate and ventilatory functions of lung. *Indian Journal of Physiology and Pharmacology, 36*, 105-108.

Khalsa, S. (2004). Bibilometirc study on therapeutic interventions of Yoga. *Indian Journal of Physiology and Pharmacology, 48*(3), 269-285. Retrieved from http://www.ijpp.com/vol48_3/vol48_no3_spl_invt_art.pdf

Khanam, A. A., Sachdeva, U., Guleria, R., & Deepak, K. K. (1996). Study of pulmonary and autonomic functions of asthma patients after yoga training. *Indian Journal of Physiology and Pharmacology, 40*(4), 318-324.

Khatri, K., Goyal, A. K., Gupta, P. N., Mishra, N., & Vyas, S. P. (2008). Plasmid DNA loaded chitosan nanoparticles for nasal mucosal immunization against hepatitis B. *International Jouranl of Pharmacology, 354*(1-2), 235-41.

King, D. B. (2009). A Viable Model and Self-Report Measure of Spiritual Intelligence. *International Journal of Transpersonal Studies, 28*, 68-85.

Kjaer, T. W., Bertelsen, C., Piccini, P., Brooks, D., Alving, J., & Lou, H. C. (2002). Increased dopamine tone during meditation-induced change of consciousness. *Cognitive Brain Research, 13*, 255-259.

Konar, D., Latha, R., & Bhuvaneswaran, J. S. (2000). Cardiovascular responses to head-down-body-up postural exercise (Sarvangasana). *Indian Journal of Physiology and Pharmacology, 44*(4), 392-400.

Kulkarni, D. D., & Bera, T. K. (2009). Yogic exercises and health – a psycho-neuro immunological approach. *Indian Journal of Physiology and Pharmacology, 53*, 3–15.

Kuntsevich, V., Bushell, W. C., & Theise, N. D. (2010).Mechanisms of Yogic Practices in Health, Aging, and Disease. *Mount Sinai Journal of Medicine, 77*, 559–569

Langhorst, J., Mueller, T., Luedtke, R., Franken, U., Paul, A., & Scand, J. (2007). Effects of a comprehensive lifestyle modification program on quality-of-life in patients with ulcerative colitis: a twelve-month follow-up. *Gastroenterology, 42*(6), 734-45.

Lehrer, P., Sasaki, S. & Saito, Y. (1999). Zazen and cardiac variability. *Psychosomatic medicine, 61*, 812-821.

Lipton, L. (2008). Using yoga to treat disease: an evidence based review. *Journal of the American Academy of Physician Assistants, 21*, 38–41.

Macy, D. (2008). 'Yoga in America' market study practitioner spending grows to nearly $6 billion a year. *Yoga Journal: press release.* Retrieved May 6, 2011 from http://www.yogajournal.com/advertise/press_releases/10

Makwana, K., Khirwadkar, N., & Gupta, H. C. (1988). Effect of short term yoga practice on ventilatory function tests. *Indian Journal of Physiology and Pharmacology, 32*(3), 202-8.

Manocha, R., Marks, G. B., Kenchington, P., Peters, D., & Salome, C. M. (2002). Sahaja yoga in the management of moderate to severe asthma: a randomised controlled trial. *Thorax., 57*(2), 110-5.

McCaffrey, R., Ruknui, P., Hatthakit, U., & Kasetsomboon, P. (2005). The effects of yoga n hypertensive persons in Thailand. *Holistic Nursing Practice, 19*, 173–180.

McCall, T. (2009).*Yoga as Medicine: The Yogic Prescription for Health and Healing*: Bantam. Retrieved from www.DrMcCall.com

Michalsen, A., Grossman, P., Acil, A., Langhorst, J., Lüdtke, R., Esch T, … Dobos, G. J. (2005). Rapid stress reduction and anxiolysis among distressed women as a consequence of a three month intensive yoga program. *Medical Science Monitor, 11*, 555–561.

Moadel, A. B., Shaw, C., Wylie-Rossett, J., Harris, M. S., Patel, S. R., Hall, C. B. & Sparano, J. A. (2007). Randomized controlled trial of yoga among a multiethnic sample of breast cancer patients: Effects on quality of life. *Journal of Clinical Oncology, 25*(28), 4387-4395.

Modeling the impact of a comprehensive wellness program. (2010). *Enhancing corporate performance by tackling chronic diseases.* Retrieved May 4, 2011 from at https://members.weforum.org/pdf/Wellness/BCG-Report.pdf

Mohandas, E. (2008). Neurobiology of spirituality. In A. R. Sing and S. A. Singh (Eds), Medicine, mental health, science, religion, and well being, MSM, 6 Jan- Dec 2008.

Monro, R., Nagarathna, R. & Nagendra, H. R. (1995). *Yoga for common ailments.* New York/London: Simon & Schuster.

Murugesan, R., Govindarajulu, N., & Bera, T. K. (2000). Effect of selected yogic practices on the management of hypertension. *Indian Journal of Physiology and Pharmacology, 44*(2):207-10.

Nagarathna, R., & Nagendra, H. R. (1985). Yoga for bronchial asthma: a controlled study. *British Medical Journal, 291*(6502), 1077-1079.

Nagendra, H. R., & Nagarathna, R. (1986). An integrated approach of yoga therapy for bronchial asthma: A 3-54-month prospective study. *Journal of Asthma, 23*(3), 123-37.

Narendran, S., Nagarathna, R., Narendran, V., Gunasheela, S. & Nagendra, H. R. (2005). Efficacy of yoga on pregnancy outcome. *The Journal of Alternative and Complementary Medicine, 11*(2), 237–244

Nayak, N. N., & Shankar, K. (2004). Yoga: a therapeutic approach. *Physical Medicine & Rehabilitation Clinics of North America, 15*, 783–98.

Newcombe, S. (2007). Stretching for health and well-being: Yoga and women in Britain, 1960-1980. *Asian Medicine, 3*, 37-63.

Ornish, D. (2009). Intensive life style changes and health reform. *The Lancet Oncology, 10*, 198-199.

Ornish, D., Scherwitz, L. W., Billings, J. H., Brown, S. E., Gould, K. L., Merritt, T. A., …Brand, R. J. (1998). Intensive lifestyle changes for reversal of coronary heart disease. *JAMA 280*, 2001–2007.

Ornish, D., Scherwitz, L. W., Doody, R. S., Kesten, D., McLanahan, S. M., Brown, S. E., & Gotto, A. M. (1983). Effects of Stress Management Training and Dietary Changes in Treating Ischemic Heart Disease. *JAMA, 249*(1), 54-59.

Osterziel, K. J., Rohring, N., Dietz, R., Manthey, J., Hecht, J., & Kubler, W. (1988). Influence of captopril on the arterial baroreceptor reflex in patients with heart failure. *European Heart Journal, 9*, 1137–1145.

Pandya, P. (2006). *Antarjagat Ke Yatra Ka Jnana-Vijnana* (Science of Inner Journey). Haridwar, India: Vedmata Gayatri Trust.

Pruzan, P. & Pruzan, M. K. (2001). *Leading with wisdom: Spiritual based leadership in business.* New Delhi: Response Books from SAGE.

Pullen, P. R., Thompson, W. R., Benardot, D., Brandon, L. J., Mehta, P. K., Vadnais, D. S., …Khan, B. V. (2010). Benefits of yoga for African American heart failure patients. *Medicine and Science in Sports and Exercises, 42*(4):651-7.

Ramsay, H., Scholarios, D. & Harley, B. (2002). Employee and high-performance work system: testing inside the black box'. *British Journal of Industrial Relations, Worker.* Ithaca, NY: Cornell University Press.

Raub, J. A. (2002). Psychophysiologic effects of Hatha Yoga on musculoskeletal and cardiopulmonary function: a literature review. *Journal of Alternative and Complementary Medicine, 8*(6), 797-812.

Riley, D. (2004). Hatha yoga and the treatment of illness. *Alternative Therapy and Health Medicine, 10*(2), 20-1.

Ritz, T. (2001). Relaxation Therapy in adult asthma. Is there new evidence for its effectiveness? *Behavior Modification, 25*, 640-666,

Ross, A. & Thomas, S. (2010). The Health Benefits of Yoga and Exercise: A Review of Comparison Studies. *The Journal of Alternative and Complementary Medicine, 16*(1), 3–12. doi: 10.1089=Acm.2009.0044

Saper, R., Eisenberg, D., Davis, R., Culpepper, L., & Phillips, R. (2004). Prevalence and patterns of adult yoga use in the United States: Results of a national survey. *Alternative Therapy & Health Medicine, 10*, 44–48.

Sathyaprabha, T. N., Murthy, H., & Murthy, B. T. (2001). Efficacy of naturopathy and yoga in bronchial asthma--a self controlled matched scientific study. *Indian Journal of Physiology and Pharmacology, 45*(1), 80-86.

Satyananda, S. (2002). *The Four Chapters on Freedom.* Bihar, India: The Yoga Publication Trust.

Selvamurthy, W., Sridharan, K., Ray, U. S., Tiwary, R. S., Hegde, K. S., Radhakrishan, U., & Sinha, K. C. (1998). A new physiological approach to control essential hypertension. *Indian Journal of Physiology and Pharmacology, 42,* 205–213.

Siegel, D. J. (2009). Mindful awareness, mindsight and neural integration. *The Humanistic Psychologists, 37,* 137- 158.

Singh, N. (2009, October). Yog Ne Napi Puri Dharti. *Kadambini, 12 (49),* 18-23.

Singh, S. M., Longmire, W. P. Jr., & Reber, H. A. (1990). Surgical palliation for pancreatic cancer. The UCLA experience. *Annals of Surgery, 212, 132-139.*

Sivananda, S. (2003). *The Bhagavad Gita* (11th ed.). Uttarakhand, India: The Divine Life Society.

Sovik, R. (2000). The science of breathing- the yogic view. *Progressive Brain Research, 122,* 491-505.

Spicuzza, L., Gabutti, A., Porta, C., Montano, N., & Bernardi, L. (2000). Yoga and chemoreflex response to hypoxia and hypercapnia. *Lancet, 356*(9240), 1495–1496.

Stanescu, D. (1990). Yoga breathing exercises and bronchial asthma. *Lancet, 336*(8724), 1192.

Stanescu, D. C., Nemery, B., Veriter, C., & Marechal, C. (1981). Pattern of breathing and ventilator response to CO_2 in subjects practicing hatha-yoga. *Journal of Applied Physiology, 51,* 1625-1629.

Sterling, P. (2004). Principles of allostasis: Optimal design, predictive regulation, pathophysiology, and rational therapeutics. In Schulkin, J. (Ed.), *Allostasis, Homeostasis, and the Costs of Physiological Adaptation* (pp. 17–64). Cambridge: Cambridge University Press.

Stück, M., Meyer, K., Rigotti, T., Bauer, K., & Sack, U. (2003). Evaluation of a yoga based stress management training for teachers: Effects on immunoglobulin A secretion and subjective relaxation. *Journal for Meditation and Meditation Research, 3,* 59-68.

Taimni, I. K. (1961). *The science of yoga.* Madaras, India: The Theosophical Publishing House.

Vahia, N. S., Vinekar, S. L. & Doongaji, D. R. (1966). Some ancient Indian concepts in the treatment of psychiatric disorders. *British Journal of Psychiatry, 112*(492), 1089-1096.

Vaze, N. & Joshi, S. (2010). Yoga and Menopausal Transitiion. *Journal of Mid-life Health, 1*(2), 56-58. doi: 10.4103/0976-7800.76212

Vedanthan, P. K., Kesavalu, L. N., Murthy, K. C., Duvall, K., Hall, M. J., Baker, S., Nagarathna, S. (1998). Clinical study of yoga techniques in university students with asthma: a controlled study. *Allergy and Asthma Proceedings, 19*(1), 3-9.

West, J., Otte, C,. Geher, K., Johnson, J. & Mohr, D. C. (2004). Effects of Hatha yoga and African dance on perceived stress, affect, and salivary cortisol. *Annals of Behavioural Medicine, 28,* 114–118.

Wolfson, N. (n. d). *Yoga journal, incorporating yoga: In boardrooms from Manhattan to Silicon Valley, the mantra "let's do lunch" is being replaced by "let's do yoga."* Retrieved May 17, 2010 from http://www.yogajournal.com/lifestyle/294.

Yadav, R. K., & Das, S. (2001). Effect of yogic practice on pulmonary functions in young females. *Indian Journal of Physiology and Pharmacology, 45*(4), 493-6.

Zohar, D. (2005). Spiritually intelligent people. *Leader to leader journal, 38,* 45-51.